Handbook of Culture, Therapy, and Healing

Handbook of Culture, Therapy, and Healing

Edited by

Uwe P. Gielen
St. Francis College

Jefferson M. Fish
St. John's University

Juris G. Draguns
The Pennsylvania State University

LEA LAWRENCE ERLBAUM ASSOCIATES, PUBLISHERS
2004   Mahwah, New Jersey   London

Senior Consulting Editor:	Susan Milmoe
Editorial Assistant:	Kristen Depken
Cover Design:	Sean Trane Sciarrone
Textbook Production Manager:	Paul Smolenski
Full-Service Compositor:	MacAllister Publishing Services
Text and Cover Printer:	Hamilton Printing Company

This book was typeset in 10/12 pt. Palatino Roman, Italic, Bold, and Bold Italic.

Lawrence Erlbaum Associates, Inc., Publishers
10 Industrial Avenue
Mahwah, New Jersey 07430
www.erlbaum.com

Library of Congress Cataloging-in-Publication Data

Handbook of culture, therapy, and healing/edited by Uwe P. Gielen, Jefferson M. Fish,
  Juris G. Draguns.
    p. cm.
  Includes bibliographical references and index.
  ISBN 0-8058-4924-6
    1. Cultural psychiatry--Handbooks, manuals, etc. 2. Psychiatry,
  Transcultural--Handbooks, manuals, etc. 3. Psychotherapy--Cross-cultural
  studies--Handbooks, manuals, etc. 4. Healing--Cross-cultural studies--Handbooks,
  manuals, etc. I. Gielen, Uwe P. (Uwe Peter), 1940- II. Fish, Jefferson M. III. Draguns,
  Juris G., 1932-

RC455.4.E8H366 2004
362.2--dc22   2003049523

Books published by Lawrence Erlbaum Associates are printed on
acid-free paper, and their bindings are chosen for strength and durability.

Printed in the United States of America
10 9 8 7 6 5 4 3 2

To my students.
—Uwe P. Gielen

To my family, Dolores, Krekamey, Chris, Jordan, and Jaden.
—Jefferson M. Fish

To my family, Marie, Julie, and George.
—Juris G. Draguns

Contents

Preface

In recent years, students of psychology, anthropology, psychiatry, sociology, comparative religion, nursing, and other disciplines have converged in recognizing health and disease as the long-term outcomes of a complex process of biopsychosocial interactions. Therapy, healing, and counseling typically take place in a psychosocial field shaped by culturally constituted forces. This volume brings together the work of well-known scholars from psychology, anthropology, psychiatry, and related disciplines. It is partially based on a workshop organized by us under the auspices of the New York Academy of Sciences. The contributors focus on the interaction of cultural, social, psychological, and biological variables as they influence therapy, counseling, and psychological healing. The volume includes broadly conceived theoretical and survey chapters as well as detailed descriptions of specific healing traditions in Asia, the Americas, Africa, and the Arab world. Other chapters focus on multicultural considerations, specific populations such as refugees, and the integration of traditional and modern forms of counseling and healing. Taken together, the chapters provide a broad overview of Western and non-Western healing, psychotherapeutic traditions, and counseling traditions as these span the divide between psychosocial, anthropological, medical, and religious approaches. The emphasis throughout the book is on social interaction between healers, therapists, counselors, and their clients, as well as on the cultural belief systems shaping these interactions.

Historically speaking, the world's first healers served simultaneously as religious specialists, healers, diviners, and psychotherapists. In contrast to modern divisions between body, mind, and soul (if any!), they perceived both the patient and themselves as inhabiting a unitary world of visible and invisible forces and beings that could induce health or sickness, growth or fragmentation, good or evil. In the course of history, Western medicine lost sight of this unitary vision. Instead, a secular, mechanistic world view came to dominate the training of allopathic physicians who looked upon the body as complex machinery in need of fixing. Interpersonal and intrapsychic considerations, in turn, were mostly handed over to psychiatrists and psychologists whose position on the medical totem pole was low or precarious. Neither physicians nor psychologists understood how much their conceptions of healing were influenced by cultural belief systems and expectations.

In contrast to these earlier, acultural viewpoints, this volume is based on the assumption that culture influences pervasively:

- What we experience as distressing, how we label our distress, to what and to whom we attribute the distress, whether or not we believe that invisible beings and forces are part of the origins of the distress and its treatment.

- To whom, if anyone, we communicate our suffering; whom we consult in the hope of alleviating our distress; whom we regard as appropriate healers, therapists, and counselors; what we expect from them and how we experience our interactions with them; whom we regard as appropriate participants in the healing process.
- Whether healing takes place publicly or privately, what we consider to be a successful outcome or cure, how our bodies react to the encounters with healers, whether or not we choose to continue a given treatment, whether we take our pills or throw them away, and many other health-related actions, beliefs, and feelings.

However, although both healers and their clients are immersed in their culture, this does not mean that culture determines everything: Humans are at the same time biological creatures with distinctive predispositions and vulnerabilities that are the outcome of millions of years of evolution, differentiation, and adaptation. Two chapters in this volume, respectively by Horacio Fabrega, Jr. and by Michele Hirsch, pay special attention to the interaction of biological processes, psychological processes, and sociocultural systems.

This volume is intended for all those in the healing and helping professions: clinical, counseling, school, and other applied psychologists; therapists with other professional backgrounds; psychiatrists and other physicians; social workers; pastoral, educational, and guidance counselors; members of the allied health professions; medical anthropologists; members of the clergy; cross-cultural, cultural, and multicultural psychologists; and all their students. We hope that on reading this book, they will better understand how their services fit into the global panorama of distress, its conceptualization, and its treatment. They can also use it as a reference volume in order to arrive at a sense of the belief systems that clients from diverse cultural backgrounds might bring to therapy, counseling, and healing sessions. In addition, the volume will prove useful to nonpractitioners with a scholarly interest in, or curiosity about, systems of healing and counseling around the world. They will be able to sample a significant variety of belief systems and the modes of intervention that stem from them. In the process, we expect that they will acquire both factual information and a comparative appreciation of the diversity of these approaches.

Several recent volumes on multicultural counseling have adopted a cookbook format. Following several introductory chapters, they guide the reader to interpersonal encounters in which a counselor from a mainstream American cultural background is confronted with the task of counseling culturally distinctive clients, usually from African American, Hispanic, Asian American, Native American, and other backgrounds. Our volume diverges from such an approach in two ways. First, we have adopted a global approach rather than dealing with specific subcultures thought to be different from the mainstream culture. We believe that the worldwide perspective adopted in this volume is uniquely suited to help the reader step back from the various American viewpoints that surreptitiously continue to dominate even those multicultural counseling books that attempt to present a variety of culturally divergent perspectives. Second, we have refrained from including chapters that purport to teach how to counsel clients of specific cultural backgrounds. Instead, we set the goal of elucidating the *general* nature of cultural influences in healing and counseling situations.

Our decision to adopt a global perspective was shaped in part by our formative experiences. Uwe P. Gielen, a specialist in culture and developmental psychology, grew up as an internal refugee in Germany, immigrated to the United States, and has done fieldwork in the Himalayas and elsewhere in Asia. Jefferson M. Fish, a specialist in culture and therapy, has served as a Fulbright scholar and visiting professor in Brazil where he trained clinical psychologists to function as therapists in cultural settings quite different from those prevailing in his native New York. Juris G. Draguns, a specialist in culture and psychopathology, was born in Latvia, attended high school in Germany, immigrated to the United States, and has held visiting appointments at universities located on four continents. Thus, an awareness of the importance of cultural factors in counseling and healing has come to us as a result of personal experience and has become an integral part of our subjective outlook and our professional *modus operandi*.

The chapter authors represent a veritable Who's Who of researchers interested in the cultural basis of worldwide healing systems. Their cultural and professional origins range widely from Taiwan to Sicily, from India to Europe, from Japan to Canada, from Saudi Arabia to the United States. The contributors include cross-cultural psychologists, psychiatrists, counselors and therapists, medical anthropologists, proponents of indigenous healing methods, peace psychologists, psychoanalysts and behaviorists, and both theoreticians and practitioners. The reader will thus encounter a broad variety of perspectives, yet the contributions share a concern with the intertwining of culture and the tangle of psychosocial processes that forge a bond between healer and client.

Because both distress and healing are basic human experiences, they touch our existential roots. Consequently, healing in all its varieties has been a part of the human journey for many thousands of years. Healers in the shamanistic tradition were probably the first in counteracting human distress. Consequently, they played a central role in their respective societies. Many of them were charismatic if sometimes fearful figures, and even today their modern descendants—priests, physicians, psychologists, counselors, charismatics, *curanderos*, witch doctors, and numerous others—are surrounded by a special aura. This aura does not reflect the special qualities of the healer, but instead it expresses the intense hopes, fears, and expectations of deeply distressed clients, regardless of whether the healer is a *curandero* displaying his skills in the Andean highlands or a psychoanalyst interpreting the confusing dreams of an unhappy New York lawyer.

Studying healing across cultures, then, brings us face to face both with the unending variety of culturally shaped ways of life and with some fundamental existential concerns that humans everywhere seek to understand. We invite the reader to follow us on an imaginary journey around the globe, a journey that calls into question one's habitual ways of thinking, poses conceptual demands and challenges, and requires a readiness to perceive unity in variety and variety in unity. Welcome to the transcultural world of healing, therapy, and counseling!

—Uwe P. Gielen
—Jefferson M. Fish
—Juris G. Draguns

List of Contributors

Ihsan Al-Issa, PhD, The International Arab Psychological Association, Toronto, Canada

Abdulla Al-Subaie, MD, Medical School, King Saud University, Riyadh, Saudi Arabia

Joseph F. Aponte, PhD, Department of Psychology, University of Louisville, Louisville, Kentucky

Cecilia Askeroth, Department of Psychology, St. Francis College, New York City, New York

Frederic P. Bemak, PhD, Counseling and Development Programs, George Mason University, Fairfax, Virginia

Dimitry Burshteyn, PhD, Siena College, Loudenville, New York

Rita Chi-Ying Chung, PhD, Counseling and Development Programs, George Mason University, Fairfax, Virgina

Juris G. Draguns, PhD, Department of Psychology, The Pensylvannia State University, University Park, Pennsylvania

Andrea Einhorn, White Plains, New York

Horacio Fabrega, Jr., MD, Department of Psychiatry, University of Pittsburgh, Pittsburgh, Pennsylvania

Kaja Finkler, PhD, Department of Anthropology, University of North Carolina, Chapel Hill, North Carolina

Jefferson M. Fish, PhD, Department of Psychology, St. John's University, New York City, New York

Sandra T. Francis, PhD, University of the Sciences in Philadelphia, Philadelphia, Pennsylvania

Uwe P. Gielen, PhD, Department of Psychology, St. Francis College, New York City, New York

Michele Hirsch, PhD, Department of Psychology, St. Francis College, New York City, New York

Rashmi Jaipal, PhD, Department of Psychology, Bloomfield College, Newark, New Jersey

Wolfgang G. Jilek, MD, Department of Psychiatry, University of British Columbia, Vancouver, British Columbia, Canada

Joan D. Koss-Chioino, PhD, Department of Anthropology, Arizona State University, Tempe, Arizona

Ching-Tse Lee, PhD, Department of Psychology, Brooklyn College, The City University of New York, New York City, New York

Ting Lei, PhD, Social Science Department, Borough of Manhattan Community College, The City University of New York, New York City, New York

Carlinda Monteiro, Christian Children's Fund, Luanda, Angola

Raymond Prince, MD, McGill University, Montreal, Quebec, Canada

Jeffrey B. Rubin, PhD, Harlem Family Institute, New York City, New York

Linda K. Sussman, PhD, Department of Anthropology, Washington University, St. Louis, Missouri

Junko Tanaka-Matsumi, PhD, Department of Psychology, Kwansei Gakuin University, Nishinomia City, Japan

Michael Wessells, PhD, Department of Psychology, Randolph-Macon College, Ashland, Virginia

Handbook of Culture, Therapy, and Healing

Approaches to Culture, Healing, and Psychotherapy

Juris G. Draguns
The Pennsylvania State University

Uwe P. Gielen
St. Francis College

Jefferson M. Fish
St. John's University

CULTURE, HEALING, AND PSYCHOTHERAPY: THEIR CHARACTERISTICS AND INTERRELATIONSHIPS

The subject of this book concerns the relief of mental suffering and physical distress by means of healing and psychotherapy, and the manner in which these objectives are pursued in a wide array of cultures around the world. To this end, our first task is to introduce, anchor, and pinpoint the three key terms in the title: culture, healing, and psychotherapy.

Culture

Definitions of culture abound. Our preference is to introduce culture, with Melville Herskovits (1949), as the part of the environment that has been generated or created by human beings. Social scientists are in agreement that culture encompasses concrete, visible, and tangible products created by human action, as well as that which Hofstede (1991) has called "software of the mind" (p. 4): the systems of communication and the preserved experience of prior generations, and also the shared values and beliefs that, at the same time, represent templates for future action. Cultures differ then not only in their artifacts, but in their languages, subsistence and production systems, and philosophies of life, both implicit and explicit. Closer to the major objective of this volume, it is reasonable to expect that cultures have shaped the healing and psychotherapeutic practices that have evolved within them.

Healing

Healing is an age-old practice found in virtually all cultures across space and time. No culture stands by idly in the face of human suffering; all human societies have evolved methods aimed at restoring physical health, promoting psychological contentment, and achieving spiritual serenity. Healing as a concept then refers to the aggregate of techniques used to make human beings whole again by counteracting distress in the body, mind, and spirit. In traditional cultures, healers tended to address the gamut of human dysfunction. In the modern era, this holistic orientation to healing has been increasingly compromised and strained, if not irretrievably lost. Fragmentation and specialization have supplanted undifferentiated unity as subdisciplines within and outside medicine; psychology, counseling, nursing, and religious ministry complement each other's services and often minister to, and even compete for, the same clients. Systems of alternative medicine have evolved, largely in order to restore coherence to the human strivings for promoting health and overcoming illness. As several chapters in this volume make clear, practitioners of alternative medicine are widely represented and consulted both within the United States and elsewhere.

In philosophy, René Descartes drew a sharp line between the body and the mind. In the ensuing centuries, the secularization of Western civilization largely banished spiritual problems from the purview of scientifically based biomedical and psychological interventions, thereby extending separation of church and state to the individual on the intrapsychic plane. In her chapter in this volume, Michele Hirsch further develops some aspects of this theme.

Psychotherapy

In response to the compartmentalization of human experience, the enterprise of psychotherapy has come into being. It may be provisionally defined as "a method of working with patients/clients to assist them to modify, change, or reduce factors that interfere with effective living" (Fabrikant, 1984, p.184). A crucial aspect of psychotherapy is that it "involves the interaction between psychotherapist and patients/clients in the process of accomplishing its goals" (Fabrikant). In this sense of the term, the advent of psychotherapy as a specific modality of the treatment of human distress can be traced to the last decade of the nineteenth century. As the founder of psychoanalysis, Sigmund Freud is widely regarded as a pivotal figure in this development, although no single person can be identified as its inventor, inaugurator, or first known practitioner. Instead, the advent of psychotherapy can be viewed as the outgrowth of the prevailing zeitgeist, which placed emphasis on introspection, individualism, and the extension of scientific practices to mental and subjective phenomena.

Within a more general framework, however, it must be recognized that psychotherapy has existed across space and time, much as has healing. In fact, psychotherapeutic interventions are deeply embedded in the traditional healing arts. Prince (1980) was able to discern a number of universal components of psychotherapy in interventions practiced across cultures in all of the world's regions. These features include a worldview shared by the healer and the sufferer, the ability to provide a culturally meaningful explanation of distress or dysfunction, and the exercise of social influence through suggestion and other means. Overshadowing these external features, however, Prince highlighted the mobilization of the sufferer's endogenous self-healing or self-corrective mechanisms, often in the form of altered states of consciousness, as the most important and universally valid ingredient of psychotherapy.

In his scholarly volume, *Care of the Psyche: A History of Psychological Healing*, the medical historian Stanley W. Jackson (1999) has traced essential elements of psychological healing in the Western tradition from antiquity to modern times. According to him, "talking cures" have traditionally included an emphasis on the healer-sufferer relationship; an authoritative and attentive healer; and his or her use of reward or punishment, suggestion and persuasion, explanation, interpretation, and guidance. The healer offers consolation and comfort to the sufferer, and provides support for the client's efforts "to get things out." Confession, confiding, and changes in the client's self-understanding and self-observation have also been essential features of successful psychotherapeutic interventions over the centuries. It should be added that many of these therapeutic processes can also be found in non-Western healing encounters, although cultural influences and expectations typically determine which of these elements are assigned primary importance and which of them are relegated to the tacit background for the encounter between healer and sufferer.

Healing and Psychotherapy Within and Across Cultures

All psychotherapy aims at the relief of personal suffering and distress (Prince, 1980). It attempts to achieve this general objective by means of techniques and interventions that make sense and can be integrated with the preexisting corpus of culturally shared knowledge in the milieu in which they are applied (Torrey, 1972). Thus, interventions that may work in the culture in which they were developed often fail when transferred across cultural barriers. In a culturally diverse society, this state of affairs is often observed when techniques that are demonstrated to be effective within the mainstream segment of the population are extended and applied without modification to members of ethnocultural minority groups. High drop-out rates early in therapy, before any gains are realized, are a frequent result of such interventions (Sue & Sue, 1977). Moreover, psychotherapy, as well as healing, only encompasses interventions that are designed for the suffering person's benefit in order to bring about improvement in his or her well-being. Therefore, social influence techniques that do not posit this goal are consensually relegated outside of psychotherapy, from torture and brain-washing to sorcery and purification for the group's good and not the individual's.

Once the potential relevance of culture in psychotherapy is acknowledged, a host of questions arises. What is the relative weight of culture in determining the effectiveness of psychotherapy, its conduct, and style? What specific cultural dimensions matter in paychotherapy, in what way, and to what extent? Which of the many psychotherapies currently practiced are applicable across ethnic lines, and which are not? Which psychotherapies require modification and how can its degree and nature be established and tested for efficacy? Furthermore, what can we learn from the accounts of psychotherapy from other cultural traditions? What can we adapt from these interventions and apply in our own cultural milieu? How can traditional and modern therapies be creatively combined and integrated in their application to underserved and isolated cultural groups? Finally, what generic features can be identified on the basis of a panoramic view of psychotherapy around the world? Some of these questions are posed and partially answered in the chapters of this book, but most of them are many steps removed from a definitive, empirically based resolution. Collectively, these questions may guide the field for decades to come.

The relationship between psychotherapy and healing remains to be addressed. Healing is the more inclusive activity, psychotherapy the more specific. Perhaps the classical formulation by Jerome Frank (1961) is helpful in making this distinction. Psychotherapy is healing through persuasion, broadly understood as the sum of methods that counteract demoralization, which is the common feature that brings clients to psychotherapy. Healing is a term that is applicable to the techniques, presented in several chapters of this book, that straddle the fence between the bio-medical and the psychological. Michele Hirsch's chapter conceptually addresses the issue of how healing occurs. Specifically, anthropological observations are integrated with the findings of psychoneuroimmunology and the role of expectation and belief in producing biochemical change from illness to health. Jefferson Fish tackles the same problem in his chapter, but does so from a somewhat different point of view as he attempts to specify the psychological and sociocultural commonalities in healing. Two chapters by Ting Lei and his team of collaborators provide substantial information not yet available elsewhere on indigenous Chinese healing procedures and their effects on a variety of psychophysiological indicators. In her chapter, Rashmi Jaipal shares information on the Indian view of mental health and healing. The conception of bal-ance as the main feature of health anticipates Western homeostatic formulations. Moreover, the Indian view avoids the problems that arise when an impenetrable wall is posited between the mind and body, as was historically the case in the West. The chapter by Ihsan Al-Issa and Abdulla Al-Subaie on Arab societies also provides copi-ous illustrations of physical ailments helped by psychological means and of psycho-logical symptoms relieved by biological interventions.

Similarly, chapters about several other regions of the world reveal how porous the boundary is between mental and spiritual healing, not only in Arab countries and in India, but also among the Salish Indians of Canada, as described in the chapter by Wolfgang Jilek, and among spiritual healers of Mexico, which is the topic of Kaja Finkler's chapter. Skepticism will no doubt be aroused by the claims of successful intercession with the spirit world and other non-naturalistic occurrences. Pending clarification, one might accept verified descriptive accounts of such phenomena and maintain skepticism regarding traditional within-culture explanations. The challenge to which the chapters' authors have already responded is to integrate the observed effects with the sum total of relevant information that bears on the observed phe-nomena.

PSYCHOTHERAPY AND HEALING IN CULTURE: HISTORY, PRESENT SITUATION, FUTURE PROSPECTS

Historical Origins

Observations of culturally distinctive healing practices are scattered throughout ethnographic descriptions and psychiatric reports of many decades. Yet a coherent body of literature did not begin to emerge until the second half of the twentieth cen-tury. It is perhaps not coincidental that professional interest in this topic was sparked by the early stirrings of the community mental health movement. Thus, Alexander and Dorothea Leighton were involved both in pioneering the epidemiological approach to communities in Nova Scotia (Leighton, Harding, Macklin, MacMillan, & Leighton, 1963) and in extending these explorations to the Yoruba in Nigeria (Leighton, Lambo, Hughes, Leighton, Murphy, & Macklin, 1963). In the process, the Leightons encountered and observed the operations of local healers or witchdoctors whose diagnostic practices and therapeutic interventions sometimes overlapped with and diverged from the familiar procedures of modern Western psychotherapists. What the Leightons and their coworkers confronted was a coherent healing system that was partially based on the accumulated observations and experience by the current practitioners and their predecessors, as well as on the traditions and beliefs shared within the culture in question. Their observations and those of their contemporaries marked the beginning of taking local healers seriously as mental health practitioners within the framework of their culture. A prominent Nigerian psychiatrist, T. A. Lambo (1964), emerged as an articulate mediator between the two systems of care and treatment and was instrumental in incorporating healers into the therapy programs of a Nigerian psychiatric hospital. Another influential contributor was Ari Kiev (1962) whose descriptions of Voodoo practices in Haiti and among West Indian immigrants in London were focused upon the interplay of magical and naturalistic interventions in bringing about therapeutic change. His compendium of clinical reports of interventions embedded in the traditions of different cultures (Kiev, 1964) was widely read by American and other Western psychotherapists. It helped bring about a decentering of outlook in the American community of mental health professionals and called into question the existence of optimal treatment approaches that work in all cultures. Extensive observations in Indonesia and elsewhere were gathered over several decades by Wolfgang Pfeiffer (1994), a German psychiatrist who articulated a number of commonalities, as well as contrasts, among traditional and modern interventions. According to Pfeiffer, culturally patterned techniques aim at and result in integration into the group rather than the individuation of a unique person, a Western tradition that has been traced to the Renaissance, Reformation, and Enlightenment (Murphy, 1978).

Among contemporary psychotherapists who emphasize the cogency of indigenous beliefs and practices is the Parisian psychoanalyst, Tobie Nathan (1994), who rejects the imposition of any extraneous conceptual framework in treating patients who come from radically different cultures. Instead, he advocates accepting cultural reality as it appears to the client and promoting therapeutic change within his or her pre-existing network of cognitions and convictions.

In this book, the chapter by Raymond Prince takes us back to the time and place of the discovery of indigenous healing. It is based on the report of clinical observations and experiences over three years during which Prince was a government psychiatrist in Nigeria in the early 1960s. A participant in the early efforts to study and learn from native healers on par with Leighton and others, Prince was surprised to find that insight played a minor role, if any, in bringing about clinical improvement and the disappearance of presenting symptoms. Moreover, nondirective techniques, recently introduced at the time, were found to be ineffective in the Nigerian setting. What worked instead was forceful suggestion, reinforced by the accoutrements of a culturally sanctioned role. Because of its historical importance, we, as editors, encouraged Prince to modify his original report minimally in order to preserve the freshness and immediacy of his observations, which Prince proceeded to conceptualize in accordance with the theories available at the time.

Since then, progress in the field has proceeded from case to case, building upon the field experience of earlier observers. New interventions, combining the traditional and the modern, have often been applied on a trial-and-error basis. In the typical case, the documentation has been in the form of a descriptive naturalistic study in which evidence and inference are sometimes hard to separate. Culture's influence upon psychotherapy was first noted in remote settings exotically different from the Western therapists' point of view. During the last three and four decades, culture's impact upon therapy has been scrutinized in a much wider set of milieus, above all within the culturally diverse nations in North America and elsewhere.

Current State of Evidence: Predominantly Descriptive

We have endeavored to include in this volume a cross section of recent reports on the points of contact among healing, psychotherapy, and culture. Unfortunately, not all regions of the world are represented, but we have striven to maximize geographic and cultural variety across nations, as well as within multicultural North America. Reflecting the current state of methodology, the information in the bulk of the chapters is qualitative rather than quantitative. In a relatively new, yet burgeoning field, this state of affairs reflects the current realities of data gathering. Phenomena must be observed and described before scores and ratings can be meaningfully imposed on them and before any meaningful comparisons can be executed. Thus, there is a continuing need for recording factually the operations and the context of indigenous Japanese therapies such as Morita and Naikan, as Junko Tanaka-Matsumi has done in her chapter. Similarly, in the chapter on Navajo dance, Sandra T. Francis has combined field interviews with films, sacred texts, and the accounts of other anthropologists, yet she has refrained from imposing an external frame of reference. Kaja Finkler's chapter on the spiritualist healers in Mexico takes a further step and inquiries into the effectiveness of these interventions. To this end, Finkler has amassed an impressive amount of information on the rationale and nature of spirtualists' procedures, the relationship between the practitioner and the patient, and the recruitment into the healing role. Since the spiritualist's career unfolds in time, information is presented on these healers as persons, and not just as agents of interventions. Joan D. Koss-Chioino's chapter concerns a similar topic as she asks what experiences matter in starting a woman on her way toward a calling as healer in Puerto Rico. Answers to this question are sought in the context of detailed autobiographical information Koss-Chioino was able to obtain, and recurrent themes are identified.

Four chapters consist of a major review of literature. Joseph F. Aponte's chapter seeks to specify the manner in which the culture of four major ethnic groups in the United States impinges upon treatment operations, process, and outcome. Fred Bemak and Rita Chi-Ying Chung survey in their chapter the interaction of several relevant factors in devising and implementing psychotherapeutic services for traumatized refugees. Ting Lei, Cecilia Askeroth, and Ching-Tse Lee have provided a thorough introduction to the theories and methods of Chinese healing. Ihsan Al-Issa and Abdulla Al-Subaie address both indigenous Arab therapies and the adaptations of Western techniques that have been applied in Arab countries.

From Qualitative Description to Quantified Research: Harbingers of an Emerging Trend?

Research based on statistical analysis is not entirely absent from this volume. In her chapter on therapies developed in Japan, Junko Tanaka-Matsumi has sought to include objective outcome data, but did not find them. She was, however, able to caution against some apparent incipient misconceptions. Quantitative information was adduced to demonstrate that Naikan and Morita are far from being the most prominent therapies in their country of origin, even though they have a distinctive role to pay, mostly as adjuncts to more familiar and universal modes of therapy.

Proceeding from their description of approaches to healing that originated in China, Ting Lei, Cecilia Askeroth, Andrea Einhorn, and Ching-Tse Lee embarked upon a major undertaking: the meta-analysis of outcome research on the gamut of methods they reviewed. The realization of this ambitious objective was stymied by the low quality of the available outcome data, and the size of effect of the various treatments could not be determined. Nonetheless, useful incremental information was obtained by means of criteria-based meta-analysis. Thus, the effectiveness of acupuncture in China was found to be equal to that in Russia, but clearly superior to the results obtained in England and the United States, a finding that in part makes sense and in part raises questions still to be answered.

Traditional Healers: Their Role and Their Characteristics

What native healers do and what they are like have been topics of fascination and speculation for a long time. Although, in the older writings, shamans and other healing practitioners have often been dismissed and denigrated in a blanket fashion as psychotic, malevolent, and ignorant, the newer trend sometimes veers in the direction of positive but undifferentiated characterization. Beyond these dichotomous views, the question is often asked: What is the role of the healers in implementing comprehensive community-based programs in locales where healers' services are known and available? Indigenous healers have often been idealized, yet they remain underutilized.

The chapter by Wolfgang G. Jilek reports on an innovative project in which Salish Indian dance ceremonials were integrated into a multimethod program designed to counteract depression rooted in alienation from traditional values. In another part of the world, local healers were integrated in an attempt to rehabilitate underage soldiers who were forced to fight in the civil war in Angola and to return them to their families and communities whenever possible, as described in the chapter by Michael Wessells and Carlinda Monteiro.

The formative events and influences that impelled future healers to embark on their paths toward these practices are elucidated in the chapters by Joan D. Koss-Chioino and Kaja Finkler. Koss-Chioino introduces another theme: that the healing arts provide an avenue of fulfillment and self-enhancement for women whose occupational and educational opportunities have been severely restricted by tradition. Indeed, it is remarkable that the bulk of the relevant literature is focused on male healers, even though several healing traditions have provided women with an occupational and social niche.

Barely addressed in the several chapters is another controversial aspect of healing activities, particularly prominent in cultures in which shamanistic tradition is represented and magic is an important part of modus operandi. Healers are often trusted and sought out for help, yet they are also feared because of their perceived special powers for good or ill. Brodwin (1996) describes the mixture of awe and fear with which the Voodoo priests are perceived in Haiti. The attitude of benevolence that we postulated as sine qua non of healing and psychotherapy is not present in pure form in many healing traditions.

More recently, Krippner (2002) systematically analyzed several historically influential Western perspectives for the understanding of shamans and, by implication, of other healers who minister to the psychological and spiritual needs of their community and enjoy a privileged status in exchange. Within their cultures, shamans are thought to possess special powers that enable them to provide highly valued healing services. Krippner's conclusion is that several of the explanations advanced have partial validity, but that none of them fully account for the phenomena of healing as practiced in numerous traditional cultures. Thus, shamans are definitely not charlatans, yet a part of their modus operandi involves tricks and sleights of hand, which may enhance the effectiveness of their healing influence. Benedict's (1934) hypothesis that one society's madmen may be another society's healers has been refuted on the basis of studying medicine men in several traditional societies in Mexico, Nepal, Siberia, and the United States. Projective test protocols and results of diagnostic interviews converge in suggesting the absence of serious mental disorder in shamanistic healers, sometimes accompanied by indications of greater freedom of expression and creativity. Reports of modified states of attention and consciousness among shamans are both varied and numerous, yet they do not support the existence of a uniquely shamanistic mode of consciousness. Krippner hypothesized that the suppression of traditional and public shamanistic rituals such as dancing, chanting, and drumming has led contemporary shamans to concentrate on internal bodily and mental states. In their ambiguous and often marginalized status,

> more often than not, shamans engage in trickery, improvise and engage in unpredictable behavior, embrace the fluidity of different planes of human existence, and exhibit ambiguous sexuality. In their efforts to share esoteric knowledge with their community, it is essential for shamans to deconstruct order, especially if a person's or a community's rigidy and inflexibility have blocked adaptation and growth. (Krippner, 2002, p. 970)

Krippner describes shamans as precursors of psychotherapists, but also of magicians, physicians, performers, and storytellers. Thus, the role of healers in their societies is inclusive, complex, and multifaceted; it encompasses therapeutic activity, but goes beyond it in a variety of directions. In Krippner's view, the intensive study of shamans' operations holds the promise of enriching the understanding of neuropsychology of consciousness, the psychology of social influence and modeling, and the cultural plasticity of psychological therapy.

Responding to Unique Stresses in Space and Time: The Detraumatizing Function of Cultural Healing and Therapy

Two of the chapters deal with unique and tragic developments and the aftermath of human suffering that they engender. Fred Bemak and Rita Chi-Ying Chung respond to the challenge of helping the providers of mental health services serve the needs of refugees who have fled war, oppression, and sometimes genocide, and do so in a culturally sensitive fashion. In a concrete and specific situation, that of prolonged civil strife in Angola, both the problem and the solution were embedded in culture. As Michael Wessells and Carlinda Monteiro report, the recruitment of soldiers in their early teens was seen as less of a violation of age norms than it would be in many countries. Yet finding a place for them in their families was deemed to be virtually essential for social and psychological survival in a tightly integrated, sociocentric culture. This unique and novel challenge was effectively met, and many ex-child soldiers were successfully rehabilitated. Moreover, this objective was attained by blending the activities of traditional cultural agents with interventions that were developed and applied outside the culture.

FROM OBSERVATIONS TO EXPLANATIONS: RAISING CONCEPTUAL ISSUES PERTAINING TO CULTURE, HEALING, AND THERAPY

Five of the chapters are primarily theoretical. Within an evolutionary frame of reference, Horacio Fabrega inquires into the origins of psychopathology in relation to the emergence of culture and plausibly traces the likely evolution of sickness and healing. Linda Sussman's contribution pertains to the specific role of culture in defining illness, interpreting its meaning, and managing its course. Although illness is probably a panhuman universal concept, culture enters into the progression of illness at the earliest possible moment and shapes its experience at all steps until termination, which is also culturally determined. Michele Hirsch's chapter espouses a biopsychological perspective on cross-cultural healing and revisits the age-old issue of the body/mind connection in light of the recent advances in psychoimmunology and of the recrudescence of interest in the placebo response. Jefferson M. Fish in his chapter also searches for cross-cultural constancy in therapy and healing. As a result of this effort, he identifies six shared themes that he concedes may in part reflect current globalizing trends. Others, however, are likely to be more fundamental, traceable to the shared challenges of human existence. In the context of building bridges between disparate conceptual systems, Jeffrey B. Rubin explores the potential common ground between psychoanalysis and Buddhist practice and thought. Equally important are the divergences and contrasts between these two conceptions of the human condition. Yet the chapter ends on a hopeful note, emphasizing complementarity rather than mutual exclusiveness.

Toward Comparative Research on Psychotherapy and Culture

The final chapter, by Juris G. Draguns, stands apart from the rest of the book. For one, it has little to say about the broader enterprise of healing and concentrates on the as-yet barely initiated task of research on psychotherapy across cultures. To this end, the five cultural dimensions identified and investigated by Hofstede (2001) are extended to the arena of psychotherapy. Predictions are advanced pertaining to the possible relevance of these characteristics in the conduct and experience of psychotherapy. Implicit in this chapter is the belief of the comparability of many, though not all, features of psychotherapy across culture lines, especially when cultures of modern nation-states are studied.

Yet some say that such an effort is misguided and doomed to failure due to the inherent incompatibility of the phenomena of psychic healing and therapy in very different cultural milieus. Certainly, it is conceded that a formal comparative study of a limited number of variables squeezed into a tight statistical research design does not do justice to the richness, complexity, and uniqueness of the raw data of psychotherapy within their unique cultural context. However, all social science disciplines advance by pooling a multiplicity of imperfect methods initiated from a variety of vantage points. Thus, although large-scale quantitative methods are advocated, it is recognized that the potential of the traditional descriptive case study is by no means exhausted. Several of the chapters included in this volume exemplify the application of qualitative research methods at their best.

JUSTIFYING THE STUDY OF HEALING AND PSYCHOTHERAPY IN RELATION TO CULTURE

There remains the final question: Why study healing and psychotherapy in and across cultures? The potential users of such information range from busy practitioners in multicultural environments to theoreticians concerned with the universality of crucial ingredients in psychotherapy to program planners charged with developing effective mental health services for culturally diverse or culturally different populations.

Moreover, the extent of cultural malleability of psychotherapy is the subject of considerable fascination and curiosity for many sophisticated and informed persons in and around the several social science disciplines and helping professions.

On a global basis, the World Health Organization has sponsored the expansion of mental health services to a variety of sites where they hitherto did not exist (Desjarlais, Eisenberg, Good, & Kleinman, 1995). These services have to be culturally accommodated to their communities in order to produce workable results and to be acceptable to their clientele (Higginbotham, 1984). Even therapy dyads have been construed as involving negotiation between the therapist and the client in which culturally mediated expectations and experiences are likely to play an important part (Kleinman, 1978). With the influx of migrants, refugees, and sojourners into North America and Western Europe, the challenge is to devise and implement flexible and culturally fitting services, quite often for severely traumatized victims of persecution and war. As an ambitious, but not utopian, objective, one can envisage the emergence of a unique worldwide network for exchanging useful information on psychotherapy and culture, with mutual and multilateral learning across regions, countries, and cultures. As yet, such a network does not exist, but the information contained in this volume may help culturally concerned therapists inch closer to this goal.

On a more general plane, four general conclusions appear to be warranted on the basis of the contributions included in this volume:

1. Culture does matter in the delivery of mental health and related services to the clients. As pointed out by several authors in this book, culture is crucial in defining, conceptualizing, and treating illness, disorder, or dysfunction.

2. Despite highly different trappings, certain commonalities are discernible in widely different cultural settings. Apart from globalization, which exercises a pull toward uniformity both in the experience of human distress and in the treatment of it, these shared elements may constitute the panhuman components of helpful intervention for those human problems that are beyond the sick person's available coping resources.

3. Treatment situations and therapy dyads provide glimpses into important, although often implicit and subtle, features of the culture. Therapy and healing may reflect culture, but the pathway from the technique or ritual to its cultural source or meaning is often tortuous and difficult to trace.

4. The field is at an early stage of linking cultural dimensions with indicators of psychotherapy. At this point, the potential exploration of this long neglected subject rests on a substantial amount of descriptive information about healing and therapy, which is exemplified in part by the reports and accounts included in this volume.

REFERENCES

Benedict, R. (1934). Culture and the abnormal. *Journal of General Psychology, 10,* 59–82.

Brodwin, P. (1996). *Morality and medicine in Haiti: The contest for healing power.* New York: Cambridge University Press.

Desjarlais, R., Eisenberg, L., Good, B., & Kleinman, A. (1995). *World mental health: Problems and priorities in low-income countries.* New York: Oxford University Press.

Fabrikant, B. (1984). Psychotherapy. In R. J. Corsini (Ed.), *Encyclopedia of psychology* (Vol. 3, pp. 184–186). New York: Wiley.

Frank, J. D. (1961). *Persuasion and healing: A comparative study of psychotherapy.* New York: Schocken Books.

Herskovits, M. (1949). *Man and his works.* New York: Knopf.

Higginbotham, H. N. (1984). *Third world challenge to psychiatry: Culture accommodation and mental health care.* Honolulu, HI: University of Hawaii Press.

Hofstede, G. (1991*). Cultures and organizations: Software of the mind.* London: McGraw-Hill

Hofstede, G. (2001). *Culture's consequences: Comparing values, behaviors, institutions, and organizations across nations* (2nd ed.). London, England: Sage.

Jackson, S. W. (1999). *Care of the psyche: A history of psychological healing.* New Haven, CT: Yale University Press.

Kiev, A. (1962). Psychotherapy in Haitian Voodoo. *Transcultural Psychiatric Research Review, 12,* 57–59.

Kiev, A. (1964). *Magic, faith, and healing.* New York: Free Press of Glencoe.

Kleinman, A. (1978). Clinical relevance of anthropological and cross-cultural research: Concepts and strategies. *American Journal of Psychiatry, 135,* 427–431.

Krippner, R. (2002). Conflicting perspectives on shamans and shamanism: Points and counterpoints. *American Psychologist, 57,* 962–978.

Lambo, T. A. (1964). Patterns of psychiatric care in developing African countries. In A. Kiev (Ed.), *Magic, faith, and healing* (pp. 443–453). New York: Free Press of Glencoe.

Leighton, A. H., Lambo, T. H., Hughes, C. C., Leighton, D. C., Murphy, J. M., & Macklin, D. B. (1963). *Psychiatric disorders among the Yoruba.* Ithaca, NY: Cornell University Press.

Leighton, D. C., Harding, J. S., Macklin, D. B., MacMillan, A. M., & Leighton, A. H. (1963). *The character of danger: Psychiatric symptoms in selected communities.* New York: Basic Books.

Murphy, H. B. M. (1978). The advent of guilt feelings as a common depressive symptom: A historical comparison on two continents. *Psychiatry, 41,* 229–242.

Nathan, T. (1994). *L'influence qui guérit* [*The healing influence*]. Paris: Odile Jacob.

Pfeiffer, W. M. (1994). *Transkulturelle Psychiatrie: Ergebnisse und Probleme* [*Transcultural psychiatry: Findings and problems*] (2nd ed.). Stuttgart, Germany: Thieme.

Prince, R. H. (1980). Variations in psychotherapeutic procedures. In H. C. Triandis & J. G. Draguns (Eds.), *Handbook of cross-cultural psychology. Volume 6. Psychopathology* (pp. 291–350). Boston: Allyn & Bacon.

Sue, D. W., & Sue, D. (1977). Barriers to effective cross-cultural counseling. *Journal of Counseling Psychology, 24,* 420–429.

Torrey, E. F. (1972). *The mind game: Witchdoctors and psychiatrists.* New York: Emerson Hall.

Culture, Therapy, and Healing: Basic Issues

Culture and the Origins of Psychopathology

Horacio Fabrega, Jr.
University of Pittsburgh

This chapter explores intellectual territories in the social and biological sciences that are important to cross in order to reach an optimal, culturally appropriate, and theoretically compelling understanding of mental illness that can be represented in a system of diagnosis, classification, and healing (Fabrega, 2002).

There are many specific and general terms for describing the psychological, social, and physiological disturbances ordinarily designated as mental illness, emotional illness, and psychiatric disorders. Specific terms include, for example, anxiety, depression, dementia, mania, psychosis, and personality disorders. Many types of conditions that encompass problems of personal experience and behavior are referred to collectively as psychopathology. Other familiar, general terms are mental illness, social maladjustment, and emotional health problems. Looking beyond contemporary diagnoses, we encounter terms such as insanity, madness, craziness, and the like, often used by social historians, that describe particular types of psychopathology viewed in a social context.

The cultural enterprise in human psychology must be taken seriously because any society shows and recognizes the totality of mental health issues that are covered by my chosen general term "psychopathology." Consequently, it needs to be acknowledged at the outset, that this usage represents an analytical, theoretical, scientific, and, in this sense, etic, perspective.

The term etic, from phonetic, indicates an external, scientific frame of reference and contrasts with emic, from phonemic, which involves an intracultural point of view. In a cultural-anthropological formulation, etic signifies the analyst's scientific point of view regarding a phenomenon (e.g., what a pattern of belief or social practice is interpreted by the analyst to imply or mean). An emphasis on an emic point of view draws attention to what a social practice as a pattern of belief means in the culture of the group being studied.

PROLEGOMENON: THE WESTERN, MEDICAL, AND PRAGMATIC IMPERATIVE ON THE UNIVERSALITY OF SICKNESS AND HEALING

An initial problem that must be identified and then set aside stems from the fact that my approach in this chapter is historically and culturally specific. Although it is couched in a scientific frame of reference and allegedly etic, it is also emic. The history and culture of my society has produced a knowledge base, conceptual categories, and educational institutions that in turn determined my approach. Concerns about problems of mental health and illness, or psychopathology, go back to the roots of our civilization in the Mediterranean region of Europe during antiquity, when medicine as a body of theory and practice took shape. The history of mental illness and of psychiatry can be traced to political, economic, and medical developments in Anglo-European societies involving conceptions of mental illnesses or disorders that were adopted in order to be consistent with general medicine where diseases were conceptualized as natural objects possessing their own identity and natural history.

In Anglo-European societies, there were important historical and cultural developments in the understanding of mental illness in the late 18th century and especially the 19th century. During this era, evocatively captured by intellectual and social historians like Michel Foucault, Roy Porter, Robert Castel, and Andrew Scull, psychopathology was defined as a social and highly visible public health and medical problem. The discipline and profession of psychiatry evolved as the appropriate one to handle such a problem (Fabrega, 1994, 1995, 1997).

Thus, Anglo-European societies produced the human beings whose problems were categorized as psychopathology, as well as the frame of reference that provided the concepts, idioms, and vocabularies with which the problems were analyzed. In the distinctive context of social, political, intellectual, and cultural concerns of the period, and of the complex sociodemographic and ecological changes taking place, a certain people were set apart as troubled and in need of attention, provided with public and private care, and confined to spaces where their behavior could be controlled and observed.

This project, in many ways a social mandate, consolidated the psychiatric enterprise as a species of the medical genus and as a profession. The types of psychopathology described in the dominant diagnostic systems of Anglo-European societies, enshrined in *the International Classification of Diseases (10th edition)* and *DSM-IV* systems of diagnosis, are children of the larger medical enterprise that consolidated itself in the 19th century and went on to evolve into an international configuration during the late 20th century. The medical framing of psychopathology, of course, is simply one of many approaches to mental health problems; other forms of healing exist, but they need not march under the medical banner of psychiatry.

Today, then, it is crucial to realize that distinctive historical, political, ecological, demographic, and cultural factors shape the window through which one peers at psychopathology. In other words, the mental health professions through which attempts are now made to heal peoples of diverse cultures have practical and pragmatic roots in and are keyed to the assortment of problems of living in a distinctive ecology and the cultural urban psychology of urban settings in modern Anglo-European societies.

Nonhuman Primate Studies

Descriptions of the social life of nonhuman primates, especially chimpanzees, who constitute the closest living evolutionary relatives of *Homo sapiens*, disclose that they are subject to disease, pathology, and injury (Goodall, 1986). Although this is hardly surprising, what is more relevant is that when stricken, their social behavior appears to reflect an awareness of being in an altered state or condition of sickness and healing (Boesch, 1992). They show manifestations of disease and loss of energy, motivation, debility, and pain in a socially meaningful way that appears to communicate a condition of suffering and a need for healing. Chimpanzees also nurture those who are sick and to whom they are closely bonded, cleaning their wounds and offering assistance. Ethologists have recognized this phenomenon when diseased chimpanzees seek and use special plant specimens in ways that suggest medicinal self-healing. All of these observations and interpretations about sickness and healing are proffered with an appreciation of the fact that chimpanzees are highly social and respond to conspecifies in meaningful ways (de Waal, 1996). For chimpanzees, certain injuries and diseases of the medical domain are on the threshold of constituting a symbolic, protocultural category.

Based on such observations, one can suggest that diseased and injured chimpanzees show and communicate sickness and ultimately participate in forms of healing. Consequently, one can surmise that the last common ancestor of *Homo sapiens* and the Pongid line showed behaviors analogous to what we humans call sickness and healing. Although sickness and healing behaviors are culturally shaped and constructed in humans, one can argue that their roots are actually homologous to those of the Pongids and, presumably, the earliest hominids, and that they could reflect the operation of what Tooby and Cosmides (1992) refer to as a psychological adaptation (Fabrega, 1997).

Human Studies

Some of the fossil remains of Neanderthals, a group of archaic humans whose origins preceded the advent of *Homo sapiens,* show evidence of healed fractures and arrangements of these fossils that suggest burial practices (Gamble, 1993; Stringer & Gamble, 1993; Trinkaus & Shipman, 1992). This raises the question of medical practices and a possible symbolic awareness of death. Thus, it is possible that sickness and healing behaviors were part of the behavioral ecology and culture of these groups. Although prehistory disease and pathology were common eventualities, paleoanthropologists and medical ecologists have been able to estimate the level of disease and the epidemiological profile of human populations in relation to ecology and social organization and complexity (Cohen, 1989).

Ethnographies of sociocultural anthropologists reveal that all extant social groups, from the most elementary nomadic, foraging hunter-gatherers to the more complex sedentary, agricultural tribes and prestates, possessed systems of knowledge about medical problems and culturally elaborated modalities of therapy. Scholars from many disciplines have shown that complex civilizations of Mediterranean Europe, India, China, Tibet, Mesoamerica, and the ancient Near East had elaborate knowledge structures pertaining to sickness and healing (Fabrega, 1997; see also the Chapters 12, 16, and 19 in this volume).

All of the literate great traditions of medicine have conceptualized medical problems in a holistic and functional way. In other words, they handled bodily ailments and manifestations on par with psychological and emotional problems. Physical health problems and mental health problems were explained and dealt with therapeutically within a common rationalized frame of reference that encompassed what can be termed ethno- or cultural forms of anatomy, physiology, pharmacology, and psychology. Problems of health were acknowledged from the standpoint of the individual's needs. In other words, his or her personal and social circumstances were critically relevant to the equation that explained sickness, suffering, and rationalized therapies. In this context, a functional approach to disease is comprised of herbal medicines and procedures applied to the body, advice and counseling on living practices and moral dilemmas, curing rituals, and attempts to persuade and help resolve social conflicts inevitably entangled in scenarios of sickness and healing. They were all part of the holistic, integrated approach to suffering and to its therapy.

THE EVOLUTIONARY STUDY OF PSYCHOPATHOLOGY

Problems of Defining Psychopathology

Human problems marked by compelling personal suffering universally elicit compassion and are consistently interpreted as "sickness." For reasons connected to cultural and historical traditions, these problems are classified as physiological as compared to psychosocial. According to many experts, this classification would already constitute an undesirable medicalizing of the topic of cultural therapy.

It is necessary to take one step further in this medicalization and refer to psychosocial behavior problems as forms of psychopathology, or what otherwise are known as mental health problems. Consistent with an evolutionary analysis, this term is efficient and easily applicable in a purely nominal sense to the kinds of major developments that involve cognition, language, and culture—all of which are at the heart of the "psycho" part of psychopathology. Considering this chapter's evolutionary frame of reference, one must rely on a broad definition that distinguishes specific processes in animals, especially nonhuman primates, as well as humans.

Psychopathology can be defined as forms of altered psychosocial behavior of organisms or individuals, almost invariably associated with disorders of bodily function, discomfort, and pain that are productive of personal suffering and pose a potential cost to their fitness. Generally, the term fitness identifies an adequate coping mechanism in a particular sociocultural context, or a specific biological one in terms of one's ability to survive and reproduce. Suffering and fitness, then, are the key aspects of psychopathology viewed in an evolutionary context, which is not inconsistent with a clinician's point of view. It must be reemphasized that this definition is analytical because it is based on scientific knowledge from the social and biological sciences. In this sense, the definition is also etic. It portrays cultural variability and relativism within the framework of social construction that interprets disturbances of personal experience, behavior, and bodily functions.

This definition brings us into a consistent relationship with ethologists, comparative psychologists, veterinary specialists, and perhaps even with animal psychologists. When psychopathology is deconstructed, a range of manifestations appears to include certain aspects of animal distress and impaired well-being, the many symptoms of mental illness that psychiatrists and clinical psychologists study, the impairments in social living, and their potential deleterious consequences. Subsequently, the latter incorporate the potential interference of subsistence pursuits, social relations, mating, reproducing, parenting, and longevity. These factors are central to the evolutionary account of social behavior considered as a cluster of traits of organisms and individuals. It should be noted that because of the way psychopathology has been defined, it also constitutes a variety of sicknesses with special characteristics examined in a later section of this chapter.

The Problem of Speciesism and Anthropomorphism

To study and make scientific sense of the social and communicative behavior patterns of animals, particularly those of the higher primates whose capacities are more closely related to *Homo sapiens*, means to plunge deeply into philosophical quandaries. When certain questions pertaining to health, particularly to a level of well-being and possible suffering, are added, these quandaries seem magnified. In this case, one seems to be exporting concepts derived from the study of humans to animals whose nature and adaptation should be analyzed by means of objective, impersonal concepts and a scientific theory. Evolutionary theory analyzes such things as the relative effectiveness of the use of resources, success in reproduction, interspecific and intraspecific competition, reciprocal altruism, inclusive fitness, and mortality. However, this approach overlooks the possibility of an organism suffering because of poor health. Biologists, veterinary specialists, comparative psychologists, and paleoanthropologists use the terms anthropomorphism and speciesism to refer to inappropriate application of human traits to animals. (Dawkins 1980, 1990).

Although this topic remains philosophically complex, it is blunted in the case of the nonhuman primates, especially chimpanzees, whose cognitive and cultural capacities are widely appreciated and have received much attention (de Waal, 1996). Comparative psychologists have been able to study higher primates in various natural and controlled laboratory conditions in order to clarify in what ways it is appropriate to ascribe to them such human qualities as self-awareness, intentionality, deception (termed Machiavellian intelligence), and mental attribution. Similarly, biologists and veterinary specialists have argued strongly for the appropriateness of considering questions of suffering and well-being within a general biological and evolutionary frame of reference. When one pursues the implications of these topics, namely, the problems of social behavior and biological fitness on the one hand, and matters involving well-being and suffering on the other, one is not far removed from the common meaning of etic concepts such as pathology and even psychopathology. A strict evolutionary approach differs from a clinical one.

Problems with the Concept and Definition of Culture

The concept of culture plays a critical role in the social and biological sciences and is, of course, vital to the discussions included in this volume. In this chapter, the term culture represents the system of symbols and their meaning by means of which members of a group make sense of their world, program subsistence activities in their habitat, and rationalize social action. Therefore, culture refers to a system of information that groups have evolved for their members to learn, and which is passed on within and across generations. In this context, a capacity for language serves as a form of cognition and communication and constitutes an integral part of culture.

In a strict scientific sense, the concept of culture poses some problems, especially when one concentrates on human behavior in an evolutionary framework (Parker & Russon, 1996). The exact cultural attributes are all heavily contested questions about which cultural anthropologists, biological anthropologists, and evolutionary psychologists have different answers (Foley, 1987, 1995). Specific examples include whether the higher apes show cultural attributes, how and when they were acquired in the line of evolution stretching from the earliest hominids (the "ape end" of the evolutionary continuum), to the advent of *Homo sapiens* (the "modern human" end of that continuum), and even whether the concept of culture itself has scientific probity. One common and defensible position is that human cognition and culture, including a language capacity, constitute attributes of what Donald has referred to as the modern mind, and that these, together with related traits and properties of *Homo sapiens*, have an evolutionary history (Donald, 1991). At some point during human evolution (with a highly disputed date), organisms acquired characteristics such as a capacity to represent the external world, think and communicate by means of language (preceded, perhaps, by a protolanguage of sorts), explain their place in the scheme of things and maintain a group identity through myths and by means of ritual, and acquire verbally transmitted knowledge structures about natural history and practical affairs of living (for background, see Bickerton, 1990, 1995; Donald, 1991; Dunbar et al., 1995; Foley, 1987, 1995; Knight, 1991, 1995).

As a consequence of the process of enculturation, conceived in this context as a progressive incorporation of a capacity for language, cognition, and culture, organisms which we can now begin to refer to as individuals and persons came to learn about and conceptualize natural history and the ecology. An expansion of culture led to integrated conceptions pertaining to disease, injury, and pathology, and, as a result, better ways to cope with these eventualities. Sickness and healing phenomena, which one can trace back to the ape end of the evolutionary continuum, became elaborated and socially constructed. One can assume that these developments entailed the recognition of sickness and suffering in relation to personal and group crises requiring intervention or healing. The actual impairments and disabilities associated with pain, suffering, the morbidity of disease, and the possibility of losing life became part of the organism's existented response, and ways of handling this incorporated in group's medical knowledge.

Problems with the Concept of Psychopathology

How groups deal with sickness dominated by psychosocial disturbances compared to how they deal with those dominated by physiological ones can pose a conceptual problem in cultural psychiatry and medical anthropology. A similar problem exists in return to evolutionary studies. When syndromes of psychopathology include prominent bodily manifestations and associated suffering/distress, handling them under the rubric of sickness/healing and conceptualizing them as part of the medical equation are not particularly difficult to understand (Fabrega, 1997). However, from an evolutionary point of view, it is more difficult to understand syndromes of psychopoathology that, on the one hand, were dominated by and/or limited to purely social and psychological behaviors that did not appear to constitute physical states of disease, while, on the other hand, their manifestations involved self-interested actions that were socially divisive (e.g., hostility, sexual possessiveness and jealousy, failure to reciprocate and share, antisocial actions, etc.). A cross-cultural emic shows that these types of antisocial behaviors are not usually interpreted in ways that suggest psychopathology (i.e., as forms of distress, suffering, or maladaptation that suggest sickness and for which healing is deemed appropriate). In addition, where contemporary societies attempt to equate forms of social deviance and antisociality with mental illness this gives rise to controversy (Kittrie, 1971). In short, one can infer that to conceptualize all forms of contemporary psychopathology (especially those giving rise to socially divisive behaviors) as having their roots in human evolution creates intellectual tension. Nevertheless, since psychopathology is usually associated with distress and is further discussed in the context of an individual's psychosocial behavior, one's analysis can proceed to link responses to psychopathology to those of sickness and of occasional healing efforts. It is also the case, of course, that even socially divisive forms of psychopathology have been brought under the explanatory scheme of evolutionary psychology and psychiatry, as is the case with antisocial behavior (Fabrega, 2002).

Frequently, psychopathology incorporates problems involving altered states of consciousness, including trance and possession, and these also seem counterintuitive in a nonhuman context. With respect to the latter, the anthropologists Goodman (1988, 1990) and Oubré (1997) have conjectured that resorting to ritual actions and the capacity to enter and make cultural sense and use of altered states of consciousness were part of the prehistoric behavioral equation (Ludwig, 1968). In coping with the dilemmas of self-awareness, implications of being as compared to nonbeing or death, and the need to maintain a group identity, organisms/individuals along the line extending from protoculture to culture probably began to engage in patterns of behavior that included repetitive motor sequences, rhythmic chanting, and ritualized postures serving as stimuli to induce altered states of consciousness. Thus, it is likely that during evolution, prehistoric altered states of consciousness involving trance and possession were part of a symbolic coping repertoire that may have colored incidents of psychopathology.

Setting altered states of consciousness aside, it is with respect to types of purely social and psychological forms of potential psychopathology, particularly when devoid of bodily/physiological manifestations, that the concept of psychopathology presents intellectual quandaries for one intending to apply it to nonhuman groups. To connect this point to the previous discussion, it is precisely with respect to predominantly social and psychological behavior problems that the quandary of speciesism and anthropomorphism, in accordance with the interpretation of behavior of animals and higher primates, and by extension, protocultural and protohuman groups of organisms, presents itself most acutely. Psychopathology encompasses a great deal more than what one can comfortably handle by means of a concept such as sickness and healing and what one can attribute to the mode of behavior of a group of protohuman organisms or individuals. This brings us to the issue of the exquisitely human and cultural connotative implications of the concept of psychopathology, which will be discussed later.

THE BIOLOGICAL EVOLUTION OF PSYCHOPATHOLOGY

The Character of the Evolutionary Terrain

There is comparatively little ethnographic data about sickness, healing, and psychopathology among contemporary hunter-gatherers (Fabrega, 1997), although it enables one to claim that such medical- and mental-health-related phenomena are well represented in these groups (Simons & Hughes, 1985). There is much controversy about whether the culture and the way of life of contemporary hunter-gatherers preserve characteristics of prehistoric foragers, especially certain salient attributes of the kind of life that existed when modern humans evolved in response to the so-called environment of evolutionary adaptedness (Lee & DeVore, 1968; Price & Brown, 1985). In this regard, one prevalent and highly influential generalization states that hunter-gatherers offer the best possible glimpse of what life might have been like during the later phases of human evolution.

The starting point of the evolutionary terrain that pertains to sickness and psychopathology can be placed among groups of the last common ancestors of hominids and Pongids for which the behaviors and culture of chimpanzees offer the best model of what life was like. Generally speaking, the way foragers and hunters handle problems of disease, pathology, and injury more specifically allows one to place the end point of the biological evolution of sickness, healing, and psychopathology. From this point onwards, one is essentially involved in mapping the picture of the cultural evolution of these problems.

On the Phylogeny of Psychopathology

Obtaining a direct picture of what one can regard as psychopathology among pre- or protohumans is, of course, impossible. Results of studies of the natural behavior of the higher primates regarding such practices as infanticide and cannibalism encourage ethologists to raise the question of the possibility of psychosocial pathologies (Goodall, 1986). A dominant explanation of such "abnormal" behaviors is provided by evolutionary theory, especially sexual selection (e.g., males eliminate the offspring of their competitors). A competing explanation is that stress, crowding, and even human intervention enter into the group's life ways and perturbit.

Another window through which one may be afforded a look at prehistoric psychopathologies is provided by its laboratory manufacture in nonhuman primates. These include, first, the set of studies set in motion by Harlow and carried forward by his students involving social and maternal separation and the imposition of different and less pronounced forms of stress on parent-offspring relations (Harlow & Novak, 1973; Suomi 1978). These studies reveal that a variety of gross and subtle forms of what can safely be regarded as psychopathologies can be induced in nonhuman primates, and that these persist and can be shown to exist when infants reach adolescence and maturity. Second, laboratory versions of psychopathology are, of course, created by brain lesion studies of nonhuman primates (Franzen & Myers, 1973). Various forms of gross psychological ineptitude, social behavioral avoidance and timidity, and more subtle personality disturbances, have been produced as a consequence of lesions to selected regions of the brain (Fabrega, 2002). Third, and finally, there exists the myriad other types of animal models of psychopathology that have been devised to study the natural history and response to treatment of psychotic-like states, syndromes resembling autism, and varieties of mood disorders, including depression and anxiety (Kaplan, 1986).

All of the preceding are examples of psychopathology produced or manufactured in the laboratory. In "real life," the serious ones would inevitably culminate in the organism's failure to compete, look after itself, reproduce, and simply thrive. The more subtle forms produce behavioral changes of the sort likely to interfere negatively in the organism's social behavior by rendering the animal impulsive, timid, overly anxious, easily prone to regress, and socially compromised. Such changes also lead generally to lower positions in the ranking system.

Some psychiatrists and psychologists, most notably Crow (1991, 1993a, 1993b), Gardner (1982), Marks (1987), Wenegrat (1984, 1990), Gilbert (1992a, 1992b), Bailey (1987), Stevens and Price (1996), and Sloman and Gilbert (2000) have provided general and comprehensive formulations about the origin of distinctive types of psychiatric disturbances based on ideas of evolutionary theory. To these theorists, contemporary psychiatric disturbances constitute exaggerations or perturbations of naturally adaptive programs of behavior that played vitally important roles during human evolution (i.e., that might have been positively selected for) and/or that are the result of mutations that are maintained in human populations (i.e., that have not been selected out) because the traits themselves of associated ones in other systems of function provide fitness advantages through heterozygosity and/or heterosis.

The preceding summarizes the explanatory schemes and related body of data that one can use to argue for something like the biological evolution of psychopathology. The material discloses that higher primates are genetically and biologically prone to develop behavioral disturbances in the context of stress and/or injury to the central nervous system. In most instances, if such pathologies were to arise naturally, organisms would be unable to survive or be rendered so compromised as to fare less well in their group. With respect to happenings in natural communities of primates, a biologist would probably explain the *consequences* of such psychopathologies in terms of the theory of evolution. For example, environmental pressures, predation from social carnivores, disease, and injury are harsh realities of a brutish nature and can be expected in the course of events to not only challenge and stress, but also traumatize members of primate communities. The result of this will be conditions of sickness, including syndromes of psychopathology not unlike those manufactured in the laboratory as models of mental illness and observed in natural communities of social primates by ethologists and primatologists (see Fabrega, 2002, for review). A strict evolutionary accounting of these conditions, including their causation and consequences or natural history, would draw on ideas of competition, natural selection, and adaptation. Recently, the idea that disorders, including psychiatric disorders, constitute harmful dysfunctions (i.e., disturbances in the realization of natural biological functions that are harmful to the individual) has been argued forcibly and also critiqued (see Fabrega, 2002, for review).

A clinician interested in an evolutionary understanding of the origins of human psychopathology is left with several questions. Why does the potential for such disturbances to occur in primates exist? Is an explanation that the disorders arise merely as a passive consequence of severe disruptions in the organism's evolved mechanisms and routines of adaptation (e.g., either its social environment and/or its apparatus) sufficient? Is behavior in an evolutionary context to be conceptualized as holistic and the manifestations of these disturbances as merely a consequence of breaking apart such a holistically programmed organism? Can one hypothesize that such disorders reflect the integration of a number of traits, each of which has a genetic basis, and that these traits are implicated in and can help explain the bases for some of the major psychiatric disturbances? During the course of evolution when language, cognition, and culture were emergent phenomena in the hominid line, how might such naturally occurring forms of psychopathology have been handled as social phenomena? At what point during evolution did psychopathologies come to be handled less in the brutish ways of natural selection and more in terms of cultural factors that involved values, moral traditions, and systems of social governance that reflected a humane and moral understanding and interpretation of the afflicted individual? Some of the possible answers to these questions are looked at later (see also Fabrega, 2002).

Comment

During the last several decades, the theory of human evolution has become increasingly more influential in the study of human behavior, sparked in part by the publication and popularization of Wilson's (1975) *Sociobiology: The New Synthesis*. Studies in ethology, comparative psychology, behavioral ecology, and then primatology provided the background and helped articulate a framework for conceptualizing human behavior as a product of natural selection. Social and psychological behavior, like features of morphology and physiology, came to be considered legitimate traits of the phenotype and were conceptualized as a product of the evolutionary process. This is exemplified by the subdisciplines of evolutionary psychology and evolutionary psychiatry, each of which has now standard textbooks for students of the respective parent disciplines (see Fabrega, 2002, for review). Developmental studies in particular have been influenced by the attention paid to seemingly innate, biologically prepared routines pertaining to the acquisition of interpersonal attention and attunement, language, social cognition, and the theory of mind.

The respective doctrines influenced by the evolutionary theory examine human social behavior, including psychopathology, as the result of selective influences that operated in ancestral environments or so-called ultimate causes of behavior that were designed by natural selection in the environment of evolutionary adaptiveness. In psychology, an increasing number of constructs pertaining to the interface of brain and behavior (variously termed psychological adaptations, algorithms, or infrastructural mechanisms), are posited as influencing, producing, mediating, governing, and/or determining behavior—depending on the orientation and emphasis of the researcher. Much controversy and contention is quite obviously associated with the evolutionary perspective because it appears to challenge and contradict strongly held notions about the unique character of human beings and culture.

Most recently, and in relation to the doctrine of innate, naturally designed psychological mechanisms or algorithms, the idea has been put forth that psychopathology (or in the language of the respective theoreticians, psychiatric disorders) constitutes, in effect, examples of harmful dysfunctions of natural mechanisms. Persons, in other words, are the embodiment of evolutionary mechanisms that have definable, natural biological functions shaped in ancestral environments. It is the breakdown of these mechanisms and the failure to realize the respective functions in association with the production of harm to the person that qualify the resulting syndrome of behavior as a disorder or variety of psychopathology. The strengths and weaknesses of the harmful dysfunction slant on psychopathology are not central to the present discussion. Evolutionary psychiatrists and psychologists certainly think as though psychopathology constitutes a harmful dysfunction, but they also appear to think that some examples of so-called psychopathology are really adaptations that have either gone awry or are misapplied in the contemporary environment. Complex issues in cognitive psychology, cultural anthropology, and evolutionary biology are implicated in these discussions, but they can be put aside here (Fabrega, 2002).

The important point is to emphasize that evolutionary biology has a claim to be represented in a system of understanding pertaining to mental health and illness. In other words, if one hopes to arrive at a way of understanding and representing psychopathology in a fully satisfactory way, then one must traverse the evolutionary terrain, cross the intellectual hurdles it poses to understanding, and take away from this challenge insights and knowledge learned by traversing its epistemic landmarks. What these evolutionary principles and landmarks consist of and how they should be represented in a system of diagnosis and classification should occupy the minds of those intending to derive a prudent psychiatric nosology or theory of understanding, diagnosis, and classification of psychopathology.

THE EMERGENCE OF CULTURE AND PSYCHOPATHOLOGY

General Considerations

What exactly took place during prehistory that culminated in the establishment of a human cultural way of life constitutes an enormously complex and controversial question about which a great deal has been written. It is asserted by some that higher primates, particularly chimpanzees, display learned traditions and ways of doing things that could pass as culture (Parker & Russon, 1996). This position underscores the view that culture is an overused, empirically weak concept that is best approached as referring to a cluster of traits (e.g., tool use, language, stable heterosexual bonding, rituals, and beliefs) that human communities display, and each of the traits should be viewed as having its own evolutionary history. Such a partible, gradualist perspective holds that the emergence of culture was a slow process that was not necessarily marked by any definitive Rubicon-like landmark. At the other extreme are those keeping with a *punctualist point of view*, who contend that the emergence of a cultural way of life necessarily tied very closely to the evolution of language, with all of this constituting a major transformative event.

Leaving aside the possibility of a single, major mutation or physical change, the evolution of language was undoubtedly extended in time and naturally selected. It ushered in a new, unique way of life consisting of what is termed a "symbolic niche" (Carruthers, 1996; Chase & Dibble, 1987; Noble & Davidson, 1996; Pfeiffer, 1982). In other words, it established a totally different conceptual way of life (from earlier hominids) that featured individuals living in communities of rules and contracts, notions of personal and social identity clearly profiled, patterned obligations to one another constituting a social order, and myths, systems of beliefs, and rituals that rationalized the position of the group in the world. An interesting version of this position is that of Knight (1991), who holds that much of culture can be explained by processes involving female bonding, synchronous control of menstruation, and contracting with males for supply of meat in exchange for sexual favors.

Fundamentally, the topic of the emergence of culture can be viewed as simply another version of the topic of human evolution with all of its complexity and contestation. However, most paleoanthropologists and archeologists hold the view that something dramatic and fairly unique happened during the transition between the Middle and Upper Paleolithic era about 40,000 years ago. Archeological remains point to a symbolic capacity and approach to life, something that is viewed as categorically different from the preceding Neanderthals and other archaic humans and later varieties of *Homo erectus*. Pfeiffer (1982) referred to this phase of evolution as producing a creative explosion in order to emphasize the way of life of the earliest Upper Paleolithic peoples, whose remains consist of imaginative cave paintings, sculptured objects made of stone and bone, and evidence of organized living arrangements. In general, timing and pace of the processes that culminated in the evolution of language, cognition, and culture are highly complex and contested among biological anthropologists, archeologists, and evolutionary biologists and psychologists.

Effects of the Emergence of Culture on Sickness and Healing

It is not too difficult to formulate a general scenario of how the emergence of culture affected the character of sickness and healing. Practical knowledge that could be learned by trial and error and accumulated in a group was made available. A lore or perspective about sickness and healing was made possible. In other words, illness theories, healing schedules, and what anthropologists term explanatory models and idioms of distress and affliction together made sickness and healing a more or less tangible, socially identified, and cultural reality.

A cultural way of life also imparted a greater social and existential significance to ensembles of sickness and healing. The implications of disease/pathology/injury, which individuals could suffer visibly and possibly not recover from, was made a palpable reality in the group. It enabled a more elaborated and conceptual approach with groups having knowledge available to them that had accumulated over generations about the character of sickness and about procedures and medicines that could heal, alleviate pain, and restore health.

Anthropologists believe that tied to the emergence of culture is a cosmological orientation; a capacity for religious, supernatural, or numinous experiences; and abilities to make use of altered states of consciousness via dancing and ritualized motor routines in a group setting (Boyer, 1994; Oubré, 1997). Practical, mundane knowledge of sickness and healing was conjoined with esoteric, sacred knowledge and with associated religious/supernatural experiences in which trance and possession constituted embryonic ceremonies having diverse functions in the group. Among these functions, one can safely surmise, were the reversal of disease/pathology/injury in a defined individual or individuals and the maintenance and the protection of health of all group members.

Effects of the Emergence of Culture on the Character of Psychopathology

Formulating a realistic scenario of how the emergence of culture affected the character of psychopathology and its handling is a far more difficult undertaking. It is useful to merely summarize briefly some of the relevant issues to better grasp this problem. First, there is the matter of causation. Here it is best to assume 1) a baseline of genetic vulnerability that became incorporated into human populations and that constituted the accumulation of earlier attempts to cope socioecologically and behaviorally with selective forces of the environment; 2) the possibility of disease and physical trauma, the direct or indirect consequences of which could alter brain function; and 3) the inevitability of strains and stressors related to having to compete and survive both in a group and in a harsh, demanding habitat. These scientifically construed factors can be regarded as the fundamental conditions that prevailed throughout prehistory and that caused varieties of psychopathologies to be inevitable, recurring eventualities in hominid and human groups. Given this baseline, and looking at things from the point of view of the group members, a symbolic approach to life (constituted in culture and language) meant that all sorts of imagined, remembered, and anticipated incidents and agents could be brought into a picture of psychological distress that contributed to an incident of psychopathology. Such things as worries, doubts, fears, suspicions, a sense of profound emptiness, despondency at the loss of valued objects, jealousies, temptations to transgress, and unfounded beliefs all became possible sources of mental agony and behavioral alterations that served to undermine adaptive coping.

Second, there is the matter of manifestations. The psychological consequences of culture and symbolization meant that all incidents of psychopathology could be permeated by the range of distressing concerns that become possible when individuals exist and relate to one another and to themselves in fantasy and imagination, that is to say, in terms of the inner worries and preoccupations reviewed earlier. All of these concerns were realized in explanations and cognized emotions associated with the altered behavior and experiences that make up an episode of psychopathology. Then they were enacted and played out in meaningful, interpretable social psychological behavior routines. Such emotional manifestations of culture, language, and cognition were naturally added to the range of disturbances of social behavior of hominids and earlier varieties of *Homo* that manifested themselves in impairments of traditional biological pursuits involving foraging, cooperation and competition, mate selection, parenting, warding off predators, and competing with other groups of hominids, earlier varieties of *Homo*, and/or *Homo sapiens*.

Third and last, there is the matter of handling social responses. From the standpoint of the evolution of language, cognition, culture, and especially psychopathology, how are the signs and symptoms of psychopathology interpreted by a member of the group and how are they handled? This issue is perhaps the most complex and difficult to conceptualize and make sense of in evolutionary terms. As indicated earlier, less of a problem is created by incidents of psychopathology associated with prominent bodily/physiological symptoms and suffering and/or with manifestations of social and cognitive dilapidation (i.e., grossly psychotic states). This suggests that general biological approaches involving responses to sickness and associated practices involving healing held sway (Fabrega, 1997). Indeed, any incidents of psychopathology (irrespective of associated bodily/physiological symptoms) in which behavioral manifestations were not socially divisive or antisocial in nature (that is, behaviors that pointed inwardly and negatively to the individual and reflected his or her personal distress) were probably handled in terms of existing conventions pertaining to sickness and healing and do not pose serious problems to one seeking to understand the origins of psychopathology. These were essentially social psychological syndromes featured by prominent indicators of suffering and pain, regardless of how these were culturally/symbolically configured and enacted.

Other varieties of contemporary psychopathology pose more of a problem to an individual intending to clarify how the emergence of language, cognition, and culture may have affected the interpretation of psychopathology as a social phenomenon. I have in mind those varieties of psychopathology in which behavioral manifestations pointed negatively outwards, such as psychopathologies manifesting themselves by suspicion, distrust, social antagonisms, antisocial behavior, social exploitation, sexual coercion, and social as well as sexual violence. These are manifestations that even in modern medical psychology, psychiatry, and mental health practice more generally create intellectual and moral tensions, as discussed earlier. From an evolutionary standpoint, they have been explained in different ways, for example, as features of natural strategies or natural functions, as evolutionary residuals rooted in biological functions, and as aberrations or dilapidations of natural functions. These varieties of psychopathology are more difficult to explain in terms of ideas pertaining to sickness and healing, in other words, as naturally eliciting support, consolation, forms of tolerance, and outright healing. Some of these socially divisive forms of psychopathology invariably bring the individual into positions of conflict with group mates and lead to social isolation, retaliatory punishment and violence, and/or banishment. The result can be misery and suffering for the person showing the "psychopathology" as well as impaired biological fitness. And although many individuals who show such behavioral pathologies may have been abused, exploited, and generally mistreated (and their behavior a result of this), their sense of suffering and misery is often screened and concealed. Frequently, it is not easy to erase the impression that the "afflicted persons" are following selfish interests, pursuits, and social agendas.

In summary, syndromes or ensembles of behavior featured by such things as prominent displays of or predispositions toward hostility, suspiciousness, antisociality, pride and vanity, social arrogance, grandiosity, social and sexual exploitation, and violence, as well as socially aversive and divisive behavior, create tensions for one intending to achieve a broad understanding of psychopathology. Although these syndromes are conceptualized and handled today as treatable conditions, and in this sense as falling within the rubric of psychiatric disorder, it is hard to visualize them as objects of treatment in ancestral environments. The social behavior content of the syndromes blurs the line that separates the "natural" morality of suffering and ailment from the "natural" censure and punishment of the antisocial, a region of behavior that can be accommodated within evolutionary biology and psychology but creates tension in the attempt to integrate these sciences with traditional concerns of the clinician (Fabrega, 2002).

Many of these antisocial varieties of psychopathology are handled today as aspects of personality disorders. Nonetheless, although one must insist that configurations of personality and its aberrations are culturally constructed, even native, culturally constructed varieties of personality aberrations or "disorders" are unlikely to have been handled as forms of personal affliction and sickness/healing when they impacted negatively upon group mates. The handling of personally enhancing, selfish, and socially divisive manifestations of psychopathology as forms of sickness for which healing is "natural" constitutes a chapter in the later cultural evolution of psychopathology.

It needs to be emphasized that any and all of the varieties of psychopathology, as well as ensembles pertaining to sickness and healing more generally, that have been discussed in relation to the emergence of culture could have been and frequently were associated with altered states of consciousness. Altered mental states, including trance and possession, could form a part of a picture of sickness and psychopathology, or of a healing response (either on the part of the "patient" or his/her healing audience). Clearly, in no way can one maintain even today that all syndromes of behavior featured by altered states of consciousness are psychopathological. Moreover, this applies even more so to what probably transpired during the transition to a cultural/symbolic way of life, when recourse to the controlled use of such altered states of consciousness was arguably likely to have been more common. Altered states of consciousness, particularly when they involved making connections with religious/cosmological agents and themes, probably confounded and ambiguated the interpretation of psychopathology in emergent communities of modern humans, in some instances blurring the sickness/healing part and in others the personally aggrandizing and socially divisive part.

THE CULTURAL EVOLUTION OF SICKNESS, HEALING, AND PSYCHOPATHOLOGY

On the Nature of Cultural Evolution

In a general way, cultural evolution implies changes in the way of life and thinking of a people that take place across time. More specifically, it includes the kinds of intellectual, political, economic, social, ecological, scientific, and technological changes that have taken place since the Upper Paleolithic era when modern humans first became dominant. In a more technical sense, the term cultural evolution is used to refer to the process that brought about such changes, conceptualized now in terms analogous to those of biological evolution. Whereas biological evolution involves the changes in the character and spread of genetic traits or units of information (conceptualized as genes, with variation, natural selection, and inheritance as key features of the process of evolution), cultural evolution involves changes in the character and spread of cultural traits or units of information, (conceptualized as memes, with variation, (now) cultural selection, and spread within and across generations as key features of the process). The relationship between biological traits, genetic traits as compared to cultural evolution, and the nature of the differing influences that the effects of these processes have on social and psychological behavior is complex and very contestable (Boyd & Richerson, 1985; Campbell, 1960, 1965, 1975; Cavalli-Sforza & Feldman, 1981; Lumsden & Wilson, 1981).

Two Ways of Visualizing Cultural Evolution

At least two ways exist in which one can make sense of the process of cultural evolution. Anthropologists and sociologists have described phases that capture salient characteristics that societies have undergone since the emergence of modern humans (Sanderson, 1990). For example, one scheme involves family-level societies, village-level societies, chiefdoms, prestates, states, civilizations and empires, modern European societies, and postmodern European societies (Fabrega, 1997; Johnson & Earle, 1987). Each of these types of society, which can be characterized in terms of size, complexity, mode of subsistence, level of technology, and political economic structures, as well as cultural/symbolic resources and mentalities, is held to capture a particular phase of cultural evolution. Differences would occur in the kinds of persons and social relations constructed in these societies; the forms of work and occupation that pattern daily lives; the kinds of rules, obligations, and laws that maintain order and organization; and the types of leisure pursuits that are available. Meanings of symbols are emphasized in this approach.

Another way in which one can make sense of cultural evolution is to describe the kinds of social and historical processes and transformations that have taken place since the emergence of culture. This involves taking account of such things as changes in social ecology, the mode of subsistence, demography, political economic organization, the system of communication and the storage of information and literacy, the level of industrialization, the development of science and technology, forms of government, and civil participation in the workings of society. Rather than concentrating on distinctive types of society, one concentrates on the processes that have transformed small-scale, nomadic societies into increasingly more complex ones in terms of sociological characteristics as per roles, social practices, institutions, and the like. Such sociological changes have the effect of altering ways of feeling and thinking. Both ways of making sense of cultural evolution are obviously interrelated and presuppose each other.

Effects of Cultural Evolution on Sickness, Healing, and Psychopathology

How cultural evolution has affected the character of sickness, healing and psychopathology represents a very complex topic in the social sciences (Fabrega, 1997). The process of social evolution itself has been taken up by sociologists and essentially involves analyzing and chronicling the factors that have contributed to bringing about increases in the size, social stratification, and political-economic organization in societies culminating in modern, capitalist societies (Sanderson, 1990). For purposes of understanding sickness/healing and psychopathology, it is best to handle this topic abstractly in a global way and concentrate on modern, contemporary developments.

As implied earlier, the advent of science and the evolution of European medicine during the late eighteenth and nineteenth centuries created what social historians of medicine term the modern concept of disease. This development emphasized that problems of sickness and healing became centered on disease as a specific, ontologically identified "thing" and on treatment directed at either removing, undoing, or neutralizing the effects of disease. This model of sickness and healing contrasts sharply with the functional approach of the great traditions of medicine (and indeed, of most earlier approaches and of those of contemporary nonindustrial societies) in which a psychosomatic and somatopsychic integrated view of the person prevailed (see Chapters 12, 13, 15, 16, and 19). In this holistic view, organic or bodily manifestations of sickness and the character of an individual's life, habits, and behaviors were given salient consideration. In the modern conception, manifestations of sickness and efforts at healing were aimed at disease entities, and psychological symptoms or manifestations were viewed as resulting from brain pathologies. At the same time, dualism was given a major emphasis, with the mental realm of symptoms and maladies taking on heightened concern (Porter, 1987; see also Chapter 5 in this volume).

As alluded to earlier in the chapter, reform movements in Anglo-European societies tackled the vexing social problems posed by the rise and concentration of persons who were seriously mentally ill and in need of institutional care. What had been a concern of many social disciplines and institutions became strongly medicalized. The movement toward medicalization was reflected in the creation of the "science" of psychopathology, an enterprise aimed at rigorously describing and classifying manifestations of mental illnesses that were presumed to be rooted in the brain. Because the character of mental illness was held to be reflected in mental phenomena and because science aims at "carving nature at its joints," the science of descriptive psychopathology dutifully aimed at uncovering, labeling, and codifying the way mental experiences and mental processes (i.e., thinking, emotion, and will) were altered by the disease of the brain that explained mental illnesses (Fabrega, 1993a, 1993b, 1994, 1995).

The approach to diagnosis and the system of classification of psychiatric disorders that is dominant in psychiatry today, and employed by many clinical psychologists as well, is largely a product of this biomedical, disease-oriented way of thinking. Today a medical approach to diagnosis and clinical accounting is complemented by an increasing reliance on neuroscientific and psychopharmacological approaches to treatment. Contemporary and mainstream (e.g., official, establishment) psychiatry is governed by a universalistic approach to psychopathology. In other words, a basic assumption is that the disorders categorized and described in the *DSM IV-R* constitute "natural objects" that are common across cultural groups and historical epochs.

PROBLEMS ASSOCIATED WITH A UNIVERSALISTIC ACCOUNT OF PSYCHOPATHOLOGY

Are Psychiatric Disorders Biomedical Entities or Cultural Constructions?

Strong exponents of biomedical psychiatry, relying on the logic of the science of descriptive psychopathology, believe that psychiatric disorders constitute naturalistic entities that are describable in a suitable language or calculus that can be unproblematically applied across human populations regardless of cultural differences. To them, the essence of these disorders resides in disturbances of the brain viewed as a neuroscientific object. Genetic factors, molecular biological processes, and neurologically situated "lesions," processes, and/or mechanisms account for the manifestations of behavior disturbances of "mental illnesses" that the science of psychopathology describes and codifies. The measurement and ascertainment of these neural properties of psychiatric disturbances is accomplished by means of special laboratory tests and procedures.

Contemporary neurobiological psychiatry holds that diagnosis will eventually depend on the application of laboratory methods and tests. Although diagnosis still is dependent on the analysis and interpretation of behavioral manifestations, it should be possible (the theory postulates) to objectively codify these in the language or calculus of descriptive psychopathology and so evolve a universal taxonomy. Criteria for the objective diagnosis of psychiatric disorders have been standardized and are widely circulated and used.

In contrast to the official, standard picture of diagnosis, culturally oriented clinicians maintain that psychiatric disorders constitute cultural constructions to an indeterminate extent. A distinctive set of cultural categories, assumptions, and values—one that has produced distinctive psychologies and approaches to behavior, emotion, and personal identity—lies embedded in the official system of diagnosis. This is the culture of middle-class, Anglo-European populations of the modern era. Members of other national, cultural, and ethnic groups manifest different psychologies, different ways of experiencing and expressing emotions, and different ways of behaving, and hence it is natural that they should conceive of and show psychopathology in distinctive ways. According to culturally oriented clinicians, a diagnosis of psychopathology requires taking into account the different social and cultural backgrounds of the person.

Do the Neurosciences and Psychopharmacology Suffice for Treatment?

In the United States, the practice of psychiatry is being carried out more and more through the use of psychotropic agents. Even when these are not used or when adjunct forms of therapy are deemed appropriate, objective and standardized protocols of psychotherapy have been developed. There is a movement in clinical psychiatry and psychology to devise suitable protocols and criteria for the treatment of specific psychiatric disturbances that complement the objective description and criteria used in diagnosis.

In contrast to the objective, standard, and biomedical view of treatment, culturally oriented clinicians maintain that attention to the cultural background and orientation of any individual burdened by psychopathology is a requirement of therapy. To be effective, therapy must make use of techniques, methods, agents, and modalities of interpersonal engagement that make sense given the cultural background of the person needing therapy. If resorting to psychotropic agents is deemed necessary, then it must be undertaken 1) with an appreciation of differences in pharmacological effects produced by drugs as a consequence of cultural, ethnic, and/or racial differences (i.e., an informed ethnopsychopharmacology), and 2) with an appreciation of what use of a drug means, and how the effects of a drug are likely to interpreted, given the cultural understanding of the person needing therapy.

The Need for a Cultural Approach to Diagnosis and Therapy

Culturally oriented clinicians constituted a culture and diagnosis group that advised the framers of the latest version of the *Diagnostic Manual in Psychiatry* (Mezzich, Kleinman, Fabrega, & Parron, 1996). This group was active in emphasizing the limitations of a culture-free approach to diagnosis, therapy, and the necessity of taking into consideration cultural factors affecting experience and behavior at every level and at every stage of the clinical practice enterprise. The group made recommendations of proposed protocols of diagnosis prepared by various committees empowered to develop the criteria of diagnosis for the major classes of psychiatric disorders. Overall, the recommendations included the following:

1. How the various criteria for diagnosis of each of the psychiatric disturbances can be obscured and confounded as a function of the cultural background of the person, and proposing ways of describing criteria in a way that take into account ethnic differences

2. Describing forms of maladaptive behavior or culture-specific syndromes of psychopathology that are found in different ethnic groups that do not easily map onto the categories of the official manual of diagnosis

3. Recommending the use of a special axis, as an addition to the standard multiaxial system of diagnosis, that addresses salient cultural characteristics of the person that may figure importantly in diagnosis and the conduct of therapy

4. Making available manuals that illustrate graphically the cultural history, as opposed to "natural history," of different varieties of psychopathology. This includes such things as how different disturbances originate, unfold, manifest, reach clinical establishments, and respond to interventions rendered by well-meaning clinicians who all too often are not conversant with the cultural background of their clients. It also includes the meanings that individuals and their families attach to psychopathology, professional intervention, outpatient contracting, and inpatient hospitalization.

It was pointed out earlier that cultural factors play an influential role in how human behavior problems are conceptualized and handled. The Western practical imperative is a cultural construction of psychopathology meant to be universally applicable in all societies. Because of political economic developments of world history and medicine that are germane to globalization, colonization, and domination, it actually operates today as an increasingly universal system for understanding mental illness.

Cultural factors influence psychopathology in all societies and are perhaps most graphically illustrated in non-Western ones where one finds wholly different traditions and worldviews that affect personal experience and behavior. Workers in the old fields of culture and personality and cross-cultural psychology occupied themselves with these problems of cultural relativism in relation to mental illness, as do workers of the newer field of cultural psychology. Parenthetically, knowledge in comparative social and cultural history now affords a glimpse, however general and imprecise, of what traditional Chinese psychiatry and Ayurvedic psychiatry were like (see Chapters 12, 13, and 16). Adopting a counterfactual perspective for the moment, one can conjure up in one's mind what world systems of classification and diagnosis of psychopathology would have been like if Chinese and Indian societies, and not societies imbued with elements of Western civilization, had gained ascendancy in world politics and economics.

It is a truism that local understanding of self, appropriate social behavior, emotions, and what anthropologists term the behavioral environment are influential and indeed determinative of how behavior, including psychopathology, is construed. What is configured and handled as normality or abnormality, on the one hand, and as medical, religious, or political, on the other, is determined by systems of meaning glossed by our concept of culture. There is no reason to anticipate that the same assumptions about behavior, including striking behavioral anomalies or eccentricities that Western diagnostic systems qualify as medical or illness related and define under psychopathology, will be found cross-culturally. Other systems of understanding behavior, normality, abnormality, sickness, or nonsickness cannot be expected to exactly parallel ours. Thus, the Western practical imperative, when applied to members of societies governed by different cultures, and obviously also to nonmainstream members of communities or subcultures in contemporary pluralistic societies, cannot be made to operate effectively unless these contrasting systems of meaning are taken into consideration. This is long-winded way of saying simply that what psychopathology is, how it is configured and handled in a community, and how best one may bring to bear resources of healing and restoration requires taking into consideration cultural systems of meaning and conventions about personal experience and behavior.

One should conceptualize culture as a part of biology and evolution (Fabrega, 2002). This view complements views already covered, involving the idea that cultural factors influencing human psychology, including human psychopathology, have a universal, innate, biological, and evolutionary justification and entitlement. The defining properties of *Homo sapiens* have a phylogenic basis: language, cognition, and culture, and the sense of social identity and history that they articulate. In other words, they are not merely added on at the end of the process of biological evolution, as it were; they are not merely the result of crossing an archeological or genealogical Rubicon after biological evolution was completed. Rather, one can argue that these distinguishing human traits have a slow, gradual evolutionary history; thus, human psychologies have a biological evolutionary basis. Moreover, and this is a key assumption, one can postulate that human psychologies are necessarily also cultural psychologies. It is the nature of natural selection to produce ways of thinking, feeling, and behaving that necessarily incorporate local conventions of meaning about social reality, the cosmos, spirituality, and the natural and supernatural world. In short, there is no inconsistency in claiming that human behavior, and psychopathology along with it, are both universal and culture specific.

In summary, if one wants to achieve a suitable system for understanding and representing psychopathology, it is imperative that one has an appreciation of the important role of cultural factors in influencing the character of personal experience and social behavior. In deriving a suitable psychiatric nosology, then, in addition to having to take into consideration practical, Western ideas, directives, and evolutionary derived mechanisms, one must also take into consideration conventions embodied in systems of meaning associated with language, culture, and cognition. Psychiatric disorders and varieties of psychopathology generally have to be conceptualized as in some way culturally specific, but in doing so one is also following generalizations from the study of biological evolution and its continuity in cultural evolution.

REFERENCES

Bailey, K. G. (1987). *Human paleopsychology: Applications to aggression and pathological processes*. Hillsdale, NJ: Erlbaum.

Bickerton, D. (1990). *Language and species*. Chicago: University of Chicago Press.

Bickerton, D. (1995). *Language and human behavior*. Seattle: University of Washington Press.

Boesch, C. (1992). New elements of a theory of mind in wild chimpanzees. *Brain and Behavioral Sciences*, 15(1), 149–150.

Boyd, R., & Richerson, P. J. (1985). *Culture and the evolutionary process*. Chicago: University of Chicago Press.

Boyer, P. (1994). *The naturalness of religious ideas: A cognitive theory of religion*. Berkeley, CA: University of California Press.

Campbell, D. T. (1960). Blind variation and selective retention in creative thought as in other knowledge processes. *Psychological Review, 67*, 380–400.

Campbell, D. T. (1965). Variation and selective retention in sociocultural evolution. In H. R. Barringer, G. I. Blanksten, & R. W. Mack (Eds.), *Social change in developing areas: A reinterpretation of evolutionary theory* (pp. 19–49). Cambridge, England: Schenkman.

Campbell, D. T. (1975). On the conflicts between biological and social evolution and between psychology and moral tradition. *American Psychologist, 30*(12), 1103–1126.

Carruthers, P. (1996). *Language, thought and consciousness: An essay in philosophical psychology.* Cambridge, England: Cambridge University Press.

Cavalli-Sforza, L. L., & Feldman, M. W. (1981). *Cultural transmission and evolution: A quantitative approach.* Princeton, NJ: Princeton University Press.

Chase, P. G., & Dibble, H. L. (1987). Middle paleolithic symbolism: A review of current evidence and interpretations. *Journal of Anthropological Archaeology, 6,* 263–296.

Cohen, M. N. (1989). *Health and the rise of civilization.* New Haven, CT: Yale University Press.

Crow, T. J. (1991). The origins of psychosis and "The Descent of Man." *British Journal of Psychiatry, 159* (Suppl. 14), 76–82.

Crow, T. J. (1993a). Origins of psychosis and the evolution of human language and communication. In N. Brunello, J. Mendlewicz, & G. Racagni (Eds.), *New generation of antipsychotic drugs: Novel mechanisms of action* (Vol. 4, pp. 39–61). New York: Karger.

Crow, T. J. (1993b). Sexual selection, Machiavellian intelligence, and the origins of psychosis. *The Lancet, 342,* 594–598.

Dawkins, M. S. (1980). *Animal suffering: The science of animal welfare.* New York: Chapman and Hall.

Dawkins, M. S. (1990). From an animal's point of view: Motivation, fitness, and animal welfare. *Behavioral and Brain Sciences, 13,* 1–61.

de Waal, F. D. (1996). *Good natured: The origins of right and wrong in humans and other animals.* Cambridge, MA: Harvard University Press.

Donald, M. (1991). *Origins of the modern mind: Three stages in the evolution of culture and cognition.* Cambridge, MA: Harvard University Press.

Dunbar, R., Knight, C., & Power, C. (1999). *The evolution of culture.* New Brunswick, NJ: Rutgers University Press.

Fabrega, H., Jr. (1993a). Toward a social theory of psychiatric phenomena. *Behavioral Science, 38,* 75–100.

Fabrega, H., Jr. (1993b). A cultural analysis of human behavioral breakdowns: An approach to the ontology and epistemology of psychiatric phenomena. *Culture, Medicine and Psychiatry, 17,* 99–132.

Fabrega, H., Jr. (1994). International systems of diagnosis in psychiatry. *Journal of Nervous and Mental Disease, 182*(5), 256–263.

Fabrega, H., Jr. (1995). Cultural and historical challenges to the psychiatric enterprise. *Comprehensive Psychiatry, 36*(5), 377–383.

Fabrega, H., Jr. (1997). *Evolution of sickness and healing.* Berkeley, CA: University of California Press.

Fabrega, H., Jr. (2002). *Origins of psychopathology: The phylogenetic and cultural basis of mental illness.* New Brunswick, NJ: Rutgers University Press.

Foley, R. A. (1987). *Another unique species: Patterns in human evolutionary ecology.* New York: John Wiley and Sons.

Foley, R. A. (1995). *Humans before humanity: An evolutionary perspective.* Cambridge, MA: Blackwell.

Franzen, E. A., & Myers, R. E. (1973). Neural control of social behavior: Prefrontal and anterior temporal cortex. *Neuropsychologia, 11,* 141–157.

Gamble, C. (1993). *Timewalkers: The prehistory of global colonization.* Cambridge, MA: Harvard University Press.

Gardner, R. (1982). Mechanisms in manic-depressive disorder: An evolutionary model. *Archives of General Psychiatry, 39,* 1436–1441.

Gilbert, P. (1992a). *Depression: The evolution of powerlessness.* New York: Guilford Press.

Gilbert, P. (1992b). *Human nature and suffering.* New York: Guilford Press.

Goodall, J. (1986). *The chimpanzees of Gombe: Patterns of behavior.* Cambridge, MA: Harvard University Press, Belknap Press.

Goodman, F. D. (1988). *Ecstacy, ritual and alternate reality: Religion in a pluralistic world.* Bloomington, IN: Indiana University Press.

Goodman, F. D. (1990). *Where the spirits ride the wind: Trance journeys and other ecstatic experiences.* Bloomington, IN: Indiana University Press.

Harlow, H. F., & Novak, M. A. (1973). Psychopathological perspectives. *Perspectives in Biology and Medicine, 16,* 461–478.

Johnson, A. W., & Earle, T. (1987). *The evolution of human societies: From foraging group to agrarian state.* Stanford, CA: Stanford University Press.

Kaplan, J. R. (1986). Psychological stress and behavior in nonhuman primates. In G. Mitchell & J. Erwin (Eds.), *Comparative primate biology: Vol. 2A. Behavior, conservation, and ecology* (pp. 455–492). New York: Alan R. Liss.

Kittrie, N. N. (1971). *The right to be different.* Baltimore, MD: Johns Hopkins Press.

Knight, C. (1991). *Blood relations: Menstruation and the origins of culture.* New Haven, CT: Yale University Press.

Lee, R. B., & DeVore, I. (Eds.). (1968). *Man the hunter*. Chicago: Aldine.

Ludwig, A. M. (1968). Altered states of consciousness. In R. Prince (Ed.), *Trance and possession states* (pp. 69–95). Montreal, Canada: R. M. Bucke Memorial Society.

Lumsden, C., & Wilson, E. O. (1981). *Genes, mind, and culture*. Cambridge, MA: Harvard University Press.

Marks, I. M. (1987). *Fears, phobias, and rituals: Panic, anxiety, and their disorders*. New York: Oxford University Press.

Mezzich, J. E., Kleinman, A., Fabrega, H., Jr., & Parron, D. L. (Eds.). (1996). *Culture and psychiatric diagnosis: A DSM-IV perspective*. Washington, DC: American Psychiatric Press.

Noble, W., & Davidson, I. (1996). *Human evolution, language and mind: A psychological and archaeological inquiry*. Cambridge, England: Cambridge University Press.

Oubré, A. Y. (1997). *Instinct and revelation: Reflections on the origins of numinous perception*. Amsterdam, The Netherlands: Gordon and Breach Science.

Parker, S. T., & Russon, A. E. (1996). On the wild side of culture and cognition in the great apes. In A. E. Russon, K. A. Bard, & S. T. Parker (Eds.), *Reaching into thought: The minds of the great apes* (pp. 430–450). Cambridge, England: Cambridge University Press.

Pfeiffer, J. E. (1982). *The creative explosion. An inquiry into the origins of art and religion*. Ithaca, NY: Cornell University Press.

Porter, R. (1987). *Mind-forg'd manacles: A history of madness in England from the restoration to the regency*. London, England: Athlone Press.

Price, T. D., & Brown, J. A. (1985). Aspects of hunter-gatherer complexity. In T. D. Price & J. A. Brown (Eds.), *Prehistoric hunter-gatherers: The emergence of cultural complexity* (pp. 3–20). New York: Academic Press.

Sanderson, S. K. (1990). *Social evolutionism: A critical history*. Cambridge, MA: Blackwell.

Simons, R. C., & Hughes, C. C. (Eds). (1985). *The culture-bound syndromes: Folk illnesses of psychiatric and anthropological interest*. Boston: D. Reidel.

Sloman, L., & Gilbert, P. (2000). *Subordination and defeat: An evolutionary approach to mood disorders and their therapy*. Mahwah, NJ: Erlbaum.

Stevens, A., & Price, J. (1996). *Evolutionary psychiatry: A new beginning*. New York: Routledge.

Stringer, C., & Gamble, C. (1993). *In search of the Neanderthals: Solving the puzzle of human origins*. New York: Thames and Hudson.

Suomi, S. J. (1978). Male sexual behavior by incompetent monkeys: Neglect and abuse of offspring. *Journal of Pediatric Psychology, 3*(1): 28–34

Tooby, J., & Cosmides, L. (1992). The psychological foundations of culture. In J. H. Barkow, L. Cosmides, & J. Tooby (Eds.), *The adapted mind: Evolutionary psychology and the generation of culture* (pp. 19–136). New York: Oxford University Press.

Trinkaus, E., & Shipman, P. (1992). *The Neanderthals: Of skeletons, scientists, and scandal*. New York: Random House, Vintage Books.

Wenegrat, B. (1984). *Sociobiology & mental disorder: A new view*. Menlo Park, CA: Addison-Wesley.

Wenegrat, B. (1990). *Sociobiological psychiatry: Normal behavior and psychopathology*. Lexington, MA: Lexington Books.

Wilson, E. O. (1975). *Sociobiology: The new synthesis*. Cambridge, MA: Harvards University Press/Belknap.

The Role of Culture in Definitions, Interpretations, and Management of Illness

Linda K. Sussman
Washington University, St. Louis

Through the process of enculturation, individuals learn how to view the world, experience it, and behave in it. All human societies experience illness, and each culture has devised its own ways of dealing with it. Medical systems are integral parts of the sociocultural systems in which they exist. Beliefs and practices related to illness and healing are inextricably linked to other components of the culture, such as social organization, religion, the economic system, and values. With the ever-increasing ethnic diversity—or multicultural character—of our own population and rapid advances in medical technology that constantly confront us with new options, often leading us to reexamine our expectations, goals, values, and definitions, the importance of culture in illness definition and management has become increasingly recognized.

Despite the fact that the content of medical systems varies greatly across cultures, several characteristics and components are common across all medical systems. I shall briefly describe some of these common attributes. Then, drawing largely on my own work in Madagascar, Mauritius, and the United States, I shall discuss three sociocultural factors and their impact on illness definition, interpretation, and management: medical beliefs, social structure and organization, and cultural values and history. Finally, recognizing that the biomedical system itself is a culturally derived system, I shall utilize the results of six years as a participant-observer in a health intervention project to demonstrate how the different "cultural lenses" of medical specialists, researchers, and patients may result in diverse perceptions of illness and conflicting treatment goals.

MEDICAL SYSTEMS IN CROSS-CULTURAL PERSPECTIVE

What is culture, anthropologically speaking? The following excellent description was written by C. Helman in his book for health care professionals, *Culture, Health and Illness*:

> Culture is a set of guidelines (both explicit and implicit) which individuals inherit as members of a particular society, and which tells them how to *view* the world, how to experience it emotionally, and how to *behave* in it in relation to other people, to supernatural forces or gods, and to the natural environment. . . . To some extent, culture can be seen as an inherited "lens," through which the individual perceives and understands the world that he inhabits, and learns how to live within it. Growing up within any society is a form

of *enculturation*, whereby the individual slowly acquires the cultural "lens" of that society. Without such a shared perception of the world, both the cohesion and continuity of any human group would be impossible.

One aspect of this "cultural lens" is the division of the world, and the people within it, into different *categories*. . . . For example . . . "kinsfolk" or "strangers," "normal" or "abnormal," "mad" or "bad," "healthy" or "ill." And all cultures have elaborate ways of moving people from one social category into another (such as from "ill person" to "healthy person"), and also of confining people—sometimes against their will—to the categories into which they have been put (such as "mad," "disabled" or "elderly"). (Helman, 1994, pp. 2–3)

Shared Elements of Medical Systems

Beliefs and practices related to illness reflect the cultural lens through which members of the society view the world. They do not exist as isolated so-called folk beliefs, folk remedies, or superstitions removed from the wider cultural context.

Within a society, the medical system is a cultural system just like the religious, political and economic systems. It is composed of all the health knowledge, beliefs, skills, and practices of members of the group. It "includes the ways in which people have become recognized as 'ill,' the ways that they present this illness to other people, the attributes of those they present their illness to, and the ways that the illness is dealt with" (Helman, 1994, p. 7), as well as "patterns of belief about the causes of illness; norms governing choice and evaluation of treatment; socially-legitimated statuses, roles, power relations, interaction settings, and institutions" (Kleinman, 1980, p. 24). Most complex societies are composed of members of ethnic and religious minorities, including recent immigrants from other cultures. Each group may possess its own cultural beliefs, norms, and practices, while individual members of the group may become acculturated to varying extents to the culture of the larger society.

Despite the great diversity of medical beliefs and practices throughout the world, a number of components have been found to be common to all. These include the following:

- Conceptual components
  - An *illness classification system*, composed of labels for various symptoms and illnesses (nosology)
  - A system of *beliefs concerning the possible causes* of illness (etiology)
  - A means of *attributing cause and labels* (diagnosis) to specific episodes
  - A set of *appropriate treatments* for specific illnesses
  - *Expectations* regarding the course of the illness and treatment outcome (prognosis)
- Personnel
  - *Healing specialists* who possess specialized knowledge or power, are usually respected members of the community, and have a set of paraphernalia for diagnosis and treatment that set them apart from other members of the community
- Behavioral components
  - *Norms regarding treatment-seeking and illness management*—criteria for defining oneself as ill and labeling others as "sick," culturally appropriate sick role behavior, and expectations regarding the identities of those responsible for making health care decisions and caring for the sick

- *Norms regarding consultations with healing specialists* include appropriate content (e.g., physical symptoms; feelings, social relations, or moral dilemmas; context in which symptoms developed), modes of interaction (e.g., formal questions/answers, patient narratives, physical examinations, ritual ceremony), the location of consultation, the identification of individuals who may or should attend consultations, the role of the healing specialists (e.g., expert, authority, counselor, advisor), the nature of specialists' advice, and the method and amount of payment (e.g., cash, livestock, food; mandatory or voluntary; payment given for each consultation or after a cure has been effected).

Within a society, there are laymen and there are healing specialists who adhere to a particular therapeutic system. In most societies today, a number of different therapeutic systems coexist, although one system may dominate. This is called *medical pluralism*. The United States is an example of a society with a plural medical system in which biomedicine dominates but coexists with other systems, such as chiropractic and osteopathy, Chinese medicine and acupuncture, faith healing, herbalism, homeopathy, and healing traditions of ethnic minorities.

In societies with plural medical systems and a polyethnic population, the situation may be fairly complex. The theories and practices of each of the healing systems (e.g., of biomedicine, chiropractice, and homeopathy) differ to varying extents from each other as do the medical beliefs and practices of lay members of ethnic groups. Of particular importance is the finding that several different therapeutic systems may be used by an individual either for different illnesses or for a single illness with little or no perceived ideological conflict (e.g., Bailey, 1991; Clark, 1970; Counts & Counts, 1989; Crandon-Malamud, 1991; Etkin, Ross, & Muazzamu, 1990; O'Connor, 1995; Press, 1969; Reeve, 2000; Scott, 1974; Snow, 1974, 1977; Sussman, 1980, 1981, 1983, 1988, 1992b; Trotter & Chavira, 1981; Woods, 1977).

The Health-Seeking Process—The Lay Perspective

The customary view is that professionals organize health care for lay people. But typically lay people activate their health care by deciding when and whom to consult, whether or not to comply, when to switch between treatment alternatives, whether care is effective, and whether they are satisfied with its quality. In this sense, the popular sector functions as the chief source and most immediate determinant of care. (Kleinman, 1980, p. 51)

Among laymen, most illness beliefs and health-seeking behavior patterns are not formally learned in school but, starting in childhood, are picked up piecemeal from experience, observation, and teaching within the household and social group. They continue to be learned and modified over one's lifetime as experiences with illness accumulate. The amount and sources of knowledge may vary considerably among cultural and subcultural groups (Agee, 2000).

Illness is first experienced by individuals, their households, and families, and it is usually within this context that illnesses are managed, with or without the advice or help of a healing specialist. In fact, most illness episodes in Western and non-Western societies are treated within the lay sector with no recourse to specialists (Kleinman, Eisenberg, & Good, 1978; Zola, 1972). Kleinman (1980), for example, found that in two districts of Taipei, 93 percent of all illness episodes in a one-month period were first treated in the family, and 73 percent of all episodes were treated exclusively in the family. Cross-culturally, most illnesses and conditions requiring special care are recognized, interpreted, and managed by a lay "therapy management group" (Janzen 1978, 1987), the composition of which varies from culture to culture (e.g., the individual patient, nuclear family, mother and grandmother, paternal kin, extended family). This group may obtain advice and suggestions from others in its "therapeutic network," composed of culturally appropriate informal and formal sources of advice and care.

The health-seeking process is a decision-making process engaged in by lay individuals (Chrisman, 1977; Gibbs, 1988; Kleinman, 1980; Mechanic, 1962, 1968, 1982; Sussman, 1992a; Sussman, Robins, & Earls, 1987). It includes decisions about the need for care and associated role changes, choices concerning the source of care, and ongoing health maintenance decisions. It is a dynamic process and may be conceptualized as involving the following steps (Fig. 3.1) (Sussman, 1992a):

1. The presence of symptoms, or physical or other changes
2. Perceive and attend to those symptoms or changes
3. Interpret and label them
4. Decide to treat (or not)
5. Delineate and evaluate the options, including self-treatment and no treatment
6. Choose treatment or source of care
7. Act upon choice and treat or seek care
8. Evaluate the outcome, and then either:
9. a. Continue the same treatment or source of care, with ongoing evaluation (steps 8–9) or
   b. Cease current treament/care and
      i. Cease treatment-seeking or
      ii. Delineate/evaluate other care options and choose care (steps 5–9) or
      iii. Reinterpret and relabel symptoms or changes (steps 3–9)

For acute or self-limiting illnesses, this process may be relatively short and uncomplicated. For chronic illness and symptoms, it may be quite complex and represent a lifetime of trying different sources of care, modifying treatment regimens, and evaluating outcomes.

Context of the Health-Seeking Process

The health-seeking and health maintenance process is shaped by the interaction of individual, social, cultural, and societal factors (Sussman, 1992a). These are represented by four concentric circles in Fig. 3.2. The inner circle represents the *individual*,

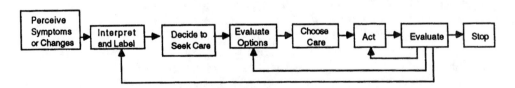

FIG. 3.1.   Health-seeking process.

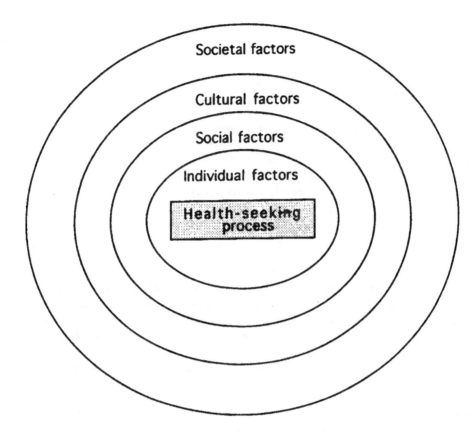

FIG. 3.2. Context of the health-seeking process.

who is imbedded in a *social group*, that is imbedded in the *culture* of the (minority) group, that in turn is imbedded in the *society* that represents the social, political, and economic realities of the society at large. It is important to realize that although these levels are separated conceptually, they are, in fact, inextricably linked and there is constant interaction and feedback among all levels.

A major emphasis of this model is that individuals reflect the layers of influence that surround them. Learning and development are ongoing, and changes in one level of the model may result in changes in other levels. Changes, for example, in a nation's health care policy may lead to changes in patient behavior; alternatively, changes in patient choices and expectations may lead to changes in physician behavior or health care policy.

Individual factors may include health status, personal resources, knowledge, and experience. Social factors refer to the composition of groups of kin and friends, the frequency of contact with them, the nature of the relationships, and their rights and obligations. Societal factors (sometimes referred to as structural factors) particularly relevant to health care and illness management include the health care system itself (distribution, cost, quality, and policies), the economic system, (the distribution and abundance of resources and social welfare policies), and demographics (including educational attainment and occupational status, the geographical distribution of the groups, and local neighborhood resources. Though all of the factors are clearly important and intertwined, in this chapter I focus on cultural factors. These include shared group norms of thought and behavior, values, and preferences, as well as shared history.

SOCIOCULTURAL FACTORS AFFECTING ILLNESS DEFINITION, INTERPRETATION, AND MANAGEMENT

In this section I discuss how medical belief systems, social structure and organization, and cultural values and history shape illness definition, interpretation, and management. These provide the lens through which patients and families of different cultural groups perceive and interpret symptoms and illness, and the context in which they decide whether or not to seek care, choose sources of care, develop treatment goals and expectations, evaluate treatment, and decide whether to continue, cease, change, or supplement care.

Medical Belief Systems

Medical belief systems provide individuals with a coherent explanatory framework in which to view illness. This framework guides the interpretation of symptoms, decisions to seek care, decisions about where to seek care, the ways in which symptoms are presented to physicians and other healing specialists, and the evaluation of treatment outcomes. In speaking about the lay belief system of African Americans who had been socialized in the rural South and maintained kin ties there, Snow, for example, notes that

> It is a coherent medical system and not a ragtag collection of isolated superstitions. If the underlying premises are accepted, it makes just as much sense to the believer as the principles of orthodox medicine do to the graduate of an accredited medical school. (1974, p. 83)

In all medical classification systems, symptoms are generally attributed to causes upon which treatment is based. Although medical belief systems may differ considerably from culture to culture, two themes that exist in many systems are the belief in multiple causes of illness and the belief that illness reflects and is caused by some type of imbalance or disharmony. These themes are highly prevalent worldwide and among ethnic groups in the United States.

Multicausal Belief Systems   The concept that illness may be caused by multiple factors is found in many medical belief systems throughout the world. By this I do not mean that illness may be caused by germs, exposure, or heredity, but that different categories of factors may cause illness and that different types of treatment or healers are effective in treating different causes.

Among the most widespread is the belief that illness (and other forms of misfortune) may be caused by either *natural* or *unnatural* (or *supernatural*) factors and agents. This has been reported in Africa (e.g., Etkin, Ross, & Muazzamu, 1990; Janzen, 1978; Janzen & Prins, 1981; Ngubane, 1977; Sussman, 1981, 1983, 1992b) and Asia (e.g., Beals, 1976; Carstairs, 1955; Kleinman, 1980; Topley, 1976), as well as among many groups in North and South America (e.g., Bailey, 1991; Brodwin, 1996; Clark, 1970; Heyer, 1981; Hill, 1973, 1976; Scott, 1974; Shutler, 1977; Snow, 1974, 1977, 1978, 1993; Staiano, 1981; Young, 1981).

Natural illnesses may result from constitutional weaknesses or exposure to forces of nature such as cold air, germs, or impurities in air, food, and water. In many cultures they are viewed as part of the world as God, the creator, intended it to be. God is thus viewed as part of the natural world or as the creator, and source, of the natural world. In fact, in several cultures, natural illnesses are referred to as "illnesses of God" (e.g., Brodwin, 1996; Janzen, 1978; Sussman, 1981, 1983, 1988, 1992b).

Unnatural and/or supernatural illnesses often represent some sort of upset in the natural order and frequently result from impaired social relations. The most common causes of these illnesses are witchcraft and sorcery. These illnesses are thus frequently caused by some malign human intervention calling upon supernatural resources. Among some groups, divine retribution (such as punishment by the ancestors or saints) for improper behavior toward other people, deceased ancestors, or other spiritual beings may be included in this category, or in a category of *supernatural* illnesses. Possession by various types of spirits, often not the fault of the victim, would also fall under this category.

In Mauritius and Madagascar, there are multicausal belief systems—actually quite similar to each other in many respects. In Mauritius, both Creoles of African origin and Indo-Mauritians believe in two major types of illness: "Illnesses of God" (*malade Bondieu*) that are naturally caused, and illness caused by sorcery (Fig. 3.3) (Sussman, 1981, 1983). Most Indo-Mauritians and a minority of Creoles also believe that illness may result from punishment from saints or gods, usually for not fulfilling a promise or a vow to a Hindu deity. (In addition, most Mauritians believe in another form of illness, "Fright," which results if an individual sees a dead soul.) In Southwest Madagascar, the Mahafaly believe that there are "Illnesses of God" (*arety Zanahary*) that are again naturally caused, "Illnesses of the Ancestors" caused by displeased ancestors, "Illnesses of Spirits" usually resulting in spirit possession, and "Illnesses of Man" caused by sorcery (man) (Table 3.1) (Sussman, 1992b). In both systems, one may be punished by illness if one does not behave in ways demanded by the gods, ancestors, and social group.

Belief Systems Based upon the Concept of Balance Another widespread theme in medical belief systems is the concept of balance, in which health is viewed as a manifestation of proper balance or harmony and ill health as a result of imbalance or

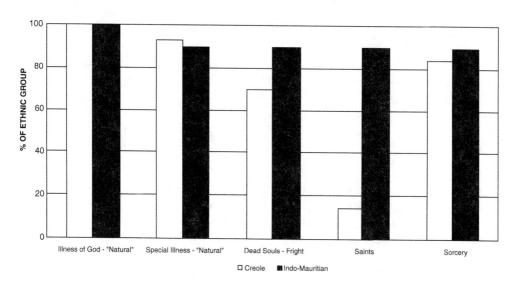

FIG. 3.3. Categories of illness recognized by two ethnic groups on Mauritius.

TABLE 3.1
Categories of Illness Recognized in Southwest Madagascar

Illness Category	Cause of Illness
Illness of God	God ("Natural")
Illness of Spirits	Spirit possession or spirit attack
Illness of the Ancestors	Displeased ancestors
Illness of Man	Sorcery

disharmony. This theme is found in such diverse regions as Latin America, North America, Asia, and Africa (e.g., Beckerleg, 1994; Greenwood, 1981; Harwood, 1971; Helman, 1994; Kleinman, 1980; Lang, 1989, 1990; Luecke, 1993; Ngubane, 1977; Shutler, 1977; Topley, 1976; Young, 1981; see also Ching-Tse Lee and Lei, Jaipal, Gielen, & Francis, this volume). In some belief systems, the balance required for health involves mainly physical and behavioral factors, whereas in others optimal health is maintained only when there is balance, order, or harmony in the physical, social, and spiritual, or moral, spheres of life. Traditional Chinese medicine and Indian Ayurveda are examples of such systems. A number of belief systems in Asia, North Africa, and Latin America emphasizing the role of balance in health classify illnesses, conditions, foods, and medicines into categories of hot and cold.

Hot/Cold Theories. The hot/cold systems of disease etiology and classification found in Latin America are largely derived from the humoral theory of disease developed in the fifth century B.C. by Hippocrates and elaborated by Galen in the second century A.D. According to this theory, health was viewed as a state of balance among four humors: blood, phlegm, black bile, and yellow bile. Health was manifest in a warm, moist body. Illness, on the other hand, was manifest in an excessively dry, wet, hot, or cold body that was caused by humoral imbalance (Harwood, 1971).

The Spanish and Portuguese later carried the system to the New World in the sixteenth and seventeenth centuries (Helman, 1994), and variations of it were incorporated into Latin American medical practices and beliefs and continue to persist today (e.g., Clark, 1970; Harwood, 1971; Young, 1981). Harwood (1971) found that this system is firmly rooted among New York City Puerto Ricans. Illnesses are grouped into hot and cold, and foods and medicines are categorized as hot, cold, or cool. Cold illnesses are treated with hot medicines and foods, and hot illnesses with cool medicines and foods. This system, however, exhibits considerable vitality because new medicines and foods are being incorporated into the system according to their effects on the body. Penicillin, for example, is classified as hot because it can cause symptoms such as rash or diarrhea, which are hot. Drugs that may cause effects such as muscular spasms, however, would be classified as cold.

The Influence of Medical Beliefs on Illness Management—Some Examples
Clearly, medical belief systems are of utmost importance in decision-making regarding health and illness management, and they influence all steps in the health-seeking and health-maintenance process (see Table 3.2).

Symptom Perception and Interpretation. Perceptions and interpretations of symptoms are shaped by beliefs about their etiology, treatability, and curability. First to con-

TABLE 3.2
How Medical Beliefs Shape Health Behavior

1. Symptom perception and interpretation:	Does the patient view the symptoms as abnormal? Can an individual conceptually be "ill" in the absence of symptoms?
2. Treatment options and choices:	Who can effectively treat this illness?
3. Treatment expectations, goals, evaluation, and adherence:	Does the treatment conflict with the patient's concept of the illness and its appropriate care? What are the treatment goals of the patient? What criteria are being used to evaluate treatment?

sider is whether the person views the symptoms as abnormal and as requiring any treatment at all. For example, in many regions of the world diarrhea is quite common in infants and children. Although oral rehydration therapy is inexpensive and widely available, its use is rejected by many for diverse reasons. Mull and Mull (1988) found that some rural Pakistani mothers viewed diarrhea in their infants as normal and not requiring treatment; some believed that it would be dangerous to try to stop it because the "heat" in it could be trapped and spread to the brain, causing fever. Also, it is important to remember that what is viewed as normal for one age or gender group may not be normal for others.

Biomedically defined psychological or emotional disorders may not be viewed by lay individuals as abnormal or in need of medical treatment, especially if the symptoms are mild. For example, analysis of data from a national psychiatric epidemiolgical household survey indicated that African Americans were less likely to seek medical care for mild symptoms of depression than Whites, but they sought care with equal frequency if they experienced severe symptoms (Sussman et al., 1987). While a number of factors may be involved in this lack of treatment-seeking, two possibly important factors might be that mild depressive symptoms could be viewed as normal among African Americans if individuals are experiencing difficulties in their lives and that it might not seem appropriate to see a medical doctor about such symptoms (feelings and emotions), although others in one's social group might be consulted.

What about instances in which an asymptomatic individual has been medically diagnosed as having a disease? The question to consider under these circumstances is whether a person can conceptually be "sick" in the absence of symptoms. Such distinctions between lay and clinical views have been addressed in sociology and anthropology through the concepts of disease, illness (Eisenberg, 1977; Mechanic, 1962), and sickness (Young, 1982). Whereas *disease* is a biologically defined pathological bodily state, *illness* refers to an individual's experience of a disvalued change of state that may include symptoms or disease. *Sick* is a socially bestowed label and culturally defined role assigned to individuals. Given these definitions, an individual can have a disease, but not have an illness and not be sick. Conversely, an individual can have an illness and be sick, but not have a disease.

Treatment Options and Choices.   Next to consider is who or what healing system the person believes can effectively treat the illness. In the earlier example from Pakistan, some respondents believed the diarrhea was caused by imbalances requiring traditional treatment with cold substances rather than with hot biomedical medicines (Mull & Mull, 1988). In Madagascar, each type of illness requires a different type of

TABLE 3.3
Categories of Illness That Can Be Diagnosed or Treated by
Each Type of Healer in Southwest Madagascar

Healer	Illness of God	Illness of Spirits	Illness of the Ancestors	Illness of Man (Sorcery)
Biomedical practitioner	X			
Herbalist	X			
Home treatment	X			
Medicine man		X		X
Healer possessed by a spirit		X		
Lineage head			X	

healer (Table 3.3). Moreover, specific symptoms do not necessarily correlate with particular causes, and divination (performed either by a male relative or by a diviner) is the primary means of determining cause (Sussman 1992b; Sussman & Sussman, 1977). Illnesses resulting from angered ancestors or caused by spirit possession, for example, will not respond to biomedical treatment. The former can be cured only by appeasing the ancestors in a ritual conducted by the head of the lineage. Spirit possession may be manifest by many different symptoms but often involves changes in behavior or mood, general malaise, and recurrent somatic symptoms such as headache and faintness, or sudden symptoms such as partial paralysis or mutism. Spirit possession may be diagnosed by a diviner or medicine man and some types of spirits may be appeased and then exorcised by medicine men during rituals that could take place over several weeks. Possession by other types of spirits must be positively diagnosed and treated by a healer possessed by a similar spirit. In these cases, the spirit is not exorcised but is appeased by the patient and patient's family, who are instructed by the spirit about the types of gifts it desires and the taboos that must be observed. The spirit will then remain with the patient but no longer cause symptoms. The terms of the "cure" are worked out by the spirit possessing the patient (while the patient is in a trance) and the spirit that possesses the healer (while the healer is in a trance). The spirits then instruct those present at the healing ceremony about what the patient and family are required to do (Sussman, 1992b).

Individuals in societies with plural medical systems may utilize more than one type of healing system either for a particular illness episode or for different illness episodes over a lifetime. To a great extent, although not exclusively, decisions regarding the type of care to seek are guided by medical beliefs. One pattern of utilization that has been reported in many societies involves the use of different types of care for illnesses with different causes. This has been termed *compartmentalization*. This is illustrated by the medical beliefs and appropriate treatment resources in Madagascar (Table 3.3) and in Mauritius (Table 3.4).

A second pattern is one in which health care options are positioned in a hierarchy of resort (Schwartz, 1969), with options being sought in a particular order, according to culturally based criteria. Different types of care are sought consecutively until, hopefully, the desired outcome is achieved. This pattern of utilization is consistent with medical systems in which it is believed that illness may have many causes and that there is a cure for every illness if the right practitioner can be found (e.g., Beals, 1976; Snow, 1974; Staiano 1981). This also applied to Mauritius (Sussman, 1981, 1983) where responses of an illness to particular treatments were utilized to make further

TABLE 3.4
Categories of Illness That Can Be Diagnosed or Treated by
Each Type of Healer in Mauritius

Healer	Illness of God	Special Illness of God	Dead Souls Fright	Saints	Sorcery
Biomedical practitioner	X				
Herbalist	X	X			
Home treatment	X				
Specialized healer		X			
Sorcerer			X	X	X
Hindu maraz			X	X	X
Tamil poussari			X	X	X
Catholic priest	X		X	X	X

diagnostic judgements. Treatments appropriate for natural illnesses were usually sought first. If the illness was not cured by such treatment, this provided grounds for suspecting it to be an unnatural illness (also see, e.g., Ngubane, 1977; Snow, 1977; Staiano, 1981; Sussman, 1992b; Yoder, 1981). In such societies, there is a tendency to reject notions concerning the chronicity or incurability of particular diseases.

A third pattern of health care utilization involves the concurrent or complementary use of two or more systems of care. For example, an individual may consult both a physician and an *espiritista*. Or a patient may consult a physician and follow the bio-medical regimen while also taking herbal remedies prepared at home. One reason for this might be to counteract presumed ill effects of one of the treatments: If a physician prescribes a hot medication, a patient may at the same time take a cool herbal tea to counteract the heat. A common variation of this pattern, especially among those with chronic diseases, is to alternate care between two systems. For example, in Mauritius it is very common for individuals with chronic illnesses requiring ongoing medica-tion, such as diabetes and hypertension, to alternate between taking physician-prescribed medication and herbalist-prescribed remedies or homegrown remedies in order to rest the body from strong biomedical medicines and their side effects (Sussman 1980, 1988).

Complementary treatment from two distinct therapeutic systems may also be sought in order to address multiple causes of an illness—such as an underlying super-natural cause and a resultant physical cause. For example, in Mauritius, individuals may consult sorcerers to remove magical objects from their bodies that were placed there by sorcery against them and simultaneously consult biomedical physicians to heal the physical injury caused by the magical objects. A typical case involved a woman diagnosed by a physician as having severe bleeding ulcers that were not responding well to treatment. A sorcerer was consulted who diagnosed the underly-ing cause as a magical thorn inserted into her stomach through sorcery. He was employed to remove the thorn and conduct a ritual to prevent further magical inser-tions, thereby enabling biomedical treatment to be effective (Sussman, 1983).

Finally, medical beliefs shape treatment expectations, goals, evaluation, and adher-ence. Here it is important to determine whether the actual treatment is congruent or conflicts with the person's concept of the illness, its appropriate care, and its cure. Lay concepts of a particular disease may differ significantly from specialist concepts. Nevertheless, it is the lay concepts that shape patient treatment expectations, goals, and evaluation, and in large part lay concepts determine whether particular treatment recommendations make sense to patients. Unless the underlying assumptions of patients concerning the disease are understood by healing specialists, patients and healers may be operating within different conceptual systems. In many ways, they may be using the same words but speaking different languages. Once again, the example of diarrhea in Pakistan serves to exemplify this issue. Many of the mothers viewed diarrhea as a hot illness requiring treatment by cold foods, herbs, and remedies. Most Western medicines, however, were classified as hot and therefore biomedical recommendations to use oral rehydration therapy were rejected as inappropriate (Mull & Mull, 1988).

Treatment Expectations   Beliefs about the cause of an illness and its natural progression largely determine expected outcomes of treatment. If it is believed that an illness is the result of divine retribution or witchcraft, expectations from biomedical treatment may, for example, be quite low since it logically follows that medical treatment will have little effect. Likewise, if sorcery is the underlying cause of an illness, then biomedicine could not work until the sorcery is dealt with first.

Treatment goals, closely linked to expectations, also reflect medical beliefs. In situations where patient and physician are from different sociocultural backgrounds, distinctions between physician and patient goals may be considerable (e.g., Raymond & D'Eramo-Melkus, 1993).

In the United States, the treatment goals of patients and physicians frequently conflict. For example, Hopper and Schechtman (1985) found that among low-income, predominantly African American individuals under medical care for diabetes, the phrase, "treatment will help," meant to the overwhelming majority that treatment would make them feel better or decrease the frequency or severity of symptoms; only 4 to 5 percent viewed "helping" as lowering or controlling blood sugar levels, which was the goal of the physician.

Snow (1974) describes an example of how differing concepts of "stroke" held by a physician and an African American woman were related to conflicting treatment goals and led to the rejection of medical treatment. Characteristics of the blood are significant in many medical systems (Helman, 1994; Snow, 1977). This is reflected in the many different ways in which blood is described in medical systems throughout the world: high vs. low blood, thick vs. thin blood, hot vs. cold blood, living vs. sleeping blood, impure vs. pure blood, dirty vs. clean blood, new vs. used blood, good vs. bad blood. Moreover, among some groups, blood is not believed to be regenerative, which could certainly lead to a reluctance by patients to part with their blood for testing.

The woman described by Snow had had a light stroke and was recuperating at home, sitting up in bed. She believed that stroke was caused by "high blood," or too much blood that boiled up and gave her "blood on the brains" (Snow, 1974, p. 92). Sitting up, she thought, would make the blood go back down more quickly. She had thrown away the medication prescribed by a physician because he had told her that she would have to take it all her life. Since she believed "high blood" to be a temporary condition, her reaction was, "Now that don't make no sense" (Snow, 1974, p. 92) and she was considering a home remedy to bring the high blood down.

Throughout human history and across cultures, medical systems have focused predominantly on curing illness and reducing pain. Chronic illness represents a special and, to many lay people around the world, a rather peculiar case of illness in that the goal of biomedical treatment is not a cure but rather lifelong management. This is not necessarily accepted by laymen in many cultures as a treatment goal. For example, in Mauritius it was generally presumed that there should be a cure for every illness; one just had to find the right kind of healer who possessed the right kind of knowledge or power to cure it. Moreover, Mauritians generally expected biomedicine to cure ailments quite quickly—within weeks—but tended to allow other types of healers, especially religious healers and sorcerers, several months.

Treatment evaluation and adherence to prescribed regimens are closely linked to each other. Although treatment evaluation may at first appear to be a straightforward appraisal of "Does it work?" it is also a culturally based process (Etkin, 1988). Treatment is evaluated according to its effectiveness in meeting treatment goals, its perceived necessity and importance vis-à-vis treatment expectations, and its logic vis-à-vis the medical belief system of the patient.

Patients, who are active in managing illness but may have treatment goals different from those of the physician, will in many cases alter the treatment regimen to fit their needs, lifestyles, and goals without informing the physician. Roberson (1992) found this to be the case among rural African Americans with chronic illnesses. She notes that although many of the individuals she studied would be seen by their physicians as noncompliant, they, in fact, "saw themselves as managing their chronic illnesses and treatment regimens effectively" (Roberson, p. 24).

Prescribed regimens may be totally rejected as senseless, ineffective, or objectionable, or may be altered according to the expectations, goals, and beliefs of patients and their therapy management groups. One criterion frequently utilized to evaluate treatment is the presence or absence of side effects. Biomedical medication is viewed as quite powerful by patients around the world—perhaps too powerful or potent to be taken over the long term. However, herbal and other traditional remedies are seen as acceptable and useful for long-term treatment. This has been reported, for example, by Puerto Rican patients with diabetes (Quatromoni, Milbauer, Posner, Carballeira, Brunt, & Chipkin, 1994) and by Mauritians with hypertension and diabetes (Sussman, 1983). Similar attitudes have been reported toward asthma medication among patients in the United States. For example, in a health education project for African American children with asthma, 54 percent of the children's parents believed upon enrollment in the program that long-term medication may be harmful for children, and 52 percent agreed that asthma medications make children jumpy or nervous (Sussman, 1992c, 1997).

In addition to evaluating explanations of illness and the actual effectiveness of a specific treatment, patients and their families also evaluate treatment and medical encounters according to whether they meet prevailing cultural norms of interaction and expectations regarding the role of healing specialists. For example, Clark notes that Mexican-Americans

> who expect a curer to be warm, friendly, and interested in all aspects of the patient's life find it difficult to trust a doctor who is impersonal and "clinical" in his manner. Nor do they accept his authority to "give orders." He may suggest or counsel, but an authoritarian or dictatorial approach on his part is resented and rejected. His behavior, culturally sanctioned in his own society, is often interpreted by Spanish-speaking patients as discourtesy if not outright boorishness. (Clark, 1970, pp. 230–231)

Similarly, O'Connor (1995), who studied Hmong refugees (mainly from Laos) in Philadelphia, demonstrates how physician behavior perceived to be coercive and authoritarian by Hmong patients and their families may contribute to decisions to refuse treatment, even for severe illness.

> Though some of the younger men in the family felt that the evaluation itself could do no harm, the older men (and in general the majority of the decision-making body) felt that pursuit of the evaluation would involve a significant risk of being coerced into the transplant itself: "since . . . they are the doctor[s], right; so they say things; scare us, right?; . . . to make [us] decide to say yes". . . . Family members decided instead to remove him from the hospital against medical advice, and to take him home for family-based care. (O'Connor, 1995, p. 96)

O'Connor notes that the family strongly disliked the "intense pressure for rapid and compliant decisions" (p. 96). This behavior was seen as coercive and served to intensify feelings of distrust. The family also felt uneasy about acting on the opinions of the resident who was quite young since "the Hmong strongly associate wisdom with age and experience" (p. 96).

In summary, most lay medical belief systems reflect an eclectic approach to health and healing. A wide array of causes are recognized and a number of diverse types of healing specialists are accepted as legitimate. Individuals working within the system are pragmatic and eclectic, base their judgements and evaluation on empirical observations (made, of course, through their cultural lens), and may utilize, simultaneously or sequentially, a diversity of healing specialists and remedies representing different theories and ideologies (e.g., Beals, 1976; Clark, 1970; Etkin et al., 1990; Reeve, 2000; Sussman, 1981, 1983, 1988; Trotter & Chavira, 1981). Medical belief systems, while internally coherent, are not closed and static. They are, rather, open and changing. New elements—theories of causation, illness categories, illness labels, and forms of treatment—may be and are incorporated into them, but they are incorporated in forms congruent with the underlying values and principles of the system as a whole.

Social Structure and Organization

> People in Sal si Puedes do not act as isolated individuals in medical situations. In illness as well as in other aspects of life, they are members of a group of relatives and compadres. Illness is not merely a biological disorder of the individual organism—it is a social crisis and period of readjustment for an entire group of people. (Clark, 1970, p. 203)
>
> . . . The authority of the family group also supersedes that of the professional medical workers. Opinions of doctors and nurses certainly influence family decisions, but they are not accepted as absolute fact. (Clark, 1970, p. 205)

Social structure and organization play a significant role in illness interpretation and management. It is overwhelmingly within the context of the family and household that illness is recognized and managed throughout the world. The conditions of individuals are assessed and individuals are labeled by the social group as "sick," thereby assigning individuals to the "sick role" and granting them culturally defined rights, privileges, and obligations of that role. The lay "therapy management group" (Janzen, 1978, 1987) makes decisions regarding the seeking of care and the following of particular treatment regimens, and specific individuals are delegated the task of caring for sick members of the group. Social structure and organization provide the means for implementing cultural beliefs, norms, and values through the delineation of those individuals responsible for the various aspects of illness management. In some cultures, it is the ill individual who is predominantly responsible for making decisions regarding treatment-seeking and care, whereas in others the authority of the family or social group may supersede that of the individual and of the healer.

Decision-Makers and Caregivers   Across cultures, peoples organize themselves into groups in diverse ways, and the roles and statuses of individuals within those groups also vary. In the United States, we tend to assume that individual patients, as long as they are physically and mentally able, are in charge of their illness management. In the case of children, we assume that the parent(s) are responsible for management decisions. However, worldwide, this is not necessarily the case, and family groups and responsibilities extend well beyond the household and nuclear family. For example, regarding a Hmong patient and family in Pennsylvania, O'Connor (1995) states

> The self is collectively developed and conceived, within the structure and mutual obligations of multigenerational family relations and clan affiliation. In traditional Hmong terms, there is no equivalent to the willful, self-interested, and individuated self that is so deeply ingrained and idealized in contemporary American culture. The consent form that Mr. L. would have to sign for transport and evaluation for liver transplant could indeed by signed by him. But the act of consent that could occasion this signature had, in fact, little to do with him personally. Within his cultural framework, momentous decisions can only be made collectively, by a meeting of all relevant family members. Each family member has the right and duty to express his or her thoughts on the matter, and the opinions and concerns of all then form the basis of a general discussion.
>
> The decision-making process includes consideration of effects of actions upon individual members and upon the entire family network. . . . In the end it is the male family elder (or elders) who brings together all of the sentiments expressed and comes to a decision by which everyone will abide. The person whom the decision will most directly affect (as seen from the individualist American perspective, or as encoded in the bioethical principle of patient autonomy) does not have private rights in such matters that can override an elder's decision. (p. 85)

The potential complexity of the decision-making process can be seen from the following example from Southwest Madagascar. In this culture, nuclear families are grouped into extended kin groups based upon biological relationships through males. An adult male will typically live in a household with his wife (wives) and unmarried children. This same adult male, if his father is deceased and if he is the eldest male child, may head a kin group composed of his wife (wives), his children, his unmarried sisters and their resident children, his mother, his widowed paternal aunts, his younger brothers and their wives and children, and so on. This male is furthermore a member of a larger, patrilineal lineage, whose head is the eldest male in the most senior generation, traced back through males. The head of the lineage is the ritual leader for the lineage and, ultimately, is responsible for making important decisions about lineage members. Although minor daily health care decisions are usually left to individual female and, then, male heads of household, those regarding more serious illness or expensive treatment options may be made by the head of the extended kin group or even by the head of the lineage. To make matters more complicated, whereas males, and the heads of their extended kin groups, are usually responsible for their wives' well-being, in cases of serious illness, the woman's father and, possibly the head of her patrilineal lineage, must be notified and brought into the decision-making process since they, ultimately, are responsible for her, although they may live in distant villages.

Social structure and organization therefore determine to a great extent the identity of those individuals who have the authority to make health care decisions. Furthermore, health care decision-makers frequently turn to an array of individuals for advice in times of illness. The identities of formal and informal sources of health care advice ("therapeutic networks") are also influenced by cultural norms and may consist of parents and other relatives, friends, other health care professionals such as pharmacists and nurses, priests and ministers, and other knowledgeable community members. Popular literature may also be another important source. Even for patients of the majority culture in the United States, biomedical practitioners may be only one of several sources of advice concerning health and illness management. Then, after a decision has been made to seek care and follow a particular treatment regimen, the identity of those who will assume the responsibility for care is largely determined by cultural norms and the roles and statuses of individuals within the group.

Cultural Values and History

Medical beliefs and social orders reflect a larger system of cultural values. Moreover, the history of a cultural group, and of a minority group vis-à-vis the majority, may play a significant role in the development of cultural values and health care norms and beliefs.

Gender-Related Values   In some cultures there is a preference for offspring of one gender. Among some peoples, this may be exhibited as a mild preference; among others it may be quite marked (e.g., Miller, 1981) as substantial benefits may hinge upon the gender of a child. In some groups, such as the Mahafaly of Southwest Madagascar, the rights and status of a woman may depend upon both bearing a son and having that son survive into adulthood.

Such preferences may influence treatment-seeking, illness management, and even nurturing decisions resulting in differential access to food (Miller, 1981; Williams, Baumslag, & Jelliffe, 1994). Although in some cultures these practices may not be normative, cultural values may nevertheless lead to differential care of sons and daughters, especially when resources are scarce. Similarly, these values, linked to the differential status of men and women, may play a part in decisions regarding the care given to and resources expended on adult members of various subgroups (Williams et al., 1994).

Values Related to Generation and Birth Order   The status and roles of members of different generations or of siblings occupying particular positions in the birth order may also have an impact on decisions regarding illness management. Where elders are highly respected and hold positions of high status, many economic and human resources may be expended to maintain their health. Likewise, children holding a specific place in the birth order, often first sons, may be given preferential treatment. However, if productivity and full functioning of the elderly in the society are valued, health conditions obviating the ability to play a productive role in society may lead to the acceptance of death as superior to life-maintenance efforts.

Affirmation or Rejection of Ethnic Identity   Medical beliefs and practices may be utilized by individuals or nations to declare something about themselves (e.g., Bailey, 1991; Beckerleg, 1994; Carrier, 1989; Crandon-Malamud, 1991; Shutler, 1977). Peoples may affirm pride in their cultural heritage by endorsing traditional healing practices and consuming particular foods. Alternatively, the rejection of traditional beliefs and practices and the acceptance and use of those of the majority culture, or of Western culture, may reflect a desire to demonstrate one's level of acculturation to the majority culture or Western culture, one's education, one's status, or one's acceptance into mainstream society. Another issue faced by members of minority groups is that of "double consciousness and double self-identity" described as the desire or attempt to be American while retaining one's ethnic identity and not being viewed as "white" (Kumanyika, Morssink, & Agurs, 1992). This may result in ambivalence toward treatment regimens and programs and alternation between adherence and nonadherence.

Medical beliefs and practices are integral parts of the cultural heritage of patients. They frequently reflect deep-seated moral and social values, worldviews, and religious beliefs that transcend specific beliefs about human anatomy, physiology, and pathology. However, one must refrain from stereotyping individuals based on their apparent ethnic background because some individuals may, through their medical beliefs and practices, be attempting to assert their *dis*similarity from others with their ethnic background.

History of a Group   The history of a group may be particularly relevant to current medical beliefs, patterns of health-seeking, and attitudes toward particular types of healing specialists. For example, the ancestors of present-day African Americans, forcefully removed from their homelands, social groups, and cultural resources, and until quite recently denied access to the same medical care as Whites, had to develop their own unique system of medical beliefs and treatment methods based on diverse medical systems from Africa and available knowledge and resources in their new environment (Bailey, 1991; Jordon; 1979; Snow, 1974, 1977; Spector, 1979). These developed over time and, although resulting in response to conditions not of their own making, came to be parts of African American culture.

Likewise, slaves received the least desirable foods and found ways to survive on them, preserve them, and make them palatable. Particular food items and dishes then also became part of African American cultural traditions. They may serve as markers of membership in the group and could also be viewed as symbolizing the history and strife of the group. Culturally insensitive attempts by White middle-class health care professionals to alter diet and patterns of use of biomedical care may quite understandably be viewed by African Americans as debasing their cultural traditions and as blaming these traditions, originally developed as adaptive responses to White oppression, for their current health states.

Native American groups similarly experienced extensive oppression at the hands of Whites settling their homelands. In speaking of the causes and development of diabetes among tribe members, the Dakota, for example, tend to view the disease not only as the result of specific dietary practices and physical conditions (e.g., obesity) of individuals, but also within the social and historical perspective of the tribe, of Native Americans in general, and of their interactions with Whites (Lang, 1989, 1990). Diabetes is seen as a new illness that has been brought to them by the White man. As for African Americans, attempts by biomedical practitioners, representatives of White society, both to implicate diet in the development of disease and to change the diet, originally imposed on them by Whites but now an integral part of current traditions, may not be well accepted by Native Americans. Dietary changes are rarely followed by Dakota individuals with diabetes; in fact, they are viewed as yet "another 'imposition' on Indian people by a non-Indian world" (Lang, 1989, p. 320).

Diet is so intimately intertwined with religion, politics, social structure, and centuries of history that medical advice that appears to place blame on the victims for their illness because of poor diet and obesity is unlikely to succeed. As Lang (1989) states, food reflects one's orientation: "community solidarity vis-à-vis other Dakota communities of the region, Dakota identity vis-à-vis other Native American groups, . . . and Indian identity vis-à-vis white society. Foods likewise provide a means by which Dakota make connections with an idealized past" (pp. 319–320).

The history of interactions of a group with the society and, in particular, with biomedicine lives on through generations. This is clearly demonstrated in a study by Agee (2000) comparing the passing on of knowledge about menopause among African American and Euro-American women and decisions regarding treatment-seeking and the use of *hormone replacement therapy* (HRT). In speaking of the African American women in her sample, she states that "many expressed that their collective history as African American women shaped important aspects of their contemporary identity as well as their interactions with the health care system" (p. 80). Most of the African American women, even those who had consulted physicians about menopause, chose not to use HRT, and about two-thirds of those interviewed

> intimated a distrust of the medical system that informed their decisions about HRT. Women framed this distrust by talking about the history of medical mistreatment of African Americans in the area. . . . This history includes the inhumane treatment of African Americans in the basement of the local hospital during segregation. . . . Even after desegregation of the hospital, similar treatment of African Americans continued. (p. 89)

Such mistreatment was actually witnessed by some of the women both before and after desegregation and is part of their personal experience as well as family experience through the generations. Agee states that "for African American women aware of biomedical practices that have attempted to limit their power and their knowledge of their bodies, being wary of biomedicine and other institutions built on knowledge/power relations informed by racist ideologies is essential survival" (p. 90).

ARE SCIENCE AND MEDICINE IMMUNE TO CULTURE AND VALUES?

In the previous sections, I have mainly addressed the cultural beliefs of peoples living in other societies or of members of minority groups of non-European ancestry living within the United States. However, are we, as scientists, researchers, and physicians, culture-free and value-free? In at least the social sciences, it is a predominant view that perceptions of reality are shaped by culture, or, stated differently, that reality is in essence culturally constructed (see Berger & Luckmann, 1967). Furthermore, science and biomedicine are products of a culture and society, represent particular worldviews, and are guided, explicitly and implicitly, by sets of values. As succinctly described by O'Connor (1995), "worldviews determine the character of what is real or true, and how it is reliably to be known" (p. 7). In order to demonstrate how science and medicine are culturally constructed and embedded in values, I briefly examine how, in our own society, the cultural lenses of medical practitioners, researchers, and patients may result in diverse perceptions of illness and conflicting treatment goals and needs.

This discussion is based on six years of observations as a participant-observer of an asthma education program for low-income Black Americans in an urban setting. The prime motivating factor for developing the program, conceived of by a physician and a psychologist, was the excess morbidity and mortality from asthma among African American children and, specifically, a succession of five deaths of adolescents from asthma in a single city. Analyses of medical reports and autopsies in the five cases led to the following findings: a) all were African American, b) two-fifths had no prescribed corticosteroids in their systems, indicating that they were not taking their medications, c) four-fifths had zero or low theophylline levels, indicating that they had not taken their medications, and d) families appeared not to appreciate the seriousness of asthma. The conclusion reached was that African American children and their families needed to be educated about how dangerous asthma was and about how to care for their asthma because, it was assumed, they were not properly treating the disease.

Therefore, the goal of the project was to educate patients, their families, and the community, using community members as teachers, project leaders, and planners, about the correct way to treat asthma. Since the treatment of asthma is highly individualized, this basically consists of staying away from avoidable things that might bring on asthma attacks (e.g., smoke, dust, pets, and roaches), seeing the doctor regularly, and following the doctor's recommendations (in all but the mildest of cases, this could involve the regular daily preventive use of one or several medications). Although participants were chosen on the basis of morbidity in the previous year, the sample was quite diverse in terms of morbidity just prior to enrollment into the program (Sussman, 1992c). No segment of the original program was directed at physicians, nor was there any medical evaluation of the appropriateness of prescribed treatment.

Assumptions About Minority Patients

The first assumption made about the "target" population (minority groups in the United States, notably Blacks, Hispanics, and Native Americans) by the funding institution and researchers was that this was a "hard-to-reach," "resistant" group (Sussman, 1992c). Therefore, it would be difficult to have an impact on them, and the researchers would need to find new, creative, acceptable ways of reaching those in need of help. On what, however, is this assumption based?

It was based on the following combination of observations, assumptions, conclusions, and logic:

- Morbidity and mortality rates for asthma are higher among African Americans than Whites (observation).
- Researchers made the tacit assumption that African Americans (and other minority groups) and Whites are adequately homogeneous within their groups and sufficiently different from each other on some set of factors, traits, or characteristics that are in some way directly related to asthma and health.
- Medical researchers began with the belief that asthma is a medically controllable chronic disease and asthma symptoms are preventable.
- Although a higher percentage of African Americans have incomes below the poverty line, adequate medical treatment was presumed to be available to most.

- Therefore, it was reasoned, morbidity and mortality rates must be higher because African American patients and their families are not caring for it appropriately.
- They are not caring for asthma appropriately because they must be resistant to seeking appropriate medical care and to adhering to treatment recommendations.
- They could be resistant or nonadherent for a number of reasons including: distrust of doctors; low educational levels and, hence, lack of understanding; misperceptions based on unsound "folk" beliefs and practices; social and familial problems reflected in higher prevalence rates of such things as "dysfunctional" families and drug abuse; and negligence or not caring.

In short, researchers and funding institutes designing interventions for minority populations frequently begin with the premise that asthma morbidity and mortality rates are high among African Americans because patients are resistant. The premise that the population is resistant is then supported by the fact that asthma morbidity and mortality rates are higher among African Americans than Whites.

Although resistance to seeking or giving appropriate care is cited as the major "cause" of poor health outcomes, do the data support this premise and do they support the previous assumptions? Clearly, the existing epidemiological data do indicate higher morbidity, mortality, and prevalence rates for asthma among Black Americans than Whites (Carr et al., 1992; Weiss, Gergen, & Crain, 1992; Weiss & Wagener 1990). Interestingly, prevalence rates, not just morbidity and mortality rates, are also higher among African Americans and, obviously, are not related to patterns of care or resistance to treatment. Moreover, most prevalence and morbidity statistics are based on previously medically diagnosed cases, meaning that in order to be identified as a "case," one needs to have sought or received medical care for the condition.

Data collected from research participants at enrollment into the educational program do not lend strong support for many of the previous conclusions. Although we do not have comparative data for White Americans, the sample of African Americans was quite heterogeneous in a variety of important characteristics despite the fact that the selection criteria were based on morbidity in the previous year (as measured by the utilization of health care resources) and area of residence (neighborhoods chosen because they contained high percentages of African Americans and relatively high percentages of households below the poverty line). Not only was current morbidity quite heterogeneous, with 35 percent having symptoms at least 3 days during the week preceding enrollment and 38 percent having had no symptoms during that time, but socioeconomic status and household composition were also quite diverse. No commonly used demographic variables (e.g., education, socioeconomic status, household composition, or even age of the child), attitudes, knowledge, or use of care satisfactorily explain the variation in morbidity in the sample. Moreover, those factor(s) that might distinguish this sample as a whole from a sample of White Americans with asthma were not immediately apparent—except, probably, lower mean household income and darker skin color (Sussman, 1997).

Eligible households were recruited from selected neighborhoods, and participants agreed to do nothing other than be interviewed every three months by telephone, be informed about program activities, and allow their medical records at hospitals, clinics, and private physician offices to be audited. They were not required to attend program activities. Interestingly, among this supposedly "hard to reach" or "resistant " group, 94 percent of those contacted agreed to participate. Retention rates were also surprisingly high: over 3 years approximately 2 percent dropped out, 2 percent moved out of town, and an additional 3 percent were lost to follow-up as a result of mobility within or out of the city. Moreover, participation in programs and activities was remarkably high with 65 percent of the households in the target neighborhoods attending some project activity or class and 25 percent of the households either helping to plan or implement an activity (Sussman, 1997).

A clear implication of this, I believe, is that most African American parents are concerned about and interested in their children's health; they are not neglectful and oblivious to the health problems of their children, and they believe it is an important issue. (Indeed, it would be a unique anthropological finding to discover an entire group of people who did not care for their children!) Parents in the program were eager to learn about the "medical facts" about asthma and its appropriate care and were appreciative of the fact that the physicians and nurses in the program were interested in their children. We could conclude that people agreed to be in the study and participate in the program because we had somehow found the key to lowering their resistance and increasing their trust and interest. However, this is unlikely, especially given the initial response rate of 94 percent in which people agreed to participate before they had had any contact with the program. These findings do not support the "negative" stereotypes of the "health behavior" of lower-income African Americans and the assumption that this population is resistant and the cause of its own ills (Sussman, 1992c, 1997; see also Page and Thomas, 1994).

Assumptions About Patients and Physicians

The language and terms used to describe categories of individuals can yield information on underlying assumptions and values held by the speakers. I now briefly examine the language used to describe patients and physicians in order to elucidate some of the assumptions underlying this project and illustrate that, indeed, medical interventions are not value-free but reflect a world seen through a learned biomedical cultural lens.

The assumption regarding the relationship between morbidity and illness management was that almost everyone can control and prevent asthma symptoms with proper medical care and home management. Furthermore, if symptoms are infrequent (and, hence, "prevented"), this can be accomplished only through proper medical care and home management. On the other hand, if symptoms are frequent, then the management/treatment plan prescribed by the physician is not being followed.

If children are not doing well and continue to have symptoms but do not take medication or seek "appropriate" care, the assumption is that there are barriers preventing appropriate disease management—logistic, economic, social or cultural barriers—that, when removed, will allow patients to seek and follow treatment as they really would like to but cannot. There is little focus on the physician or the system as contributing to what are viewed as "inappropriate" health-seeking patterns. The major emphasis in minority health interventions has generally been placed on patients and laymen. Presumed nonadherence among minority families with children with relatively high morbidity rates in the United States has increasingly been responded to by physicians, clinics, and hospitals with threats to parents, accusing them of neglect. Unfortunately, this is often done without trying to gain an adequate understanding of the situation, why it arose, and what can be done. A response to this by the family sometimes is to leave the geographic area or to try to avoid further contact with the physician or facility, which is then viewed as an authority figure and adversary—a representative of the system.

Although the prevalence, morbidity, and mortality rates are higher among African American than White Americans, defining this group as a whole as at high risk is based on nothing more than skin color and represents a form of latent racism (Sussman, 1997; see also Harrison, 1998; Smedley 1993, 1998). The population in the program, for example, was extremely diverse in beliefs, management practices, demographics of income and education, and household composition. Given the epidemiological data, the appropriate question would be "what could 'race' have to do with it?" Asthma morbidity is not biologically correlated to melanin, so what is the pathway between "race" and "high asthma morbidity?"

Although the predominant view within biomedicine is that those who have lower incomes, less education, and live in female-headed households have poorer health outcomes, in the sample of program participants, morbidity did not correlate with any of these variables. In fact, analyses of the data yielded no clear explanations for why some children were doing well and others were not. However, one question not examined was whether there were differences by the type of treatment or the type of health care provider.

Comparative Validity of Patient and Physician Beliefs

If one examines the language and terms used to denote patient and physician knowledge, experience, and behavior, one finds that for those looking through the biomedical lens, patients are characterized as having *beliefs*, *attitudes*, and *holding misconceptions*, whereas physicians and researchers are described as *possessing knowledge*. This usage of terms and the assumptions underlying it naturally lead designers of medical interventions to want to "educate" patients and their families—enlighten them to the "truth," the "real facts." If knowledge is given to them, it is thought that they will unquestioningly accept it because there is either a void waiting to be filled or space filled with uninformed cultural falsehoods waiting to be replaced by the truth.

What is the difference between knowledge, beliefs, and facts? Interestingly, in most articles in medical publications, references must be no more than three to four years old. Why is this the case? It is because research findings are quickly outdated and ideas, theories, concepts, and treatments are constantly modified. Committees are appointed to periodically set and modify guidelines for the most up-to-date treatment of various diseases. These guidelines are especially useful for general practitioners who do not have time to read up on the latest treatment for every disease. Last year's "truth" becomes replaced with this year's "truth" and "facts" (see also O'Connor, 1995). Patients with chronic diseases and those who have had these diseases in their families over generations experience the diseases over long periods of time, observe their treatment by physicians, and note that today doctors tell you to do this now, last year they told you to do that, and next year they will tell you to do something else! The view within science and medicine is that through research theories are constantly being tested and refined, bringing us ever closer to the truth. Although this may be the case, it still leaves open the question concerning the difference between facts, knowledge, and beliefs, and the relative validity and value accorded to them.

Diverse Models of Asthma, Its Care, and Goals of Treatment

Basically, medical specialist researchers, general practitioners, and patients in the program tended to hold quite different views of asthma and its care (Sussman, 1997).

Medical Specialists When the program began, specialists saw asthma as consisting of a combination of bronchospasms and inflammation in response to environmental irritants, allergens, and other stimuli such as exercise, respiratory infections, and strong emotions. It was believed to run in families but probably also require environmental factors to activate the onset of the disease. It was seen as a chronic illness requiring ongoing management, treatment, and monitoring. Management consisted of daily use of prophylactic medications (except in cases of very mild asthma) and environmental control to reduce exposure to irritants and allergens, the most emphasized being smoke, dust, furry and feathered pets, cockroaches, mold and mildew, and strong odors from products such as cleaning agents and perfumes. The goal of treatment was to prevent the onset of symptoms, which is accomplished by keeping the airways open and not inflamed. Often several medications were prescribed for daily use, several times per day, and the treatment guidelines at that time specified that routine checkups be performed four times per year.

It is believed that, if treated properly, the disease can be fully controlled so that most children can engage in most activities and remain symptom free. If symptoms do occur, however, they should be controllable with medications that patients have in their possession. In general, medications are believed to cause no major side effects and pose no danger. Usually only when prednisone, an oral steroid, was prescribed (to treat an acute, serious attack) were possible side effects explained.

General Practitioners Although there was considerable variation, general practitioners generally held a model of asthma similar to that of specialists. In practice, however, their treatment did not always reflect the "state of the art." They were less likely to prescribe daily medications, more likely to prescribe medication to be taken as needed, and less likely to prescribe anti-inflammatory medications. In fact, a surprisingly small percentage of participants had been prescribed any type of daily preventive medication (40 percent), and very few indeed had been prescribed anti-inflammatory agents (the "state of the art" treatment) along with the usual bronchodilators (Sussman, 1997).

Moreover, none followed the guidelines (NIH, 1991) of seeing asthma patients quarterly for routine care and some did not usually make appointments for checkups. The guidelines further specified that after an acute episode, the child should always see the doctor within 72 hours for follow-up. However, in general, if the parent reported that the child was doing well, physicians usually thought it unnecessary for an actual office visit.

Although some physicians and clinics had the facilities to treat acute symptoms (nebulizers), many did not. The latter usually referred symptomatic patients to an emergency room for care. In practice, many general practitioners were, then, in fact, treating asthma episodically, not encouraging routine care, and referring people to the emergency room for acute care with little or no follow-up. In fact, many patients were seldom seen for asthma because the message to them was that office visits were not appropriate for acute care, follow-up visits after acute care were not necessary if the child was not having symptoms, and there was no need for routine care except to renew prescriptions (Sussman, 1997).

Some of the general practitioners felt that asthma was frequently difficult to treat, that symptoms and attacks were not necessarily predictable, and that some of the medications prescribed by specialists for daily use were too strong or unnecessary. At another site, it was discovered that some general practitioners and pharmacists had advised their patients not to take the medications prescribed by specialists (Sussman, 1997).

Parents and Children with Asthma   There was considerable variation among the participants in the study, but some concepts were quite common. Basically, asthma was believed to run in families and was seen as an episodic illness that flares up every now and then. As such, the tendency was to treat it when symptoms occurred. Factors and conditions that were reported most frequently as important in triggering asthma attacks were changes in season, changes in weather, colds and respiratory infections, and excessive exercise. Although not addressed in the interview because they were not viewed by biomedicine as particularly important, factors such as impurities and chemicals in food, air pollution, and food allergies were believed by many community members (with whom we met in focus groups) to be important factors in bringing on asthma symptoms.

It was believed that some stimuli could be avoided, but others were unavoidable (seasonal and temperature changes) and uncontrollable. A high percentage of parents had rather low expectations from medical treatment: They did not think that much could be done to prevent asthma symptoms from occurring (59 percent) and thought that children with asthma simply could not do all the things that other children do (51 percent), despite medical care. It was generally accepted that people with asthma will at least occasionally wheeze and have attacks requiring acute care. In fact, one way to control or prevent the onset of symptoms was to restrict the physical activity of children because this frequently brought on symptoms (Sussman, 1992c, 1997). This view is in direct opposition to the view of asthma held by asthma specialists.

Many (54 percent) voiced concern over the long-term use of medication by children as well as the fear of developing a tolerance for the medications, necessitating higher and higher doses. Side effects that were sometimes very troublesome were acknowledged or experienced by many (52 percent) (Sussman, 1992c, 1997). The goal of treatment from the parents' perspectives was in most cases to stop symptoms when they occurred and then to cut back or stop the use of medication whenever possible. This is quite different from the specialists' goal of preventing symptoms altogether through the daily use of medications.

It was recognized that the airways closed up during asthma attacks, and it was believed that there was an excessive buildup of phlegm during these times that needed to be cleaned out. Many home remedies were geared toward cleaning out the phlegm. Colds and cold air were also seen as important factors contributing to asthma attacks. Although the interviews were not adequate to examine the concepts of asthma in detail, these concepts do fit well with Snow's (1977) description of African American beliefs concerning the way the body functions.

Treatment Goals   Obviously, it is ultimately the patient and family who decide how to treat an illness. Advice from health care professionals, family members, friends, and priests or ministers and knowledge from one's own experience may all be taken into account when making a decision. Considerable disparity exists between the models and messages that would be received from asthma specialists, general practitioners, and the lay population (the social group-family and friends) (Fig. 3.4). In the medical community, it is usually the patient who is blamed for not seeking routine care, for not seeking acute care quickly and going for follow-up care, for not taking appropriate medications, and for treating asthma episodically. As a result, the goal

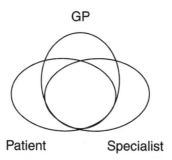

FIG. 3.4. Concepts of asthma and its care held by patients, general practitioners, and specialists.

of most programs and interventions is to change patient behavior (see, e.g., Hunt & Arar, 2001; Trostle, 1988). However, as can be seen from this example, much of the behavior of patients and their parents was probably reinforced (or was originally influenced) by messages being sent to them by medical practitioners and by their own experiences over time.

Given the cultural value placed on science and high social status, and the low value associated with low socioeconomic and minority status, patients from these groups and their families are sometimes pigeonholed into "high risk" groups by well-meaning, caring practitioners and researchers. They are also stereotyped, their observations and experiences are invalidated or at least devalued, and they are blamed for their illness. Assumptions made about them by scientists, researchers, or physicians are not even necessarily consciously recognized because they are such an integral part of the culture and society, and because science is accorded such authoritative status; they are contained in the view of the world as seen through the Western cultural biomedical lens. As such, the assumptions are neither questioned nor put to empirical test.

Four major themes are emphasized throughout this chapter.

- What are frequently termed "folk beliefs" are not isolated beliefs and practices, holdovers from different times and places. Rather, medical belief systems are coherent, logical systems of beliefs, practices, norms, and values. Although the importance of culture in shaping medical beliefs and practices of other groups is being increasingly acknowledged in biomedicine today, there is a disturbing trend toward blaming the "culture" of minority groups for the high prevalence, morbidity, and mortality rates of various diseases among these groups. In a way, a form of cultural determinism is replacing, or joining, biological determinism in explaining epidemiological data (see Harrison, 1998; Park, 1996). This then sometimes leads to the misguided goal of wishing to educate culture out of people. Hopefully, I have conveyed and substantiated the fact that culture is not just a factor that affects illness interpretation and management, but rather that it shapes it and guides it. We view, define, and manage illness according to our cultural framework—our cultural lens. Therapy is developed and its effectiveness is evaluated within our cultural framework, and decisions and the identities of those who make decisions are congruent with cultural values. For example, do we pursue life for life's sake? Does there come a time to die because one is of no use to society or a burden to one's family? Is a boy more valued than a girl and thus more likely to receive medical care? Culture permeates our view of reality: Reality is culturally constructed.

- People who are ill, along with individuals in their social group, are active; they use their own knowledge and experience and seek that of others in attempts to make sense of illness and to find relief and a cure. Although they may not consistently or completely follow treatment regimens advised by biomedical practitioners, and hence may be labeled as "nonadherent" or "negligent," they are most likely doing things—other things—and may consider themselves and be considered by others in their group to be responsibly managing their illness.

- Lay medical belief systems are open and dynamic, constantly changing, adapting to new conditions, incorporating new elements, and even modifying old elements as long as they do not directly require the rejection of beliefs and values underlying the system. New elements tend to be integrated into medical systems in forms congruent with the existing system; they rarely completely replace existing elements. Moreover, most permit, and many encourage, individuals to be pragmatic and eclectic in their quests for a cure.

- So much variation exists between individuals within groups, and so many factors (individual, social, economic, and political, as well as cultural) exist that may shape illness management, that an oversimplified characterization of cultural groups, or stereotyping, is misleading and counterproductive. Therefore, in this chapter I strive to convey an appreciation for the many lenses through which an illness may be viewed and for an understanding of the multiple sociocultural issues and processes that may shape and underlie individual health decisions and illness management practices.

REFERENCES

Agee, E. (2000). Menopause and the transmission of women's knowledge: African American and white women's perspectives. *Medical Anthropology Quarterly, 14,* 73–95.

Bailey, E. (1991). *Urban African American health care.* Lanham, MD: University Press of America.

Beals, A. R. (1976). Strategies of resort to curers in South India. In C. Leslie (Ed.), *Asian medical systems: A comparative study* (pp. 184–200). Berkeley, CA: University of California Press.

Beckerleg, S. (1994). Medical pluralism and Islam in Swahili communities in Kenya. *Medical Anthropology Quarterly, 8*(3), 299–313.

Berger, P., & Luckmann, T. (1967). *The social construction of reality.* Garden City, NY: Doubleday.

Brodwin, P. (1996). *Medicine and morality in Haiti: The contest for healing power.* Cambridge, England: Cambridge University Press.

Carr, W., Zeital, L., & Weiss, K. B. (1992). Asthma hospitalization and mortality in New York City. *American Journal of Public Health, 82,* 59–65.

Carrier, A. H. (1989). The place of Western medicine in Ponam theories of health and illness. In S. Frankel & G. Lewis (Eds.), *A continuing trial of treatment: Medical pluralism in Papua New Guinea* (pp. 155–181). Dordrecht, The Netherlands: Kluwer.

Carstairs, G. M. (1955). Medicine and faith in rural Rajasthan. In B. D. Paul (Ed.), *Health, culture, and community: Case studies of public reactions to health programs* (pp. 107–134). New York: Russell Sage Foundation.

Chrisman, N. J. (1977). The health-seeking process: An approach to the natural history of illness. *Culture, Medicine & Psychiatry, 1*(4), 351–377.

Clark, M. (1970). *Health in the Mexican-American culture: A community study* (2nd ed.). Berkeley, CA: University of California Press.

Counts, D. R., & Counts, D. A. (1989). Complementarity in medical treatment in a West New Britain Society. In S. Frankel and G. Lewis (Eds.), *A continuing trial of treatment: Medical pluralism in Papua New Guinea* (pp. 277–294). Dordrecht, The Netherlands: Kluwer.

Crandon-Malamud, L. (1991). *From the fat of our souls: Social change, political process, and medical pluralism in Bolivia*. Berkeley, CA: University of California Press.

Eisenberg, L. (1977). Disease and illness: Distinctions between professional and popular ideas of sickness. *Culture, Medicine & Psychiatry, 1,* 9–23.

Etkin, N. L. (1988). Cultural constructions of efficacy. In S. van der Geest & R. Whyte (Eds.), *The context of medicines in developing countries* (pp. 299–326). Dordrecht, The Netherlands: Kluwer Academic.

Etkin, N. L., Ross, P. J., & Muazzamu, I. (1990). The indigenization of pharmaceuticals: Therapeutic transitions in rural Hausaland. *Social Science and Medicine, 30*(8), 919–928.

Gibbs, T. (1988). Health-seeking behavior of elderly Blacks. In J. S. Jackson (Ed.), *The Black American elderly* (pp. 282–291). New York: Springer.

Greenwood, B. (1981). Cold or spirits? Choice and ambiguity in Morocco's pluralistic medical system. *Social Science and Medicine, 15B,* 219–235.

Harrison, F. V. (1998). Introduction: Race and racism. *American Anthropologist, 100*(3), 609–631.

Harwood, A. (1971). Hot-cold theory of disease: Implications for treatment of Puerto Rican patients. *Journal of American Medical Association, 216,* 1153–1158.

Helman, C. G. (1994). *Culture, health and illness: An introduction for health professionals* (3rd ed.). Oxford, England: Butterworth-Heinemann.

Heyer, K. W. (1981). *Rootwork: Psychosocial aspects of malign magical and illness beliefs in a South Carolina Sea Island community*. Unpublished doctoral dissertation, University of Connecticut, Storrs.

Hill, C. E. (1973). Black healing practices in the rural South. *Journal of Popular Culture, 6,* 849–853.

Hill, C. E. (1976). A folk medical belief system in the rural South: Some practical considerations. *Southern Medicine, 16,* 11–17.

Hopper, S. V., & Schechtman, K. B. (1985). Factors associated with diabetic control and utilization patterns in a low-income, older adult population. *Patient Education & Counseling, 7,* 275–288.

Hunt, L. M., & Arar, N. H. (2001). An analytical framework for contrasting patient and provider views of the process of chronic disease management. *Medical Anthropology Quarterly 15,* 347–367.

Janzen, J. M. (1978). *The quest for therapy in Lower Zaire*. Berkeley, CA: University of California Press.

Janzen, J. M. (1987). Therapy management: Concept, reality, process. *Medical Anthropology Quarterly (NS), 1*(1), 68–84.

Janzen, J., & Prins, G. (Eds.). (1981). Causality and classification in African medicine and health. Special issue, *Social Science & Medicine, 15B*(3).

Jordon, J. W. (1979). The roots and practice of voodoo medicine in America. *Urban Health, 8,* 38–41.

Kleinman, A. (1980). *Patients and healers in the context of culture*. Berkeley, CA: University of California Press.

Kleinman, A., Eisenberg, L., & Good, B. (1978). Culture, illness, and care: Clinical lessons from anthropologic and cross-cultural research. *Annals of Internal Medicine, 88,* 251–258.

Kumanyika, S. K., Morssink, C., & Agurs, T. (1992). Models for dietary and weight change in African-American women: Identifying cultural components. *Ethnicity & Disease, 2*(2), 166–175.

Lang, G. C. (1989). "Making sense" about diabetes: Dakota narratives of illness. *Medical Anthropology, 11,* 305–327.

Lang, G. C. (1990). Talking about a new illness with the Dakota: Reflections on diabetes, food and culture. In R. H. Winthrop (Ed.), *Culture and the anthropological tradition: Essays in honor of Robert F. Spencer* (pp. 283–318). Lanham, MD: University Press of America.

Luecke, R. (Ed.). (1993). *A new dawn in Guatemala: Toward a worldwide health vision*. Prospect Heights, IL: Waveland Press.

Mechanic, D. (1962). The concept of illness behavior. *Journal of Chronic Diseases, 15,* 189–194.

Mechanic, D. (1968). *Medical sociology: A selective view*. New York: The Free Press.

Mechanic, D. (Ed.). (1982). *Symptoms, illness behavior and help-seeking*. New York: Prodist.

Miller, B. D. (1981). *The endangered sex: Neglect of female children in rural North India*. Ithaca, NY: Cornell University Press.

Mull, J. D., & Mull, D. S. (1988). Mothers' concept of childhood diarrhoea in rural Pakistan: What ORT program planners should know. *Social Science & Medicine, 27,* 53–67.

National Institutes of Health, 1991. *Guidelines for the diagnosis and management of asthma*. National Asthma Education and Prevention Program Expert Panel Report 1. National Heart, Lung, and Blood Institute. Washington, DC: NIH.

Ngubane, H. (1977). *Body and mind in Zulu medicine: An ethnography of health and disease in Nyuswa-Zulu thought and practice*. London: Academic Press.

O'Connor, B. B. (1995). *Healing traditions: Alternative medicine and the health professions*. Philadelphia, PA: University of Pennsylvania Press.

Page, H. E., & Thomas, B. (1994). White public space and the construction of white privilege in U.S. health care: Fresh concepts and a new model of analysis. *Medical Anthropology Quarterly, 8*(1), 109–116.

Park, K. (1996). Use and abuse of race and culture: Black-Korean tension in America. *American Anthropologist, 98*(3), 492–505.

Press, I. (1969). Urban illness: Physicians, curers, and dual use in Bogota. *Journal of Health and Social Behavior, 10*(3): 209–218.

Quatromoni, P. A., Milbauer, M., Posner, B. M., Carballeira, N. P., Brunt, M., & Chipkin, S. R. (1994). Use of focus groups to explore nutrition practices and health beliefs of urban Caribbean Latinos with diabetes. *Diabetes Care, 17*(8), 869–873.

Raymond, N. R., & D'Eramo-Melkus, G. (1993). Non-insulin-dependent diabetes and obesity in the black and Hispanic population: Culturally sensitive management. *Diabetes Educator, 19*(4), 313–317.

Reeve, M. E. (2000). Concepts of illness and treatment practice in a caboclo community of the Lower Amazon. *Medical Anthropology Quarterly, 14*, 96–108.

Roberson, M. H. B. (1992). The meaning of compliance: Patient perspectives. *Qualitative Health Research, 2*, 7–26.

Schwartz, L. R. (1969). The hierarchy of resort in curative practices: The Admiralty Islands, Melanesia. *Journal of Health and Social Behavior, 10*, 201–209.

Scott, C. S. (1974). Health and healing practices among five ethnic groups in Miami, Florida. *Public Health Report, 89*, 524–532.

Shutler, M. E. (1977). Disease and curing in a Yaqui community. In E. H. Spicer (Ed.), *Ethnic medicine in the Southwest* (pp. 169–237). Tucson, AZ: University of Arizona Press.

Smedley, A. (1993). *Race in North America: Origin and evolution of a worldview*. Boulder, CO: Westview Press.

Smedley, A. (1998). "Race" and the construction of human identity. *American Anthropologist, 100*(3), 690–702.

Snow, L. F. (1974). Folk medical beliefs and their implications for care of patients. *Annals of Internal Medicine, 81*, 82–96.

Snow, L. F. (1977). Popular medicine in a Black neighborhood. In E. H. Spicer (Ed.), *Ethnic medicine in the Southwest* (pp. 19–95). Tucson, AZ: University of Arizona Press.

Snow, L. F. (1978). Sorcerers, saints and charlatans: Black folk healers in urban America. *Culture, Medicine & Psychiatry, 2*, 60–106.

Snow, L. F. (1993). *Walking over medicine*. Boulder, CO: Westview Press.

Spector, R. (1979). *Cultural diversity in health and illness*. New York: Appleton-Century Crofts.

Staiano, K. V. (1981). Alternative therapeutic systems in Belize: A semiotic framework. *Social Science & Medicine, 15B*(3), 317–332.

Sussman, L. K. (1980). Herbal medicine on Mauritius. *Journal of Ethnopharmacology, 2*(3), 259–278.

Sussman, L. K. (1981). Unity in diversity in a polyethnic society: The maintenance of medical pluralism on Mauritius. *Social Science & Medicine, 15B*, 247–260.

Sussman, L. K. (1983). *Medical pluralism on Mauritius: A study of medical beliefs and practices in a polyethnic society*. Unpublished doctoral dissertation, Washington University, St. Louis.

Sussman, L. K. (1988). The use of herbal and biomedical pharmaceuticals on Mauritius. In S. van der Geest & R. Whyte (Eds.), *The context of medicines in developing countries* (pp. 199–216). Dordrecht, The Netherlands: Kluwer Academic.

Sussman, L. K. (1992a). Discussion: Critical assessment of models. In D. M. Becker, D. R. Hill, J. S. Jackson, D. M. Levine, F. A. Stillman, & S. M. Weiss (Eds.), *Health behavior research in minority populations: Access, design, and implementation* (pp. 145–149). National Institute of Health Publication, No. 92–2965.

Sussman, L. K. (1992b). *Medical beliefs and practices among the Mahafaly of Southwest Madagascar*. Sixth International Congress on Traditional and Folk Medicine. Austin, TX, December.

Sussman, L. K. (1992c). *Hard-to-reach and resistant populations: Misguided concepts in health-related interventions and research*. Annual Meeting of the American Anthropological Association. San Francisco, December.

Sussman, L. K. (1997). *Asthma among Black Americans: Diverse perspectives*. Joint Annual Meeting of the Society for Applied Anthropology and the Society for Medical Anthropology. Seattle, March.

Sussman, L. K., Robins, L. N., & Earls, F. (1987). Treatment-seeking for depression by black and white Americans. *Social Science & Medicine, 24*(3), 187–196.

Sussman, R. W., & Sussman, L. K. (1977). Divination among the Sakalava of Madagascar. In J. Long (Ed.), *Extrasensory ecology* (pp. 271–291). New York: Scarecrow Press.

Trotter, R. T., & Chavira, J. A. (1981). *Curanderismo: Mexican American folk healing*. Athens, GA: University of Georgia Press.

Topley, M. (1976). Chinese traditional etiology and methods of cure in Hong Kong. In C. Leslie (Ed.), *Asian medical systems: A comparative study* (pp. 243–264). Berkeley, CA: University of California Press.

Trostle, J. A. (1988). Medical compliance as an ideology. *Social Science and Medicine 27*, 1299–1308.

Weiss, K. B., Gergen, P. J., & Crain, E. F. (1992). Inner-city asthma: The epidemiology of an emerging U.S. public health concern. *Chest, 101*(6), Supplement 362S–367S.

Weiss, K. B., & Wagener, D. K. (1990). Changing patterns of asthma mortality: Identifying target popula-tions at high risk. *Journal of American Medical Association, 264,* 1683–1687.

Williams, C. D., Baumslag, N., & Jelliffe, D. B. (1994). *Mother and child health: Delivering the services* (3rd ed.). New York: Oxford University Press.

Woods, C. M. (1997). Alternative curing strategies in a changing medical situation. *Medical Anthropology, 1*(3): 25–54.

Yoder, S. (1981). Knowledge of illness and medicine among Cokwe of Zaire. *Social Science & Medicine, 15B,* 237–246.

Young, A. (1982). The anthropologies of illness and sickness. *Annual Review of Anthropology, 11,* 257–285.

Young, J. C. (1981). *Medical choice in a Mexican village.* New Brunswick, NJ: Rutgers University Press.

Zola, E. (1972). Studying the decision to see a doctor. *Advances in Psychosomatic Medicine, 8,* 216–236.

Cross-cultural Commonalities in Therapy and Healing: Theoretical Issues and Psychological and Sociocultural Principles

Jefferson M. Fish
St. John's University
New York City

Let us imagine how a modern university hospital might look to anthropologists from Mars studying healing shrines in an industrialized society. They would learn that the local medical school is reputed to be a site of amazing cures . . . certain areas were open to the public and other areas . . . were reserved exclusively for the performance of arcane healing rituals . . . These special-purpose rooms contain spectacular machines . . . Those who tend and control these machines speak a special language that is unintelligible to the layperson and prominently display on their person healing amulets and charms . . . The operating rooms are the holy of holies . . . So jealously guarded are the mysteries of the operating room that patients are rendered unconscious before they are allowed to enter them.

   In evaluating the reports of the cures that occur in such a shrine, anthropologists might be as impressed with the features that mobilize the patient's expectant faith as with the staff's rationale for the treatments administered.
   —Jerome D. Frank and Julia B. Frank, (*Persuasion and Healing*, 1991, pp. 108–109)

PROCESS AND CONTENT

Does Psychology Have Any Content?

A cross-cultural perspective requires us to ask fundamental questions about the nature of psychology. In this case, in order to discuss cross-cultural commonalties in therapy and healing, we must first make a distinction between psychological processes and psychological content, so that we know what we are looking for.

   If psychology is the science of behavior, then—at least with regard to our own species—it aims at making generalizations about the behavior of all human beings. For this reason, the anthropologist George Peter Murdock suggested that it is the function of psychology to describe behavioral processes and of anthropology to describe the cultural conditions under which those processes lead to different forms of behavior (Murdock, 1972). Another way of putting this would be to say that psychology describes the processes, and anthropology fills in the content.

   Issues of culture need to be taken into account, however, even when studying such presumably universal human processes as perception, cognition, or learning. For example, in the course of formal education, children learn to think in different ways, and psychologists can study those thought processes. But in cultures that have no schools—the condition of all of our species for the first 95 percent of its existence, and the condition of much of the world today—people are not exposed to or instructed in such thought processes, and therefore never acquire them (Ogbu, 2002). For example, arithmetic reasoning is not a concept easily applied to cultures that count "one, two, many." Still, once culture is taken into account by considering the varied conditions under which human psychological processes develop differentially, it becomes possible to make important generalizations about such processes.

The Recapitulation Fallacy

Once we move from process to content, though, the possibility of making any significant generalizations would seem to evaporate.[1] Although Freud (and later Jung, on a grander scale with his archetypes) postulated universal content, such as the Oedipus complex and dream symbols, such assertions foundered on the inability to explain how humans acquired such content (quite apart from issues of verifiability and accuracy). Freud's reliance on recapitulation theory, in which the stages of psychological development were seen as corresponding to stages in human history, was essentially Lamarckian and has been shown to be false by modern genetics (Fish, 1996a; Gould, 1981, 1987). In other words, even if many generations of men did actually rise up to kill their fathers in the distant past, such acts would have had no effect on the genes they passed on to their children, and could not, therefore, have led to the creation of the Oedipus complex.

The recapitulation fallacy is sometimes seen in a new guise in modern biologized explanations for patterns of behavior that can more parsimoniously be understood as having arisen through social circumstances. Thus, personality traits like altruism, or social customs, like the Eskimo abandoning sick elders to die, are explained by persuasive stories of how genes for altruism or elder abandonment proliferate through natural selection. However, the same stories can easily be modified to show how people learn and pass on the information that it is advantageous to treat others nicely—or to abandon even esteemed others when group survival is at stake—without postulating the existence of genes to accomplish the task. Cultural transmission has the advantage over genetic transmission of being much more rapid and of allowing different groups to develop quite opposite patterns of behavior in adaptation to very different environments.

B. F. Skinner (1974) has suggested that there is a parallel between the way in which the environment selects the behavior of individual organisms (through reinforcement) and the way in which natural selection operates at the species level. Thus, if one wished to postulate genetic explanations for patterns of behavior, one could refer to the genes that presumably underlie the social learning process. In other words, postulating genes for the general process of social learning requires fewer assumptions than postulating genes—via speculative evolutionary explanations—for a series of specific forms of social behavior.

Furthermore, therapy is a recently invented Western institution, about 100 years old, while anatomically modern humans have been around for about 200,000 years—190,000 of which were spent as hunters and gatherers. Thus, any distinctively human psychological content that might exist would be adapted to forms of social interaction far removed from managed care and the 50-minute hour.

---

[1]A controversial book that might take exception to this statement is Donald Brown's *Human Universals* (1991). Many of Brown's proposed universals can be disputed, and others—his "near universals"—might less charitably be called "non-universals." Even if one were to accept many of his proposed universals, however, they are at such a level of generality (e.g., the use of language or the existence of kin categories) as to be irrelevant to therapy.

Dealing with Unacceptable Difference

It is worth noting in passing that, although all cultures deal with physical handicaps, illness, deviant behavior, and other abnormalities, "therapy and healing" is only one of five different ways of dealing with people who are temporarily or enduringly different. Societies may do the following: (a) Kill, injure, imprison, or otherwise punish such people. (b) Isolate them—for example, by creating leper colonies. (c) Deliberately ignore them or their abnormalities. (d) Reward or attempt to capitalize on their "infirmity"—for example, by viewing epilepsy as an ability to contact the spirit world. (e) Attempt to assist them, or ameliorate or cure their "illness."

It is important to recognize that all of these options are exercised by the world's cultures, and that Western societies implement all five. Furthermore, these interventions may be combined, and different groups of people may even differ as to which is or are intended. For example, would group homes for mentally retarded adults be classified as (b), (c), or (e)—or as two or all three of these possibilities? The retarded adults, their families, the staff of the group home, the agency employing them, and neighbors—to mention some of the principal groups—might all have differing views as to what is being accomplished and why.

In the situation of the "involuntary commitment" of the "mentally ill," the case is even more complicated, in that what is referred to as "therapy and healing" (e) sometimes may actually represent (a), punishment, in disguise (Szasz 1970, 1974), not to mention (b) or (c). For this reason, although this chapter, and indeed this volume, is ostensibly about the fifth alternative, we should remain alert to other less acknowledged "cross-cultural commonalties" in dealing with unacceptable difference.

Ethnocentrism

In addition to avoiding the postulation of a biological basis for cross-cultural commonalties in therapy and healing, we also have to avoid the fallacy of ethnocentrism. Ethnocentrism, in which people mistakenly view their own shared cultural perspective as reflecting objective reality, is the cultural counterpart of egocentrism in which an individual mistakenly views his or her own individual psychological perspective as objectively accurate.

ETICS AND EMICS

Ethnocentric bias is unavoidable because all adults, including mental health professionals, were enculturated long before they were in a position to consider theoretical issues in the social sciences. For this reason, and in order to minimize an otherwise unavoidable ethnocentric bias, anthropologists make use of the distinction between etics and emics (Harris, 1980, 1999). These concepts were first introduced by the linguist Kenneth Pike (1954, 1967) and are derived from the endings of the linguistic terms phonetics and phonemics.

Definitions and Applications

Phonetics is the study of the actual physical sounds of speech as the vocal apparatus produces them, so its principles and findings apply universally to all languages. Phonemics is the study of the units of meaning (phonemes) that are associated with particular ranges of sounds in a given language. Thus, phonemes vary from one language to another. For example, English divides the range of vowel sounds in the words "sit" and "seat" into two phonemes, while French has only one.

In a similar way, *etics* deals with objective information that is physically observable, or with conceptual abstractions that can be applied to all cultures; etic descriptions are made from the perspective of a scientific observer and can be used in the construction of scientific theories. *Emics*, on the other hand, deals with meanings within a given culture; emic descriptions are formulated from the perspective of participants within a culture (Harris, 1999). As a result, one can make etic comparisons or generalizations across many cultures, but emic comparisons must be limited to a small number of cultures whose features can be examined in fine-grained detail.

For example, "the number of males and females in the United States" is etic, but "the number of men and women in the United States" is emic, since age, or undergoing a social ritual, or other variable factors might determine who qualifies for manhood or womanhood in different cultures. In other words, one can make etic comparisons between the number of males and females in different cultural groups, but not emic comparisons between the number of men and women in different groups, because the cultural meanings of "man" and "woman" vary. Here is another example: "The protein content of a group's diet" is etic, but which plants and animals they consider food is emic. Furthermore, the same or cognate linguistic term can have different meanings in different cultures. For example, the avocado is a vegetable in the United States and a fruit [fruta] in Brazil, which indicates that the cognates *fruit* and *fruta* have different emic meanings in English and Portuguese[2] (Fish, 1995b).

Thus, the search for cross-cultural commonalties in therapy and healing is a search for etically grounded generalizations based on shared conditions of life and human circumstances. Can such generalizations be made without falling into the recapitulation trap, otherwise postulating biological causes, or ethnocentrically treating American (or Western) emic categories as if they were universal? (Cross-cultural psychologists recognize that it is possible to operationally define a particular concept [e.g., borderline personality disorder] that comes from a particular culture [e.g., the United States today] in such a way that it can be imposed on other cultures of which it is not a part for the purposes of gathering comparative data. Such a concept is referred to as an *imposed etic* [Berry, 1969].)

Many sociocultural anthropologists are either skeptical about the existence of important cross-cultural etic generalizations or feel their time can be spent more productively in activities other than seeking them out. They pursue an emic strategy and attempt to understand each culture from within. In the case of therapy, one can describe the emic world of another culture, what behavior its members view as worthy of change and why, what they do to change it and why, and how they understand the varying outcomes of their efforts. Such emic descriptions give us a glimpse of a significant aspect of another cultural world—but are not intended to generalize beyond that world. Even the culture next door might view apparently similar undesired circumstances quite differently, might do quite different things to improve the situation, or might do similar things for very different reasons.

Consider the example of shamanism, which has many features in common with therapy (Dobkin de Rios, 2002; Krippner, 2003; Money, 2001). Many traditional cul-

---

[2]Because most of my cross-cultural experience, including most of my cross-cultural clinical experience, has been in Brazil, most of the examples presented in this chapter are Brazilian ones. Those interested in additional discussion of therapy-related topics in a Brazilian context can find them in *Culture and Therapy: An Integrative Approach* (Fish, 1996a).

tures have healing rituals that are dramatic (or appear so to Western eyes) and in which the suffering individual undergoes physically and/or emotionally stressful treatments and expresses intense emotion. What are we to make of this cross-cultural commonality?

We want to avoid the fallacy of viewing American culture or Western culture as reality, and therefore inaccurately viewing ethnocentric emic explanations as universal. For example, if we were to view the intense emotional experience as some sort of abreaction or expression of repressed material, we would be passing off an unverifiable Western (psychoanalytic) explanation as a universal one (similar to the group's own explanation in terms of spirits or other unverifiable elements).

On the other hand, as is discussed further in this chapter, one might make sense of the process in terms of response expectancies (Kirsch, 1990, 1999; Weinberger & Eig, 1999) and placebo effects (Fish, 1973; Frank, 1961, 1973; Frank & Frank, 1991; Kirsch, 1990, 1999; Pentony, 1981). Here, the observable credibility of the ritual, strengthened by its emotional intensity, can be explained in terms of experimentally documented psychological processes to produce a generalized explanation for positive psychological change. (Even in this case, one would have to confirm the operation of these principles in cultures very different from those found in industrialized societies. For example, this cross-cultural verification has been accomplished for color categorization [Berlin & Kay, 1969]. Unfortunately, however, this is not yet the case for the great majority of what are considered to be experimentally well-established psychological processes or principles.)

Issues in Making Generalizations

Since we have narrowed our focus to etics, one might ask why it is that we would want to make universal generalizations about therapy principles. One goal might be to identify and categorize procedures in other cultures that seem strange to us, and to try to understand how and why they are reported to work. For example, we might want to make use of elements that work in other cultures in our own therapy. In contrast, we might want to know which of our therapeutic approaches might work best in other cultures, especially Nonwestern ones, or we might want to try to figure out how we could modify our therapeutic procedures so that they can be of use in those other cultures. (Naturally, plants or other substances unknown to Western medicine that are used as part of healing rituals might well have important pharmacological effects and are also worthy of investigation. But the discussion in this chapter is limited to psychological treatments. Also, although our focus is on therapies, we should not forget that other cultures may divide healers into different categories from those we are accustomed to (e.g., an herbalist who makes medicines, a diviner who makes diagnoses and/or predicts the future, a healer who treats people, a *bruxa* who casts spells, and a *curandero* who heals [Torrey, 1986]).

These kinds of questions would suggest that our interests encourage us to limit the scope of our etic generalizations in several ways. If we want to apply principles from other cultures—especially nonliterate ones—to our own, then we are likely to look in their therapies for the operation of general principles of social influence that have been established by Western science. This is because the alien cultural specifics would likely seem irrelevant or misleading to Western clinicians, and because of this they would be unlikely to attempt to understand how exotic-appearing elements function in order to seek out new general principles of social influence. It is interesting to observe that the search for new drugs among the medicines of non-Western healers is an acceptable scientific enterprise, but the psychological counterpart to that search has only been rarely pursued (for example, see Chapters 14 and 15 in this volume). Psychologists' assumption that there is nothing to discover would seem to imply that, at least in this area, psychology is more ethnocentric than medicine, and that both disciplines share a folk belief that the study of biological determinants of behavior is somehow more scientific than the study of social determinants of behavior.

If instead we want to promote the cultural diffusion of most of our therapies, then we would primarily be interested in dealing with nation states that have a system of higher education, including formal training in Western medicine and psychology. This is because such therapies are so saturated with decades of formal training and are so much a part of the fabric of highly differentiated professional role relationships in complex societies that they would be inaccessible to nonliterate members of simpler cultures, such as hunter-gatherers. In fact, for non-Westerners, the process of undergoing the extensive training necessary to become a therapist can be understood as a de facto voluntary acculturation to Western values and habits of thought. (Of course, even hunter-gatherers might happily incorporate elements of Western therapies without accepting, or even understanding, the complex cultural systems of which they are a part. For example, they might perform their healing rituals with the sick person lying on a couch instead of on a mat. Western therapists might not view this change as a great success, despite the satisfaction of the group that adopts the practice. This adoption of therapeutic elements out of their cultural context is comparable to the use of techniques from simpler cultures by Western therapists, especially New Age therapists [McGuire, 1988]. Here, as well, Western therapists are quite happy to appropriate elements from other cultures' healing systems, but may be less concerned with shamans' reactions concerning the inappropriateness of their use.)

In other words, our desire to spread Western "scientific" ways of understanding and changing behavior predominates over the desire to learn from non-Western ones. Rather, the desire to learn from those approaches is secondary, and involves their etic translation into already discovered general principles of psychology that are supposed to apply to all humans. This is in contrast to the strategies of either stopping at their emic description in a particular culture or trying to generalize discoveries from that culture into new general principles.

Nothing is inherently wrong with such an approach, as long as its Western bias is understood. It does mean, however, that the search for cross-cultural commonalties in therapy and healing has to be viewed as occurring in the context of current global transformations. These include the end of the Cold War and colonialism, the information revolution and instantaneous worldwide communication, increased global trade and international travel, and the increased importance of multinational corporations and other transnational institutions, all of which accompany the diffusion of Western values and cultural forms. Cross-cultural psychologists are increasingly taking such factors into account, usually under the rubric of "globalization" (Arnett, 2001, 2002).

SIX COMMONALTIES IN SEARCH OF A THEORY[3]

In considering cross-cultural commonalties in therapy and healing, I was able to identify six themes as unifying (if not necessarily universal) elements that bring some etic

---

[3]With apologies to Pirandello (1922/1958).

order to an otherwise bewildering range of cultural practices. These include current global trends (a), social science principles (b and c), the interactional perspective (d), and psychological principles and processes (e and f). In a sense, the first theme describes the current global conditions that create the context for the other five conceptual themes.

Industrialization and Globalization

The first theme, which was just alluded to, is changes in culture as a result of industrialization and globalization. This includes the spread of Western cultural forms, including medicine and therapy, with some cultural diffusion in the other direction as well, as can be seen in this volume (Appadurai, 2000; Giddens, 2000).

Consider the global spread of American fast-food restaurant chains. (I like this analogy between food for the body and food for the soul, especially because the diffusion of brief therapy, with which I am involved, can be seen as a counterpart to the diffusion of fast food. I should mention in passing that brief therapy—defined as lasting no more than 10, or perhaps 20 sessions—might have a special appeal for non-Western cultures that transcends its lower cost. That is, people in these cultures may be less willing to share intimate personal details with an impersonal therapist. Thus, brief therapy's focus on results both minimizes embarrassing personal disclosures and also shortens the loss of face involved in consulting a therapist for one's personal problems. In any event, in comparing brief therapy to fast food, I would like to view it as more of a low-fat, nutritionally sound salad bar than a dispensary of psychic bacon double cheeseburgers.)

Fast-food chains did not exist in my post-war New York City childhood, and before they displaced French bistros, they displaced American luncheonettes. The education of women, their mobilization in the workforce, demographic increases in the numbers of two-career families, the high divorce rate, single-parent families, and adults living alone, along with the shortage of time for housework (including cooking) and the lengthening work week (leaving harried parents less time to prepare meals, not to mention increasing their vulnerability to children's demands for advertised freebies that accompany the burgers), are some of the social forces that have led to the success of the fast-food formula in both the United States and France.

Thus, the spread of this American social form can be seen as part of worldwide economic transformations that occurred first in the United States, rather than simply as American cultural imperialism. To the extent to which these forces are at work elsewhere, as growing middle classes around the world become part of a global economy, they become a partial explanation for the spread of fast-food chains to developing countries as well. And the same forces that are pressing for fast food for increasing numbers of the world's people are pressing for fast therapy to assuage their discontents.

Naturally, the American import has to be adapted to local cultural conditions in order to succeed. For example, Brazilians are concerned about dirt—corresponding to Americans' preoccupation with germs—and don't like to touch their food, which they consider dirty. Thus, when the Subway chain came to Brazil, they found that they had to wrap their sandwiches to protect their customers' hands, and Brazilians eat their fast-food french fries with toothpicks for the same reason. Some Brazilian supermarkets, another imported institution, even provide gloves of plastic film so that customers don't have to touch the produce. On the other hand, a Brazilian, unlike an American, will readily take a bite out of someone else's partially eaten sandwich or piece of fruit, indicating that the Brazilian folk concept of dirt (*sujeira*) is different from the American folk concept of germs.

In the same way, when American therapies are exported to Brazil, they undergo similar cultural adaptations. For example, I supervised and lectured on behavior therapy, viewed as an up-to-date scientific import, to Brazilian clinical psychologists in the mid-1970s. In doing so I discovered that, when therapists taught parents to reward their children for desired behavior, they had them use blue token reinforcers for boys and pink ones for girls. This color-coding of the tokens exemplified the importance of acknowledging the greater sex role differentiation in Brazilian culture than in American culture.

Here is another example. During the same period, Brazil's first token economy—an import of American psychology's scientific technology—was set up in the psychiatric unit of a Brazilian hospital run by spiritists (Ayllon & Azrin, 1968). I have written elsewhere about "Brazilian dual consciousness (the official bureaucratic way of doing things versus the informal . . . way of getting things done)" (Fish 1996a, pp. 208–209). In this case, Brazilian psychiatric inpatients were having their prosocial behaviors conditioned by a token economy (official science) at the same time that they were receiving guidance from mediums about overcoming the causes of their distress in the spirit world (going around the rules and making use of powerful unofficial contacts).

These two intellectual worlds seemingly operated on parallel tracks without causing cognitive dissonance for the participants. For example, the token economy did not appear to disturb the spirits, nor did the psychologists investigate the impact of the spirits on the response to token reinforcers. In fact, the hospital itself was spiritist only in an unofficial sense. Its formal stance was that patients were free to consult spiritual advisors of their choice, so the spiritist component of treatment could be treated officially as a demographic coincidence, based on patients' religious preferences, rather than medical policy. Thus, although the rules of the game of the token economy were the same as in the United States, the cultural context within which the game was played, and to which it was adapted, transformed it significantly.[4]

Industrialization and globalization are also relevant to the social context of problems and healing. In the developed world, they raise issues of overcoming the alienation found in individualistic cultures. This leads to a willingness to adopt a variety of alternative worldviews stressing holism and connectedness as a way to overcome the shortcomings of individualism (McGuire, 1988). In addition, participants in a mobile work force, who also lack an extended kin network, may find that participation in religious, healing, or therapeutic organizations is a way of mobilizing group support in a lonely world. Meanwhile, around the planet, but especially in traditional cultures, the rapid rate of change and disruption of traditional role relationships brought about by globalization has both created many personal problems and

---

[4]The following imperfect ethnocentric analogy that occurs to me illustrates the difference between the rules of the game and the cultural context within which it is played. The analysis, which is imperfect because Brazilians take their soccer very seriously, is of a major league baseball game with wild parties going on in the dugouts, and the batter, with lipstick on his face, blowing kisses to the fans between pitches. Perhaps it is this dual consciousness, along with the lack of a firm separation between work and play, that led Charles De Gaulle to remark haughtily that "Brésil n'est pas un pays sérieux" (Brazil is not a serious country). Brazilians, on the other hand, view Americans and their inability to simultaneously hold conflicting ideas or go around irrational rules as rigid, inflexible, and lacking in creativity.

increased openness to Western therapies, at least among educated, affluent, and Westernized elites who participate in the global economy.

Finally, it should be pointed out that cultural diffusion often takes place in a complex back-and-forth pattern. For example, African Americans have adopted hairstyles they consider "African," which have then been imitated by African elites because they consider them American. In a similar manner, any cultural elements that Western therapies adapt from non-Western culture areas can diffuse back to those areas as part of an imported Western therapeutic package. For example, I have argued elsewhere (Fish 1995a, 1995c) that solution-focused therapy (de Shazer, 1982, 1984, 1985, 1988, 1989, 1991, 1994; de Shazer et al., 1986; Fish, 1996b, 1997) is a Western therapy with significant East Asian influences (especially regarding acausal thinking) that shows signs of gaining acceptance in that region.

Social Structure, Economics, and Power

The second theme is that problem behavior is often created by (and helped by taking into account) social structure as well as economic and power relations in the larger society and its institutions.

To begin with, gross inequalities of wealth and power exist that, although pronounced in the developed world, are extreme elsewhere. Studies of happiness have shown that, "once people are able to afford life's necessities, increasing levels of affluence matter surprisingly little" (Myers & Diener, 1995, p. 13). It is true that cultures differ in how happy their people are, as well as in how important personal happiness is thought to be, and the definition of "life's necessities" is cultural and varies from place to place. Nevertheless, it is also true that in poor countries the majority of people lack what they consider to be basic necessities. As a result, any benefits they might receive if therapy were made available to them pale in comparison to their greater needs for food, clothing, shelter, personal safety, and rudimentary health care and education.

Tom Lehrer (1959) spoke of a physician who "became a specialist, specializing in diseases of the rich" (track 6). That pretty much describes the case of therapy, not to mention medicine, in much of the world. In Brazil, for example, where the need for public health measures is obvious, the rural poor receive virtually no services, some of the urban poor have the option of waiting in long lines for many hours to get perfunctory health care of poor quality, and the rich indulge themselves with cosmetic surgery and psychoanalysis.

Popular culture recognizes these differences in treatment—as in the following joke from the era when sex therapy (Masters & Johnson 1970) arrived in Brazil:

> A man comes for his first appointment to a sex therapy clinic. While he is in the waiting room, he sees a beautiful young woman escort another man to her treatment room. A while later, an ugly old woman escorts a second man to her room. After the door closes, he asks the secretary to explain the difference. She says, pointing toward the second door, "He's with the national health plan."

Power relations also come into play in problems arising from politics at work (e.g., getting an ulcer from office politics, or getting depressed after being fired), or politics within the family (e.g., conflict between the parents leading them to discipline their children inconsistently, resulting in behavior problems), or conflicts between the demands of family and work (e.g., anxiety over having to choose between keeping one's job and staying married). When power relations are central, therapy can be seen as resembling diplomacy, and the best emotional outcomes result from an explicitly or implicitly negotiated "treaty" that the opposing parties see as preferable to continued conflict.

When thinking in terms of social structure and power, it is also important to recognize that therapy is an institution whose practice is encouraged, channeled, constrained, and impeded by other social institutions. These include, with variations from country to country, various levels of government; legislatures and the licensing, malpractice, and other therapy-related laws they produce; the courts; insurance companies or other economic parties to therapeutic arrangements; the structure and curricula of university-based and other training programs; and the formal and informal organization of service delivery settings, such as schools, clinics, and mental hospitals.

Cultural Factors

The third theme is the understanding that problem behavior and its solutions are expressive of culturally determined patterns of normative and deviant behavior (e.g., Westerners view a consistent self as more important for psychological well-being than East Asians [Suh, 2002]), and of beliefs about how behavior changes.

It should be remembered that beliefs that are considered exotic and magical in the West are ordinary and practical to those who hold them. The decision in another culture to undergo a dramatic and dangerous healing ritual to rid oneself of evil illness-causing spirits is essentially the same as the decision in our own culture to undergo a dramatic and dangerous operation to rid oneself of a brain tumor.

This practicality can be seen among the Krikati Indians of central Brazil. A tribe of several hundred hunter-gatherer-horticulturists, their life is organized around complex social ceremonies, rather than procuring harvests, game, or healing through supernatural means. They recognize that neighboring tribes are more adept at healing than they, and they make pragmatic use of shamans passing through their village, as they do of Western medicine when it is available. When left to their own devices, they have an experimental attitude toward seeing what works. Two examples of their treatments are a man with vertical scratches on his forehead to treat headaches, and a woman who boiled a bulbous (i.e., swollen in appearance) plant root to see if the liquid would help her son's swollen glands.

The Interactional Perspective

The fourth theme, the contribution of systems theory (Fish, 1992; Hoffman, 1981; Nichols & Schwartz, 2004; Watzlawick, Weakland, & Fisch, 1974), is the ability to view the problem behavior of an individual as part of a larger interactive social matrix. Systems theory is not so much a psychological theory as an attempt to understand and change behavior at the interactional level, rather than solely at the individual level. Thus, people's problems can be understood as embedded in interactional networks consisting of repetitive sequences of behavior among various individuals. Alterations in those sequences can then lead to nonproblem behavior, and restructuring hierarchical relationships can relieve conflicting demands on triangulated third parties (Haley, 1963, 1973, 1980, 1984, 1987; Madanes, 1981, 1984; Minuchin, 1974; Minuchin & Fishman, 1981; Palazzoli, Bascolo, Cecchin, & Prata, 1978; Papp, 1983).

Although the work system and other social groups (in cultures that have them) can create and perpetuate difficulties, it is the family, however it may be defined and constituted, that is the center of the most important affect-laden interactions.[5] (Although this may be even more true in traditional cultures than in the industrialized West, the family may also, in some cultures, be so central as to exclude an outsider, like a therapist, from a position of influence on important matters. This suggests that there is a limit to the cultural variability across which therapies can be transported, even if a culturally sensitive attempt is made to adapt them.)

Consider the case of a couple whose child has behavior problems resulting from inconsistent discipline. Let us suppose that the father and mother cannot agree on how to act because the mother's mother is pressuring her to bring up her child in one way, while the father's mother is pressuring him in a different direction. In the United States, to change the child's problematic American behavior, a family therapist would most likely pursue a strategy of getting the parents to exclude the grandparents from child-rearing decisions, so that they could then agree on and implement a mutually acceptable plan of action. In some Asian cultures, in contrast, to change child behavior considered unacceptable, a family therapist might try to get the grandparents to agree among themselves, so they could communicate a consistent message to the parents who could then implement it. Thus, different cultural norms would lead to different strategies for different behavior, but in both cases the transformation from a hierarchy that is dysfunctional (as judged by the norms of its own culture) to an internally consistent one can be seen to lead to the resolution of the child's culturally unacceptable behavior.

As this example illustrates, although the systemic approach opens up new possibilities for therapeutic interventions, it also raises theoretical, clinical, and ethical issues that go beyond those usually considered in individual treatment.

Expectancy and Placebo

The fifth theme is the role of expectancy in both producing and changing behavior. This applies especially to expectancies regarding involuntary behavior. Thus, the anticipatory fear of becoming afraid triggers anxiety, whereas confidence that one will not be fearful decreases it. Similarly, pessimism about not being able to overcome sadness makes one more unhappy, whereas confidence that the sadness will end has the opposite effect.

In response expectancies, we have a psychological means for understanding and making therapeutic use of the placebo effect, hypnosis, and other means of persuasion and expectancy alteration (Fish, 1973; Frank, 1961, 1973, Frank & Frank, 1991; Kirsch, 1990, 1999; Pentony, 1981). The power of expectancy to alter behavior (especially "involuntary" behavior) helps us to understand why different psychological therapies, and even ones based on mutually contradictory rationales, can have positive effects, as can various forms of shamanism and religious healing.

For example, some Brazilian social scientist friends and I accompanied my anthropologist wife, Dolores Newton, to an Umbanda spiritist meeting in São Paulo in the

---

[5]An important exception to this generalization is the large and increasing number of homeless children in many countries who grow up among and can be said to be raised by homeless peers. In those cases where social institutions intervene to help these children (as opposed to imprisoning or killing them), the pattern seems to be to remove them from the streets or to provide services for them despite their homelessness. I am not aware of programs of systemic therapy aimed at improving the child-rearing function of informally constituted groups of street children.

mid-1970's. (Believers consult spiritist mediums for help with personal and physical problems, as they might a therapist or physician.) During these religious services, which include extended periods of dancing to percussive rhythms, participants are possessed by spirits from Brazil's past, either of old slaves or of Indians. Because this was a night when the Indian spirits were going to make their presence felt, and my wife's specialty is Brazilian Indians and other native peoples of the New World, our friends wanted to get her reaction to the experience. After it was over, they asked her if the trance behavior of the participants reminded her of that of Brazilian Indians. She said that it did not, but that it did resemble that of North American Indians as portrayed in Westerns.

Such observations support the etic generalization that the kinds of religious healing that take place under such circumstances result from the culturally specific beliefs and expectancies of the participants, as well as from the emotional persuasiveness of the experience, which is also culturally specific. This is in contrast to the otherworldly forces to which the participants themselves attribute change (and to equally unverifiable psychoanalytic explanations such as the expression of repressed impulses while in an altered state of consciousness). For example, Torrey (1986) emphasizes the importance of the shared worldview of (a) the patient and healer, (b) the personal qualities of the healer, and (c) the client's sense of mastery as important elements along with the patient's expectations. It is easy to understand how the first three influence those expectations. In addition, we may be interested in the interactions among expectancies, the placebo effect, and various physiological processes. This topic is pursued by Hirsch in Chapter 5 in this volume.

Naturally, from within a given culture, emic explanations are still preferred. One of my Brazilian students asked, "We understand what you are saying about expectancy, but ... what if spirits really do exist?" In a similar way, an American might ask, "We understand what you are saying about expectancy, but ... what if unconscious impulses really do exist?"

Learning and Cognition

The sixth theme is that general psychological principles of learning and cognition apply cross-culturally to changing behavior, even though the cultural content may vary dramatically. Thus, principles of reinforcement, extinction, shaping, and modeling can be presumed to apply across cultures (though, as mentioned, this generality needs to be empirically confirmed) and may be seen to operate in a variety of therapeutic or healing circumstances. For example, assuming that a fear is culturally inappropriate, gradually and persistently approaching the feared object, as opposed to avoiding it, will help to overcome the fear. However, what that fear might be, and who and what it might take to get the fearful person to participate, are examples of culturally variable content. Even here, though, the altered expectancy ("I won't be afraid of X") that results from successfully approaching the feared object plays an important role as well (Kirsch, 1990; Schoenberger, 1999).

In the same way, cognitive therapists (e.g., Beck, 1976; Ellis, 1962) have argued that getting people to change culturally inappropriate, upsetting cognitions will lead to their becoming less upset. Once again, though, the content of those cognitions and the rhetorical means needed to change them, as well as the social role of the rhetorician and the culturally appropriate context for persuasion, vary widely. (Thomas Szasz [1974, 1978] and Jerome Frank [Frank & Frank, 1991] have discussed in great detail the pervasive role of rhetoric and persuasion in psychotherapy. In addition, an important part of the reason that cognitive change has its effect is that new beliefs alter individuals' expectancies regarding their own behavior [Kirsch, 1990, 1999].)

In summary, then, this chapter attempted to make a number of cross-cultural generalizations about therapy and healing. In order to do so, and to avoid a number of theoretical and ethnocentric pitfalls, it was necessary to explore a number of issues concerning process and content, and etics and emics. Once relevant distinctions were made, six themes were identified that bring into focus significant commonalties among the otherwise diverse and changing practices of therapy and healing around the world. These commonalties can be seen in part as reflecting the global homogenization of cultures. And they suggest the need for empirical verification of the cross-cultural generality of basic psychological processes, especially since the cultural variability against which these processes must be evaluated is rapidly diminishing.

ACKNOWLEDGMENT

I would like to thank Dolores Newton for her helpful suggestions.

REFERENCES

Arnett, J. J. (2001). *Adolescence and emerging adulthood: A cultural approach.* Upper Saddle River, NJ: Prentice Hall.

Arnett, J. J. (2002). The psychology of globalization. *American Psychologist, 57*(10), 774–783.

Appadurai, A. (Ed.). (2000). *Globalization.* Durham, NC: Duke University Press.

Ayllon, T., & Azrin, N. H. (1968). *The token economy: A motivational system for therapy and rehabilitation.* New York: Appleton.

Beck, A. T. (1976). *Cognitive therapy and the emotional disorders.* New York: International Universities Press.

Berlin, B., & Kay, P. (1969). *Basic color terms.* Berkeley, CA: University of California Press.

Berry, J. W. (1969). On cross-cultural comparability. *International Journal of Psychology, 4,* 119–128.

Brown, D. E. (1991). *Human universals.* New York: McGraw-Hill.

de Shazer, S. (1982). *Patterns of brief family therapy.* New York: Guilford Press.

de Shazer, S. (1984). The death of resistance. *Family Process, 23,* 11–21.

de Shazer, S. (1985). *Keys to solution in brief therapy.* New York: Norton.

de Shazer, S. (1988). *Clues: Investigating solutions in brief therapy.* New York: Norton.

de Shazer, S. (1989). Resistance revisited. *Contemporary Family Therapy, 11*(4), 227–233.

de Shazer, S. (1991). *Putting difference to work.* New York: Norton.

de Shazer, S. (1994). *Words were originally magic.* New York: Norton.

de Shazer, S., Berg, I. K., Lipchik, E., Nunnally, E., Molnar, A., Gingerich, W., et al. (1986). Brief therapy: Focused solution development. *Family Process, 25,* 207–221.

Dobkin de Rios, M. (2002). What we can learn from shamanic healing: Brief psychotherapy with Latino immigrant clients. *American Journal of Public Health, 92*(10), 1576–1581.

Ellis, A. (1962). *Reason and emotion in psychotherapy.* New York: Lyle Stuart.

Fish, J. M. (1973). *Placebo therapy.* San Francisco: Jossey-Bass.

Fish, J. M. (1992). Discontinuous change. *Behavior and Social Issues, 2*(1), 59–70.

Fish, J. M. (1995a). Does problem behavior just happen? Does it matter? *Behavior and Social Issues, 5*(1), 3–12.

Fish, J. M. (1995b). Mixed blood. *Psychology Today, 28*(6), 55–61, 76, 80.

Fish, J. M. (1995c). Solution focused therapy in global perspective. *World Psychology, 1*(2), 43–67.

Fish, J. M. (1996a). *Culture and therapy: An integrative approach.* New York: Jason Aronson.

Fish, J. M. (1996b). Prevention, solution focused therapy, and the illusion of mental disorders. *Applied and Preventive Psychology, 5,* 37–40.

Fish, J. M. (1997). Paradox for complainants? Strategic thoughts about solution-focused therapy. *Journal of Systemic Therapies, 16*(3), 266–273.

Frank, J. D. (1961). *Persuasion and healing: A comparative study of psychotherapy*. Baltimore, MD: Johns Hopkins.

Frank, J. D. (1973). *Persuasion and healing: A comparative study of psychotherapy* (2nd ed.). Baltimore, MD: Johns Hopkins.

Frank, J. D., & Frank, J. B. (1991). *Persuasion and healing: A comparative study of psychotherapy* (3rd ed.). Baltimore, MD: Johns Hopkins.

Giddens, A. (2000). *Runaway world: How globalization is reshaping our lives*. New York: Routledge.

Gould, S. J. (1981). *The mismeasure of man*. New York: Norton.

Gould, S. J. (1987). Freud's phylogenetic fantasy. *Natural History, 96*(12), 10–19.

Haley, J. (1963). *Strategies of psychotherapy*. New York: Grune & Stratton.

Haley, J. (1973). *Uncommon therapy: The psychiatric techniques of Milton H. Erickson, M. D*. New York: Norton.

Haley, J. (1980). *Leaving home*. New York: McGraw-Hill.

Haley, J. (1984). *Ordeal therapy: Unusual ways to change behavior*. San Francisco: Jossey-Bass.

Haley, J. (1987). *Problem solving therapy* (2nd ed.). San Francisco: Jossey-Bass.

Harris, M. (1980). *Cultural materialism: The struggle for a science of culture*. New York: Vintage Books.

Harris, M. (1999). *Theories of culture in postmodern times*. Walnut Creek, CA: AltaMira Press.

Hoffman, L. (1981). *Foundations of family therapy*. New York: Basic Books.

Kirsch, I. (1990). *Changing expectations: A key to effective psychotherapy*. Pacific Grove, CA: Brooks/Cole.

Kirsch, I. (Ed.). (1999). *How expectancies shape experience*. Washington, DC: American Psychological Association.

Krippner, S. (2003). What psychologists might learn from the study of shamans and shamanism. *Psychological Hypnosis, 12*(1), 5–10.

Lehrer, T. (1959). In Old Mexico. On *An evening wasted with Tom Lehrer* [33 rpm. record]. Cambridge, MA: Tom Lehrer, TL 202.

Madanes, C. (1981). *Strategic family therapy*. San Francisco: Jossey-Bass.

Madanes, C. (1984). *Behind the one-way mirror: Advances in the practice of strategic therapy*. San Francisco: Jossey-Bass.

Masters, W. H., & Johnson, V. E. (1970). *Human sexual inadequacy*. Boston: Little, Brown & Co.

McGuire, M. B. (1988). *Ritual healing in suburban America*. New Brunswick, NJ: Rutgers University Press.

Minuchin, S. (1974). *Families and family therapy*. Cambridge, MA: Harvard University Press.

Minuchin, S., & Fishman, H. C. (1981). *Family therapy techniques*. Cambridge, MA: Harvard University Press.

Money, M. (2001). Shamanism as a healing paradigm for complementary therapy. *Complementary Therapies in Nursing and Midwifery, 7*(3), 126–131.

Murdock, G. P. (1972). Anthropology's mythology. The Huxley memorial lecture, 1971. *Proceedings of the Royal Anthropological Institute of Great Britain and Ireland for 1971* (pp. 17–24).

Myers, D. G., & Diener, E. (1995). Who is happy? *Psychological Science, 6*(1), 10–19.

Nichols, M. P., & Schwartz, R. C. (2004). *Family therapy: Concepts and methods* (6th ed.). Boston: Allyn & Bacon.

Ogbu, J. U. (2002). Cultural amplifiers of intelligence: IQ and minority status in cross-cultural perspective. In J. M. Fish (Ed.), *Race and intelligence: Separating science from myth* (pp. 241–278). Mahwah, NJ: Erlbaum.

Palazzoli, M. S., Boscolo, L., Cecchin, G., & Prata, G. (1978). *Paradox and counter-paradox*. New York: Jason Aronson.

Papp, P. (1983). *The process of change*. New York: Guilford Press.

Pentony, P. (1981). *Models of influence in psychotherapy*. New York: Macmillan.

Pike, K. L. (1954). *Language in relation to a unified theory of the structure of human behavior, Vol. 1*. Glendale, CA: Summer Institute of Linguistics.

Pike, K. L. (1967). *Language in relation to a unified theory of the structure of human behavior*. The Hague, The Netherlands: Mouton.

Pirandello, L. (1922/1958). Six characters in search of an author. In E. Bentley (Ed. & Trans.), *Naked masks: Five plays by Luigi Pirandello* (pp. 211–276). New York: Dutton.

Schoenberger, N. E. (1999). Expectancy and fear. In I. Kirsch (Ed.), *How expectancies shape experience* (pp. 125–144). Washington, DC: American Psychological Association.

Skinner, B. F. (1974). *About behaviorism*. New York: Knopf.

Suh, E. M. (2002). Culture, identity consistency, and subjective well-being. *Journal of Personality and Social Psychology, 83*(6), 1378–1391.

Szasz, T. S. (1970). *The manufacture of madness: A comparative study of the Inquisition and the mental health movement*. New York: Harper & Row.

Szasz, T. S. (1974). *The myth of mental illness: Foundations of a theory of personal conduct*. New York: Harper & Row.

Szasz, T. S. (1978). *The myth of psychotherapy: Mental healing as religion, rhetoric, and repression.* Garden City, NY: Doubleday Anchor.

Torrey, E. F. (1986). *Witchdoctors and psychiatrists: The common roots of psychotherapy and its future.* New York: Harper & Row.

Watzlawick, P., Weakland, J. H., & Fisch, R. (1974). *Change: Principles of problem formation and problem resolution.* New York: Norton.

Weinberger, J., & Eig, A. (1999). Expectancies: The ignored common factor in psychotherapy. In I. Kirsch (Ed.), *How expectancies shape experience* (pp. 357–382). Washington, DC: American Psychological Association.

A Biopsychosocial Perspective on Cross-Cultural Healing

Michele S. Hirsch
St. Francis College

How is it that the majority of humans seeking relief from disease and illness improve their health status after being treated? This question requires a complex answer given the diversity of healing methods that are employed across different cultures. Perhaps some underlying mechanisms are operating in these various treatments. If not, the many healing traditions that have been documented across the world would have been abandoned long ago.

In order to fully comprehend how healing occurs, a multidisciplinary approach encompassing the fields of anthropology, psychology, biology, and sociology is necessary. Although each of these disciplines has contributed to our understanding of health, illness, and healing, the knowledge that each has obtained, until fairly recently, has remained largely compartmentalized and pigeonholed, with little dialogue occurring between disciplines.

It is the goal of this chapter to provide an interdisciplinary review of the mechanisms and processes that scientists understand and believe play a role in illness, health, and healing. You may notice that the flavor of this chapter is distinctly different from the others in this volume. It is not possible to present what are believed to be the underlying, interrelated key systems and mechanisms in the healing process without discussing the latest developments in biomedicine. A brief medical history and introduction to biomedicine are given from a traditional, Western perspective in order to give you an appreciation of the progression of our current scientific working knowledge on the healing process (you will note that Western medicine has provided its fair share of obstacles). Specific cross-cultural healing philosophies and techniques are presented in the following chapters. Hopefully, this chapter will provide you with a deeper biopsychosocial conceptualization of the more nontraditional (non-Western) healing approaches that exist in our world today.

HISTORY OF WESTERN MEDICINE

Hippocrates has been described as the father of medicine, or at least of Western medicine as we know it today. His work that focused on how the body and mind work in concert is cited as being one of the earliest of what today we would call holistic thinking about the mind-body connection. One major contribution for which Hippocrates is credited is his thoughts on the four humors (yellow bile, black bile, blood, and phlegm), or the fluids that he believed circulated in the body. Hippocrates stated that in order to preserve good health, both physically and mentally, it is necessary to have the right balance of the humors present in the body. The type of illness, disease, or mental unrest present in an individual is dependent on how the humors are imbalanced. This was one of the first lines of reasoning to posit that in addition to physical determinants of diseases, there are physical determinants of psychological states.

This holistic view no longer predominated during the Middle Ages, which stretched roughly from the fifth century to the fifteenth century. During this period in history, the Catholic Church gained power and was the mainstay of everyday life. Philosophically, and theoretically, medicine took on religious overtones. Sermons of medieval Christianity taught "that sickness is a divine visitation, intended as punishment for sin or a stimulus to spiritual growth. The cure, in either case, would seem to be spiritual rather than physical" (Lindberg, 1992, p. 320). For example, Baum, Gatchel, and Krantz (1997) note: "The plagues that devastated Europe during the Middle Ages were not well understood at the time. We now know that they were caused by pathogens, but explanations for the disease were more spiritual or animistic at the time!" (p. 5). For illnesses that were better understood at the time, practical methods of healing (i.e., herbs or midwifery) were viewed as legitimate and were applied by local healers or by monks (Lindberg, 1992).

Yet another shift in the mind-body view of health and illness occurred during the Renaissance. Dualism, a term used to describe a viewpoint that emphasizes that body and mind are separate and independent entities, grew in favor during this time. At the forefront of science was the field of physical medicine; the use of autopsy and the advent of the microscope enabled physicians to focus on biological causes of disease (Baum et al., 1997). Thus, the biomedical model became the core of physical medicine with its dualistic philosophy toward health and illness. The biomedical model eschews that mainly biological agents are responsible for illness. Implicit in the model is that psychological and social variables play a less significant role in the cause, maintenance, and treatment of illness.

A more holistic view of the mind-body relationship began to take hold in the late nineteenth century during the early psychosomatic movement. The work of Freud and other researchers focused on the idea that internal or unconscious conflicts could be expressed through physical symptoms. Once again, the view that events produced by the mind and the body are closely related began to be considered.

HOW WESTERN THINKING MAY HAVE SLOWED MEDICAL PROGRESS

The role that Western history has played in our current thinking about medicine and mind-body interactions has been widely acknowledged (e.g., Engel, 1977; Moerman, 1983; Myers & Benson, 1992). Until the turn of the twentieth century, before scientists possessed the technology to advance the biomedical field, doctors and physicians practiced their trade by observing their sick patients to determine what in that individual's environment might be contributing to his or her ailment. That is, biopsychosocial factors were believed to interact with one another to produce illness. Physicians diagnosed and treated their patients on an individual-by-individual basis. There was no disease model to dictate a diagnosis or how the course of treatment should proceed. It was the individual as a whole who was considered by the treating physician.

With the advent of the disease-specific model in the late 1800s and early 1900s, the medical field underwent a major shift. During this time (the dawning of the biomedical model) understanding the disease process became focused on qualities of reductionism, materialism, and universalism:

> The former emphasis on body systems as a whole gave way to the tendency to reduce systems to smaller parts, each of which could be considered separately. Simultaneously, focus shifted from individual patients to universal aspects of disease pathology. Finally, a powerful materialism took the place of the earlier tendency to see nonmaterial factors—moral, social, behavioral, and psychological—as meaningful." (Myers & Benson, 1992, p. 6)

A by-product of this shift in medical thought was that the medical world began to ignore or leave behind psychological processes that had once been acknowledged by medical science. Thus, there was in a sense a trade-off: Western medicine witnessed great therapeutic gains from focusing on biological processes, while psychosocial variables, with respect to medical interventions, fell by the wayside. Indeed, for many years psychology has been considered a "soft" science that lacks hard evidence. For this reason, the field of Western medicine "lost" part of its original design and appeal in healing individuals, the physician-patient relationship where the individual, not the illness or disease, was the focus of treatment.

Disease theory brought about enormous, undeniable change in Western medicine. Etiology, diagnosis, and cure became the predominant factors on which medical practitioners focused when treating physically ill patients. Touch, placebo (discussed in detail later in this chapter), and the interpersonal relationship between practitioners and patients (also discussed later in this chapter) were, for all practical purposes, abandoned. Benson and Friedman (1995) noted the imbalance of health care in most industrialized nations. Using a three-legged stool metaphor where pharmaceuticals, surgery, and psychological and behavioral care each represent one of the three legs, they contend that the latter leg has lagged considerably behind the two former. Although we have made great strides with the development of effective drugs and technologically advanced equipment and techniques, how this care has been delivered to patients has been less than optimal.

As a result of the impersonal nature of health care, many individuals are not satisfied with the current state of affairs in Western medicine. Data (Eisenberg et al., 1993) indicate that some of these disgruntled patients are choosing alternative, or complimentary, therapies in addition to, if not in place of, traditional, or Western, medicine. Time-tested, traditional techniques such as acupuncture, meditation, and chiropractic are being sought out. The appeal of these therapies is that the whole person is the focus of treatment, not just the disease or the illness. The importance of this trend lies in the premise that a person's beliefs and expectations of illness and health, which are influenced by both psychological and sociological factors, can directly interact with their health status.

In recent years, however, there has been a slow and resistant movement back toward a less dualistic, more holistic philosophy in Western medicine (e.g., Susman, 2001). This movement has undoubtedly come about due to our greater understanding of non-Western healing techniques, which have as a basic tenet that the mind and body are inseparable and operate in unison. The remaining sections of this chapter aim to review what we know about the mind-body relationship in health and illness, the importance of an interdisciplinary understanding of holistic treatment approaches, which incorporate both the practitioner's and the patient's culturally bound beliefs and expectations, and the need for further dialogue and research across disciplines in regard to improved comprehension of the nonspecific efficacious aspects of treatment.

MEDICAL ANTHROPOLOGY, MEDICAL SOCIOLOGY, AND UNDERSTANDING HEALTH, ILLNESS, AND HEALING

A basic understanding of cultural processes is necessary for this discussion since psychological and social processes, as well as biological processes, play a role in health, illness, and healing. Medical anthropologists have been studying the relationship of cultural beliefs and subsequent related medical problems. Clinically applied medical anthropology, a subfield of medical anthropology, encompasses the direct application of medical interventions within a culturally sensitive context. Since, as is detailed in this chapter, the practice of healing and culture are inextricably linked together, clinically applied anthropology serves a useful, necessary function in the realms of health, illness, and healing.

Medical sociology, similar in orientation to medical anthropology but different in its underlying philosophy, is another important field that contributes to our knowledge of culture and healing. Health education, studying how a society's attitudes and beliefs can influence an individual's health, and understanding the social context of health care and the setting in which delivery of care is given are the mainstays of medical sociology. Because both medical sociology and medical anthropology (discussed in Chapter 3 in further detail) are concerned with culture and health, there are occasions whereby the two disciplines intersect. By nature, then, they are complimentary.

To appreciate health, illness, and healing, one should understand the cultural context in which they occur. Indeed, criticism has been levied upon researchers who have attempted to explain healing in terms of just psychological and physiological processes (Kleinman, 1981). Cultural relativism, the understanding that what takes place within a particular culture is relative to that culture in terms of its beliefs, values, and norms (Hahn, 1999), is directly applicable here. For example, it has been demonstrated that how individuals from different cultures will respond to sham alcohol (which they believe is real alcohol) reflects how their respective culture believes individuals under the influence of alcohol behave (MacAndrew & Edgerton, 1969). In the same vein, when considering different cultural views of therapeutic interventions, it has been noted that "some patient groups expect rapid relief from their symptoms[;] others are more sensitive to the potentially detrimental side effects of Western medicines. Still others, because multiple herbal ingredients are usually prescribed in their country, often perceive the use of multiple drugs as more efficacious than single-drug therapy" (Balant & Balant-Gorgia, 2000, p. 51). Even psychotherapy as a healing modality must be considered within a cultural context (Wampold, 2001).

CULTURE AND SOCIAL SUPPORT AS MEDIATING VARIABLES IN HEALING

Specific to the discussion of healing from a biopsychosocial perspective, medical anthropology and medical sociology have made contributions by examining how social support within particular cultures exerts great influence on healing an individual.

Our current understanding of the importance that interpersonal relationships play in healing partly developed as an outgrowth of studies that focused on social support as a mediating variable in the maintenance of health. The Roseto studies are an example of how a community can buffer the effects of risk factors for heart disease. Immigrants from the town of Roseto in the province of Foggia, Italy, settled in Pennsylvania where, since at least 1912, they remained a tightly woven community until the last few decades. Until the 1960s, entrance into the community was achieved only through marriage to an Italian from Roseto. In the 1960s, Bruhn, Wolf, and colleagues (Bruhn, Chandler, Miller, Wolf, & Lynn, 1966) noted that male Roseto residents experienced a very low mortality rate from myocardial infarction and began a series of longitudinal studies of this ethnically homogenous group. In one of the follow-up studies, Wolf (1992) observed that although male Roseto residents experienced the same risk factors for heart disease, namely smoking and diet, the males from Roseto died at half the rate of comparable males in an adjacent town.

However, over the last 30 years these differences in rates of heart attacks and sudden deaths have diminished for Roseto residents. Researchers involved in this project (Bruhn, Philips, & Wolf, 1972, 1982; Egolf, Lasker, Wolf, & Potkin, 1992; Wolf, 1992) have documented that the underlying reason for this health change was that, whereas once the negative effects of stress and social changes were buffered by social support and close family ties, Roseto residents have become increasingly "Americanized" since the 1960s. Intermarriage, eating out, and several other major lifestyle changes have been implicated in the loss of protection from coronary heart disease and related deaths. These data from the Roseto community, which illustrate the relationship between acculturation and increased rates of myocardial infarction, lend credence to the importance of social support in the maintenance of health. In addition, they suggest that a critical element of healing approaches may be social support and interpersonal interactions.

Other cultures have been studied, such as the Kalahari !Kung, the Zinacanteco (Mexican Indians), and Navaho Native Americans, where group solidarity is central in the healing process (i.e., Kinsley, 1996). The following highlights the community-individual relationship as it pertains to a healing practice of the !Kung, a nomadic, hunter-gatherer society, who reside in the Kalahari desert of Southern Africa: "Their healing dances restore vigor to each member of the group and to the group as a corporate body. Individual health is dependent on the health of the whole community" (Kinsley, 1996, p. 81). (See also Chapter 8 on the role of dance in Navaho healing in this volume.)

Social support has been shown to have beneficial effects for metastatic breast cancer. In a prospective study (Spiegel, Bloom, Kraemer, & Gottheil, 1989), patients who participated in a one-year intervention program, which included weekly support group meetings, had significantly longer survival rates than control participants. Furthermore, social support positively affects an adjustment to cancer as well as survival time (Spiegel, 1997).

It would seem that healing begins at an external, interpersonal level, which is used to mobilize social support and encourage group solidarity. The process then becomes more internal with psychological and physiological mechanisms interacting, which may directly influence the immune system and the patient's health. Improvement in health would reinforce the patient's, the healer's, and the group's view of the healing process, lending credence to the healing process used and increasing the likelihood that it be used again. Although simplistic, this type of model seems to outline our current thinking on the intricately tied biopsychosocial mechanisms that must be considered together as a whole when considering how healing occurs.

The interpersonal relationship between healer and patient may even have a deeper function in the process of healing than the role of social support. There has been renewed interdisciplinary interest in the role of placebos, and social relationships have been implicated as being an element in the nonspecific aspect of a placebo's efficacy.

HISTORY OF PLACEBOS

Before the rigorous scientific method of today's research standards existed, the placebo effect was alive and well, and well noted by medical texts and physicians practicing eighteenth-, nineteenth-, and very early twentieth-century medicine (Kaptchuk, 1998; Myers & Benson, 1992). Indeed, before the existence of efficacious drugs and surgery, physicians relied upon placebos to heal their patients.

The term placebo has come to be synonymous with a fake or sham drug. Certainly, placebos have received a reputation as being ineffective, deceptive annoyances:

> When doctors who are not involved in a therapy under trial learn that it turns out to be a placebo, they howl with laughter. When you are the subject in a trial and discover that you have reacted to a placebo, as I have, you feel a fool. When you are the proponent or inventor of a therapy, whether based on contemporary rationale or old-fashioned faith, you are resentful of the need for placebo testing. (Wall, 1996, p. 166)

However, as detailed in the following sections, there is something in the nonspecific aspects of being given a placebo that usually seems to bring about desired effects. Thus, in looking toward the future of Western medicine, the question of whether placebos should continue to be viewed as ineffective mock drugs as opposed to being embraced as effective, integral parts of medical interventions is one that still remains unanswered at this time.

PLACEBO EFFECT

The placebo effect has received renewed attention in recent years. Although it once was viewed as problematic in research studies, it has been argued that the placebo effect was instead something to be embraced (Moerman, 1983). The bulk of twentieth-century medical research has made it a goal to eliminate placebo effects in order to achieve a more scientifically pure study, and in doing so has missed the opportunity to better understand *all* the components of healing, not just the effectiveness of the drug in question (Moerman, 1991). In other words, it may benefit the medical field to understand how the nonspecific aspects of medical interventions translate into physiological changes.

This brings into question the supposed scientific nature of the randomized double-blind controlled study. The goal of placebo-controlled studies is to find out whether a new drug/treatment is significantly better than a placebo. Because beliefs and expectations may produce differential placebo effects, there exists the possibility for the same drug to produce substantially different rates of healing across individuals. If controlled studies of a drug produce different rates of healing, then perhaps in addition to focusing on the effectiveness rate of the drug itself, patients' cultural beliefs and expectations should also be considered (Brody, 1983).

The resurgent interest in the placebo effect has been the impetus for many new and some controversial studies (e.g., Kirsch & Sapirstein, 1998). Many sources on the topic (e.g., Benson, 1995; Kirsch, 1985, 1990, 1997; Moerman, 1983, 1991) state that the placebo effect is a real component in healing and that the healing process is much more complicated than simply using drug therapy to cure an infection or accepting a vaccine to prevent an illness. The idea that other variables, in addition to medical intervention, play a role in healing is not new. For centuries, when psychosocial factors were considered integral to diagnosis and treatment, placebos were deliberately used in the effort to alleviate the suffering of individuals. Again, although the process is not fully understood, placebos seem to translate themselves into physical, biochemical changes.

One example of a placebo that has been documented as being substantially influenced by culture and ethnicity is that of pharmacological drugs. For example, Smith, Lin, and Mendoza (1994) found that Whites viewed white capsules as analgesics, and black capsules as stimulants, while Black subjects viewed the white capsules as stimulants and the black capsules as analgesics. In a study conducted in Amsterdam, researchers reported that red, orange, and yellow drugs were associated with stimulant effects and blue and green drugs were associated with tranquilizing effects (de Craen, Roos, Leonard de Vries, & Kleijnen, 1996). Although there is a substantial body of knowledge concerning the mechanisms responsible for ethnic and cultural variations in the pharmacological effects of drugs, several researchers (e.g., Balant & Balant-Gorgia, 2000; Lin, Anderson, & Poland, 1995) have made the point that understanding the impact of cultural and ethnic psychosocial variables on drug responses warrants further consideration.

Great strides are being made to understand the psychological and physical effects of placebos. At the same time, Harrington (1997) has acknowledged that a bridge is needed to link together both the natural scientist's and the medical anthropologist's views of placebos and how they work. Indeed, the idea that the placebo effect is due to associative learning (see the following section) is not so different from the idea that the placebo effect originates from cultural meaning and symbols. She astutely points out that placebo effects ". . . certainly function as a powerful reminder to thoughtful scholars and researchers that our minds, brains, and bodies navigate a far more seamless reality than we, in our insular academic departments, know how to study" (p. 8). That is, whereas our bodies operate in a holistic, nondualistic manner, the varying disciplines that study the interrelationships of the mind and the body tend to pigeonhole the knowledge they obtain. It has only been in approximately the last 20 years that researchers have begun to adopt an interdisciplinary approach to this topic.

PLACEBO EFFECT AS CLASSICAL CONDITIONING

Placebos have been explained in terms of classical conditioning models (e.g., Ader, 1988; Ader & Cohen, 1991; Wickramasekera, 1980). Using the classical conditioning paradigm, the unconditioned stimuli represent the active ingredients in a drug, which produce the unconditioned response or healing effects. The conditioned stimuli are present when patients experience the delivery of the drug: pills, tablets, syringes, medicinal liquids, the person who delivers the drug, or even perhaps a more benign item, such as the white lab coat that medical personnel typically wear. Then, according to Pavlovian (Pavlov, 1927) conditioning, by virtue of the conditioned stimuli being paired with the unconditioned stimuli, the conditioned stimuli alone will produce the same response as the unconditioned stimuli did alone. When this occurs, the unconditioned response is now called the conditioned response to denote that the response was initiated by a variable that usually would not produce such a response. Thus, it was postulated that a placebo response could be elicited, once the patient has associated the drug (unconditioned stimuli) with the mode of delivery (conditioned stimuli), by the administration of a substance.

Robert Ader and Nicholas Cohen first began this line of inquiry (see Ader & Cohen, 1975) after Ader noticed something unusual during a single conditioning trial taste aversion study (Ader, 1996). Rats were given saccharine-flavored water to drink and after varied amounts of the water had been consumed, they were injected with cyclophosphamide, a nausea-inducing immunosuppressive substance. Later, during extinction trials, the rats were no longer being injected, but they still received the saccharine-flavored drinking water. Remarkably and unexpectedly, these rats began to die at the same rate as the rats that were actively being injected, with mortality being a direct function of the amount of saccharine water consumption. Ader (1974) concluded that the rats had associated the water with the effects of the injected drug. Thus, this was one of the first demonstrations, albeit by accident, of the immune system's capability to be influenced by and to be responsive to a placebo substance.

Although this explanation of classical conditioning seems to adequately explain how the placebo effect operates, classical conditioning may be more complex than the mechanistic reflex tradition commonly espoused. Repeated pairings of the conditioned stimuli with the unconditional stimuli to produce a desired response will eventually result in the conditioned stimuli eliciting the same response in the absence of the unconditioned stimuli (Rescorla, 1988). A more complex process is in effect, which requires "the learning of relations among events" (Rescorla, 1988, p. 153). Specifically, it can be argued that associative learning does not always occur when a conditioned stimuli is paired with a unconditioned stimuli. As Rescorla points out, "conditioning depends not on the contiguity between the cs and the us but rather on the information that the CS provides about the US" (p. 153). For example, Kamin (1968) showed that for animals that had prior experience with a unconditioned stimuli, conditioning to a conditioned stimuli was satisfactorily demonstrated. However, when he repeated the experiment with animals that had no prior experience with the unconditioned stimuli, conditioning to another stimulus was not nearly as successful. A final important point that Rescorla makes is the following:

> Pavlovian conditioning is not a stupid process by which the organism willy-nilly forms associations between any two stimuli that happen to co-occur. Rather, the organism is better seen as an information seeker using logical and perceptual relations among events, along with its own preconceptions, to form a sophisticated representation of its world. (p. 154)

In terms of healing, then, this helps explain why placebos are at least in part culture bound and have been known to produce differential effects in different populations of people. Differences in individuals' preconceptions and world representations may affect how they respond to stimuli in the environment. That is, through the process of associative learning, individuals become conditioned to both the entire ritual and the environment in which healing occurs (Wickramasekera, 1980).

EXPECTANCY THEORY

Research in the area of expectancy theory, in relation to placebo effects, is growing. As discussed, classical conditioning models (e.g., Ader, 1988; Ader & Cohen, 1991; Wickramasekera, 1980) and further expansion of them (Rescorla, 1988) have been used to explain the process of placebos. However, more recent studies (Kirsch, 1990; Montgomery & Kirsch, 1997; Price et al., 1999) are suggesting that even more specific variables can be associated with the classical conditioning paradigm, namely expectancies, which operate as mediating factors in placebo analgesia. That is, classical conditioning is not a sufficient factor on its own for placebo effects to occur.

Montgomery and Kirsch (1997) investigated the notion that instead of the stimulus substitution model of classical conditioning being at the heart of placebo responses, expectancies generated by conditioning trials would produce conditioned placebo effects. They based their methodology on that of the work of Voudouris and others (Voudouris, Peck, & Coleman, 1985, 1989, 1990), who demonstrated placebo pain responses via classical conditioning. Subjects were exposed to a series of conditioning trials of nociceptive (painful) stimulation after a placebo "anesthetic" cream was applied to the site of the electrical stimulation. What the subjects did not know in the Voudouris, Peck, and Coleman studies was that once the cream was applied, the intensity of the electrical stimulation was decreased for some subjects and increased for others. Data suggested that both increases and decreases in nociceptive stimulation were capable of producing placebo responses. Montgomery and Kirsch added an informed group to the Voudouris, Peck, and Coleman design. These subjects were told that the intensity level of the stimulation would be decreased. Interestingly, in subsequent test trials the uninformed subjects demonstrated placebo analgesia, while the informed group did not. As expected, informed subjects had lowered expectancies for the analgesia despite the fact that they had the same number of conditioning trails as the uninformed subjects. Thus, Montgomery and Kirsch were able to establish that expectancies, not stimulus substitution, mediated the placebo response for their subjects.

Additionally, Price and colleagues (1999), in a study assessing factors that contribute to the magnitude of placebo analgesia, found that expectancies, not desire for relief, played a role in the magnitude of placebo analgesia. This lends further support to the notion that the strength of placebo analgesia is based upon both conditioning and expectancy for pain reduction.

CULTURE AND MEANING—PUTTING PLACEBOS INTO CONTEXT

Placebos are "culture-bound;" both the cultural and social settings in which the placebo is given play a role in the placebo's efficacy (Helman, 1994). Thus, not all placebos will have equal potency, if any potency at all, across all cultural groups. Both the healer and patient enter the healing environment with expectations and, as Montgomery and Kirsch (1997) and Price et al. (1999) have demonstrated (see section on Expectancies), the placebo effect is mediated by these expectations. Expectancy and belief can be culture specific. Medical anthropologists, who view symbolism and ritual as central components of healing, argue that these factors are intrinsic to expectancy and meaning. This directly relates to cultural relativism previously discussed.

Depending on the culture in question, patients and healers may have as the basis of their relationships a more mystical or rational view of illness and health. However, it is the relationship itself, where both of these individuals share a common culture and a worldview of life, that gives placebos the ability to produce effects. Not only does the patient have his or her preconceived expectation, the healer also conveys expectations to the patient, if not direct feelings, ideas, or instructions. This is evident in the doctor-patient relationship in Western medicine (Helman, 1994).

Moreover, Arthur Kleinman and his colleagues have focused their research on cross-cultural understandings of health and illness. Hahn and Kleinman (1983) address the power of belief and expectations and conclude that " . . . the healing powers of beliefs and expectations, those socially given and created in a society's ethnomedicine, constitute the vast and neglected, even stigmatized processes referred to as the 'placebo phenomenon'" (p. 17). Kleinman, Eisenberg, and Good (1978) underscore the importance of communication between practitioner and patient in what was termed the "cultural construction of clinical reality." Specifically, practitioners should attempt to assess patients' perspectives and beliefs about the nature of the presenting problem and then incorporate this information into treatment recommendations. In terms of placebo effects, this would help reaffirm the patient's expectancy for healing.

PSYCHONEUROIMMUNOLOGY

As mentioned before, despite the seemingly expansive literature on the efficacy of placebos, the exact biopsychosocial mechanisms by which placebos operate are still not fully understood. Researchers, in only the last 20 years, have been attempting to uncover this mystery. One area of study that seems to hold promise in our better understanding the underlying mechanisms of placebos is that of psychoneuroimmunology.

Psychoneuroimmunology is a relatively new field of study. It involves the interrelations of mind and body, which mutually influence one another. Specifically, mental processes, neurologic processes, and immune processes (discussed later), which were each once thought to operate autonomously (see Moyers, 1993, p. 240), are now known to engage in dialogue and communicate with each other (Ader, 1996; Ader, Cohen, & Felten, 1995). A body of literature is being produced that questions our ability to perhaps control illness and promote healing (the immune system) via psychological means. That is, researchers are currently grappling with the puzzle of understanding exactly *how* psychological and social mechanisms translate into physiological changes, which then influence the health of humans.

Before one can truly appreciate the complex nature of the physiology of health and the results of studies that implicate the role of psychological and social variables in being able to influence human physiological systems, a fairly simple working understanding of the immune system is needed. The following sections serve as a basic overview to orient the reader to the immune and neuroendocrine systems.

BASIC MECHANISMS OF THE IMMUNE SYSTEM

One of the most complex systems of the human body is the immune system. Its main function is to protect us against pathogens. Pathogens are any type of foreign or nonself microorganisms that have entered the body, such as bacteria, fungi, viruses, transplanted tissues, allergens, and toxic substances. Although the skin is the largest immune organ, cuts and lesions may allow pathogens to enter the body. They may also enter the body through inhaling them in the air or through the mouth via foods we eat or liquids we drink. Although the body does have in place several mechanisms to destroy these pathogens (i.e., cilia and mucus lining the respiratory tract and gastric processes in the digestive system), some nevertheless evade these defenses. When this occurs, our immune system begins its complex and comprehensive task of activating an immune response in order to kill or inactivate the pathogen.

The immune system is akin to the circulatory system. It operates via the lymphatic system, a noncentralized group of organs that work in concert to destroy renegade and mutant cells. Organs such as the spleen, the thymus, lymph nodes, and bone marrow all play a role in the production and maintenance of highly specialized immune system cells. Although it is beyond the scope of this chapter to detail all the intricacies of the lymphatic system, Brannon and Feist (1997) provide a good review.

Before the immune system can mobilize against a pathogen, the microorganism must be recognized as foreign to the body. That is, the immune system has the daunting task of constantly discriminating between what is part of the body, or self, and what is not, or nonself. All cells of the body are coded by an array of protein molecules that function as a "self" marker. Foreign microorganisms also have protein molecules, but they are different than those of the body cells; thus, they can be identified as nonself. Altered body cells, such as cancer cells, undergo protein changes and also become classified as nonself. Nonself proteins are called antigens. Immune system cells interact in a communication network that relays information about surrounding organisms within the body's environment. An immune response is triggered when an antigen is discovered.

Before detailing the immune response, it is important to make a distinction between nonspecific immunity and acquired immunity. Nonspecific immunity is defined as the immune system's ability to respond to new antigens, ones that the body has not yet encountered. Once an antigen has been "discovered" and attacked, specific cells (T and B cells discussed later) develop a memory for that antigen. Thus, prior exposure to both illnesses and vaccines (where a harmless version of a virus is introduced) plays a role in acquired immunity. Should that antigen reappear in the body again, it is easily recognized by the memory cells and a swift attack is initiated to destroy it.

When an antigen is recognized, the immune system mobilizes and the resulting drama is termed an immune response. Highly specialized white blood cells, called leukocytes, mediate this complicated defense response. There are three classes of leukocytes: lymphocytes, monocytes, and granulocytes. Lymphocytes are categorized as B or T cells. T lymphocytes are produced in the thymus (hence the "T") and are the major players of cell-mediated immunity. T cells have both a stimulatory effect function (helper T cells) and a restrictive effect function (suppressor T cells) on B cells. A third type of T cell is capable of producing cytotoxic cells, which play a more direct role in killing antigens. Natural killer (NK) cells, believed to be a precursor of the mature T cell not yet exposed to the target antigen, are also classified as lymphocytes. Tumor growth and metastasis are probably kept in check by NK cells. B cells carry out humoral, or circulatory, immunity. When an antigen is recognized, B lymphocytes produce plasma cells, which in turn produce antibodies (immunoglobins) that are secreted into the bloodstream. The antibodies are synthesized by different immunoglobins so that they can combine with the antigen that initiated the immune response. The major classes of immunoglobins are IgG, IgM, IgA, IgD, and IgE; each performs a slightly different function.

Bone marrow gives rise to monocytes, which only circulate in the bloodstream for about 8 to 10 hours. Upon leaving the bloodstream, they enter tissues and mature into larger cells better able to engage in phagocytosis (destruction of cells and particulate via chemotaxis, attachment, engulfment, and/or intracellular events) called macrophages. Granulocytes are named for the presence of intracytoplasmic granules whose function is to cut through, or lyse, the cellular membrane of the target cells.

THE "NEURO" IN PSYCHONEUROIMMUNOLOGY

It is equally important to comprehend how the immune system can be influenced by psychological and social variables. Researchers believe two main interrelated systems allow for brain-immune system communication: the sympathetic-adrenomedullary (SAM) system and the hypothalamic-pituitary-adrenocortical (HPA) system. Both of these systems are activated when the body encounters sympathetic nervous system (fight or flight) arousal. In short, once activated, these systems then stimulate parts of the endocrine system. Thus, the endocrine system is one of the known intermediaries between psychological variables and immune system changes. It works in concert with the nervous system in sending messages to the various parts of the body. In so doing it has been referred to as a "second nervous system" (Baum et al., 1997). In fact, the two are so intimately tied together that they have been likened as one system: the neuroendocrine environment (Ader et al., 1995).

The endocrine system consists of glands, including the pituitary, adrenals, gonads, and thyroid, which produce and then release hormones into the circulating bloodstream. Hormones are chemical messengers that help regulate organs and structures throughout the body. To accomplish this, the hormones travel in the bloodstream until they reach their destination, where they bind to the targeted organ to deliver their message. This enables communication between organs that are not in close physical proximity with one another. For example, adrenal hormones (i.e., epinephrine or cortisol) are known to affect the cardiovascular system and other endocrine organs, as well as the immune system. Receptors for hormones exist within the lymph system, bone marrow, thymus, and spleen. Most recently, receptors for hormones have been found on lymphocytes, monocytes/macrophages, and granulocytes. In addition, bidirectional pathways exist between the endocrine and immune system (Ader et al., 1995). Thus, the ability for hormones to enable organ-to-organ, organ-to-immune, and immune-to-organ system interactions throughout the body is immense.

The more purely neurological aspects of immune mediation have been the recent focus of researchers' attention as well (Ader et al., 1995). There are now known bidirectional pathways between the brain and the immune system. Moreover, it has been proposed that the neocortex of the brain may be a link between psychosocial factors and immune system functioning. This is important in that the neocortex has a "central role . . . in the perception and interpretation of environmental circumstances, including stressful life experiences" (Ader et al., 1995, p. 100).

Taken together, immune, neurological, endocrine, and psychological processes are highly interactive and undeniably interrelated. The following section provides a brief description of how scientists have been able to test these system interactions.

MEASURING IMMUNE SYSTEM FUNCTIONING

Immunocompetence is the term used to describe optimal immune system functioning. A state of immunosupression or immunocompromise exists when the immune system is not operating effectively. Researchers in the field of psychoneuroimmunology assess the effects of various variables on the immune system. However, the cells of the immune system organs cannot easily be accessed. In order to assess an individual's immunocompetence at any point in time, scientists can assay blood, saliva, and/or urine samples for immune system components. It has only been in the last 15 years that technology has allowed researchers to directly test assumptions about the relationship between emotional states and physical health (Salovey, Rothman, Detweiler, & Steward, 2000).

Researchers observe the cells that they have obtained and look for specific immune cell activity. How the cells are activated, their cytotoxicity, and how they transform and mobilize themselves are of interest to psychoneuroimmunology-related studies. Additional specific measures include "the ability of lymphocytes to kill invading cells (lymphocyte cytotoxicity), the ability of lymphocytes to reproduce when artificially stimulated by a chemical (mitogen), [and] the ability of certain white blood cells to ingest foreign particles (phagocytotic activity)" (Taylor, 1999, p. 430).

STUDIES DEMONSTRATING THE PSYCHOSOCIAL ASPECTS OF PSYCHONEUROIMMUNOLOGY

As noted earlier in this chapter, social support/interpersonal relationships can play an important role in mediating the effects of negative events on one's health. One of the contributions that psychoneuroimmunology has made in this area is that a large number of studies have reaffirmed the connection between social relationships and health. In their review of modifying variables of stress and immunity, Hall, Anderson, and O'Grady (1994) acknowledge that psychosocial factors influence how a stressor can affect one's physiological states. Just a few years earlier, Hall and O'Grady (1991) concluded that an individual's belief that results of a psychosocial intervention will be beneficial is a necessary underpinning for the intervention's efficacy.

Kiecolt-Glaser and her colleagues have conducted numerous studies examining the relationship between stress, psychosocial functioning, and immune system functioning (see Kiecolt-Glaser, 1999, for a more extensive review). Some of her earliest studies in this area focused on the variable of loneliness. For example, preliminary work with medical students suggested that loneliness might compromise the immune system (Kiecolt-Glaser, Garner, et al., 1984). Similar results were found with psychiatric patients who reported higher levels of loneliness than those who were reportedly less lonely (Kiecolt-Glaser, Ricker, et al., 1984). A more recent study has revealed that mean salivary cortisol levels, as assessed several times per day, correlated with reports of chronic loneliness (Cacioppo et al., 2000).

Further exploration has revealed that the quality of the interpersonal relationship is an important factor. When exposed to stressors, an unsatisfactory interpersonal relationship was found to be related to decreased percentages of T-helper lymphocytes and decreased NK cells. In addition, assayed NK cells showed decreased functioning abilities (Kennedy, Kiecolt-Glaser, & Glaser, 1988). In another study, Kiecolt-Glaser et al. (1987) matched women who had been separated from their spouse for one year or less to married women. They again found compromised immune system functioning in the women who were separated.

Although these studies provide evidence for the relationship between negative psychosocial variables and impaired immune system functioning, there is still a need to demonstrate that positive health changes in individuals with compromised, immunosuppressed, or immunodysregulated systems can occur. One study that meets this need is a Venezuelan study, which examined the impact of a psychosocial intervention based on the concepts of psychoneuroimmunology on the management of asthma in children between the ages of 6 to 15 years (Castés et al., 1999). Participants were from the village of San Pedro on Coche Island, where asthma is a major health problem. In addition to antiasthmatic medicine, the experimental group received a psychosocial intervention that utilized psychoeducation about the mechanisms of the allergic response; relaxation and guided imagery; workshops, group activities, and family participation to improve self-esteem; and counseling sessions for the mothers or legal guardians of the children that mainly addressed secondary gains from illness, as well as self-esteem and other issues regarding their children's asthma. Control participants received only antiasthmatic medication. All participants were clinically evaluated (pulmonary function and immunological evaluations) for six months prior to intervention and during the six-month intervention period. Participants who received the psychosocial intervention showed significant improvement in clinical, pulmonary, and immunological parameters (despite reduced bronchodilator inhaler use) whereas no significant changes occurred in the control subjects. Interestingly, specific IgE antibody levels to the most important allergen for this population were significantly reduced in the experimental participants. This was in contrast to total IgE antibody levels, which remained unchanged. Furthermore, the children in the experimental group demonstrated significant increases of NK cells, so much so that post-intervention levels matched those of a nonasthmatic sample of children. Overall, these results suggest that psychosocial intervention not only enabled the asthmatic children to decrease asthma crises and use of bronchodilators, but that it produced specific immune system improvements.

THE FUTURE OF BIOPSYCHOSOCIAL PROCESSES IN HEALTH AND HEALING

Western medicine has, in a sense, blind-sighted itself by discounting the contributions of psychosocial factors in its biomedical orientation. With the adoption of a reductionist, universal, materialisitc view of medicine (Myers & Benson, 1992), Western medicine lost its (w)holistic approach toward treating the patient, not just the patient's illness. It is interesting, as you will discover from other chapters in this volume, that some older, non-Western therapeutic approaches (e.g., traditional Chinese, Ayurveda, and Tibetan medicine) have always embraced a holistic approach in their respective philosophies. It is perhaps even more interesting to witness modern Western medicine rethink its own philosophy and begin to rediscover the elements of holistic treatments in response to a disgruntled patient population tired of being perceived as "diseases" instead of individuals worthy of interpersonal interactions and human contact.

The psychoneuroimmunology and placebo literatures will hopefully continue to provide new and exciting evidence that there are connections between an individual's psychology and culturally bound beliefs and expectations with their health status. Indeed, psychoneuroimmunology is flourishing (for a review, see Kiecolt-Glaser, McGuire, Robles, & Glaser, 2002). This is evidenced by the creation of medical journals (e.g., *Brain, Behavior, and Immunity; Journal of Neuroimmunology;* and *Psychosomatic Medicine*) dedicated to the science of better understanding the interplay between disciplines such as psychology, sociology, anthropology, neurology, endocrinology, and immunology, and by the optimistic international researchers who contribute to these scholarly endeavors.

However, it should be noted that despite the evidence for placebo effects in the human healing process, enthusiasm for more research in this area has wavered. Several noted researchers in this area have stressed the importance of further investigating the placebo effect. Benson (1995) acknowledges that physicians should have a better understanding of placebo effects so that they can be incorporated into modern medical treatments. More recently, Moerman and Jonas (2000) have made the case that the overall benefits of a research agenda on placebo effects are evident in terms of health care costs, scientific understanding, and policy consequences. Additionally, Benson and Friedman (1995) declare that the attitudes of clinicians, patients, policy makers, and insurers must change.

Finally, in terms of the role culture plays in health and illness, the importance of interdisciplinary training and research for medical sociologists needs to be further emphasized (Coe, 1997). Gains within the sociological realm of understanding the complex nature of human behavior will further elucidate how we approach health and illness. This point is well taken given the dearth of medical training programs around the world that address the role of culture. Recently, a Birmingham, England-based research group (Loudon, Anderson, Gill, & Greenfield, 1999) conducted an international search for medical school programs that included training on cultural diversity, including racial and ethnic diversity. Using online databases, online data sets, manual searches of medical journals, and the knowledge of medical experts, they found that only 17 programs (13 in North America) addressed cultural diversity. As a result, they stress that given the growing sensitivity toward multiculturalism and the unquestionable role of culture in health, adequate training should be available to practitioners to heighten their cultural sensitivity.

REFERENCES

Ader, R. (1974). Letter to the Editor: Behaviorally conditioned immunosuppression. *Psychosomatic Medicine, 36,* 183-184.

Ader, R. (1988). The placebo effect as conditioned response. In R. Ader, H. Weiner, & A. Baum (Eds.), *Experimental foundations of behavioral medicine: Conditioning approaches* (pp. 47-66). Hillside, NJ: Erlbaum.

Ader, R. (1996). Historical perspectives on psychoneuroimmunology. In H. Friedman, T. W. Klein, & A. L. Friedman (Eds.), *Psychoneuroimmunology, stress, and infection* (pp. 1-24). Boca Raton, FL: CRC Press.

Ader, R., & Cohen, N. (1975). Behaviorally conditioned immunosuppression. *Psychosomatic Medicine, 37,* 333-340.

Ader, R., & Cohen, N. (1991). The influence of conditioning on immune responses. In R. Ader, D. L. Felton, & N. Cohen (Eds.), *Psychoneuroimmunology* (2nd ed., pp. 611-646). San Diego, CA: Academic Press.

Ader, R., Cohen, N., & Felten, D. (1995). Psychoneuroimmunology: Interactions between the nervous system and the immune system. *The Lancet, 345,* 99-103.

Balant, L. P., & Balant-Gorgia, E. A. (2000). Cultural differences: Implications on drug therapy and global drug development. *International Journal of Clinical Pharmacology and Therapeutics, 38,* 47-52.

Baum, A., Gatchel, R. J., & Krantz, D.S. (1997). *An introduction to health psychology* (3rd ed.). New York: McGraw-Hill.

Benson, H. (1995). Commentary: Placebo effect and remembered wellness. *Mind/Body Medicine, 1,* 44-45.

Benson, H., & Friedman, R. (1995). The three-legged stool. *Mind/Body Medicine, 1,* 1-2.

Brannon, L., & Feist, J. (1997). *Health psychology: An introduction to behavior and health* (3rd ed.). Pacific Grove, CA: Brooks/Cole.

Brody, H. (1983). Does disease have a natural history? *Medical Anthropology Quarterly, 14,* 3, 19-22.

Bruhn, J. G., Chandler, B., Miller, M. C., Wolf, S., & Lynn, T. N. (1966). Social aspects of coronary heart disease in two adjacent, ethnically different communities. *American Journal of Public Health: Nations Health, 56,* 1493-1506.

Bruhn, J. G., Philips, B. U., & Wolf, S. (1972). Social readjustment and illness patterns: Comparisons between first, second and third generation Italian-Americans living in the same community. *Journal of Psychosomatic Medicine, 16,* 387-394.

Bruhn, J. G., Philips, B. U., & Wolf, S. (1982). Lessons from Roseto 20 years later: A community study of heart disease. *Southern Medical Journal, 75,* 575-580.

Cacioppo, J. T., Ernst, J. M., Burlson, M. H., McClintock, M. K., Malarkey, W. B., Hawkley, L. C., et al. (2000). Lonely traits and concomitant physiological processes: The MacArthur social neuroscience studies. *International Journal of Psychophysiology, 35,* 143-154.

Castés, M., Hagel, I., Palenque, M., Canelones, P., Corao, A., & Lynch, N. R. (1999). Immunological changes associated with clinical improvement of asthmatic children subjected to psychosocial intervention. *Brain, Behavior, and Immunity, 13,* 1-13.

Coe, R. M. (1997). The magic of science and the science of magic: An essay on the process of healing. *Journal of Health and Social Behavior, 38,* 1-8.

de Craen, A. J., Roos, P. J., Leonard de Vries, A., & Kleijnen, J. (1996). Effect of colour of drugs: Systematic review of perceived effect of drugs and of their effectiveness. *British Medical Journal, 313,* 1624-1626.

Egolf, B., Lasker, J., Wolf, S., & Potvin, L. (1992). The Roseto effect: A 50-year comparison of mortality rates. *American Journal of Public Health, 82,* 1089-1092.

Eisenberg, D. M., Kessler, R. C., Foster, C. Norlock, F. E., Clakins, D. R., & Delbanco, T. L. (1993). Unconventional medicine in the United States—prevalence, costs, and patterns of use. *New England Journal of Medicine, 328,* 246-252.

Engel, G. (1977). The need for a new medical model: A challenge for biomedicine. *Science, 196,* 129-136.

Hahn, R. (1999). Anthropology and the enhancement of public health practice. In R. Hahn (Ed.), *Anthropology in public health: Bridging differences in culture and society* (pp. 3-24). New York: Oxford University Press.

Hahn, R., & Kleinman, A. (1983). Belief as pathogen, belief as medicine: "Voodoo death" and the "placebo phenomenon" in anthropological perspective. *Medical Anthropology Quarterly, 14,* 3-19.

Hall, N. R. S., Anderson, J. A., & O'Grady, M. P. (1994). Stress and immunity in humans: Modifying variables. In R. Glaser & J. Kiecolt-Glaser (Eds.), *Handbook of human stress and immunity* (pp. 183-215). San Diego, CA: Academic Press.

Hall, N. R. S., & O'Grady, M.P. (1991). Psychosocial interventions and immune function. In R. Ader, D. L. Felton, & N. Cohen (Eds.), *Psychoneuroimmunology* (2nd ed., pp. 1067-1080). San Diego, CA: Academic Press.

Harrington, A. (1997). Introduction. In A. Harrington (Ed.), *The placebo effect: An interdisciplinary exploration* (pp. 1-11). Cambridge, MA: Harvard University Press.

Helman, C. (1994). *Culture, health and illness* (3rd ed.). London: Butterworth-Heinemann.

Kamin, L. J. (1968). Attention-like processes in classical conditioning. In M. R. Jones (Ed.), *Miami symposium on the prediction of behavior: Aversive stimuli* (pp. 9-32). Coral Gables, FL: University of Miami Press.

Kaptchuk, T. J. (1998). Powerful placebo: The dark side of the randomized controlled trial. *The Lancet, 351,* 1722-1725.

Kennedy, S., Kiecolt-Glaser, J. K., & Glaser, R. (1988). Immunological consequences of acute and chronic stressors: Mediating role of interpersonal relationships. *British Journal of Medical Psychology, 61,* 77-85.

Kiecolt-Glaser, J. K. (1999). Stress, personal relationships, and immune function: Health implications. *Brain, Behavior, and Immunity, 13,* 61-72.

Kiecolt-Glaser, J. K., Fisher, L., Ogrocki, P., Stout, J. C., Speicher, C. E., & Glaser, R. (1987). Marital quality, marital disruption, and immune function. *Psychosomatic Medicine, 49,* 31-34.

Kiecolt-Glaser, J. K., Garner, W., Speicher, C. E., Penn, G. M., Holliday, J. E., & Glaser, R. (1984). Psychosocial modifiers of immunocompetence in medical students. *Psychosomatic Medicine, 46,* 7-14.

Kiecolt-Glaser, J.K., McGuire, L, Robles, T. F., & Glaser, R. (2002). Psychoneuroimmunology and psychosomatic medicine: Back to the future. *Psychosomatic Medicine, 64,* 15-28.

Kiecolt-Glaser, J. K., Ricker, D., Messick, G., Speicher, C. E., Garner, W., & Glaser, R. (1984). Urinary cortisol, cellular immunocompetency and loneliness in psychiatric inpatients. *Psychosomatic Medicine, 46,* 15-24.

Kinsley, D. (1996). *Health, healing, and religion: A cross-cultural perspective.* Upper Saddle River, NJ: Prentice-Hall.

Kirsch, I. (1985). Response expectancy as a determinant of experience and behavior. *American Psychologist, 40,* 1189-1202.

Kirsch, I. (1990). *Changing expectations: A key to effective psychotherapy.* Pacific Grove, CA: Brooks/Cole.

Kirsch, I. (1997). Specifying nonspecifics: Psychological mechanisms of placebo effects. In A. Harrington (Ed.), *The placebo effect: An interdisciplinary exploration* (pp. 166-186). Cambridge, MA: Harvard University Press.

Kirsch, I., & Sapirstein, G. (1998). Listening to Prozac but hearing placebo: A meta-analysis of antidepressant medication. *Prevention & Treatment, 1,* Article 0002a. Retrieved April 1, 2000 from the World Wide Web: http://journals.apa.org/treatment/volume1/pre0010002a.html.

Kleinman, A. (1981). *Patients and healers in the context of culture: An exploration of the borderland between anthropology, medicine, and psychiatry*. Berkeley, CA: University of California Press.

Kleinman, A., Eisenberg, L., & Good, B. (1978). Culture, illness, and care: Clinical lessons from anthropological and cross-cultural research. *Annals of Internal Medicine, 88*, 251-258.

Lin, K. M., Anderson, D., & Poland, R. E. (1995). Ethnicity and psychopharmacology: Bridging the gap. *Psychiatric Clinics of North America, 18*, 635-647.

Lindberg, D. C. (1992). *The beginnings of Western science: The European scientific tradition in philosophical, religious, and institutional context, 600 B.C. to A.D. 1450*. Chicago: The University of Chicago Press.

Loudon, R. F., Anderson, P. M., Gill, P. S., & Greenfield, S. M. (1999). Educating medical students for work in culturally diverse societies. *Journal of the American Medical Association, 282*, 875-880.

MacAndrew, C., & Edgerton, R. B. (1969). *Drunken comportment: A social explanation*. Chicago: Aldine-Atherton.

Moerman, D. E. (1983). General medical effectiveness and human biology: Placebo effects in the treatment of ulcer disease. *Medical Anthropology Quarterly, 14*, 3-15.

Moerman, D. E. (1991). Physiology and symbols: The anthropological implications of the placebo effect. In L. Romanucci-Ross, D. E. Moerman, & L. Tancredi (Eds.), *The anthropology of medicine: From culture to method* (2nd ed., pp. 129-143). New York: Bergen & Garvey.

Moerman, D. E., & Jonas, W. B. (2000). Toward a research agenda on placebo. *Advances in Mind Body Medicine, 16*, 33-46.

Montgomery, G. H., & Kirsch, I. (1996). Classical conditioning and the placebo effect. *Pain, 72*, 107-113.

Moyers, B. (1993). *Healing and the mind*. New York: Doubleday.

Myers, S. S., & Benson, H. (1992). Psychological factors in healing: A new perspective on an old debate. *Behavioral Medicine, 18*, 5-11.

Pavlov, I. P. (1927). *Conditioned reflexes*. London: Oxford.

Price, D. D., Milling, L. S., Kirsch, I., Duff, A., Montgomery, G. H., & Nicholls, S. S. (1999). An analysis of factors that contribute to the magnitude of placebo analgesia in an experimental paradigm. *Pain, 83*, 147-156.

Rescorla, R. A. (1988). Pavlovian conditioning: It's not what you think it is. *American Psychologist, 43*, 151-160.

Salovey, P., Rothman, A. J., Detweiler, J. B., & Steward, W. T. (2000). Emotional states and physical health. *American Psychologist, 55*, 110-121.

Smith, M., Lin, K. M., & Mendoza, R. (1994). "Nonbiological" issues affecting psycho-pharmacology: Cultural considerations. In K. M. Lin, R. E. Poland, & G. Nagasaki (Eds.), *Psychopharmacology and psychobiology of ethnicity. Progress in Psychiatry 39* (pp. 37-58). Washington, DC: American Psychiatric Press.

Spiegel, D. (1997). Psychosocial aspects of breast cancer treatment. *Seminars in Oncology, 24*, S1-36–S1-47.

Spiegel, D., Bloom, J. R., Kraemer, H. C., & Gottheil, E. (1989). Effect of psychosocial treatment on survival of patients with metastatic breast cancer. *The Lancet, 2*, 888-891.

Susman, E. (2001). Mind-body interaction and development biology, behavior and context. *European Psychologist, 6*, 163-171.

Taylor, S. E. (1999). *Health psychology* (4th ed.). New York: McGraw-Hill.

Voudouris, N. J., Peck, C. L., & Coleman, G. (1985). Conditioned placebo responses. *Journal of Personality and Social Psychology, 48*, 47-53.

Voudouris, N. J., Peck, C. L., & Coleman, G. (1989). Conditioned response models of placebo phenomena: Further support. *Pain, 38*, 109-116.

Voudouris, N. J., Peck, C. L., & Coleman, G. (1990). The role of conditioning and verbal expectancy in the placebo response. *Pain, 43*, 121-128.

Wall, P. D. (1996). The placebo effect. In M. Velmans (Ed.), *The science of consciousness: Psychological, neuropsychological and clinical reviews* (pp. 162-180). New York: Routledge.

Wampold, B. E. (2001). Contextualizing psychotherapy as a healing practice: Culture, history, and methods. *Applied and Preventive Psychology, 10*, 69-86.

Wickramasekera, I. (1980). A conditioned response model of the placebo effect: Predictions from the model. *Biofeedback and Self-Regulation, 5*, 5-18.

Wolf, S. (1992). Predictors of myocardial infarction over a span of 30 years in Roseto, Pennsylvania. *Integrated Physiological Behavior Science, 27*, 246-257.

II

Therapeutic Services and Multiculturalism in North America

The Role of Culture in the Treatment of Culturally Diverse Populations

Joseph F. Aponte
University of Louisville

The purpose of this chapter is to describe how culture enters into the psychological treatment of ethnically diverse populations. The chapter takes a multicultural approach rather than a cross-cultural perspective, although many of the observations are applicable to other cultures. More specifically, it focuses on four major ethnic groups (African Americans/Blacks, Hispanics/Latinos, Asian Americans and Pacific Islanders, and American Indians/Native Americans), recognizing that there is a rich diversity of other ethnic groups in this country. Although the focus of the chapter is on the treatment process, it is important to discuss two major trends that will have a direct impact on this process: changes in the ethnic profile and changes in the delivery of mental health services in the United States. Both of these changes will have an important impact on mental health services to ethnic clients.

A broad prospective is used in describing the impact of culture on the treatment process. This perspective involves the different pathways to treatment and mental health utilization rates for ethnic populations. These perspectives are integrated using Beutler and Clarkin's (1990) Differential Treatment Selection model as a mechanism for analyzing the cultural influences on the total treatment process. Throughout this discussion, the relationship between what is often labeled as sociocultural moderator variables (Aponte & Barnes, 1995; Aponte & Johnson, 2000; Dana, 1993; Sodowsky, Lai, & Plake, 1991) and acculturation is a pervasive theme. It is through acculturation, and its correlates, that culture manifests itself in the mental health service delivery and treatment process.

This chapter is directed toward mainstream mental health workers and therapists, and the standard psychotherapeutic treatments used by them, whose clients are one or more of the four previously identified ethnic groups. As Wohl (1995, 2000) points out, the mental health profession has not been very successful in recruiting and training ethnic practitioners. The prospects of that changing in the future remain dismal (Aponte & Aponte, 2000; Aponte & Clifford, 1995). Accordingly, White mainstream practitioners will invariably find themselves working with ethnically diverse clients. The discussion thus focuses on developing an appreciation for, and application of, cultural factors in the psychological treatment of ethnic clients.

MAJOR TRENDS AND THEIR IMPACT ON TREATMENT

Beginning in the 1970s, the ethnic profile of the United States began to change dramatically with the number of ethnic persons increasing and the population of this country becoming more diversified (O'Hare, 1992). This trend has continued unabated into the 1990s and into the 2000s (DeVita, 1996; American Psychological Association, 2003). During the 1980s, the delivery of health services also began to change and has continued to do so into the 1990s with the implementation of managed health care. The reorganization of the delivery of mental health services soon followed that of health services and is still in the process of evolving. Both of these trends will have a dramatic impact on the treatment of ethnic clients throughout the twenty-first century.

Changing Ethnic Profile of the United States

Although it can be argued that "racial" categories are too restrictive, illogical, and confusing (Betancourt & López, 1993; Spickard, 1992; Yee, Fairchild, Weizmann, & Wyatt, 1993), these categories are nevertheless used by the U.S. Bureau of Census and periodically will be used in this chapter. According to the 2000 census data, these ethnic populations constitute the following percentages of the total population: African-Americans—12.9 percent, Hispanics/Latinos—12.5 percent, Asian/Pacific Islanders—4.5 percent, and American Indians/Eskimos/Aleuts—1.5 percent (U.S. Bureau of Census, 2000a). In 2000, these groups constituted 31.4 percent of the population. By the year 2050, these groups will constitute an estimated 47.3 percent of the total population in the country (Aponte & Crouch, 2000).

These population changes will lead to an increased demand for an array of mental health services in all parts of the country. The increasing number of recent immigrants will also tax mental health services in a number of specific ways. Some of the issues for this group are generic to all ethnic groups, whereas others are unique to recent immigrants (Bemak & Chung, 2000; see Chapter 7, this volume). Those immigrants who come from impoverished, politically volatile, and war-torn countries present a number of economic, social, and psychological issues that pose additional and different challenges for mental health service providers (Root, 1992; Takaki, 1994).

The changing ethnic population characteristics (age, birth rates, and mortality rates) will also have a profound impact on the need for mental health services and the types of services to be provided to these groups (Aponte & Crouch, 1995, 2000). Ethnic persons tend to be young and will experience problems that are common to all young populations in addition to issues that are unique to them, such as struggles around their ethnic identity, discrimination, and violence (Aponte & Barnes, 1995; Young Porter, 2000a). Members of ethnic groups are also aging and will begin to experience increasingly some of the same problems faced by the White elderly, as well as some problems that are more profound for ethnic elderly, such as poverty (Grant, 1995).

Family structure and marriage patterns tend to be different for African Americans, Hispanics/Latinos, Asian Americans and Pacific Islanders, and American Indians (Aponte & Crouch, 2000; Wilson, Kohn, & Lee, 2000). Ethnic households tend to be larger than White households and are more likely to be headed by females, a high percentage of whom have never married (Young Porter, 2000b). Socioeconomic status (SES) and those components that are subsumed under this concept (occupational status, income, and education) are also related to ethnicity. Ethnic groups, particularly African Americans, Hispanics/Latinos, and Native Americans, tend to be overrepresented in the lower SES strata (Aponte & Crouch, 1995, 2000).

The increasing need for diversified mental health services resulting from the changing ethnic profile of the United States is obvious. Such a statement was made more than two decades ago by the President's Commission on Mental Health (1978). In addition, services need to target high-risk groups within ethnic populations such as children, adolescents, the poor, and the elderly. An array of treatments, in addition to individual therapeutic interventions, such as family approaches, group treatments, and community interventions need to be used with ethnic populations (Aponte & Crouch, 1995, 2000). Such flexibility will need to occur in an environment where dramatic changes are occurring in the delivery of mental health services.

Changes in Mental Health Services

Over the last several decades health care costs in the United States have continued to increase; so too has the number of individuals who lack health care coverage (Frank & VandenBos, 1994). Cost containment efforts have been implemented in the health arena that have led to the development of health maintenance organizations (HMOs) and related health delivery structures, such as preferred provider organizations (PPOs; DeLeon, VandenBos, & Bulatao, 1991). Approximately 140 million Americans are covered by managed mental health plans. Almost 90 percent of them are enrolled in specialized mental health plans, often referred to as "carve-outs," that specialize in providing mental health services to members of the HMOs.

The managed health care plans utilize a number of cost-cutting strategies (Hersch, 1995), including caps on the number of sessions, limits on the cost per session, increased co-payments, caps on both expenditures per year and life time, increased deductible payments, the exclusion of various types of problems or treatment modalities (e.g., marital problems or family therapy), and the utilization of case managers with limited professional training and credentials. In addition, consumer choice in selecting a mental health professional with whom to work has oftentimes been restricted to those professionals who belong to the managed mental health plan.

Over the past two decades a number of organizational structures also have evolved in order to contain mental health costs and provide more effective services. Mental health providers have become more diversified, operating within primary and speciality health care settings, such as physician offices, and nursing homes (Hersch, 1995). Diversified organizational and administrative structures, such as group practices, have also developed to provide services in a managed care environment (Belar, 1995). Changed philosophies have emerged in which the integration of physical and mental health approaches and structures for delivering these services has been developed (Hersch, 1995; Sherbourne, Hays, & Wells, 1995).

The development of other practices has dovetailed with the emergence of the above organizational structures in the managed care environment (Barlow, 1994; Clinton, McCormick, & Besteman, 1994; Schulberg & Rush, 1994). These include the development of diagnostic-related groups (DRGs), clinical practice guidelines, the manualized treatment of specific disorders, and brief, short-term, and cost-effective interventions. All mental health service providers and service recipients have been affected by these organizational and practice changes; however, ethnic populations are more at risk to be affected adversely by these changes.

As previously mentioned, a disproportionate number of ethnic persons are found at the lower SES levels (Aponte & Crouch, 1995, 2000), and as such, they are less likely to have health insurance and thus be part of managed health plans. Medicare and Medicaid's managed care umbrella of services is available to those not enrolled in private health plans who meet Medicare and Medicaid requirements (McCombs, 1997).

However, a disproportionate number of ethnic persons are also homeless (Milburn & Curry, 1995) and thus have limited access to or do not utilize private or public health and mental health services.

Those ethnic persons who are enrolled in managed mental health care plans face a number of issues that are unique to their ethnicity. Because of the service delivery, organizational, and practice changes that have emerged under managed mental health care, ethnic patients will find themselves having more difficulty paying the increased deductibles and co-payments, will be less likely to be able to select mental health professionals of their own ethnicity, and will be more likely to be treated with structured treatment packages (e.g., individual short-term therapy that adheres to clinical practice guidelines or is manualized). Some ethnic clients also prefer to work with therapists from their own ethnic group (López, López, & Fung, 1991). In addition, clinical practice guidelines and manualized treatments have routinely emerged from working only with White middle-class clients.

ROLE OF CULTURE ON ENTRY INTO THE MENTAL HEALTH SYSTEM

People enter the mental health system by a number of pathways (Draguns, 2000). People can directly come into treatment on their own because of the distress and unhappiness they are experiencing. They can be referred to treatment by employers, social service agencies, educational institutions, physicians, or other community agencies. They can be encouraged or forced to seek treatment by family and friends. The pathways to treatment and utilization patterns for ethnic clients are often different from those of their White counterparts, because of their ethnic group membership or acculturation status. In general, ethnic clients are less likely to seek services on their own and are more likely to be referred to services by other health or service organizations (Dinges & Cherry, 1995; Rogler & Cortes, 1993).

The different pathways by which ethnic clients enter the mental health system are reflected in differential mental health service utilization rates. The research findings indicate that African Americans and American Indians tend to overutilize, whereas Asian Americans and Latinos tend to underutilize mental health services (Cheung & Snowden, 1990; Snowden & Cheung, 1990; Sue, Chun, & Gee, 1995; Sue, Fujino, Hu, Takeuchi, & Zane, 1991). However, it is important to note that these are gross estimates of service utilization that are generally based on rates under treatment, which may be misleading. For example, Neighbors (1985) reported an underutilization of mental health services among African Americans; others report that these rates vary drastically by type of service (Wood & Sherrets, 1984). It is thus suggested that ethnic clients have different patterns of use and that these differences vary within ethnic groups as well (Leong, Wagner, & Tata, 1995).

The different pathways to treatment that exist among these various groups can be attributed to a number of factors, including different conceptualizations of the problem (Kleinman, 1980; Sussman, Chapter 3 in this volume); attitudes toward their symptoms and mental health service practitioners (Leong et al., 1995; Neighbors, Caldwell, Thompson, & Jackson, 1994); how the person's symptoms are expressed (Dinges & Cherry, 1995); accuracy of the diagnosis made by the referral source or gatekeeper (Good, 1993); familial tolerances for symptoms and problematic behaviors (Neal & Turner, 1991; Randall-David, 1989); use of traditional or folk practices (Koss-Chioino, 2000, also Chapter 11 in this volume); prior experiences with social service and mental health agencies (Angel & Thoits, 1987); and the availability of mental health services (Randall-David, 1989).

Some Hispanic/Latino groups, for example, categorize psychological disorders under the socially acceptable category of *nervios* (Dinges & Cherry, 1995; Draguns, 2000; Koss, 1990). The literature indicates that African Americans tend to be overdiagnosed with psychotic disorders and underdiagnosed with depressive and anxiety disorders (Neighbors et al., 1994; Paradis, Friedman, Lazar, Grubea, & Kesselman, 1992). It is reported that Asian Americans tend to tolerate psychological symptoms in their family members, often protecting them until their symptoms become severe (Randall-David, 1989). Koss-Chioino (2000) reports that ethno-medical treatments are used by between 5 percent and 23 percent of Hispanic populations in California. Native Americans have reportedly had poor experiences with social and mental health agencies, and appropriate mental health services are not always readily available to this group (LaFromboise, 1998; Penn, Kar, Kramer, Skinner, & Zambrana, 1995).

KEY CULTURAL FACTORS THAT INFLUENCE THE TREATMENT OF ETHNIC CLIENTS

In order to fully appreciate the role of culture in the psychological treatment of culturally diverse populations, it is essential to identify and discuss in more detail a number of selected key cultural factors, sometimes referred to as moderator variables in the literature (Aponte & Barnes, 1995; Aponte & Johnson, 2000; Dana, 1993; Sodowsky et al., 1991). However, before discussing these factors it is important to review the phases of second culture acquisition (Aponte & Barnes, 1995; Berry, 1980; Berry & Kim, 1988) and models of second culture acquisition (Aponte & Barnes, 1995; Aponte & Johnson, 2000; LaFromboise, Colemen, & Gerton, 1993) that directly affect and interact with these cultural factors.

Phases of Second Culture Acquisition

Acculturation can be viewed as either a unidirectional process in which a person relinquishes his or her ethnic characteristics or a bidirectional process in which the ethnic person assumes some of the characteristics of the second culture, retains his or her ethnic culture and identity, and influences or changes the second culture (Aponte & Barnes, 1995; Aponte & Johnson, 2000). Regardless of one's position on this matter, ethnic persons go through specific stages in the acculturation process. Berry and his associates identify five phases through which groups can go through, including the pre-contact phase, contact phase, conflict phase, crisis phase, and adaptation phase (Berry, 1980; Berry & Kim, 1988).

For most African Americans, this acculturation process has stretched over hundreds of years. For some Latino and Asian groups who are recent immigrants, the process is of short duration. For Native Americans, the process has included placement and forced acculturation. The culmination of this second culture acquisition can be influenced by a number of variables, such as socioeconomic status, residence (including years of residence in the United States and ethnic density of the person's neighborhoods), immigration status, and familial and social network structure (Aponte & Barnes, 1995; Aponte & Johnson, 2000; Garcia & Lega, 1979; Sodowsky & Carey, 1987). An examination of different types of acculturation follows.

Models of Second Culture Acquisition

A number of models of second culture acquisition can be found in the literature; however, this discussion will focus on the model proposed by LaFomboise et al. (1993). These authors identify five acculturation models: assimilation, acculturation, alternation, multicultural, and fusion. They go on to analyze each of these models according to contact with the culture of origin, loyalty to the culture of origin, involvement with the culture of origin, acceptance by members of the culture of origin, contact with the second culture, affiliation with the second culture, and acceptance by members of the second culture.

According to LaFromboise et al. (1993), those individuals who are assimilated would have low levels of contact, loyalty, involvement, and acceptance by members of their culture of origin. In contrast, they would also have high levels of contact, affiliation, and acceptance by members of the second culture. Additionally, assimilated individuals would be expected to have little knowledge of traditional cultural beliefs and values, thus lacking any sense of groundedness within their culture of origin. Such individuals would tend to feel disconnected from their culture of origin and experience generational friction with those members of their family who are not assimilated.

Those persons who have not assimilated into a second culture would maintain high levels of contact, loyalty, involvement with, and acceptance by members of their culture of origin. These persons would be expected to have low levels of contact, a lack of affiliation, and a lack of acceptance by members of the second culture. According to Berry and Kim (1988), such a pattern has existed in a number of countries with the existence of separation (self-imposed withdrawal from the larger society) or segregation (forced separation of ethnic groups by the larger society). Such patterns have typically led to friction between the ethnic populations and the second culture.

Role of Ethnic Identity

Acculturation and ethnic identity should not be viewed as synonymous, but as separate concepts (Aponte & Barnes, 1995; Aponte & Johnson, 2000; Kitano, 1989). Acculturation focuses on a process of change that occurs in one's values, beliefs, and behaviors as a result of contact with a second culture. Ethnic identity, on the other hand, focuses on the process of incorporating these culturally influenced beliefs and values into one's overall self-concept and identity (Helms, 1990, 1995). A number of ethnic identity models exist and, although they share similar features, they are different in focus. Whereas some models focus on the incorporation of general cultural material into the self-concept (Atkinson, Morton, & Sue, 1998), others highlight the incorporation of specific cultural material, namely the social construct of "race" and the meanings ascribed to it by society, into one's self-concept (Cross, 1991, 1995; Helms, 1990, 1995; Jackson, 1975).

The Minority Identity Model (MID) model, for example, identifies five stages (Conformity, Dissonance, Resistance and Immersion, Introspection, and Synergetic Articulation and Awareness) of the struggles of ethnic persons to understand themselves, their culture, other cultures, and the majority culture (Atkinson et al., 1998). These stages are not rigid boundaries, and ethnic persons can either stay at one stage or move from one stage to another. Individuals may have attitudes associated with more than one stage at a time and, furthermore, the prevailing stage-related attitudes and behaviors can vary according to context (Helms, 1995). Models such as the MID can help identify ethnic client attitudes and behaviors. The model also has implications for the therapeutic process since the model addresses how the ethnic client views and interacts with someone from the majority culture.

A number of ethnic identity measures have been developed for each of the major ethnic groups. Among these are the Developmental Inventory of Black Consciousness

(Milliones, 1980); the Racial Identity Attitudes Scale (Parham & Helms, 1981); the Hispanic Acculturation Identity Questionnaire (Marin, Sabogal, Marin, Otero-Sabogal, & Perez-Stable, 1987); the Suinn-Lew Asian Self Identity Acculturation Scale (Suinn, Richard-Figueroa, Lew, & Vigil, 1987); and the Rosebud Personal Opinion Survey (Hoffman, Dana, & Bolton, 1985) for American Indians. For a more detailed description of ethnic identity models and instruments, the reader is directed to Dana (1993, 1998) and Helms (1990). Such instruments can provide important information to the service provider on the ethnic person's background and current level of ethnic identity.

Other Key Cultural Factors

A number of factors are a direct result of the acculturation process (e.g., worldview, language fluency, familial and social network structure, coping styles). Other variables interact with the acculturation process (e.g., socioeconomic status, personality characteristics, racism, oppression, legal constraints) yielding values, beliefs, attitudes, and behaviors that are a by-product of this interaction. All of these factors can have a direct impact on the psychological functioning of ethnic persons, their use of mental health services, and the subsequent effectiveness of those services (Aponte, 1997; Aponte & Barnes, 1995; Aponte & Johnson, 2000; Berry & Kim, 1988; Pedersen, Draguns, Lonner, & Trimble, 2002; Sodowsky et al., 1991).

The ethnic clients' worldview, for example, is an important factor in the treatment process. Culture-specific elements of one's worldview can have an impact on entry into treatment and its subsequent course and outcome (Aponte & Barnes, 1995; Aponte & Johnson, 2000; Ivey, Ivey, & Simek-Morgan, 1997). A representative sample of culture-specific components of one's worldview might include the individual's beliefs about mental illness and emotional difficulties, beliefs about the appropriate expression of emotion, and attitudes toward authority figures. Once treatment has begun, any or all of these elements might prove to be significantly discrepant from the therapist's conceptualization of the client's psychological distress and the therapist's treatment plan.

Anderson (1991) provides an excellent overview of the worldviews and values of Black Americans. According to Anderson, there are striking differences between Afro-centric and Euro-centric values. Afro-centric values include a time focus in the present; a worldview that is systemic, holistic, spiritual, and focuses on the group/community and on harmony; an identity of self and community; the acquisition of knowledge through introspection and faith; and the transmission of knowledge through oral expression. Such values and views would be strongly influenced by the degree of assimilation into the majority culture. These values and views would also strongly influence African American views toward their psychological problems and the treatment they would receive for these problems.

Language usage and fluency are also key factors in the treatment process (Aponte & Barnes, 1995; Aponte & Johnson, 2000). These factors take on added importance in the therapeutic process with members of ethnic groups such as African Americans, who may not use standard English, and Latinos and Asians, who may not be fluent in English (Russell, 1988; Sciarra & Ponterotto, 1990). According to the 2000 Census, there were 28,340,052 persons in the United States who spoke Spanish (U.S. Bureau of Census, 2000b). Of these individuals, 49 percent are reported to speak English "less than very well." Another 6,960,065 individuals used an Asian or Pacific Island language, with 51 percent of this group speaking English "less than very well."

Those Latino clients who do not speak English well should be working with translators or bilingual mental health professionals. These clients, as well as those who are bilingual, enter into the treatment process at a disadvantage in comparison to those who can use standard English (Aponte & Barnes, 1995; Aponte & Johnson, 2000). Marcos (1976), for example, has found that clients who spoke primarily Spanish were rated as having more pathology and being more emotionally withdrawn when interviewed in English as compared to Spanish. These findings were attributed to the disruptive speech patterns and reduced expression of affect that emerge when a person is required to speak in a nondominant language (Marcos & Urcuyo, 1979).

Space does not permit the discussion of other culture-related factors; however, several comments on socioeconomic status are warranted. Research findings generally indicate that persons from low-SES backgrounds exhibit more psychopathology, utilize mental health services less, and have less successful treatment outcomes than do middle-class and upper-class persons (Aponte & Bracco, 2000; Kuraski, Sue, Chun, & Gee, 2000). As previously noted, ethnic persons are overrepresented in the lower-SES levels, and the literature does not always make a clear distinction between the effects of ethnicity and SES. Caution needs to be exercised in drawing conclusions about ethnic clients from the literature because of this potential confound.

ROLE OF CULTURE IN OVERALL TREATMENT OF ETHNIC CLIENTS

The previous discussion has focused on the major trends (i.e., changing the ethnic profile and delivery of mental health services), the role of culture on entry into the mental health system, and key cultural factors that influence the treatment of ethnic clients. After discussing phases and models of second culture acquisition, several key selected variables (i.e., ethnic identity, worldview, and language usage and fluency) were highlighted. This portion of the chapter will focus on the actual treatment of ethnic clients once they get to mental health services. The treatment model that will be used as an overall framework is a model of Differential Treatment Selection developed by Beutler and Clarkin (1990).

This integrative model for differential treatment (see Figure 6.1) includes four broad categories of factors:

- Patient predisposing variables (i.e., diagnosis, personal characteristics, and environmental circumstances)
- Treatment context (i.e., setting, mode/format, and frequency/duration)
- Relationship variables (i.e., personal compatibility matching and enhancing/maintaining alliance)
- Strategies and techniques (i.e., selecting focal targets of change, selecting level of experiences addressed, conducting therapeutic work, mediating goals/phases of treatment, and maintenance relapse prevention (Beutler & Clarkin, 1990)

Space will not permit a detailed discussion all of the components of these four variables. The remainder of this chapter focuses on the role of culture in each of the broad categories of this model.

Patient Predisposing Variables

According to Beutler and Clarkin (1990), *patient predisposing variables* are those characteristics of the patient and his or her environment at the time he or she enters into treatment. As previously noted in an earlier part of this chapter, ethnic clients are less likely to seek services on their own and are more likely to be referred to services by other health or service organizations (Aponte & Wohl, 2000; Dinges & Cherry, 1995; Rogler & Cortes, 1993). As such, the mental health service utilization pattern of ethnic clients may be affected by the diagnosis, personal characteristics, and environmental/circumstances dimensions of the patient predisposing variables (see Figure 6.1).

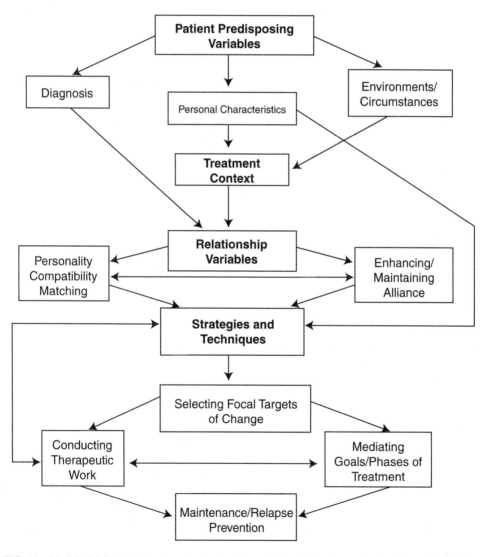

FIG. 6.1. Model of differential treatment selection. From *Systematic treatment selection: Toward targeted therapeutic interventions*, by L. E. Beutler and J. F. Clarkin, New York: Brunner/Mazel. Modified and reproduced with permission of publisher.

The psychiatric diagnosis of ethnic clients in treatment settings has been characterized by misdiagnosis, underdiagnosis, and overdiagnosis of severity of psychopathology (Good, 1993). When rigorous epidemiological studies are conducted with community samples, many differences between ethnic groups and Whites disappear. For example, the prevalence of schizophrenia has been found to be highest among African Americans and lowest among Hispanics/Latinos in comparison to Whites (Escobar, 1993; Gaw, 1993). When socio-educational status is controlled, most differences between these groups disappear (Escobar, 1993).

Recently, attention has been directed toward "culture-bound syndromes." These are characterized as recurrent and locality-specific patterns of behavior that have historically been outside conventional Western psychiatric diagnostic categories (Simons & Hughes, 1993). More recently cultural variables and the identification of "culture-bound syndromes" have been included in the American Psychiatric Association *Diagnostic and Statistical Manual*, 4th Edition (DSM-IV) (American Psychiatric Association, 1994). Such efforts to incorporate cultural variables in the diagnosis of psychiatric disorders may enhance the cultural sensitivity of diagnosticians and make the diagnostic categories more cross-culturally suitable (Wohl & Aponte, 1995).

Within the Beutler and Clarkin (1990) model, there are a number of components under the personal characteristics dimension. One particularly important component of this dimension is that of treatment specific expectations. Ethnic clients, particularly those who are minimally assimilated, have different expectations about the therapeutic process, the role of client and therapist, and the outcome of therapy (Aponte, Young, Rivers, & Wohl, 1995). These clients' treatment expectations can be determined by using Kleinman's explanatory belief model and asking a series of questions around the cause, symptoms, process, course, type, and length of treatment (Dinges & Cherry, 1995; Kleinman, 1980).

Environmental/circumstances are divided into two categories, stressors and resources. Ethnic persons, particularly those with low-SES backgrounds, tend to experience more stress than persons from middle- and upper-SES backgrounds. They also have fewer personal resources and less social supports, and are subject to more long-term personal and situational stressors (Aponte & Barnes, 1995; Aponte & Johnson, 2000; Dohrenwend & Dohrenwend, 1981; Lorion & Felner, 1986). Despite these factors, it is possible for low-SES ethnic persons to function well and to be "resilient" (Aponte & Barnes, 1995; Aponte & Johnson, 2000).

The type of resources available to ethnic populations is one of the important factors in accounting for this resiliency. Familial and social network structure is an important resource that accounts for some of the resiliency found in ethnic groups (Aponte & Barnes, 1995). African Americans, for example, have complex networks involving immediate kin, several generations of relatives, and close friends residing in the same household (Boyd-Franklin, 1990). Hispanics/Latinos and Asian Americans also rely heavily on immediate and extended family members, particularly grandparents (Lee, 1998; Martinez, 1988). Puerto Ricans have a system of *compadrazgo* (grandparents and coparents) that is built into the extended network (Ramos-McKay, Comas-Díaz, & Rivera, 1988).

Such family structures could serve to decrease role strain and the stress associated with childrearing. In fact, it has been suggested that attention to risk factors and deficit models should be shifted to a bolstering of protective factors and incorporation of the strengths of ethnic families into treatment (McAdoo, 1993). If family members are involved in treatment, strong kinship bonds and a sense of collective responsibility could greatly facilitate the treatment process. Additional strengths of many ethnic families that could also improve the effectiveness of treatment include a strong work ethic, a desire to achieve, and a strong religious/spiritual orientation (Fukuyama & Sevig, 1999; Hill, 1993).

Treatment Context

Treatment context is subdivided into three dimensions by Beutler and Clarkin (1990): setting, mode/format, and frequency/duration. Setting is further divided into restrictive (acute hospital, long-term hospital, and day hospital alternatives) and nonrestrictive (on-site and office) categories. Mode/format is divided into psychosocial mode (individual, family, and group formats) and medical/somatic modes. Frequency/duration is divided into crisis, short-term, and long-term care. Most of the available research on ethnic clients has only made comparisons between inpatient and outpatient settings and has not delineated the type and frequency of treatment (Cheung & Snowden, 1990; Snowden & Cheung, 1990; Sue et al., 1995; Sue et al., 1991). However, many treatment options, as previously noted, are clearly driven by managed care constraints.

Because of the previously mentioned cost-effective strategies implemented in the health care and mental health sectors (Hersch, 1995), a number of treatment modalities have been excluded. Current treatments tend to focus on specific problems and short-term interventions, whereas long-term care and inpatient hospitalizations have been curtailed significantly. The array of service and treatment options for all clients has been seriously constrained. However, because of the nature and complexity of mental health needs of ethnic populations and the need for a broader array of flexible services (Aponte & Crouch, 1995; Wohl & Aponte, 1995), it can be argued that managed care has had a more adverse effect on ethnic clients.

Relationship Variables

The importance of the therapeutic relationship has been underscored by a number of researchers and practitioners regardless of the theoretical orientation of the therapeutic interventions (Hays, 2001; Horvath & Luborsky, 1993; Kanfer & Schefft, 1988; Luborsky, McLellan, Diguer, Woody, & Seligman, 1997; Moursund, 1990; Teyber, 1997). Beutler and Clarkin (1990) also view the therapeutic relationship as important and break down relationship variables into two components that are particularly relevant to ethnic clients: personal compatibility matching and relationship enhancement skills (see Figure 6.1). The former includes several demographic variables (i.e., age, gender, ethnicity, and SES) and several interpersonal response patterns (i.e., interpersonal strivings, personal beliefs/values, and attributes) on which client and therapist can be matched. Relational enhancement skills include a number of components. Particularly relevant to ethnic clients is a component labeled by Beutler and Clarkin as "role induction methods" in the treatment process.

Demographic similarity between the client and therapists increased the likelihood of returning for more than one treatment session, especially among ethnic clients (Beutler & Clarkin, 1990; Terrell & Terrell, 1984). Ethnic similarity between client and therapist is often preferred by ethnic clients, and is associated with an enhanced commitment to remain in treatment (López et al., 1991; Sue et al., 1995). However, preference for an ethnically similar therapist appears to be related to a number of variables such as the client's ethnic identity, gender, level of acculturation, and trust of Whites (Bennett & BigFoot-Sipes, 1991; Helms & Carter, 1991; Sue et al., 1995; Watkins & Terrell, 1988).

Of the interpersonal response patterns, personal beliefs/values are particularly relevant in client-therapist matching for ethnic clients. Differences in beliefs/values among African Americans, Latinos, Asian Americans, Native Americans, and Whites have been noted by numerous authors (Aponte, Young Rivers, & Wohl, 1995; Atkinson et al., 1998; Dana, 1993, 2000; Gaw, 1993; Ivey et al., 1997; Seeley, 2000; Takaki, 1994; see also Pedersen et al., 2002). These differences in beliefs/values are clearly linked to ethnic identity and level of acculturation. Striking differences in beliefs/values between the client and therapist call for increased awareness and adjustments on the part of the therapist.

"Role induction methods" refer to a process that involves efforts to prepare clients for treatment by educating them about the process and outcomes of treatment before psychotherapy begins (Beutler & Clarkin, 1990). Most investigations of role induction methods have supported the value of these methods. These methods tend to improve treatment retention rates, facilitate positive perceptions of the treatment process, promote treatment compliance, and enhance psychotherapy outcomes (Beutler & Clarkin, 1990; Mayerson, 1984; Meichenbaum & Turk, 1987; Orlinsky & Howard, 1986; Wilson, 1985; Zwick & Attkisson, 1985). Most of the research in this area has, however, focused primarily on low-SES clients.

It would appear that role induction methods can be useful with ethnic clients, particularly those who are minimally acculturated. These methods include instructional methods, observational and participatory learning, and treatment contracting (Beutler & Clarkin, 1990). Although it is useful for mental health workers to educate clients about the therapeutic process, client/therapist roles, and expected outcomes, it is essential that therapists be willing and able to understand their client's explanatory belief model as previously noted and to adjust their intervention strategies and technologies accordingly (Aponte, Young Rivers, & Wohl, 1995; Aponte & Wohl, 2000; Dinges & Cherry, 1995; Kleinman, 1980; Sussman, Chapter 3 in this volume).

Strategies and Techniques

Beutler and Clarkin (1990) move beyond the predisposing and contextual factors of their Differential Treatment Selection model to focus on tailoring strategies and techniques to fit the clients presenting problems and needs. The amount of time devoted to these previously mentioned predisposing and contextual factors attests to the importance attributed to these variables in their model. Strategies and techniques refer to the complex process of conducting therapeutic work, including selecting the targets of change, the levels at which to work, and conducting the actual therapeutic work (Beutler & Clarkin, 1990).

Space does not permit a detailed discussion of the specific strategies and techniques in Beutler and Clarkin's model. The reader is directed to several works (Aponte, Young Rivers, & Wohl, 1995; Aponte & Wohl, 2000; Atkinson et al., 1998; Dana, 2000; Gaw, 1993; Ivey et al., 1997; Pedersen, 2000; Pedersen et al., 2002; Ponterotto, Asas, Suzuki, & Alexander 1995, 2001) for a more detailed discussion of therapeutic approaches that have been found to increase the effectiveness of working with ethnic clients. The remainder of this chapter will focus on two factors: credibility and giving, which are viewed as critical elements that cut across different therapeutic interventions in the application of any therapeutic strategy or technique in working with ethnic clients (Sue & Zane, 1987).

As previously noted, an ethnic client's cultural background and degree of acculturation will affect his or her attitudes toward mental health treatment (Aponte, 1997; Dinges & Cherry, 1995). For ethnic clients who are minimally acculturated, the mental health worker will have "ascribed status" because the therapist is viewed as a trained professional with authority and knowledge who commands respect (Sue & Zane, 1987). This ascribed status is initially present as the ethnic client enters treatment for the first time. This ascribed status also leads to the initial treatment strategies and techniques used by the therapist as credible by the ethnic client.

Initial ascribed status and credibility will increase the probability that the ethnic client will come back for more than one treatment session. The continued use of mental health services will be enhanced by the similarity between therapist and client on the problem conceptualization, communication style, problem-solving preference, and means of problem resolution (Sue & Zane, 1987). Such a matching of these critical factors can be achieved through the utilization of the previously identified role induction methods (Beutler & Clarkin, 1990), through the therapist adjusting or modifying his or her approaches (Aponte et al., 1995; Aponte & Wohl, 2000; Atkinson et al., 1998; Hays, 2001), or a combination of the two.

According to Sue and Zane (1987), credibility and giving emerge as the therapist develops "achieved status." Giving involves the client believing that he or she is receiving some benefit from the therapeutic process. When there are striking sociocultural differences between the therapist and client, it will be difficult for an achieved status to be obtained, and the credibility and giving components will not be present in treatment, leading to difficulty in obtaining successful therapeutic outcomes. Credibility and giving are only two variables that can contribute to successful therapeutic outcomes with ethnic clients. Sue et al. (1995) discuss in more detail the process and outcome research literature for African Americans, Latinos, Asian Americans, and Native Americans.

This chapter has highlighted the role of culture in the treatment of African Americans, Latinos, Asian Americans, and Native Americans. As noted in the chapter, two major trends will have an important impact on the treatment of ethnic clients. These trends are the changing ethnic profile of the United States and changes in the delivery of the mental health services through managed care. Culture influences all levels of the treatment process, including entry into the mental health system. It is particularly important to understand how culture influences the predisposing, relationship, and contextual factors, as well as the treatment strategies and techniques. All of these factors will have an impact on the therapeutic outcome.

ACKNOWLEDGMENTS

Appreciation is expressed to Dr. Catherine E. Aponte and Ms. Laura R. Johnson for their help and thoughtful comments on this chapter.

REFERENCES

American Psychiatric Association (1994). *Diagnostic and statistical manual of mental disorders, DSM-IV* (4th ed.). Washington, DC: American Psychiatric Association.

American Psychological Association (2003). Guidelines on multicultural education, training, research, practice, and organizational change. *American Psychologist, 58,* 377-402.

Anderson, L. P. (1991). Acculturative stress: A theory of relevance to Black Americans. *Clinical Psychology Review, 11,* 685-702.

Angel, R., & Thoits, P. (1987). The impact of culture on the cognitive structure of illness. *Culture, Medicine and Psychiatry, 11,* 465-494.

Aponte, J. F. (1997). *The role of culture in the treatment of culturally diverse populations.* Presentation at a workshop organized by the Section of Psychology of the New York Academy of Sciences, New York City.

Aponte, J. F., & Aponte, C. E. (2000). Educating and training professionals to work with ethnic populations in the twenty-first century. In J. F. Aponte & J. Wohl (Eds.), *Psychological intervention and cultural diversity* (2nd ed., pp. 250-267). Boston: Allyn and Bacon.

Aponte, J. F., & Barnes, J. M. (1995). Impact of acculturation and moderator variables on the intervention and treatment of ethnic groups. In J. F. Aponte, R. Young Rivers, & J. Wohl (Eds.), *Psychological intervention and cultural diversity* (pp. 19-39). Boston: Allyn and Bacon.

Aponte, J. F., & Bracco, H. F. (2000). Community approaches with ethnic populations. In J. F. Aponte & J. Wohl (Eds.), *Psychological intervention and cultural diversity* (2nd ed., pp. 131-148). Boston: Allyn and Bacon.

Aponte, J. F., & Clifford, J. (1995). Education and training issues for intervention with ethnic groups. In J. F. Aponte, R. Young Rivers, & J. Wohl (Eds.), *Psychological intervention and cultural diversity* (pp. 283-300). Boston: Allyn and Bacon.

Aponte, J. F., & Crouch, R. T. (1995). The changing ethnic profile of the United States. In J. F. Aponte, R. Young Rivers, & J. Wohl (Eds.), *Psychological intervention and cultural diversity* (pp. 1-18). Boston: Allyn and Bacon.

Aponte, J. F., & Crouch, R. T. (2000). The changing ethnic profile of the United States in the twenty-first century. In J. F. Aponte & J. Wohl (Eds.), *Psychological intervention and cultural diversity* (2nd ed., pp. 1-17). Boston: Allyn and Bacon.

Aponte, J. F., & Johnson, L. R. (2000). The impact of culture on intervention and treatment of ethnic populations. In J. F. Aponte & J. Wohl (Eds.), *Psychological intervention and cultural diversity* (2nd ed., pp. 18-39). Boston: Allyn and Bacon.

Aponte, J. F., & Wohl, J. (Eds.). (2000). *Psychological intervention and cultural diversity* (2nd ed.). Boston: Allyn and Bacon.

Aponte, J. F., Young Rivers, R., & Wohl, J. (Eds.). (1995). *Psychological intervention and cultural diversity.* Boston: Allyn and Bacon.

Atkinson, D. R., Morton, G., & Sue, D. W. (1998). *Counseling American minorities: A cross-cultural perspective* (5th ed.). Boston: McGraw-Hill.

Barlow, D. H. (1994). Psychological interventions in the era of managed competition. *Clinical Psychology: Science and Practice, 1,* 109-122.

Belar, C. D. (1995). Collaboration in capitated care: Challenges for psychology. *Professional Psychology: Research and Practice, 26,* 139-146.

Bemak, F. P., & Chung, R. C. (2000). Psychological interventions with immigrants and refugees. In J. F. Aponte & J. Wohl (Eds.), *Psychological intervention and cultural diversity* (2nd ed., pp. 200-219). Boston: Allyn and Bacon.

Bennett, S. K., & BigFoot-Sipes, D. S. (1991). American Indian and White college student preferences for counselor characteristics. *Journal of Counseling Psychology, 38,* 440-445.

Berry, J. W. (1980). Acculturation as varieties of adaptation. In A. M. Padilla (Ed.), *Acculturation: Theory, model, and some new findings* (pp. 9-25). Boulder, CO: Westview.

Berry, J. W., & Kim, U. (1988). Acculturation and mental health. In P. R. Dasen, J. W. Berry, & N. Sartorius (Eds.), *Health and cross-cultural psychology: Toward applications* (pp. 207-236). Newbury Park, CA: Sage.

Betancourt, H., & López, S. R. (1993). The study of culture, ethnicity, and race in American psychology. *American Psychologist, 48,* 629-637.

Beutler, L. E., & Clarkin, J. F. (1990). *Systematic treatment selection: Toward targeted therapeutic interventions.* New York: Brunner/Mazel.

Boyd-Franklin, N. (1990). Five key factors in the treatment of Black families. In G. W. Saba, B. M. Karrer, & K. V. Hardy (Eds.), *Minorities and family therapy* (pp. 53-69). New York: Haworth.

Cheung, F. K., & Snowden, L. R. (1990). Community mental health and ethnic minority populations. *Community Mental Health Journal, 26,* 277-291.

Clinton, J. J., McCormick, K., & Besteman, J. (1994). Enhancing clinical practice: The role of practice guidelines. *American Psychologist, 49,* 30-33.

Cross, W. E., Jr. (1991). *Shades of Black: Diversity of African-American identity.* Philadelphia, PA: Temple University Press.

Cross, W. E., Jr. (1995). The psychology of Nigrescence: Revising the Cross model. In J. G. Ponterotto, J. M., Casas, L. A. Suzuki, & C. M. Alexander (Eds.), *Handbook of multicultural counseling* (pp. 93-122). Thousand Oaks, CA: Sage.

Dana, R. H. (1993). *Multicultural assessment perspectives for professional psychology.* Boston: Allyn and Bacon.

Dana, R. H. (Ed.). (1998). *Handbook of cross-cultural and multicultural personality assessment.* Mahwah, NJ: Erlbaum.

Dana, R. H. (2000). *Multicultural intervention perspectives for professional psychology.* Upper Saddle River, NJ: Prentice-Hall.

DeLeon, P. H., VandenBos, G. R., & Bulatao, E. Q. (1991). Managed mental health care: A history of the federal policy initiative. *Professional Psychology: Research and Practice, 22*, 15-25.

DeVita, C. J. (1996). The United States at mid-decade. *Population Bulletin, 50* (4), 1-48.

Dinges, N. G., & Cherry, D. (1995). Symptom expression and the use of mental health services among American ethnic minorities. In J. F. Aponte, R. Young Rivers, & J. Wohl (Eds.), *Psychological interventions and cultural diversity* (pp. 40-56). Boston: Allyn and Bacon.

Dohrenwend, B. S., & Dohrenwend, B. P. (1981). Hypotheses about stress processes linking social class to various types of psychopathology. *American Journal of Community Psychology, 9*, 146-159.

Draguns, J. G. (2000). Psychopathology and ethnicity. In J. F. Aponte & J. Wohl (Eds.), *Psychological intervention and cultural diversity* (2nd ed., pp. 40-58). Boston: Allyn and Bacon.

Escobar, J. I. (1993). Psychiatric epidemiology. In A. C. Gaw (Ed.), *Culture, ethnicity, and mental illness* (pp. 43-73). Washington, DC: American Psychiatry Press.

Frank, R. G., & VandenBos, G. R. (1994). Health care reform: The 1993-1994 evolution. *American Psychologist, 49*, 851-854.

Fukuyama, M., & Sevig, T. D. (1999). *Integrating spirituality into multicultural counseling.* Thousand Oaks, CA: Sage.

Garcia, M., & Lega, L. T. (1979). Development of a Cuban ethnic identity questionnaire. *Hispanic Journal of Behavioral Sciences, 1*, 247-261.

Gaw, A. C. (Ed.). (1993). *Culture, ethnicity, and mental illness.* Washington, DC: American Psychiatric Press.

Good, B. J. (1993). Culture, diagnosis and comorbidity. *Culture, Medicine, and Psychiatry, 16*, 427-446.

Grant, R. W. (1995). Interventions with ethnic minority elderly. In J. F. Aponte, R. Young Rivers, & J. Wohl (Eds.), *Psychological interventions and culture diversity* (pp. 199-214). Boston: Allyn and Bacon.

Hays, P. A. (2001). *Addressing cultural competencies in practice: A framework for clinicians and counselors.* Washington, DC: American Psychological Association.

Helms, J. E. (1990). *Black and White racial identity: Therapy, research, and practice.* Westport, CT: Greenwood Press.

Helms, J. E. (1995). An update of Helm's White and people of color racial identity models. In J. G. Ponterotto, J. M. Casas, L. A. Suzuki, & C. M. Alexander (Eds.), *Handbook of multicultural counseling* (pp. 181-198). Thousand Oaks, CA: Sage.

Helms, J. E., & Carter, R. T. (1991). Relationships of White and Black racial identity attitudes and demographic similarity to counselor preferences. *Journal of Counseling Psychology, 38*, 446-457.

Hersch, L. (1995). Adapting to health care reform and managed care: Three strategies for survival and growth. *Professional Psychology: Research and Practice, 26*, 16-26.

Hill, R. B. (1993). Dispelling myths and building on strengths: Supporting African American families. *Family Resource Coalition Report, 12*, 3-5.

Hoffmann, T., Dana, R. H., & Bolton, B. (1985). Measured acculturation and MMPI-168 performance of Native American adults. *Journal of Cross-Cultural Psychology, 16*, 243-256.

Horvath, A., & Luborsky, L. (1993). The role of the therapeutic alliance in psychotherapy. *Journal of Consulting and Clinical Psychology, 61*, 561-573.

Ivey, A. E., Ivey, M. B., & Simek-Morgan, L. (1997). *Counseling and psychotherapy: A multicultural perspective.* Boston: Allyn and Bacon.

Jackson, B. (1975). Black identity development. *MELFORM: Journal of Educational Diversity & Innovation, 2*, 19-25.

Kanfer, F. H., & Schefft, B. K. (1988). *Guiding the process of therapeutic change,* Champaign, IL: Research Press.

Kitano, H. H. L. (1989). A model for counseling Asian Americans. In P. B. Pedersen, J. G. Draguns, W. J. Lonner, J. E. Trimble (Eds.), *Counseling across cultures* (3rd ed.) (pp. 139-151). Honolulu: University of Hawaii Press.

Kleinman, A. (1980). *Patients and healers in the context of culture.* Berkele, CA: University of California Press.

Koss, J. D. (1990). Somatization and somatic complaint syndromes among Hispanics: Overview and ethno-psychological perspectives. *Transcultural Psychiatric Review, 27*, 5-29.

Koss-Chioino, J. D. (2000). Traditional and folk approaches among ethnic minorities. In J. F. Aponte & J. Wohl (Eds.), *Psychological intervention and cultural diversity* (2nd ed., pp. 149-166). Boston: Allyn and Bacon.

Kurasaki, K. S., Sue, S., Chun, C., & Gee, K. (2000). Ethnic minority intervention and treatment research. In J. F. Aponte & J. Wohl (Eds.), *Psychological intervention and cultural diversity* (2nd ed., pp. 234-249). Boston: Allyn and Bacon.

LaFromboise, T. (1998). American Indian mental health policy. In D.R. Atkinson, G. Morton, & D. W. Sue (Eds.), *Counseling American minorities* (5th ed., pp. 137-158). Boston: McGraw-Hill.

LaFromboise, T., Coleman, H. L. K., & Gerton, J. (1993). Psychological impact of biculturalism: Evidence and theory. *Psychological Bulletin, 114*, 395-412.

Lee, E. (1998). *American-Asian families: A clinical guide to working with families*. New York: Guilford.

Leong, F. T., Wagner, N. S., & Tata, S. P. (1995). Racial and ethnic variations in help-seeking attitudes. In J. G. Ponterotto, J. M. Casas, L. A. Suzuki, & C. M. Alexander (Eds.), *Handbook of multicultural counseling* (pp. 415-438). Thousand Oaks, CA: Sage.

López, S. R., López, A. A., & Fong, K. T. (1991). Mexican Americans' initial preferences for counselors: The role of ethnic factors. *Journal of Counseling Psychology, 38,* 487-496.

Lorion, R. P., & Felner, R. D. (1986). Research on mental health interventions with the disadvantaged. In S. L. Garfield & A. E. Bergin (Eds.), *Handbook of psychotherapy and behavior change* (3rd ed., pp. 739-775). New York: Wiley.

Luborsky, L., McLellan, A. T., Diguer, L., Woody, G., & Seligman, D. A. (1997). The psychotherapist matters: Comparison of outcomes across twenty-two therapists and seven patient samples. *Clinical Psychology: Science and Practice, 4,* 53-65.

Marcos, L. R. (1976). Bilinguals in psychotherapy: Language as an emotional barrier. *American Journal of Psychotherapy, 30,* 552-560.

Marcos, L. R., & Urcuyo, L. (1979). Dynamic psychotherapy with the bilingual patient. *American Journal of Psychotherapy, 33,* 331-338.

Marin, G., Sabogal, F., Marin, B. V., Otero-Sabogal, R., & Perez-Stable, E. (1987). Development of a short acculturation scale for Hispanics. *Hispanic Journal of Behavioral Sciences, 9,* 183-205.

Martinez, C., Jr. (1988). Mexican-Americans. In L. Comas-Díaz & E. E. H. Griffin (Eds.), *Clinical guidelines in cross-cultural mental health* (pp. 182-232). New York: Wiley.

Mayerson, N. H. (1984). Preparing clients for group therapy: A critical review and theoretical formulation. *Clinical Psychology Review, 4,* 191-213.

McAdoo, J. L. (1993). Understanding fathers: Human services perspectives in theory and practice. *Family Resource Coalition Report, 12*(1), 18-20.

McCombs, H. G. (1997). *Provision of mental health services in a managed care environment: The good, the bad and the ugly.* Presentation at the Fifth Annual Conference on Behavior, Neurobiology, Substance Abuse and Culture, Los Angeles, CA.

Meichenbaum, D. J., & Turk, D. C. (1987). *Facilitating treatment adherence: A practitioner's guidebook.* New York: Plenum Press.

Milburn, N. G., & Curry, T. L. (1995). Intervention and treatment for ethnic minority homeless adults. In J. F. Aponte, R. Young Rivers, & J. Wohl (Eds.), *Psychological intervention and cultural diversity* (pp. 250-265). Boston: Allyn and Bacon.

Milliones, J. (1980). Construction of a Black consciousness measure: Psychotherapeutic implications. *Psychotherapy: Theory, Research and Practice, 17,* 175-182.

Moursund, J. (1990). *The process of counseling and therapy* (2nd ed.). Englewood Cliffs, NJ: Prentice Hall.

Neal, A. M., & Turner, S. M. (1991). Anxiety disorders research with African Americans: Current status. *Psychological Bulletin, 109,* 400-410.

Neighbors, H. W. (1985). Seeking professional help for personal problems: Black Americans' use of health and mental health services. *Community Mental Health Journal, 21,* 156-166.

Neighbors, H. W., Caldwell, C. H., Thompson, E., & Jackson, J. S. (1994). Help seeking behavior and unmet need. In S. Friedman (Ed.), *Anxiety disorders in African Americans* (pp. 26-39). New York: Springer.

O'Hare, W. P. (1992). America's minorities—The demographics of diversity. *Population Bulletin, 47* (4), 1-47.

Orlinsky, D. E., & Howard, K. T. (1986). Process and outcome in psychotherapy. In S. L. Garfield & A. E. Bergin (Eds.), *Handbook of psychotherapy and behavior change* (3rd ed.) (pp. 311-384). New York: Wiley.

Paradis, C. H., Friedman, S., Lazar, R. M., Grubea, J., & Kesselman, M. (1992). Use of a structured interview to diagnose anxiety disorders in a minority population. *Hospital and Community Psychiatry, 43,* 61-64.

Parham, T. A., & Helms, J. E. (1981). The influence of Black student's racial identity attitudes on preference for counselor's race. *Journal of Counseling Psychology, 28,* 250-257.

Pedersen, P. B. (2000). *Handbook for developing multicultural awareness* (3rd ed.). Alexandria, VA: American Counseling Association.

Pedersen, P. B., Draguns, J. G., Lonner, W. J., & Trimble, J. E. (Eds.). (2002). *Counseling across cultures* (5th ed.). Thousand Oaks, CA: Sage.

Penn, N. E., Kar, S., Kramer, J., Skinner, J., & Zambrana, R. E. (1995). Panel VI: Ethnic minorities, health care systems, and behavior. *Health Psychology, 14,* 641-646.

Ponterotto, J. G., Casas, J. M., Suzuki, L. A., & Alexander, C. M. (Eds.). (1995). *Handbook of multicultural counseling*. Thousand Oaks, CA: Sage.

Ponterotto, J. G., Casas, J. M., Suzuki, L. A., & Alexander, C. M. (Eds.). (2001). *Handbook of multicultural counseling* (2nd ed.). Thousand Oaks, CA: Sage.

President's Commission on Mental Health (1978). *Task panel reports: The nature and scope of the problem. Volume 2.* Washington, DC: U.S. Government Printing Office.

Ramos-McKay, J. M., Comas-Díaz, L., & Rivera, L. A. (1988). Puerto Ricans. In L. Comas-Díaz & E. E. H. Griffith (Eds.), *Clinical guidelines in cross-cultural mental health* (pp. 204-232). New York: Wiley.

Randall-David, E. (1989). *Strategies for working with culturally diverse clients*. Washington, DC: Association for the Care of Children's Health.

Rogler, L., & Cortes, D. (1993). Help-seeking pathways: A unifying concept in mental health care. *American Journal of Psychiatry, 150,* 554-561.

Root, M. P. P. (Ed.). (1992). *Racially mixed people in America*. Newbury Park, CA: Sage.

Russell, D. M. (1988). Language and psychotherapy: The influence of nonstandard English in clinical practice. In L. Comas-Díaz & E. E H. Griffith (Eds.), *Clinical guidelines in cross-cultural mental health* (pp. 33-68). New York: Wiley.

Schulberg, H. C., & Rush, A. J. (1994). Clinical practice guidelines for managing major depression in primary care practice: Implications for psychologists. *American Psychologist, 49,* 34-41.

Sciarra, D. T., & Ponterotto, J. G. (1990). Counseling the Hispanic bilingual family: Challenges to the therapeutic process. *Psychotherapy, 28,* 473-479.

Seeley, K. M. (2000). *Cultural psychotherapy: Working with culture in the clinical encounter*. Northvale, NJ: Jason Aronson.

Sherbourne, C. D., Hays, R. D., & Wells, K. B. (1995). Personal and psychosocial risk factors for physical and mental health outcomes and course of depression among depressed patients. *Journal of Consulting and Clinical Psychology, 63,* 345-355.

Simons, R. C., & Hughes, C. C. (1993). In A. C. Gaw (Ed.), *Culture, ethnicity, and mental illness* (pp. 75-99). Washington, DC: American Psychiatry Press.

Snowden, L. R., & Cheung, F. K. (1990). Use of inpatient mental health services by members of ethnic minority groups. *American Psychologist, 45,* 347-355.

Sodowsky, G. R., & Carey, J. C. (1987). Asian Indian immigrants in America: Factors related to adjustment. *Journal of Multicultural Counseling and Development, 15,* 129-141.

Sodowsky, G. R., Lai, E. W., & Plake, B. S. (1991). Moderating effects of socio-cultural variables on acculturation attitudes of Hispanics and Asian Americans. *Journal of Counseling & Development, 70,* 194-204.

Spickard, P. R. (1992). The illogic of American racial categories. In M. P. P. Root (Ed.), *Racially mixed people in America* (pp. 12-23). Newbury Park, CA: Sage.

Sue, S., Chun, C., & Gee, K. (1995). Ethnic minority interventions and treatment research. In J. F. Aponte, R. Young Rivers, & J. Wohl (Eds.), *Psychological interventions and cultural diversity* (pp. 266-282). Boston: Allyn and Bacon.

Sue, S., Fujino, D. C., Hu, L., Takeuchi, D. T., & Zane, N. W. S. (1991). Community mental health services for ethnic minority groups: A test of the cultural responsiveness hypothesis. *Journal of Consulting and Clinical Psychology, 59,* 533-540.

Sue, S., & Zane, W. (1987). The role of culture and cultural techniques in psychotherapy: A critique and reformulation. *American Psychologist, 42,* 37-45.

Suinn, R. M., Richard-Figueroa, K., Lew, S., & Vigil, S. (1987). The Suinn-Lew Asian Self-Identity Acculturation Scale: An initial report. *Education and Psychological Measurement, 47,* 401-407.

Takaki, R. (Ed.). (1994). *From different shores: Perspectives on race and ethnicity in America*. New York: Oxford University Press.

Terrell, R., & Terrell, S. (1984). Race of counselor, client sex, cultural mistrust level, and premature termination from counseling among Black clients. *Journal of Counseling Psychology, 31,* 371-375.

Teyber, E. (1997). *Interpersonal process in psychotherapy: A relational approach* (3rd ed.). Pacific Grove, CA: Brooks/Cole.

U.S. Bureau of Census (2000a). *U.S. Census 2000: DP-1, Profile of general demographic characteristics*. Washington, DC: U.S. Government Printing Office.

U.S. Bureau of Census (2000b). *U.S. Census 2000: DP 2, Profile of selected social characteristics*. Washington, DC: U.S. Government Printing Office.

Watkins, C. E., Jr., & Terrell, F. (1988). Mistrust level and its effects on counseling expectations in Black client-White counselor relationships: An analogue study. *Journal of Counseling Psychology, 35,* 194-197.

Wilson, D. O. (1985). The effects of systematic client preparation, severity, and treatment setting on dropout rate in short-term psychotherapy. *Journal of Social and Clinical Psychology, 3,* 62-70.

Wilson, M. N., Kohn, L. P., & Lee, T. S. (2000). Cultural relativistic approach toward ethnic minorities in family therapy. In J. F. Aponte & J. Wohl (Eds.), *Psychological intervention and cultural diversity* (2nd ed., pp. 92-109). Boston: Allyn and Bacon.

Wohl, J. (1995). Traditional individual psychotherapy and ethnic minorities. In J. F. Aponte, R. Young Rivers, & J. Wohl (Eds.), *Psychological interventions and cultural diversity* (pp. 74-91). Boston: Allyn and Bacon.

Wohl, J. (2000). Psychotherapy and cultural diversity. In J. F. Aponte & J. Wohl (Eds.), *Psychological intervention and cultural diversity* (2nd ed., pp. 75-91). Boston: Allyn and Bacon.

Wohl, J., & Aponte, J. F. (1995). Common themes and future aspects. In J. F. Aponte, R. Young Rivers, & J. Wohl (Eds.), *Psychological interventions and cultural diversity* (pp. 301-316). Boston: Allyn and Bacon.

Wood, W. D., & Sherrets, S. D. (1984). Requests for outpatient mental health services: A comparison of Whites and Blacks. *Comprehensive Psychiatry, 25,* 329-334.

Yee, A. H., Fairchild, H. H., Weizmann, F., & Wyatt, G. E. (1993). Addressing psychology's problems with race. *American Psychologist, 48,* 1132-1140.

Young Porter, R. (2000a). Understanding and treating ethnic minority youth. In J. F. Aponte & J. Wohl (Eds.), *Psychological intervention and cultural diversity* (2nd ed., pp. 167-182). Boston: Allyn and Bacon.

Young Porter, R. (2000b). Clinical issues and interventions with ethnic minority women. In J. F. Aponte & J. Wohl (Eds.), *Psychological intervention and cultural diversity* (2nd ed., pp. 183-199). Boston: Allyn and Bacon.

Zwick, R., & Attkisson, C. C. (1985). Effectiveness of a client pretherapy orientation videotape, *Journal of Counseling Psychology, 32,* 514-524.

Culturally Oriented Psychotherapy with Refugees

Fred Bemak and Rita Chi-Ying Chung
George Mason University

The United Nations (1995) has estimated that 70 to 100 million persons in the world today are displaced as a result of widespread political instability, regional and national conflicts, war, genocide, social and economic upheaval, poverty, natural disasters, deportation, and population increases. It should be noted that there is a distinction between displaced persons with regards to "forced" or "free" migration (Murphy, 1977) whereby refugees are involuntarily forced to relocate, while immigrants voluntarily choose to leave their communities or countries. Refugees consist of more than 26 million people worldwide (Balian, 1997). Despite growing numbers of refugees, many countries are increasingly reluctant to resettle them, resulting in governments more rigidly interpreting the 1951 United Nations Convention governing the determination of refugee status (Jupp, 1994).

The international dilemma is exemplified in Great Britain, where recently there has been a controversy over what constitutes refugee status. The British government has defined refugees as victims of war, excluding those suffering from economic hardship due to war, national and state conflict, and natural disasters, which is the present plight of many of the refugees. The result of this has been national debate about who is a refugee and therefore admissible to Great Britain under these terms. One serious aspect of this debate is the neglect of victims of other war atrocities, such as the widespread repeated rape of women and girls who currently do not, but could, fall into this category. The repercussion of the narrow and rigid definition of refugee status is that refugees, who are already in a vulnerable position, may experience retraumatization due to the difficulties and stringent regulations that many are subjected to in entering developed or Western countries (Baker, 1992; Cox & Amelsvoort, 1994).

Similar to the British controversy over refugee status, the ongoing international debates regarding refugees are timely given the 35 current ongoing international conflicts and 118 countries currently involved in the resettlement of refugees. With the current status of geopolitical conflict and ongoing natural disasters, it is anticipated that there will be a continuation of the displacement of refugees emigrating to other countries. Western countries like the United States, which already have almost 10 percent of the population from refugee backgrounds (Balian, 1997), may again reexamine policy and practice. Given these realities and the growing number of refugees in the United States and other resettlement countries, this chapter focuses on specific issues encountered by refugees once in the resettlement countries, an examination of refugee mental health, and a discussion on culturally responsive psychotherapy.

REFUGEE RESETTLEMENT ISSUES

Although refugees come from different home countries with dramatic variations in culture, customs, beliefs, values, social practices, and religion, they also have shared pre- and postmigration experiences. When examining premigration experiences, economic hardship, social and environmental dislocation, language and cultural adjustments, and acculturation processes, it is evident that there is a great extent of commonality in the refugee experience (Berrol, 1995). Shared premigration experiences include the exposure to the atrocities of war and other traumatic and stressful life events; forced or involuntary migration with little or no planning, preparation, or choice; refugee camp experiences; and a profound loss and separation from culture, community, friends, and family. Refugees carry these premigration experiences with them to their resettlement country, which has an impact on postmigration adjustment.

Common postmigration experiences for refugees consist of acculturating to a new society and thus encountering the psychosocial processes that are inherent in the adjustment process. Bemak (1989) outlined a three-phase refugee developmental model of acculturation with a goal of biculturalism, whereby refugees first attempt to use existing skills to master the new environment, then integrate old and new skills as they become more acculturated, and finally they combine old and new skills with a enhanced sense of the future. Acculturation only takes place when psychological safety is acquired through a mastery of culture and language, leading to the establishment of realistic future goals. This model is consistent with reports from Tayabas and Pok (1983) who identified the first one to two years of resettlement as crucial. During these initial years, refugees seek to fulfill basic needs, such as employment and housing. This period is particularly important since it is during these beginning years that refugees learn the new skills that facilitate their mastery over the new environment and establish resources from which they can draw upon in the future. During this time, not only do the refugees acquire skills, but the foundation for "learning to learn" is also established, setting the way for future psychosocial adjustment and acculturation. Cultural integration emphasizing biculturalism has been found to produce the most successful and healthy adaptation and acculturation (Berry, 1986; Wong-Reiger & Quintana, 1987).

Language Barriers

Language plays an important part in the psychosocial adjustment of refugees. The transition to a new language may symbolize a type of psychological departure from one's culture and history to the new culture. Yet learning the language of the resettlement country is imperative for successful resettlement. Language is important in that without language skills it is difficult to fully access community resources and become culturally empowered, thus creating barriers to successful adjustment (Bemak, Chung, & Pedersen, 2003). Learning a new language may be particularly frustrating for those who are illiterate in their mother language, or who have had little or no education prior to their migration. There is a high correlation between language acquisition and psychosocial adjustment to the resettlement country (Chung & Kagawa-Singer, 1993; Lin, Masuda, & Tazuma, 1982).

Family Dynamics

Difficulties in learning a new language for parents may manifest in family role reversals. Children learn the language of a new culture more rapidly than their parents, resulting in the children becoming interpreters for their parents. Becoming the interpreters exposes children to information that has traditionally been limited to adults and perpetuates a sense of dependency by parents. Furthermore, children may witness a transformation of their parents from competent and strong caretakers to depressed, helpless, and overwhelmed individuals. Confidence in their parents may therefore be undermined. In addition, children, through exposure to school and the media, may acculturate faster than their parents. Conflicts arise when children show less respect and affinity for traditional cultural values and question and challenge parents about traditional customs and practices. This dramatic change in family dynamics upsets normative standards for families and creates difficulties for both children and parents (Baptiste, 1993; Bemak & Chung, 2002). Parents may feel that they are losing authority and control over their children, and in turn, children may feel independent of parents and hence have the courage to challenge parents about traditional cultural values.

Employment

Employment is another factor related to successful psychosocial adjustment. Skills, education, and training in one's country of origin may not be transferable in the new country. It is often necessary for refugees to undergo retraining, lose professional stature, or even acquire new skills that provide a better fit with the host country's demands and employment needs. Securing gainful employment and being underemployed may cause psychological distress such as lowered self-esteem, depression, feelings of worthlessness, and a sense of lack of control over one's life and destiny (Beiser, 1987; Buchwald, Manson, Ginges, Keanne, & Kinzie, 1993; Chung & Bemak, 2000; Hinton, Tiet, Tran, & Chesney, 1997). Further, due to unemployment or underemployment of refugee men, refugee women who may have traditionally been caretakers may work to contribute to the family income. This change in traditional gender roles frequently results in conflict within the family, especially when the men are underemployed or unemployed and women are contributing financially and hence gaining independence (Chung, Bemak, & Okazaki, 1997; Chung & Okazaki, 1991).

Survivor's Guilt

Another aspect of psychosocial adjustment relates to ambivalence about the actual relocation and ensuing acculturation. The uncertainty may correlate with deeper existential questions regarding the meaning of one's existence, especially as one becomes psychologically secure enough to reflect on past experiences. One result of this reflection may be survivor's guilt. Numerous refugees have reported experiencing survivor's guilt (Brown, 1982; Lin et al., 1982; Tobin & Friedman, 1983), which leaves them with feelings of guilt about their relatives and friends who were left behind or who died as a result of the conditions in the home country. Reports in the resettlement country about the conditions in his or her home country may also contribute to survivor's guilt (Bemak, Chung, & Bornemann, 1996; Bemak, Chung, & Pedersen, 2003). With the difficulty of strong residual feelings that may interfere with learning new skills and moving ahead with one's life, survivor's guilt may be one reason for refugees' poor adaptation in the resettlement country.

REFUGEE MENTAL HEALTH ISSUES

Clearly, refugees have experienced multiple dramatic stressful life events. It has been well documented that there is a relationship between highly stressful life events and long-term effects on mental health (e.g., Davidson & Baum, 1986; Holen, 1991; Kessler, Sonnega, Bromet, Hughes, & Nelson, 1995; Kilpatrick & Resnick, 1993). It is therefore not surprising that refugees exhibit and are at risk for developing serious mental health disorders, including posttraumatic stress disorder (PTSD). Studies utilizing clinical and community populations have found that the refugee population exhibits a higher incidence of psychopathology and other psychological problems compared to the general population of the resettlement country (e.g., Bemak & Greenberg, 1994; Garcia-Peltoniemi, 1991; Kinzie, 1993; Marsella, Friedman, & Spain, 1993; Mollica & Lavelle, 1988; Weisaeth & Eitinger, 1993; Williams & Berry, 1991). It has been reported that PTSD among clinical refugee populations is at a rate of 50 percent or higher, while depressive disorders range from 42 percent to 89 percent (Bemak & Greenberg, 1994; Hauff & Vaglum, 1995; Mollica, Wyshak, & Lavelle, 1985; Ramsay, Gorst-Unsworth, & Turner, 1993; Van Velsen, Gorst-Unsworth, & Turner, 1996). Studies using community samples have found depression rates of 15 percent to 80 percent (Carlson & Rosser-Hogan, 1991; Pernice & Brook, 1994; Westermeyer, 1988).

At-risk Subgroups

Within the refugee population there are specific subgroups that have been identified as being particularly at risk for developing serious mental health disorders. Older refugees have been identified as one such group (Buchwald et al., 1993; Kinzie et al., 1990; Matsuoka, 1993; Weine et al., 1995). Older refugees entering a resettlement country carry a longer history in their country of origin and maintain more pronounced roots within their culture. This may result in greater difficulties in changing established norms, thus accentuating mental health problems associated with acculturation. Further, older men have difficulty finding jobs and may be disadvantaged in terms of having to learn a new language, acquire new skills, and attain jobs relative to their status and expectations. Hence, they tend to experience more social isolation and increased feelings of worthlessness because the pace of acculturation is slower for them (Beiser, 1987; Buchwald et al., 1993; Chung & Bemak, 2000; Hinton et al., 1997).

Rape and sexual abuse are often a by-product of war and armed conflict. Many refugee women and girls have been subjected to rape and sexual abuse during the war, while escaping, and in refugee camps (Refugee Women in Development, 1990). In addition, a large percentage of refugee women are widowed due to their husbands being killed or lost during the war, and/or they have lost their children due to starvation or death (Caspi, Poole, Mollica, & Frankel, 1998; Mollica, Wyshak, & Lavelle, 1985; Refugee Women in Development, 1990). These women also experience extreme difficulties in the adjustment to the resettlement country due to low levels of education and English proficiency, little family and emotional support, and limited access to community resources (Chung, 2000). Due to the high intensity of traumatic events experienced by refugee women, this group has been classified as a group at risk for developing serious mental health disorders (Refugee Women in Development, 1990).

Unaccompanied minors, that is, children and adolescents who were not accompanied by close family members during their resettlement are another group at risk (Nidorf, 1985; Williams & Westermeyer, 1983). This group often suffers from the loss of their parents as a result of political and social upheaval, or, if their parents are still living, feelings that they have been rejected or abandoned by their parents. Those who experience trauma during escape or in the camps may blame their parents for not protecting them and subjecting them to vulnerable and horrific situations. Certain events, such as holidays, receiving letters from home, or reports by the media may trigger increased anxiety, loneliness, homesickness, depression, or feelings of guilt (Chung & Okazaki, 1991).

Pre- and Postmigration Predictors of Psychological Distress

Several predictors identified in the research lead to mental health problems. One consistently identified major predictor of psychological distress is, not surprisingly, the experience of premigration trauma (Bemak & Greenberg, 1994; Chung & Bemak, 2002; Chung & Kagawa-Singer, 1993; Hinton et al., 1997; Mollica et al., 1998; Nicholson, 1997). Even if refugees appear to be adjusting, or have lived in the resettlement country for a period of time, trauma experienced during premigration may still have a major effect in their lives (Chung & Kagawa-Singer, 1993; Hauff & Valgum, 1995; Hinton et al., 1997). This premigration trauma, which the authors of this chapter have labeled "emotional noise," interferes with the daily functioning and activities of the refugee, resulting in associations, thoughts, and subsequent feelings attached to seemingly benign external stimuli. An example of emotional noise is the refugee who is employed in the resettlement country as a driver of a bakery delivery truck who becomes startled, fearful, and disoriented whenever he hears a car backfire. He associates this noise with gunfire and flashes back to memories of life-threatening premigration experiences. It is unclear when or what will initiate the "emotional noise," but it is highly problematic in that it creates a psychological disturbance for him that is intrusive and disorienting.

Another predictor of psychological distress relates to adults who are not in a significant relationship, that is, those who are unmarried, divorced, or widowed (Noh, Wu, Speechley, & Kasper, 1992). This may point to the need for adults to be in a significant relationship during the resettlement process in order to give and receive financial and emotional support and assistance during the complex process of acculturation. Findings have also shown that older refugees, lower socioeconomic status, low income (Chung & Kagawa-Singer, 1993), welfare dependence (Chung & Bemak, 1996), and unemployment (Hurh & Kim, 1990) are also indicators for mental health problems. The lack of financial resources enhances the hardship experienced by many refugees, especially those who are financially struggling to support their family and in some cases extended families (Chung & Bemak, 1996). Furthermore, the lack of education and proficiency in English has been shown to be predictors for mental health problems (e.g., Bagheri, 1992; Chung, Bemak, & Kagawa-Singer, 1998; Matsuoka, 1993). Lacking education, technical skills, or a profession that is transferable to the resettlement country also contributes to lower income levels and associated mental health problems. Thus, a refugee who was an engineer or physician when in his or her home country may not find equivalent employment in the resettlement country, instead finding work sorting mail in a large company office. This may be due to having nontransferable skills or the lack of language proficiency to effectively communicate in the host country.

CULTURE AND MENTAL HEALTH

Refugees are frequently from dramatically different cultures as compared to the culture of the resettlement country. Subsequently, it is critical that mental health professionals understand the cultural background of refugees so they can provide effective and culturally responsive services. This is particularly important since the refugees' beliefs about mental health may differ from Western views of mental health (Bemak, Chung, & Pedersen, 2003). Their conceptualization of mental health does not only affect their manifestation of mental health problems (Chung & Kagawa-Singer, 1993), but also their help-seeking behavior (Chung & Lin, 1994) and expectations in treatment and services (Chung, Bemak, & Okazaki, 1997). For example, refugees that come from a culture where deceased ancestors continue to provide wisdom and guidance for the living would seek out help from individuals who respected and honored their cultural belief systems, such as a spiritualist. The expectations of treatment would be for the spiritualist to assist in communicating with the ancestors to establish the cause of the problem as well as subsequent solutions.

It is essential that clinical diagnoses and interventions be consistent with the client's cultural belief system, values, and healing practices. Kleinman and Good (1985) emphasize the need to understand, accept, and confirm the client's cultural conceptualization of their problem. To be effective, Sue and Zane (1987) suggest that mental health professionals need to maintain both ascribed and achieved credibility with their refugee clients. Ascribed credibility is associated with a mental health professional's position or role, such as age, gender, or expertise. Achieved credibility, on the other hand, is associated with what the mental health professional actually does in the session to gain the trust and confidence of the client. Therefore, if mental health professionals have a low ascribed credibility with their client, they may achieve credibility by displaying cultural sensitivity.

Despite the increased attention given to culture and mental health, the basic Western psychological theories continue to focus on individualistic societies rather than on collectivistic cultures. This negates many of the cultural origins of the refugees of today, where family, community, clan, and/or tribe have far more importance than the individual. Furthermore, the Western perspective continues to dichotomize the mind and body, whereas many non-Western countries that are home to the refugees conceive of the mind and body as integral parts of the whole (Chung & Kagawa-Singer, 1995; Pedersen, 2000). The result of the merging of mind and body has a profound impact on the conceptualization of health and illness and therefore on healing. For example, many refugees come from cultures where physical aliments may be a manifestation of psychological problems, so that refugees who complain about headaches or stomach pains may actually be alluding to psychological difficulties. It has been recommended that Western mental health practitioners working with refugees redefine their cultural perspectives and view of mental health to coincide with the refugee's worldview (Kagawa-Singer & Chung, 1994; Pedersen, 1988, 1991; Sue & Sue, 1990). Similarly, it is recommended that practitioners present an openness to traditional healers and at times even forge partnerships with traditional healers to treat specific problems of the refugees (Bemak & Chung, 2002; Bemak, Chung, & Bornemann, 1996).

MULTILEVEL MODEL (MLM) OF PSYCHOTHERAPY FOR REFUGEES

Given the complexities of providing mental health services to refugees, Bemak, Chung, and Bornemann (1996) developed the multilevel model (MLM) of psychotherapy for refugees. The model takes into account the unique experiences of refugees, including premigration factors such as loss of culture, family, friends, and community; separation; transition; mental health predisposition; experience and exposure to trauma; refugee camp experience; the escape process; and circumstances leading to migration. The process of acculturation is also taken into account in this culturally sensitive model. The model includes a psychosocial adjustment to a new culture as well as assistance in defining and looking toward the future and new perspectives in the refugee's life. The model also stresses that for therapists to be one step closer in achieving culturally sensitive psychotherapy, they must not only have skills in individual, family, and/or group psychotherapy, but also an awareness of the refugee experience, as well as cultural, social, and political awareness.

The MLM is a psychoeducational model that integrates cognitive, behavioral, and affective factors with an underpinning of cultural change as a foundation for examining intrapersonal and interpersonal processes. The MLM includes four distinct yet interrelated levels that are as follows: Level I, mental health education; Level II, individual, group, and/or family psychotherapy; Level III, cultural empowerment; and Level IV, indigenous healing. Although each of the MLM levels may be a focus of psychotherapy at a given point in time, levels may also be simultaneously combined depending upon the presenting therapeutic issues of the client. Due to cultural differences between refugees and the resettlement country, as mentioned in the previous section, refugees' conceptualization and expectations of mental health will invariably differ from that of the resettlement country. Therefore, Level 1 of the MLM model advocates that mental health education is an essential first step. During this period refugee clients are educated about the expectation of psychotherapy, the role of the therapist, the intake procedure, expected normative behavior of the therapist and client, the role of the interpreter, time boundaries, usage or nonuse of medication, administrative procedure, and/or logistical concerns, such as payment, transportation, and child care. Level I provides information for refugee clients about the process, expectations, and pragmatics of psychotherapy.

Level II is based upon the Western individual, group, and family therapy model. It has been demonstrated that these traditional forms of psychotherapy are effective with several culturally diverse groups (Zane & Sue, 1991). However, to be effective in utilizing the previous techniques, it is essential that therapist be able to adapt these traditional Western interventions into a therapeutic process that is culturally adaptive to the norms, belief systems, and healing practices of the client. For example, Kinzie (1985) underscored the need to be more directive and active with Southeast Asian refugees during therapy, while Bemak and Timm (1994) suggested the use of dream work and fantasy with this population. Thus, it is suggested that individual, group, and family psychotherapy be used as a framework to develop innovative and culturally responsive therapeutic interventions.

In Level III, cultural empowerment, the model suggests that the therapist assist refugee clients in gaining knowledge and a mastery of their environment. Refugees are faced with ongoing challenges while trying to acculturate and adjust to their new environment. During the therapeutic sessions, refugee clients may present daily challenges that they are facing, such as the acquisition of public transportation passes, the location of a court office to file papers, or managing problems with a landlord.

Concerns such as these may be related to housing, employment, language skills, education, problems in accessing resources, legal issues, social services, and/or money. It is essential that mental health professionals address these issues as an integral component of mental health in order to assist with the acculturation process, staying consistent with the studies cited previously in this chapter and indicating a strong correlation between psychosocial well-being and acculturation. It is essential that these issues are addressed with the same care and concern as the deeper social and psychological problems and premigration traumas experienced by the client.

Refugees' conceptualization of mental health frequently differs from that of the resettlement country professionals, causing them to seek help outside of the mainstream service system. Level IV, indigenous healing, takes into account these differences in belief systems and practices, and incorporates traditional Western methods with the refugees' indigenous cultural healing methods. An example would be the Western mental health practitioner who works collaboratively with Buddhist monks, spiritualists, or *curanderos*, dependent on their client's belief system. An illustration of this is the community mental health center in Long Beach, California, that has a Buddhist monk as part of its mental health team. Other facilities have open lines of communication with traditional healers, and clients are referred back and forth. It is recommended that Western mental health professionals become familiar with practices beyond the traditional Western framework, and when appropriate, integrate and encourage the usage of culturally based healers in therapeutic partnerships.

A case example to illustrate the MLM is as follows: Sam (nickname) is a 35-year-old Bosnian male who has been working in an American food restaurant for the past four months. His wife, who is also Bosnian, is attending night school to become a hairdresser. They have a six-year-old daughter and are expecting their second child in three months. Sam and his family have been in the United States for one year. Although they are part of the Bosnian community, Sam reports that he feels lonely since both his and his wife's families remained in Bosnia. Recently, he has had difficulty sleeping at night and getting up in the morning for work. Sam attributes his uncharacteristic irritability and growing number of accidents at work (breaking dishes and spilling food on customers) to the lack of sleep. His supervisor at work has given him a warning, threatening that Sam could lose his job. A friend of his wife recommended that he see someone at a community mental health clinic. In the MLM model, it is important that the therapist simultaneously provide counseling for Sam while learning about the Bosnian culture, sociopolitical and historical background of Bosnia, and the cultural conceptualization and attitudes toward mental health. To prevent premature dropout, it is critical that the therapist gain credibility by demonstrating cultural sensitivity, respect, and receptivity. Psychotherapists may utilize community leaders to educate themselves and understand the context of healing for Sam. Simultaneously, therapists should acquire a familiarity with the U.S. resettlement policies that may affect their client, such as policies on reunification for family members.

The first step in the MLM model is to clearly define for Sam the process and expectations for therapy. Since many clients come to clinics with misconceptions, this is an important first step in helping Sam to understand the therapeutic process, such as what is permissible and helpful to talk about, the course of treatment, and parameters of the interaction (such as privacy).

The second stage of MLM is to employ appropriate therapeutic interventions with Sam that would most benefit his needs. In Sam's situation, intervention strategies may focus on issues such as examining life transitions that include the impending birth of a new child, recent resettlement in the United States and adjustment challenges, being home alone at night since his wife is at school studying, the loss of extended family, English language barriers, and the cultural differences and subsequent pressures of his new job in an American restaurant. This may include a combination of insight-oriented therapy as well as cognitive behavioral interventions that may assist in developing skills to handle pressures and cultural differences at work. Given the importance of social networks and community in Bosnian society, there may also be discussion about the social ramifications of Sam's staying home at night with his daughter while his wife is out, a dramatic shift from traditional gender-based role expectations that he was accustomed to in Bosnia. The restructuring of family roles and relationships has relevance for Sam's adjustment to his new life in the United States. Finally, there may be an exploration into Sam's past and the loss of family who remained in Bosnia. It is quickly ascertained in therapy that there was significant trauma associated with Sam's departure from Bosnia and that he has little knowledge about his family. Through the therapeutic process, Sam is supported in tracking his family through appropriate international agencies while simultaneously examining his guilt and concern for leaving.

In the third phase of MLM, Sam is encouraged by the therapist to maintain and honor his own culture-bound traditions and values. This is essential for someone like Sam who is immersed in a new culture that requires significant adaptation. MLM therapy supports refugees in retaining their identity within their own culture while simultaneously assisting them to achieve mastery in the new culture in order to succeed in their adaptation. Sam also indicated that he wanted to speak with one of the religious leaders of his community who was also known as a faith healer. The therapist supported this suggestion and with Sam's permission contacted the faith healer to provide some background information and establish an open line of communication. Subsequently, the therapist honored Sam's belief system and formed a working relationship with the faith healer that bound together Western mental health practice and traditional healing within the context of Sam's beliefs and culture. This method also indicates to Sam that the therapist is culturally responsive and therefore establishes credibility.

Given the ongoing wars, conflicts, and natural disasters worldwide, refugees will continue to be a global issue. Resettlement countries, such as the United States and other Western countries, cannot ignore the situation of refugees, which in turn will foster ongoing governmental debates regarding refugee policies. These policies, which will influence receptivity, acculturation processes, and, in turn, psychosocial adjustment, will have serious implications for the mental health profession that is attempting to provide culturally responsive services. It is therefore essential that mental health professionals become knowledgeable about the full scope of issues that combine to foster refugee mental health, including governmental policies, the theory and process of migration, premigration psychological history, postmigration adjustment variables, and sociopolitical and economic factors that affect migration. It is also critical that mental health professionals have the awareness and understanding to be able to fully acknowledge, receive, respect, and accept the unique experience of the refugee, including the cultural differences that exist between the refugees' and the resettlement country's culture. The previous factors are essential for culturally sensitive and effective mental health services for current and future refugees.

REFERENCES

Bagheri, A. (1992). Psychiatric problems among Iranian immigrants in Canada. *Canadian Journal of Psychiatry, 37,* 7-11.

Baker, R. (1992). Psychological consequences for tortured refugees seeking asylum and refugee status in Europe. In M. Basoglu (Ed.), *Torture and its consequences* (pp. 83-106). Cambridge, England: Cambridge University Press.

Balian, K. (1997). *Overview of issues and the United Nations role.* Paper presented at the meeting on Survivors of Torture: Improving our Understanding Conference, Washington, DC.

Baptiste, D. A. (1993). Immigrant families, adolescents and acculturation: Insights for therapists. *Marriage and Family Review, 19*(3/4), 341-353.

Beiser, M. (1987). Changing time perspective and mental health among Southeast Asian refugees. *Culture, Medicine, and Psychiatry, 11,* 437-464.

Bemak, F. (1989). Cross-cultural family therapy with Southeast Asian refugees. *Journal of Strategic and Systemic Therapies, 8,* 22-27.

Bemak, F., & Chung, R. C. Y. (2002). Counseling and psychotherapy with refugees. In P. B. Pedersen, J. G. Draguns, W. J. Lonner, & J. E. Trimble (Eds.), *Counseling across cultures,* (5th ed., pp. 209-232). Thousand Oaks, CA: Sage.

Bemak, F., Chung, R. C. Y., & Bornemann, T. (1996). Counseling and psychotherapy with refugees. In P. Pedersen, J. Draguns, W. Lonner, & J. Trimble (Eds.), *Counseling across cultures* (4th ed.; pp. 243-265). Thousand Oaks, CA: Sage.

Bemak, F., Chung, C. Y., & Pedersen, P. B. (2003). *Counseling refugees: A psychosocial approach to innovative multicultural counseling interventions.* Westport CT: Greenwood Press.

Bemak, F., & Greenberg, B. (1994). Southeast Asian refugee adolescents: Implications for counseling. *Journal of Multicultural Counseling and Development, 22* (4), 115-124.

Bemak, F., & Timm, J. (1994). Case study of an adolescent Cambodian refugee: A clinical, developmental, and cultural perspective. *International Journal for the Advancement of Counseling, 17,* 47-58.

Berrol, S. C. (1995). *Growing up American: Immigrant children in America then and now.* New York: Twayne.

Berry, J. W. (1986). The acculturation process and refugee behavior. In C. L. Williams & J. Westermeyer (Eds.), *Refugee mental health in resettlement countries* (pp. 25-37). Washington DC: Hemisphere.

Brown, G. (1982). Issues in the resettlement of Indochinese refugees. *Social Casework, 63,* 155-159.

Buchwald, D., Manson, S. M., Ginges, N. G., Keane, E. M., & Kinzie, D. (1993). Prevalence of depressive symptoms among established Vietnamese refugees in the United States. *Journal of General Internal Medicine, 8,* 76-81.

Caspi, Y., Poole, C., Mollica, R.F., & Frankel, M. (1998). Relationship of child loss to psychiatric and functional impairment in resettled Cambodian refugees. *Journal of Nervous and Mental Diseases, 186*(8), 489-481.

Carlson, E. B., & Rosser-Hogan, R. (1991). Trauma experiences, posttraumatic stress, dissociation, and depression in Cambodian refugees. *American Journal of Psychiatry, 148,* 1548-1551.

Chung, R. C. Y. (2000). Psychosocial adjustment of Cambodian refugee women: Implication for mental health counseling. *Journal of Mental Health Counseling, 23*(2), 115-126.

Chung, R. C. Y., & Bemak, F. (1996). The effects of welfare status and psychological distress among Southeast Asian refugees. *Journal of Nervous and Mental Disease, 184*(6), 346-353.

Chung, R. C. Y., & Bemak, F. (2000). Vietnamese refugees' levels of distress, social support, and acculturation: Implications for mental health counseling. *Journal of Mental Health Counseling, 22*(2), 150-161.

Chung, R. C. Y., & Bemak, F. (2002). Revisiting the California Southeast Asian mental health needs assessment data: An examination of refugee ethnic and gender differences. *Journal of Counseling and Development, 80,* 111-119.

Chung, R. C. Y., Bemak, F., & Kagawa-Singer, M. (1998). Gender differences in psychological distress among Southeast Asian refugees. *Journal of Nervous and Mental Disease, 186*(2), 112-119.

Chung, R. C. Y., Bemak, F., & Okazaki, S. (1997). Counseling Americans with Southeast Asian descent: The impact of the refugee experience. In C. C. Lee (Ed.), *Multicultural issues in counseling* (2nd ed.). (pp. 207-231). Alexandria, VA: American Counseling Association.

Chung, R. C. Y., & Kagawa-Singer, M. (1993). Predictors of psychological distress among Southeast Asian refugees. *Social Science and Medicine, 36,* 631-639.

Chung, R. C. Y., & Kagawa-Singer, M. (1995). Interpretation of symptom presentation and distress: A Southeast Asian refugee example. *Journal of Nervous and Mental Disease, 183* (10), 639-648.

Chung R. C. Y., & Lin, K. M. (1994). Help-seeking behaviors among Southeast Asian refugees. *Journal of Community Psychology, 22,* 109-120.

Chung, R. C. Y., & Okazaki, S. (1991). Counseling Americans with Southeast Asian descent: The impact of the refugee experience. In C. C. Lee & B. L. Richardson (Eds.), *Multicultural issues in counseling* (pp. 107-126). Alexandria, VA: American Counseling Association.

Cox, D. R., & Amelsvoort, A. V. (1994). *The wellbeing of asylum seekers in Australia: A study of policies and practices with identification and discussion of key issues.* Centre for Regional Social Development. Melbourne, Australia: LaTrobe University.

Davidson, L. M., & Baum, A. (1986). Chronic stress and posttraumatic stress disorders. *Journal of Consulting and Clinical Psychology, 54,* 303-308.

Garcia-Peltoniemi, R. (1991). Epidemiological perspectives. In J. Westermeyer, C. L. Williams, & A. N. Nguyen (Eds.), *Mental health services for refugees* (DHHS Publication No. ADM 91-1824), pp. 24-41. Washington, DC: U.S. Government Printing Office.

Hauff, E., & Vaglum, P. (1995). Organized violence and the stress of exile: Predictors of mental health in a community cohort of Vietnamese refugees three years after resettlement. *British Journal of Psychiatry, 166,* 360-367.

Hinton, W. L., Tiet, Q., Tran, C. G., & Chesney, M. (1997). Predictors of depression among refugees from Vietnam: A longitudinal study of new arrivals. *Journal of Nervous and Mental Disease, 185*(1), 39-45.

Holen, A. (1991). A longitudinal study of the occurrence and persistence of posttraumatic health problems in disaster survivors. *Stress Medicine, 7,* 11-17.

Hurh, W. M., & Kim, D. C. (1990). Correlates of Korean immigrants' mental health. *Journal of Nervous and Mental Disease, 178,* 703-711.

Jupp, J. (1994). Australian immigration and settlement: History and current trends. In I. H. Minas & C. L. Hayes (Eds.), *Migration and mental health: Responsibilities and opportunities* (pp. 3-11). Melbourne, Australia: Victorian Transcultural Psychiatry Unit.

Kagawa-Singer, M., & Chung, R. C. Y. (1994). A paradigm for culturally based care in ethnic minority populations. *Journal of Community Psychology, 22,* 192-208.

Kessler, R. C., Sonnega, A., Bromet, E., Hughes, M., & Nelson, C. B. (1995). Posttraumatic stress disorder in the National Comorbidity Survey. *Archives of General Psychiatry, 52,* 1048-1060.

Kilpatrick, D. G., & Resnick, H. S. (1993). A description of the posttraumatic stress disorder field trial. In J. R. T. Davidson & E. B. Foa (Eds.), *Posttraumatic stress disorder: DSM-IV and beyond* (pp. 243-250). Washington, DC: American Psychiatric Press.

Kinzie, J. D. (1985). Overview of clinical issues in the treatment of Southeast Asian refugees. In T. C. Owan (Ed.), *Southeast Asian mental health: Treatment, prevention, services, training and research* (pp. 113-135). Washington, DC: U.S. Department of Health and Human Services.

Kinzie, J. D. (1993). Posttraumatic effects and their treatment among Southeast Asian refugees. In J. Wilson & B. Raphael (Eds.), *International handbook of traumatic stress syndromes* (pp. 311-320). New York: Plenum.

Kinzie, J. D., Boehnlein, J. K., Leung, P. K., Moore, L. J., Riley, C., & Smith, D. (1990). The prevalence of posttraumatic stress disorder and its clinical significance among Southeast Asian refugees. *American Journal of Psychiatry, 147*(7), 913-917.

Kleinman, A., & Good, B. (1985). *Culture and depression: Studies in the anthropology and cross-cultural psychiatry of affect and disorder.* Berkeley, CA: University of California Press.

Lin, K. M., Masuda, M., & Tazuma, L. (1982). Adaptational problems Vietnamese refugees: Part III. Case studies in clinic and field: Adaptive and maladaptive. *Psychiatric Journal of the University of Ottawa, 7*(3), 173-183.

Marsella, A. J., Friedman, M., & Spain, H. (1993). Ethnocultural aspects of PTSD. *Review of Psychiatry, 12,* 157-181.

Matsuoka, J. (1993). Demographic characteristics as determinants in qualitative differences in the adjustment of Vietnamese refugees. *Journal of Social Service Research, 17*(4), 1-21.

Mollica, R. F., & Lavelle, J. (1988). Southeast Asian refugees. In L. Comas-Diaz & E. H. Griffith (Eds.), *Clinical guidelines in cross-cultural mental health* (pp. 262-303). New York: Wiley.

Mollica, R. F., McInnes, K., Pham, T., Fawzi, M. C. S., Murphy, E., & Lin, L. (1998). The dose-effect relationships between torture and psychiatric symptoms in Vietnamese ex-political detainees and a comparison group. *Journal of Nervous and Mental Disease, 186,* 543-553.

Mollica, R. F., Wyshak, G., & Lavelle, J. (1985). The psychosocial impact of war trauma and torture on Southeast Asian refugees. *American Journal of Psychiatry, 144,* 1567-1572.

Murphy, H. B. (1977). Migration, culture and mental health. *Psychological Medicine, 7,* 677-684.

Nicholson, B. F. (1997). The influence of premigration and postmigration stressors on mental health: A study of Southeast Asian refugees. *Social Work Research, 21,* 19-31.

Nidorf, J. F. (1985). Mental health and refugee youths: A model for diagnostic training. In T. C. Owan (Ed.), *Southeast Asian mental health: Treatment, prevention, services, training, and research* (pp. 391-429). Washington, DC: NIMH.

Noh, S., Wu, Z., Speechley, M., & Kaspar, V. (1992). Depression in Korean immigrants in Canada. II. Correlates of gender, work, and marriage. *Journal of Nervous and Mental Disease, 180,* 578-585.

Pedersen, P. B. (1988). *A handbook for developing multicultural awareness.* Alexandria, VA: American Association for Counseling and Development.

Pedersen, P. B. (1991). Multiculturalism as a generic approach to counseling. *Journal of Counseling and Development, 70,* 6-12.

Pedersen, P. B. (2000). *A handbook for developing multicultural awareness* (3rd ed). Alexandria, VA: American Association for Counseling and Development.

Pernice, R., & Brook, J. (1994). Relationship of migrant status (refugee or immigrant) to mental health. *International Journal of Social Psychiatry, 40,* 177-188.

Ramsay, R., Gorst-Unsworth, C., & Turner, S. (1993). Psychiatric morbidity in survivors of organised state violence including torture: A retrospective series. *British Journal of Psychiatry, 162,* 55-59.

Refugee Women in Development (1990). *What is a refugee?* (Available from RefWID, Washington, DC.)

Sue, D. W., & Sue, D. (1990). *Counseling the culturally different: Theory & practice* (2nd ed.). New York: Wiley.

Sue, S., & Zane, N. (1987). The role of culture and cultural techniques in psychotherapy: A critique and reformulation. *American Psychologist, 42*(1), 37-45.

Tayabas, T., & Pok, T. (1983). The arrival of Southeast Asian refugees in America: An overview. In Asian Community Mental Health Training Center (Ed.), *Bridging cultures: Southeast Asian refugees in America* (pp. 3-14). Los Angeles: Asian American Community Mental Health Training Center.

Tobin, J. J., & Friedman, J. (1983). Spirits, shamans and nightmare death: Survivor stress in a Hmong refugee. *Journal of Orthopsychiatry, 53,* 439-448.

United Nations (1995). *Notes for speakers: Social development.* New York: Department of Public Information, United Nations.

Van Velsen, C., Gorst-Unsworth, C., & Turner, S. (1996). Survivors of torture and organized violence: Demography and diagnosis. *Journal of Traumatic Stress, 9,* 181-193.

Weine, S. M., Becker, D. F., McGlashan, T. H., Laub, D., Lazrove, S., Vojvoda, D., et al. (1995). Psychiatric consequences of "ethnic cleansing": Clinical assessments and traumatic testimonies of newly resettled Bosnian refugees. *American Journal of Psychiatry, 152,* 536-542.

Weisaeth, L., & Eitinger, L. (1993). Posttraumatic stress phenomena: Common themes across wars, disasters, and traumatic events. In J. Wilson & B. Raphael (Eds.). *International handbook of traumatic stress syndromes* (pp. 69-78). New York: Plenum.

Westermeyer, J. (1988). DSM-III psychiatric disorders among the Hmong refugees in the United States: A point prevalence study. *American Journal of Psychiatry, 145,* 197-202.

Williams, C. L., & Berry, J. W. (1991). Primary prevention of acculturative stress among refugees. *American Psychologist, 46,* 632-641.

Williams, C. L., & Westermeyer, J. (1983). Psychiatric problems among adolescent Southeast Asian refugees. *Journal of Nervous and Mental Disease, 171*(2), 79-85.

Wong-Reiger, D., & Quintana, D. (1987). Comparative acculturation of Southeast Asian and Hispanic immigrants and sojourners. *Journal of Cross-Cultural Psychology, 18*(3), 345-362.

Zane, N., & Sue. S. (1991). Culturally responsive mental health services for Asian American: Treatment and training issues. In H. Myers, P. Wohlford, P. Guzman, & R. Echemendia (Eds.), *Ethnic minority perspectives on clinical training and services in psychology* (pp. 47-58). Washington, DC: American Psychological Association.

III

Traditional Healing in the Americas

The Role of Dance in a Navajo Healing Ceremonial

Sandra T. Francis
University of the Sciences in Philadelphia

Although Navajo healing ceremonials have received attention from scholars for more than 100 years, their associated dances have gone, until now, unanalyzed. In the triple role of cultural anthropologist, registered nurse, and dancer, I documented the dances of the powerful Nightway ceremony and posed basic questions about dance content and function. Using labanotation scores supplemented by information obtained from field interviews, films, sacred texts, and the anthropological literature, I addressed the following questions: What is dance (*alzhish*)? What is the ceremonial purpose of *alzhish*? How is that purpose accomplished? The focal question of my research is: How can a dance make a person well?

BACKGROUND: THE NAVAJO NATION

The Navajo Nation is located in the American Southwest. Reservation lands, covering 25,351 square miles, extend from northeastern Arizona into northwestern New Mexico and a portion of southeastern Utah. Navajos are the largest and most extensively studied tribe in the United States with a population of more than 250,000 and a history of ethnographic research spanning more than 100 years. According to tribal government estimates for 1995, approximately 159,481 members live on the reservation; 68,529 in neighboring states; and 31,546 elsewhere in the United States (Rogers, 1995). The origins of the term "Navajo" are not known, but it is possibly the Spanish rendition of a Tewa Pueblo word (Harrington, 1940, p. 518; Hewett, 1906). Navajos refer to themselves as *Diné* (plural *Dine'é*) which means roughly "the People." In this paper I will use the term "Navajo," as it predominates in the more recent literature.

Archaeological and linguistic evidence suggest a relatively late arrival in the Southwest for the Athabascan-speaking Navajos, relatives of the Apaches. Their gathering and hunting forbearers migrated from Alaska, northwestern Canada, and the Pacific Northwest and found Pueblo farmers already settled in the area. Although there is no scholarly consensus regarding the time of migration, it may have occurred between 1000 and 1525 A.D. (see Brugge, 1983, p. 489).

Navajo culture is a blend of elements, some distinctively Navajo and some adapted from other groups. Through time, Navajo contact with Pueblo, Spanish, Mexican, and Euro-American cultures resulted in considerable cultural exchange. Farming, certain ceremonial practices, and possibly weaving were learned from the Pueblos. Horses, cattle, sheep, goats, new crops, and metal tools were obtained from the Spanish. Silversmithing was learned through Mexican contact, and modern conveniences, along with educational, political, medical, and economic institutions were derived from the dominant Anglo society (Stewart, 1977, pp. 292, 296-297).

Navajos have been widely characterized as an adaptive and pragmatic people who take what is useful from other cultures without giving up traditional ways. Where health care is concerned, Navajos have certainly demonstrated a willingness to combine old and new approaches. On the reservation today the biomedical model coexists rather peacefully with traditional therapies. However, acceptance of "white man's medicine" took some time to develop.

When the first hospital was established on the reservation in 1912, the doctors encountered resistance from the population. Since patients sometimes died on the premises, hospitals were looked on as "places of death" and were feared due to the traditional taboo against contact with the dead. However, these institutions were found useful in the same regard because relatives could be sent there to die. In traditional custom, if a sick person were allowed to die at home, his or her family would be forced to abandon their dwelling to avoid the angry spirit of the deceased (Bergman, 1983, p. 672).

Navajo contacts with Western physicians were plagued with other complications as well. Typically, the physicians did not speak Navajo, nor did they understand the culture; consequently, many doctors had a poor opinion of traditional medicine and healers. Fortunately, this is no longer the case. Today, medical doctors on the reservation generally acknowledge the value of traditional healing and many will refer patients to a *hataaɬii* or medicine man to complete treatment. It has been found that patients receiving supplemental traditional therapy have a more rapid recovery, experience fewer complications, and are less likely to suffer depression after a bout with illness (Kompare, 1980). Medicine men, in turn, acknowledge the usefulness of Western medicine, but they find it effective primarily in treating symptoms. Pills, injections, and surgeries do not treat the spiritual, root cause of an illness. For that, a ceremony is needed.

TRADITIONAL HEALING: SACRED KNOWLEDGE AND RITUAL PRACTICE

The traditional system of healing rests on certain fundamental assumptions about what illness is, how it is caused, and how it should be treated. Wellness to a Navajo does not mean simply the absence of injury or disease; rather, it means living in *hózhǫ*—a state of being that has been defined as "everything that is good, harmonious, orderly, happy, and beautiful" (Witherspoon, 1975, pp. 76-77). In order to be well, the individual must live in harmony with nature, the sacred beings (Holy People or *Diyin Dine'é*), and other Navajos. When a person begins to feel "unwell"—that is, he or she may have physical or emotional symptoms, bad dreams, or bad luck—this is an indication that a mistake has been made. The individual may have broken a taboo, neglected ceremonial duties, indulged in excess, come into contact with a dangerous entity, or aroused the anger of a witch (Reichard, 1950, pp. 80-83). The patient's first step is to consult a diagnostician, an individual gifted with the ability to divine the root cause of the illness (the error that brought about the imbalance). The diagnostician will then search for similarities between the symptom picture of the patient and the condition of a hero from a body of sacred narratives and will prescribe the appropriate ceremony.

Each curing ceremony is associated with a corpus of narrative episodes.[1] Following the typical narrative format, a hero commits an error that leads to some form of hard-

---

[1]For a discussion of the structure and use of narrative texts, along with a critique of the Western misuse of these texts, see Faris, 1990, pp. 25-31.

ship. The Holy People take pity on the unfortunate earth-surface-person and conduct a ceremony to restore the hero to wholeness. The healed one is then instructed to return to his kin and teach them the ceremony so that, in the future, others may be healed.

Once a ceremony has been prescribed for a contemporary patient, there is much preliminary work to be done. The patient, along with family and clan members, must find a *hataałi* or medicine man who knows the ceremony. Lengthy negotiations are entered into and many decisions are made. It must be decided where and when to hold the event, how long the ceremony will be (from one to nine nights), and what the payment will be. A full nine-night sing is quite an expensive undertaking. The medicine man and his helpers are supplied all meals for the duration of the sing and are paid in cash, sheep, blankets, and other goods. If a public dance is held, the dance teams must be paid and the audience, which often numbers in the hundreds, must be fed.

Family members are generally willing to invest labor, money, and time in a ceremony not only out of concern for a sick relative, but for their own good as well. It is a fundamental assumption in Navajo cosmology that the individual is intimately and meaningfully connected to everything else. Therefore, if a person is not well, that person's family, clan, and community are also not well. In fact, the Navajo Nation is not well. The presence of an unbalanced, unharmonious condition impacts others and must be corrected ritually.

Navajo ceremonials are extremely complex affairs encompassing a large number of individual rites and rituals. The function of many ceremonial acts is to recreate the sacred healing episode of long ago and identify the patient with the restored hero. This is accomplished in part through the use of ceremonial objects, dry paintings, prayers, dances, and songs. The Navajo patient's role is not a passive one (as is typically the case in Western therapies); the patient, or one-sung-over, is present for and actively participates in all ceremonial rites. He or she must intone the prayers, sing the songs, and perform the ritual actions necessary for restoring order and wellness.

In the early part of this century, nearly 30 ceremonials or chantways were in use, but many have become extinct and currently fewer than a dozen are performed regularly (Kluckhohn & Wyman, 1938; Wyman, 1950, p. 351; Wyman, 1983, p. 542). Chants can be grouped according to the etiology of the illness, similarities in ritual patterns, and similarities in mythological association into Holy Way, Life Way, and Evil Way categories. These three groupings are related to the attraction of good, the treatment of accidental injuries, and the expulsion of evil respectively (Wyman, 1983, p. 542).[2] An individual chantway can be divided into three phases: During the first phase the patient is purified through sweat baths, emetics, and prayers and is made ready to receive the power of the ceremony. In the second phase, the actual transference of power occurs, and during the final phase, the patient is secluded while the power is sealed in.

It is interesting to look at Navajo ceremonialism in a regional and pan-Indian context. Even the casual observer would note similarities between the ceremonies of the Navajos and those of their Pueblo neighbors. Dry paintings, prayer stick offerings, corn pollen offerings, masked dancers, and clowns are some of the elements featured by both groups. However, there are equally obvious differences. Pueblo ceremonials are largely communal affairs performed in relation to phases of the agricultural cycle by ritual specialists who are members of a religious society. In contrast, Navajo

---

[2]See also Wyman and Kluckhohn, 1938, pp. 5-7; Reichard, 1950, pp. 322-323; Kluckhohn, 1960, pp. 69-70; Kluckhohn and Leighton, 1962, p. 220.

chantways are generally performed for the purpose of healing, and they are conducted by specialists who have undergone an apprenticeship with an established medicine man.[3] Unlike their Pueblo counterparts, Navajo healers operate independently, and most have resisted sporadic efforts to organize them into a society for the preservation of traditional medicine (Bergman, 1973).

Navajo medicine men also differ from other Native American healers with regard to the source of their power. They do not receive their power by means of hallucinogens, dreams, vision quests, or spirit possession; rather, their power is derived from their encyclopedic knowledge of ceremonial detail. This knowledge is acquired through a course of study that may be as lengthy and rigorous as that of any medical student (approximately 10 years for the major ceremonials). To be accepted as an apprentice, the individual need only show interest, but only those gifted with stamina, a strong voice, and an excellent memory are likely to succeed.

Although one does hear about medicine women from time to time, it is certain that the vast majority of practitioners are men. It should be pointed out, however, that there is no traditional prohibition against a woman becoming a hataałii. Women do serve important ceremonial functions as diagnosticians, herbalists, sand painters, and song participants.[4]

Scholars have debated the issue of how Navajo ceremonies work. The "mechanistic model" proposes that, through the correct and complete performance of ritual acts, the Holy People are controlled and compelled to sanction the healing of the patient (Kluckhohn, 1968, p. 679; Kluckhohn & Leighton, 1962, p. 221; Reichard, 1944a, 1950, pp. 126, 181, 267-276; Witherspoon, 1977, pp. 61, 77). What I have termed the "reciprocity model" emphasizes prestations and the kinship bond between the Holy People and the earth-surface-people. According to this model, healing is achieved because of the kin-based, reciprocal exchange between human and deity. In exchange for offerings of corn pollen, prayer sticks, and prayers, the Holy Ones empower the healing process (Griffin-Pierce, 1992, pp. 32-35; McAllester, 1980, pp. 231-234). Wyman's view appears to combine these two positions. He has described the ritual process as "[compulsion] by the ethic of reciprocity" (1983, p. 537; see also Francis, 1996, pp. 157-164 for further treatment of this debate).

It may be difficult for an outsider to understand how earth-surface-people can gain control over their more powerful relatives, the Holy People. However, Witherspoon points out that it was the Holy People who gave earth-surface-people the ritual means to control them when they gave Navajos ceremonial knowledge. According to Witherspoon, "Through correct ceremonial procedures, the Navajo beseech the Diyin Dine'é in ways they cannot resist" (1996). In my own research, which I will shortly discuss, I found both elements, compulsion and reciprocity, to be operating where the dances are concerned.

THE NIGHTWAY CEREMONY (TŁÉÉ'JI)

A Nightway ceremony is prescribed for diseases of the head, including decreased vision, hearing loss, and mental disturbance. It is also used for "deer sickness," which

---

[3]For broader comparative analyses of Native American religious practices in the Southwest, see Reichard, 1945 and Lamphere, 1983.

[4]Perrone, Stockel, and Krueger (1989, pp. 29-44) discuss the work of Annie Kahn, Navajo medicine woman.

may be associated with rheumatoid conditions (in Sandner, 1979, p. 45). Nightway is considered by many Navajos to be the most powerful ceremony in that it is believed to contain the combined power of all other ceremonies. Because of this great power, it is also dangerous; therefore, many taboos govern its performance. If a person has a long-term association with this ceremony (e.g., as a dancer, sand painter, or medicine man), it is probable that, somewhere along the way, that person will break one of the rules. If this occurs, the treatment of choice is Nightway because, following traditional logic, if you become ill because of Nightway, you must be cured by the same means.

Nightway is a winter ceremony, usually performed from late October to early February. The focal symbols of this ceremony are the masked representatives of a category of Holy People known as *Yé'ii* or *Yé'ii Bicheii* (YAY bah-chay). The literal meaning of Yé'ii Bicheii is "the maternal grandfathers of the giants" (Kluckholm [sic], 1923, p. 187).[5] These deities are benevolent and helpful to humans (Haile, 1947, p. 39). Through eight days and nine nights the masked dancers who represent the Yé'ii administer treatment to the patient and occasionally to the audience. The first half of the ceremony is taken up with rites of purification and exorcism; then follow ceremonial rites and song sequences, which recreate the world of the legend.

One of the sacred narratives associated with Nightway is called "The Visionary" (Curtis, 1907, pp. 111-116; Klah, 1938; Matthews, 1902, pp. 159-171, 197-212; Sapir & Hoijer, 1942, pp. 136-259; Stevenson, 1891, pp. 278-279). In this narrative, the hero's encounters with the Holy People result in his learning the Nightway ceremony, which he is then instructed to teach to his kin. Part of this acquired ceremonial knowledge pertains to dancing.

THE ROLE OF DANCE IN NIGHTWAY

Most elements of Navajo ceremonials have been documented and studied. Among these elements are *prayer* (Gill, 1977, 1980; Matthews, 1888; Reichard, 1944a), *music and song* (Boulton, 1992; Matthews, 1894; McAllester, 1954; McAllester & Mitchell, 1983), *sand painting* (Griffin-Pierce, 1992; Newcomb & Reichard, 1937; Wyman, 1960), and *myth* (Haile, 1938; Luckert, 1979; Matthews, 1887, 1902, 1907, 1994[1896]; Reichard, 1944b; Sapir & Hoijer, 1942; Wheelwright, 1942, 1949, 1956; Zolbrod, 1984). Ceremonial dancing, although described in some sources (Haile, 1947; Lyon, 1985, 1986; Matthews, 1902; Stevenson, 1891), merits further examination.

At present there are three surviving ceremonial dance complexes: the "Squaw" Dance (or, more appropriately, the Girls' Dance) of Enemyway, the Corral or Fire Dance of Mountainway, and the Yé'ii Bicheii dancing of Nightway. I chose to study the Yé'ii Bicheii complex at the advice of my Navajo teachers who considered this ceremony to be the most powerful.

Background of This Study

My study of Yé'ii Bicheii dancing was carried out intermittently from 1990 through 1996 (Francis, 1996). As a cultural anthropologist with a degree in nursing and

---

[5]As Faris (1990, p. 69–22) has observed, Kluckhohn was such an unknown at the time of the publication of his brief paper on Nightway that his name was misspelled as Kluckholm. [Faris lists the misspelling as "Klukhohm," but in my copy of this paper it is "Kluckholm."]

25 years of experience as a performer of ethnic dance, I felt well equipped to undertake this study of dance and healing. My professional background helped me establish rapport with my collaborators; ceremonial dancers related to me as a fellow performer and medicine men accepted me as a fellow health care professional. But most critical to the success of my project was that entity that propels ceremonial activity: the extended family. At the invitation of two Navajo families, I was able to document an entire nine-night Nightway and to work closely with a family of dancers who have maintained the tradition of Yé'ii Bicheii dancing through four generations.

I observed over 40 hours of dancing performed by approximately 30 dance teams. Although photography, filming, and audio taping were prohibited, my colleague Nadia Nahumck, a professional labanotator, was able to use existing film footage shot in 1963 and 1964 to create detailed Labanotation scores (American Indian Films Group; see Francis, 1996, pp. 118-119). This system enables the researcher to record movement in much the same way that words allow us to record thought and speech. Using this method, Dr. Nahmuck and I created a precise record of what the dancing consisted of—every movement, gesture, and pattern.

What Is Alzhish?

My research began with a survey of the literature. When I examined the literature on Navajo ceremonials in general and Nightway in particular, I found that, although Yé'ii Bicheii dancing had been described, it had not been analyzed (Haile, 1947; Lyon, 1985, 1986; Matthews, 1902; Stevenson, 1891). The following questions had not been addressed: What word do Navajos use to refer to that portion of a ceremony that we would call "dance?" Do Navajos have a concept that is similar to our "dance?" If so, what is the ceremonial function of dance? How is that function achieved? These questions formed the focus of my doctoral research.

Navajos do have a word, *alzhish*, which they apply to activities that Euro-Americans would call dance. Alzhish is used to refer to "human action (mainly involving movement of the feet) that is stylized, rhythmic, patterned, expressive, and accompanied by music and/or song" (Francis, 1996, p. 176). Actually, the entire Nightway ceremony is filled with patterned/stylized/expressive/rhythmic movements, but the action of the feet and the musical accompaniment appear to make the activity alzhish and not something else.

Dance is an optional and expensive element of Nightway. In reaching a decision regarding the dance option, the families I worked with considered two factors: the severity of the patient's illness and the cost of the dancing in labor, time, money, and goods. In the end they decided to include the dance rites because they wanted to provide the full, nine-night ceremonial (the strongest possible medicine), and they had the resources to do so.

The public dance events are eagerly awaited and often attract 300 to 500 spectators. The performances occur on the eighth and ninth nights of the chantway and are preceded by six days and seven nights of ceremonial activity.

Physical Setting

Every Nightway begins with the selection of a campsite and the construction of a ceremonial *hooghan*. This traditional Navajo dwelling is a many-sided structure made of wooden beams chinked with mud. A hooghan built for a ceremony will hold around 90 people rather uncomfortably. For the indoor rites, observers sit along the north and south walls on the packed-earth floor while the medicine man, his assistants, and the patient sit at the western end facing east. Several other rites, including the dancing, take place outdoors.

A large area (nearly half the length of a football field) is raked just outside the hoogan entrance to serve as the dance field. At the eastern end of the field a brush arbor is constructed where dancers can dress and warm themselves between performances. Large electric lights are sometimes set up to illuminate the field. Spectators, who bring lawn chairs and blankets for seating, assemble along the sides of the dance area around campfires.

Ceremonial Attire

The male dancers, who often perform bare-chested, wear a woven kilt, knee-high stockings, moccasins, and beautiful silver jewelry. Some wear ornate knee and elbow bands or streamers. Their ceremonial dress and paraphernalia are their property, but their masks belong to the medicine man. Females wear a woven dress with apron, moccasins, leggings, jewelry, and a distinctive Female God mask.

On the fourth night, the masks, which are treated as living entities, are laid out on the floor of the hooghan, ritually fed with corn pollen, and awakened by shaking. The masks are made of unwounded buckskin, dyed blue, and worn over the dancer's head like a bag. There are two half-dollar sized holes for the eyes and a gourd beak, rimmed in downy feathers, for a mouthpiece. Red-dyed horsetail, adorned with two eagle feathers, is used for the hair. A large wreath of spruce is worn around the neck like a collar. Male dancers carry a gourd rattle in the right hand and a bundle of spruce in the left; females carry spruce in each hand.

It should be stressed that the dancers *represent* the Holy People; they do not *become* these deities. They do not enter a trance state, nor are they possessed by the spirits of the Yé'ii. If a dancer were to experience such an altered state, he or she would be considered "out of balance" and would need to seek immediate treatment from the medicine man.

The Dances

The first dance event of the evening is the performance of the First Dancers ('Atsáłeeh). They are four in number, always males, and are usually the apprentices of the medicine man. It is said that they represent initial corn, child rain, vegetation, and corn pollen; they are also associated with thunderbirds (Klah, cited in Faris, 1990, p. 205, Matthews, 1902, p. 141). The song that they sing while dancing is extremely important and must be executed perfectly. One mistake can result in the cancellation of the entire ceremony (Matthews, 1902, p. 145).[6] The theme of this important song is plant fertility.

Before the dance performance, the medicine man and the patient administer a corn meal blessing (an extremely important act) to each dancer. Corn is the food of the Yé'ii and this offering, along with other offerings of prayer sticks, songs, and prayers, initiates a reciprocal exchange. It is understood that, if these offerings are correct, the Holy People must reciprocate by empowering the healing.

After the performance of the First Dancers, dance teams from all over the reservation perform until dawn. Their dance, which is called *na'akai*, may be done with either

---

[6]The text of this song is found in Matthews (1902, pp. 286-287).

six men or with six men and six women. Both the First Dancers and the na'akai teams accompany their dancing with gourd rattles and singing, but na'akai songs are not fixed and immutable, as is the case with the song of the First Dancers. Na'akai songs can be created anew as long as they follow a given musical format. These songs are said to be untranslatable in that they are sung in the mysterious Yé'ii language.

All Nightway dances are structurally similar: They begin with a formal, stylized introduction during which dancers face first north, then south, while making a low bow at the waist and dipping their rattles downward. The dancers are arranged in straight lines running west to east that, at a musical cue, begin to travel clockwise with a simple shuffling step.[7] When the circuit is completed, the straight line is reformed in its original position. The focus of the dancing is the patient who is seated just outside the entrance of the hoogan facing the dance field. The performances continue from dusk to dawn, but frequent breaks are taken to allow the patient and dancers time to rest. All dance teams are led by Talking God, the principal Yé'ii figure. Typically, each team will bring one or two clown dancers (Water Sprinklers) to amuse the crowd.

The Nightway Experience

A simple description of ceremonial elements cannot convey the feel of a Nightway. No one who has ever attended a performance of Nightway dancing can forget the experience; it is a sensuous one. The event takes place outdoors in the desert on a winter night under a canopy of stars. The campfires give off the pungent smell of burning cedar and fill the air with clouds of eye-stinging smoke. Hot campfire coffee is passed around, along with mutton stew and fry bread. But most memorable are the sounds: the alternating deep bass and falsetto of the Yé'ii Bicheii singing and, simultaneously, the soft chanting that emanates from the hoogan. A constant presence throughout the night is the mesmerizing sound of the dancers' gourd rattles and the rasping beat of the medicine man's basket drum. The dancers in their masks and glittering jewelry appear magical in the firelight. It is easy, even for an outsider, to forget time and place and enter the world of the legend and its account of the first Yé'ii Bicheii dance to be observed by an earth-surface-person. The patient becomes the hero, the Visionary, hidden in darkness on the rim of a canyon, watching the Holy People crisscrossing in their dance in sacred time long, long ago (Matthews, 1902, p. 160; Stevenson, 1891, p. 281).

HOW DANCE EFFECTS HEALING

The Ceremonial Function of Dance

When I first read about the ceremonial dances of Navajos, I was uncertain of their function. Descriptive passages in some sources made me wonder if the dances were purely social events or perhaps postceremonial celebrations. Kluckhohn and Leighton compared the "Squaw" Dance of Enemyway to a "debutante ball" because of its obvious courtship function (1962, p. 229). Wyman likened the Corral Dance of

---

[7]The only exception is the woman's line in the male/female version of the dance.

Mountainway to a "sacred vaudeville show" referring to the sleight-of-hand feats performed by the dance teams (1960, p. 59). When I began my field study, it quickly became apparent that, although Euro-Americans may create a distinct boundary between sacred and profane realms, Navajos do not. It is true that certain behaviors are considered inappropriate when sacred rites are being conducted, such as loud talking, laughing, or any excessive emotional display. But the fact that people are having a good time socializing during a Nightway in no way detracts from the serious, sacred nature of the event. Although the Yé'ii Bicheii dancing has entertainment value, especially with regard to the clowns who mock the dancers and the audience during a performance, the purpose of the dancing, as with all other Nightway rites, is to heal the patient.

How Dance Effects Healing

My Navajo teachers confirmed my supposition that dancing effects healing, but it was not clear precisely how that effect was achieved. Through analysis of the labanotation scores, ceremonial texts (song, prayer, and legend), interview data, and the Nightway literature, it was demonstrated that the healing work was accomplished in the following four ways:

Through the Power of Attraction   According to sacred knowledge, the appearance of the dancers mirrors the actual appearance of the Yé'ii Bicheii. The Holy People are attracted to their likenesses and are enticed to leave their homes in the canyons to attend the ceremony. They are attracted also by the offerings that are made to them. Thus, the dancers attract the Holy People and their power to the ceremony.

Through the Restoration of Orderly Conditions   The state of imbalance or disharmony that is associated with the patient's illness must be corrected before wellness can be restored. In a variety of ways, the movements of the dancers reestablish the orderly, beautiful state known as *hózhǫ́*. To understand how this occurs, we must first consider some important features of the Navajo cosmos.

The Navajo universe is structured according to principles relating to number, direction, form, and action. These entities are imbued with multiple meanings, both negative and positive. The dances are shaped by those principles having positive meanings.

Number   For example, an even number of dancers (4, 6, or 12) is used in adherence to the rule that "blessing and divinity are represented by even numbers, evil and harm by odd" (Reichard, 1950, p. 244). Number shapes the dance performance in other ways as well. Dance sets are performed four times following the conviction that four is the ritual number of completion, that is, for an action to bear results, it must be performed four times (Reichard, 1950, p. 242).

Direction   Orientation to cardinal direction is an inflexible feature of the dancing. Direction is imbued with social and sacred meanings too numerous and complex to be defined here (see McNeley, 1994, pp. 6-13), but a few associations are particularly relevant to dance. For example, dance teams invariably enter and exit the dance field from the east and the patient must be seated facing east, a direction which is associated with the rising sun, hope, newness, change, and commencement. In addition, clockwise or sunwise travel is important because it mirrors the path that the sun takes across the sky and is considered the natural or correct direction of movement (Reichard, 1950, pp. 161-170).

Form and Action   The form of the dance is also significant. When a dance line arcs to form a semicircle, there is typically a gap left between the lead and end dancers, thus creating an open circle. This obeys the rule that a circle must be left open so that harm may exit and good may enter (Reichard, 1950, pp. 89-90). And finally, the action of stepping heavily on the right foot relates to the belief that evil spirits favor stepping on the left foot (Kluckhohn & Wyman, 1940, p. 86). In sum, the movements of the dancers reestablish the positive and orderly conditions essential to harmony and wellness.

Through the Recreation of a Sacred Healing Episode   For the contemporary patient to be healed, the healing of the legend's hero must be made to happen again. What is sought is a recurrence, not a reenactment. The repetitive, focused, orderly movements of the dancers generate great power and, in essence, "bring the legend to life." This phenomenon cannot be easily grasped without some understanding of the Navajo concepts of time, repetition, and movement.

Time   To Euro-Americans time is linear, progressive, and rigidly compartmentalized. It "marches on." The present is forever occurring now; the past is behind us, and the future lies ahead. In contrast, Navajo time is cyclical and flexible in nature; it can be "telescoped or expanded" (Reichard, 1950, p. 54). Through the power of the ceremony, the past and present can converge and the healing of long ago can be brought forward. Anglos may experience something similar to Navajo "flexible time" through skillful theater or cinema performances of historical events. Let us say, for example, that you attend a religious play about Christ's healing ministry and you find the acting so powerfully convincing that your sense of time and place is suspended. If you respond to the stage performance as if the events were actually happening and you were a part of the drama of healing, then you may be experiencing something similar to a Navajo ceremony.

Repetition   Repetition also has a different meaning for Navajos, particularly in ceremonial context. Among Euro-Americans, repetition is often considered monotonous, boring, and tiring. This is not true of Native American cultures in general and Navajos in particular. Repetition results in the steady accumulation of power and, as stated by Reichard, "Repetition is compulsive and authoritative" (1950, p. 118). With every beat of the drum, shake of the rattle, and step of the dancer, power is being produced. Far from being boring, ceremonial repetition has undertones of dramatic tension and a feeling of building toward climax or completion.

Movement   The role of movement in the Navajo worldview can scarcely be overemphasized. From their verb-laden language to their seminomadic life way, Navajos demonstrate a preoccupation with action and motion. The sacred narratives are filled with references to movement. The heroes are forever journeying and it is through these wanderings that they learn lessons that ultimately benefit the People.

Movement is likewise a dominant theme in ceremonial songs, prayers, and dry paintings, but it is the role of movement in Navajo philosophy that is most important where dance is concerned. Movement is considered to be "the essence of life and being" (Witherspoon, 1977, p. 48). Put simply, it is the life force; to be without movement is to be without life. According to ethnomusicologist and authority on Navajo ceremonial music David McAllester, "Motion is a key to sacred power in Navajo thought. Wind is the basic metaphor of the power of motion. Speech, song and prayer are wind in motion shaped by the added power of human articulation" (1979, p. 30). The same logic can be applied to dance. Ceremonial dancing involves movement shaped by ritual control and is thus a vehicle for generating great power. Dance is the life force ritually controlled and directed toward the restoration of beautiful conditions or hózhǫ́. It is this force that brings the legend to life as past time and present time merge, and the patient/hero is restored.

Through the Power of Identification   Of central importance in a healing ceremony is the identification of the contemporary patient with the legendary first patient. This identification is accomplished in a number of ways:

- **Through sand painting rites**   The elaborate paintings made of crushed rock, minerals, and other substances are constructed on the floor of the hoogan. Depicted in these paintings are mythic scenes. To begin the rite of identification, the patient approaches the painting, sometimes by walking virtually in the hero's footsteps, which have been painted along the periphery. The patient then sits on the painted figure of the hero, or of a Holy Person, and the Medicine Man performs the rite of identification by touching some area of the painted figure (head, feet, arms, etc.) and then touching the corresponding area of the patient's body. The patient and the hero/Holy Person symbolically become one.
- **Through song sequences**   These sequences, which may go on all night, were the ceremonial element most eagerly anticipated by my Navajo friends. The songs evoke the world of the legend and the experiences of the hero. They transport the patient mentally and spiritually to this sacred realm.
- **Through prayers and recitations**   The patient speaks the words passed on by the hero. Although Anglos have a saying—"sticks and stones can break my bones, but words can never hurt me"—such sentiments would seem nonsensical to a traditional Navajo. Words are considered to be "speech acts;" that is, they have the power to make things happen. Through the power of words, the patient becomes the hero.
- **Through the dance event**   Although the patient does not participate in the dancing, he or she is the one danced for. The patient is present for all dance events, and all dance teams begin and end their performances facing the patient. Prior to each dance, the patient, in the role of hero, blesses (feeds) the Yé'ii representatives with corn meal, thus creating conditions for reciprocal exchange and healing.

In sum, the Yé'ii Bicheii dancers facilitate healing by attracting the Holy People and their power to the ceremonial site; correcting disorderly conditions through their properly executed movements; bringing the healing episode to life through their power-producing, life-giving movements; and representing the Holy People and accepting the offerings of the patient in the role of hero.

WHAT CAN WE LEARN FROM NAVAJO HEALERS?

It may be difficult for some Euro-American health practitioners to credit the therapeutic effectiveness of a ceremony such as Nightway. Exponents of a science-based model of health care might acknowledge the benefit of such things as herbal infusions, inhalants, and sweat baths, but the healing value of words, objects, and ritualized movements might be more difficult to accept.[8] This skeptical attitude has certainly been typical of the doctors and nurses I have worked with over the past 20 years.

Medical ethnocentrism can have serious consequences on the reservation, as I learned from two of my Navajo colleagues who are social workers. The husband and wife team expressed frustration at their failure to obtain federal funding for a program designed to help troubled families though traditional ceremonies. Although some Indian Health Service officials in charge of funding may doubt the efficacy of traditional medicine, I was able to observe the benefits at close range.

I have followed the progress of the elderly male patient whose Nightway I attended in November 1995. This man, in his late seventies or early eighties, was suffering from severe joint pain, deafness, and depression. He had been a Yé'ii Bicheii dancer for many years and was diagnosed as having "Yé'ii Bicheii sickness." This meant that he had broken one or more of the many ceremonial taboos and needed to be cured by Nightway.

Through the days and nights of the ceremony I saw a marked improvement in the patient's physical and mental condition. Four years later, his family reported that he continued to walk without a walker and that his hearing and mood remained significantly improved. Had he not shown improvement, this would have indicated that some error in diagnosis or ceremonial procedure had been committed and his illness would have been reevaluated and retreated. This is, of course, only one case, but Navajo families have hundreds of comparable success stories to share. Traditional methods persist in the twentieth century because they are often effective—they can make people well.

It is my view, as a registered nurse and anthropologist, that the Navajo health care system presents an important model for study. The holistic movement in U.S. health care is the result of an increasing awareness that our germ theory of disease and our compartmentalized approach to therapy is inadequate in many cases. What is being searched for is a means of treating a patient on all levels: physical, mental, emotional, social, and spiritual. We are searching for something that Navajos have never lost.

What can we learn from Navajo healers? Traditional Navajos believe that each patient is meaningfully connected to natural, sacred, and social realms. They also believe that all aspects of a patient's being must be treated: words, thoughts, emotions, past experiences, body, and behavior. They make kinship an important part of healing by involving caring individuals in the treatment process and restoring the patient's social place. Finally, they acknowledge the healing power of words, thoughts, objects, music, and ritual movement.

But it is the Navajo patients themselves who best express the value of traditional medicine. The following pronouncement is made by the one-sung-over at the close of a Nightway ceremony:

Happily I recover.

Happily my interior becomes cool.

---

[8]Obvious exceptions here would be the fields of psychiatry and psychology. Members of these disciplines have shown long-term appreciation for the efficacy of Navajo healing (see Bergman, 1973; Kluckhohn & Leighton, 1962; Leighton & Kluckhohn, 1947; Leighton & Leighton, 1941; Levy, 1963; Sandner, 1979).

Happily my eyes regain their power.

Happily my head becomes cool.

Happily my limbs regain their power.

Happily I hear again.

Happily for me (the spell) is taken off.

Happily I walk . . .

Impervious to pain, I walk.

Feeling light within, I walk.

With lively feelings, I walk (Matthews, 1902, p. 143).

REFERENCES

Barrett, S. (Director). (1963/1964). *Nightway films: Tape 26-645*, Berkeley, CA: American Indian Films Group University of California Production Lab.

Bergman, R. (1973). A school for medicine men. *American Journal of Psychiatry, 130* (6), 663-666.

Bergman, R. (1983). Navajo health services and projects. In A. Ortiz (Ed.), *Handbook of North American Indians* (Vol. 10, pp. 672-678). Washington, DC: Smithsonian Institution.

Boulton, L. (1992). *Navajo songs: Recorded by Laura Boulton in 1933 and 1940*. Annotated by Charlotte J. Frisbie and David McAllester. Washington, DC: Smithsonian/Folkways Recordings.

Brugge, D. (1983). Navajo prehistory and history to 1850. In A. Ortiz (Ed.), *Handbook of North American Indians* (Vol. 10, pp. 489-501). Washington, DC: Smithsonian Institution.

Curtis, E. (1907). *The North American Indian: Being a series of volumes picturing and describing the Indians of the United States, and Alaska*. F. Hodge (Ed.) Norwood, MA: Plimpton Press.

Faris, J. (1990). *The Nightway: History and a history of documentation of a Navajo ceremonial*. Albuquerque, NM: University of New Mexico Press.

Francis, S. (1996). *The Yé'ii Bicheii dancing of Nightway: An examination of the role of dance in a Navajo healing ceremony*. Unpublished doctoral dissertation, Department of Anthropology, Wright State University. Available through University Microfilms International (97-10,563) Ann Arbor, MI.

Gill, S. (1977). Prayer as person: The performative force in Navajo prayer acts. *History of Religions, 17* (2), 143-157.

Gill, S. (1980). *Sacred words: A study of Navajo religion and prayer. Contributions in intercultural and comparative studies 4*. Westport, CT: Greenwood Press.

Griffin-Pierce, T. (1992). *Earth is my mother, sky is my father: Space, time and astronomy in Navajo sandpainting*. Albuquerque, NM: University of New Mexico Press.

Haile, B. (1938). *Origin legend of the Navaho enemy way: Text and translation. Yale University Publications in Anthropology 17*. London: Yale University Press.

Haile, B. (1947). *Head and face masks in Navaho ceremonialism*. St. Michaels, AZ: St. Michaels Press.

Harrington, J. (1940). Notes on the name Navaho. Manuscript in John P. Harrington Papers. National Anthropological Archives. Washington, DC: Smithsonian Institution.

Hewett, E. (1906). Origin of the name Navaho. *American Anthropologist, 8* (1), 193.

Klah, H. (1938). *Tleji or Yehbechai myth by Hasteen Klah: Retold in shorter form from the myth by Mary C. Wheelwright. Bulletin No. 1*. Santa Fe, NM: Museum of Navajo Ceremonial Art.

Klah, H. (1942). *Navajo creation myth: The story of the emergence. Navajo Religion Series 1*. Santa Fe, NM: Museum of Navajo Ceremonial Art.

Kluckhohn, C. (1960). Navaho categories. In. S. Diamond (Ed.), *Culture and history: Essays in honor of Paul Radin* (pp. 65-98). New York: Columbia University Press.

Kluckhohn, C. (1968). The philosophy of the Navaho Indians. In M. Fried (Ed.), *Readings in anthropology* (Vol. 2, pp. 674-699). New York: Thomas Y. Crowell.

Kluckhohn, C., & Leighton. D. (1962). *The Navaho* (rev. ed). New York: Natural History Press. Originally published by Harvard University Press, 1946.

Kluckhohn, C., & Wyman, L. (1938). Navaho classification of their song ceremonials. *Memoirs of the American Anthropological Association 50*.

Kluckhohn, C., & Wyman, L. (1940). An introduction to Navaho chant practice: With an account of the behavior observed in four chants. *Memoirs of the American Anthropological Association 53*.

Kluckholm [sic], C. [Kluckhohn, C.] (1923). The dance of Hasjelti: Being an account of the Yeibitchai held at Thoreau, N.M., November 9th to 18th. *El Palacio, 15,* 187-192.

Kompare, E. (1980). In *Good medicine* [videocassette]. Pittsburgh, PA: WQED.

Laban, R. (1928). *Schrifttanz* [Writing dance]. Vienna, Austria: Universal Edition.

Laban, R. (1960). *The mastery of movement* (2nd ed., revised by L. Ullman). London: MacDonald and Evans.

Laban, R. (1966). *Choreutics*. Edited and annoted by L. Ullman. London: MacDonald and Evans.

Laban, R., & Lawrence, F.C. (1947). *Effort*. London: MacDonald and Evans.

Lamphere, L. (1983). Southwestern ceremonialism. In A. Ortiz (Ed.), *Handbook of North American Indians* (Vol. 10, pp. 743-763). Washington, DC: Smithsonian Institution.

Leighton, A., & Leighton, D. (1941). Elements of psychotherapy in Navaho religion. *Psychiatry, 4,* 515-523.

Leighton, D., & Kluckhohn, C. (1947). *Children of the people: The Navaho individual and his development.* Cambridge, MA: Harvard University Press.

Levy, J. (1963). *Navajo health care concepts and behavior*. Window Rock, AZ: U.S. Public Health Service.

Luckert, K. (1979). An approach to Navajo mythology. In E. Waugh & K. Dad Prithipaul (Eds.), *Native religious traditions* (pp. 117-131). Waterloo, Ontario: Wilfred Laurier University Press.

Lyon, L. (1985). *Nightway Nov. 9-10, 1985, Tohatchi, NM*. Unpublished paper, courtesy of James Faris, Santa Fe, NM.

Lyon, L. (1986). Notes on Nightway (Yeibichai) ceremony Nov. 1, 1986. Unpublished paper, courtesy of James Faris, Santa Fe, NM.

Matthews, W. (1887). The mountain chant: A Navajo ceremony. *Annual Report of the Bureau of American Ethnology, 5,* 385-467.

Matthews, W. (1888). The prayer of a Navajo Shaman. *American Anthropologist 1,* 149-170.

Matthews, W. (1894). Songs of sequence of the Navajos. *Journal of American Folk-lore, 7* (26), 185-194.

Matthews, W. (1902). *The night chant: A Navaho ceremony*. Memoirs of the American Museum of Natural History VI. New York: Knickerbocker Press.

Matthews, W. (1907). Navaho myths, prayers, and songs: With texts and translations. In P. E. Goddard (Ed.), *University of California Publications in Archaeology and Ethnology, 5*(2), 21-63.

Matthews, W. (1994). *Navaho legends*. Salt Lake City: University of Utah Press. Originally published in 1896. New York: Houghton, Mifflin.

McAllester, D. (1954). Enemy way music: A study of social and esthetic values as seen in Navajo Music. *Papers of the Peabody Museum of American Archaeology and Ethnology, 41*(3). Cambridge, MA: Harvard University.

McAllester, D. (1979). A paradigm of Navajo dance. *Parabola, 4*(2), 28-35.

McAllester, D. (1980). Shootingway: An epic drama of the Navajos. In C. Frisbie (Ed.), *Southwestern Indian ritual drama* (pp. 199-238). Albuquerque, NM: University of New Mexico Press.

McAllester, D., & Mitchell, F. (1983). Navajo music. In A. Ortiz (Ed.), *Handbook of North American Indians* (Vol. 10, pp. 605-623). Washington, DC: Smithsonian.

McNeley, J. (1994). The pattern which connects Navajo and Western knowledge. *Journal of Navajo Education, XII*(1): 10-13.

Newcomb, F., & Reichard, G. (1937). *Sandpaintings of the Navajo shooting chant*. New York: J. J. Augustin.

Perrone, B., Stockel, H., & Krueger, V. (1989). *Medicine women, curanderas, and women doctors*. Norman, OK: University of Oklahoma Press.

Reichard, G. (1944a). *Prayer: The compulsive word. Monographs of the American Ethnological Society 7.* New York: J. J. Augustin.

Reichard, G. (1944b). Individualism and mythological style. *Journal of American Folklore, 57,* 16-25.

Reichard, G. (1945). Distinctive features of Navaho religion. *Southwestern Journal of Anthropology, 1*(2), 199-220.

Reichard, G. (1950). *Navaho religion: A study of symbolism*. Princeton, NJ: Princeton University Press.

Rogers, L. (1995). *USA Navajo profile*. Source: 1990 Census. Division of Community Development. Window Rock, AZ: Navajo Nation Government.

Sandner, D. (1979). *Navaho symbols of healing: A Jungian exploration of ritual, image, and medicine*. Rochester, VT: Healing Arts Press.

Sapir, E., & Hoijer, H. (1942). *Navaho texts*. Iowa City, IA: Linguistic Society of America.

Stevenson, J. (1891). Ceremonial of Hasjelti Dailjis and mythical sand painting of the Navajo Indians. *Eighth Annual Report of the Bureau of American Ethnology for the Years 1886-1887* (pp. 258-285). Washington, DC: United States Government Printing Office.

Stewart, K. (1977). The Southwest. In R. Spencer et al. (Eds.), *The Native Americans* (pp. 250-311). New York: Harper & Row.

Wheelwright, M. (1949). *Emergence myth: According to Hanelthnayhe or upward-reaching rite*. Recorded by Father Berard Haile. Navajo Religion Series 3. Santa Fe, NM: Museum of Navajo Ceremonial Art.

Wheelwright, M. (1956). *The myth and prayers of the Great Star Chant and the myth of the Coyote Chant.* Navajo Religion Series 4. Santa Fe, NM: Museum of Navajo Ceremonial Art.

Witherspoon, G. (1975). The central concepts of Navajo world view (II). *Linguistics, 161,* 69-87.

Witherspoon, G. (1977). *Language and art in the Navajo universe.* Ann Arbor, MI: University of Michigan Press.

Witherspoon, G. (1996). Telephone interview, September 16, 1996.

Wyman, L., & Kluckhohn, C. (1938). Navaho classification of their song ceremonials. *Memoirs of the American Anthropological Association 50.*

Wyman, L. (1950). The religion of the Navaho Indians. In V. Ferm (Ed.), *Forgotten religions* (pp. 341-361). New York: Philosophical Library.

Wyman, L. (1960). *Navaho sandpainting: The Huckel collection.* Colorado Springs, CO: The Taylor Museum of Colorado Springs Fine Arts Center.

Wyman, L. (1983). Navajo ceremonial system. In A. Ortiz (Ed.), *Handbook of North American Indians* (Vol. 10, pp. 536-557). Washington, DC: Smithsonian Institution.

Zolbrod, P. (1984). *Diné bahane': The Navajo creation story.* Albuquerque, NM: University of New Mexico Press.

The Therapeutic Aspects of Salish Spirit Dance Ceremonials

Wolfgang G. Jilek
University of British Columbia

THE TRADITIONAL GUARDIAN SPIRIT CEREMONIAL

The southwestern part of the province of British Columbia and the western part of the state of Washington are home to the Coast Salish Indian nation. The Coast Salish have important elements of traditional culture and art in common with other North American Indian nations of the Northwest Pacific coast. However, in mythology and ritual they are close to the Salish-speaking populations of the Plateau Culture Area that extends over wide regions of interior British Columbia, eastern Washington, Idaho, and Montana. In accordance with their intermediate position, both geographically and culturally, the Coast Salish combined the Plateau tribes' quest for vision and the power of a guardian spirit that was part of the ancient North American Indian guardian spirit complex (Benedict, 1923) with the secret society feature of initiation to the winter spirit ceremonial that was typical of traditional North Pacific Indian cultures, especially of the Kwakiutl.

In the aboriginal culture of the Coast Salish, before the dominance of non-Indian governmental and ecclesiastical authorities was firmly established, the most important ceremonial of the guardian spirit complex was the winter spirit dances in which all tribes of this North American Indian nation participated, as documented in ethnographic reports (Barnett, 1938, 1955; Boas, 1894; Curtis, 1913; Duff, 1952; Eells, 1889; Elmendorf, 1960; Gunther, 1927; Haeberlin & Gunther, 1924; Hill-Tout, 1902, 1904, 1905; Jenness, 1955; Olson, 1936; Smith, 1940; Stern, 1934; Suttles, 1955; Willoughby, 1889; Wilson, 1866).

In traditional Coast Salish society, adolescents and young adults of both sexes were encouraged to show endurance on an ascetic quest in search of a guardian spirit, roaming for months, sometimes years, through forest wilderness and along ocean beaches. The tutelary spirit would eventually appear in a vision and bestow on the determined seeker an individual song with special protective powers as well as talents that would be of great benefit in later life. The future shaman's quest for healing power was characterized by longer, more demanding ordeals, and a more intensive vision experience. For those who had successfully acquired spirit powers, the advent of the ceremonial Salish winter season was heralded by a nostalgic despondency with various physical symptoms that revealed their suffering from *spirit power illness* akin to the *initiatory sickness* of the budding shaman, which is institutionalized in many tribal societies (Eliade, 1964). In traditional Salish culture, spirit power illness was a ritualized pathomorphic, but not pathological state, that indicated initiation into the winter spirit dance ceremonial in order to publicly manifest one's newly acquired spirit powers and alleviate the sickness through ritual singing and dancing in an individual style.

The Salish guardian spirit ceremonial was suppressed by government authorities together with other traditional Northwest Coast North American Indian rituals toward the end of the nineteenth century; in British Columbia, through the Canadian "Law against the Potlatch Festival and Tamanawas Dance," in Washington by decree of the U.S. Superintendent of Indian affairs. At the same time, most North American Indian children and adolescents were sent to government-sponsored and church-run boarding schools where native languages and customs were to be driven out of their young minds in order to facilitate the then-official policy of assimilation. Traditional North American Indian ceremonials were considered as heathenish by the churches, as a waste of time by the authorities, and as contrary to the interests of an expanding capitalist economy in need of constantly available and relatively cheap manpower. Suppression of the Salish guardian spirit ceremonial appeared advisable to the authorities who had been frightened by the nativistic and anticolonialist Ghost Dance movements (Du Bois, 1939; Mooney, 1896) that originated in North American Indian cult dances of the Northwest Coast (Spier, 1953). In spite of threatened legal prosecution, some Coast Salish shamans and elders secretly continued the tradition of the guardian spirit ceremonial on a small scale.

REVIVAL AND TRANSFORMATION OF THE SALISH GUARDIAN SPIRIT CEREMONIAL

In the context of the "native renaissance" (Jilek, 1978, 1992), the Coast Salish guardian spirit ceremonial was revitalized in the beginning of the 1960s, thanks mainly to the mission-like activity of a few surviving Salish elders and shamanic healers. This author and Dr. Louise Jilek-Aall were able to observe this process because of our close cooperation with traditional North American Indian healers during the 1960s, 1970s, and 1980s (Jilek & Jilek-Aall, 1978; Jilek, 1982; Jilek-Aall & Jilek, 2001). The surviving shamanic healers recognized that under drastically changed demographic and socioeconomic conditions the traditional ceremonial had to be adapted to meet the therapeutic needs of the younger North American Indian population who suffered from the psychosocial consequences of imposed acculturation. Instead of achieving the assimilation that had been the desired goal of governmental policy in the past, the forced acculturation had led to a state of deculturation among the younger North American Indian population. The results of the deculturation were reflected in a steadily growing North American Indian overrepresentation in the statistics of morbidity, alcohol abuse, proneness to suicide, and intrafamily violence. Among the younger Salish people, sociocultural deprivation and identity confusion were the basis upon which developed a syndrome of chronic dysphoric and despondent mood often associated with diverse functional complaints that I have described as *anomic depression* (Jilek, 1974, 1982). In a significant number of cases, the depression is often alternating with an alcohol-and/or drug-induced behavior disorder. In response to the needs of the younger Coast Salish, the traditional functions of the initiation to the revived guardian spirit dance ceremonial were changed by the shamanic healers and ritualists in order to serve the required socio- and psychotherapeutic purposes.

THERAPEUTIC ASPECTS OF THE INITIATION PROCESS

In the view of the Salish ritualists today, younger North American Indian people suffering from anomic depression are considered as afflicted with spirit power illness due to their alienation from traditional North American Indian spirituality under the materialistic-hedonistic influences of modern Western society. Their hope for a cure is therefore not to be found in Western-type psychological counseling, psychiatric treatment, or correctional rehabilitation programs, but in the initiation to the Salish guardian spirit ceremonial that also permits re-identification with aboriginal culture through participation in spirit dancing. Salish ritualists realized that under contemporary conditions, it is no longer possible to undertake the traditional spirit vision quest in the wilderness as forests and beaches are being encroached on everywhere. The spirit dance initiation was therefore transformed into a therapeutic process in which the initiate acquires the healing guardian spirit power when experiencing a vision in an altered state of consciousness during one winter season and then expresses it in song and dance. The following is based on this author's own observations and the information he received from Salish Indian elders and ritualists (cf. Jilek, 1982).

In order to maintain his or her well-being, the new spirit dancer will have to actively participate in the annual winter spirit dances and always observe the traditional behavioral rules: show respect for the guardian spirit ceremonial and for the elders, feel responsible for needy members of family and tribe, and lead a lifestyle that is in line with the "old Indian ways," which discourage alcohol and drug use, entirely excluding it during the ceremonial season. The psychohygienic importance of these rules is obvious, especially in view of the fact that the obligatory abstention from alcohol during the fall and winter months of the spirit dance season coincides with the peaks of general liquor consumption in the area. Initiated spirit dancers breaking these rules risk losing the guardian spirit power that is understood as promoting physical and mental health and other rewards in life; eventually they will suffer a grave, perhaps even lethal calamity as punishment by the betrayed guardian spirit. This may indeed happen in case of relapse into alcohol or drug abuse.

The central theme of spirit dance initiation is the archetypal myth of death and rebirth: The former personality with all its negative behaviors due to alienation from traditional North American Indian ways is killed, as it were, and the initiate is reborn into a new and healthier existence by acquiring his or her guardian spirit power and at the same time reclaiming a cultural identity as a proud North American Indian person. In their ceremonial speeches, the ritualists equate the individual rebirth of the initiates with the collective revival of the Salish nation and culture. The first phase of the initiation process consists in therapeutic measures aiming at personality "de-patterning" and induction of an altered state of consciousness. In a kind of shock therapy, which is more intensely administered to young males than to females, the candidates are "grabbed" and symbolically "clubbed to death" with the ritualist's power-charged staff. The novice initiates are then subjected to psychic and physiological stress in a treatment regimen consisting of periods of immobilization under sensory and sleep deprivation, alternating with sensory overload and excitation by kinetic, tactile, temperature, and acoustic stimulation. The initiates are confined to the ceremonial house, lying blindfolded in a screened-off area in intended regression as "helpless babies," guarded and attended by their "babysitters," fasting, dehydrated, and sweating under heavy blankets. They are repeatedly subjected to forced hypermotility, are chased around the ceremonial house through snow and ice-cold brooks, and are frequently exposed to intensive sound stimulation through loud singing, rattling, and rhythmic drumming. The physical analysis of rhythmic drumming, which we recorded during the initiation procedures, revealed predominant frequencies above 3.0 cps (cycles per second), that is, stimulus frequencies that are known to elicit auditory driving with theta waves in the electroencephalogram, facilitating the induction of trance states (Neher, 1961, 1962). The combined action of these somato-psychic factors sooner or later induces an altered state of consciousness (Jilek, 1989, 1996; Ludwig, 1966) in the initiates, who under the influence of collective expectation and direct individual suggestion receive in a vision experience their guardian spirit power with an individual song and dance style. Having finally "found their spirit song," the initiates sing it out loud and feel blissfully carried away by their newly acquired power when dancing through the ceremonial house for the first time, spurred on by dozens of drums, deerhoof rattles, and the chanting and clapping of the crowd.

Whereas in the aboriginal Salish culture, spirit power was acquired in an individual quest and later manifested in the initiation, today it is acquired in, and through, the initiation process that at the same time constitutes an effective treatment of the contemporary spirit illness with symptoms of anomic depression.

> One could therefore say that the newly found spirit song of the initiate can have two different meanings today; it is both an inheritance of the power quest and a birth cry. There are two different systems, one the spirit power quest, the other the initiation that consists of being killed and reborn. The song occurs at the point where the two systems merge. (Lévi-Strauss, 1974)

For their first public appearance, the initiates are attired in the traditional Salish garb and equipped with the paraphernalia of new spirit dancers, the symbolism and semantics of which I have described elsewhere in detail (Jilek, 1982, 2000). The "uniform" of today's Salish spirit dancers is still essentially the same as the ceremonial garb depicted by the early ethnographers. The costume is often adorned with miniature paddles, reminiscent of the ancient travels of Salish shamans to the other world by spirit canoe (cf. Haeberlin, 1918; Jilek, 1982). Deerhoof rattles are tied to the calves and ankles of the dancers to loudly sound their rhythmic dance steps. The headdress of the initiates is made of thick woolen strands and partly covers the face and back for their own protection, and for that of the noninitiated, from interfering spirit powers. The initiates hold on to a staff adorned with small paddles, deer hooves, cedar bark, and eagle feathers, so that all of nature's realms are represented.

Today, witnesses to the initiation also tie handkerchiefs containing quarter-dollar coins to the staff as souvenir gifts. The new dancer's staff is likened to a supportive cane but also to a canoe pole to be used when walking as if "poling upstream toward life." Before each dance round, the tightly held power-laden staff shakes and its bearer "hears the spirit song coming out of it." While dancing, the initiate leaves the staff with the "babysitters" but upon returning from the dance round immediately clings to it again for strength and protection. At the end of the initiation season, the staff is secretly hidden in a hollow cedar lest an unauthorized person mishandling this veritable representation of the archetypal Tree of Life imperils the new dancer's safety or even life. Throughout the winter season of their initiation, the new dancers are strengthened in body and mind by a combination of hardening physical training and intensive indoctrination with ceremonial lore, rules of behavior, and what may be called nativistic culture propaganda.

Coast Salish leaders and ritualists strive to revitalize the North American Indian heritage and to uphold to the young an idealized image of aboriginal culture that is in contrast to the obvious deficiencies of modern Western society (cf. Jilek, 1988). In the contemporary guardian spirit ceremonial, a ritualized pan-North American Indian culture propaganda is taking over the didactic role of traditional Salish mythology and is serving a therapeutic function by boosting the initiates' self-esteem and promoting the formation of a positive cultural identity that counteracts the ego-damaging effects of anomic depression.

Toward the end of the ceremonial winter season, the initiation process is solemnly completed with the disrobing ceremony. Witnesses are called out of the gathering of visitors from all Coast Salish tribes to document the candidates' successful cure from "spirit illness" through a duly performed initiation treatment. The new dancers shed the last vestiges of their old personality together with their uniform and are publicly presented in the crowded ceremonial house as evidence of the healing and regenerating power of the guardian spirit.

After four years of faithful participation in the guardian spirit ceremonial and observance of its rules, a human-hair headdress will be bestowed on them as an insignia of their status as mature dancers who have graduated from an animal-like level of untamed wild power to a human-like level of controlled and socialized power. The "grown-up" spirit dancers now qualify for the ownership of an individually designed rattle stick with deer hoof pendants and a human or animal head carved at the top end. During the ceremonial, even experienced spirit dancers will hold on to their rattle stick for support after their dance round and "cry like a baby because they are being born again," reliving in every winter season the death and rebirth of their original initiation.

ANNUAL THERAPEUTIC SEASON

Salish spirit dancers count their spiritual age from the date of their successfully completed initiation. Every year from autumn to spring they actively participate in the spirit dance rituals several times a week at different ceremonial houses throughout the entire Coast Salish region. Of significance for mental health is the abstention from alcohol and other substance use expected of participants throughout the ceremonial season and of all guests, family and friends of participants, at the winter dances (Jilek, 1981). A remarkable degree of physical fitness is achieved by spirit dancers of all ages and exerts a positive psychohygienic effect.

Active participants in the Salish spirit dance ceremonial are immersed in a complex therapeutic enterprise combining well-defined treatment modalities. Spirit dancers experience direct ego support from the positive attention focused on them by the elders and the audience. When possessed by guardian spirit power, every one of the dancers commands respect. The drummers have to adjust to the individual dancer's song rhythm and tune, and spectators rise from their seats in deference to the spirit power when the dancer passes by. As a ritual group therapy, the ceremonial provides participants with support, acceptance, and stimulation. Group solidarity is emphasized in the speeches of ritualists and invited guests. Besides the active spirit dancers, many other Salish men and women are involved in the ceremonial enterprise. Their help is essential: They are organizing the dances, sewing the uniforms, tending the fires, and catering the meals; the drummers beat the rhythms and sing for hours, while the "babysitters" provide care for the initiates.

Perhaps the most relevant group-therapeutic aspect of the annual ceremonial is that those who participate in it are turned from egocentric preoccupation to the pursuit of

collective goals. For the active spirit dancers, the ceremonial provides frequent opportunities for cathartic abreaction in front of an accepting and empathic audience.

Affective discharges and dramatic acting take place in the Salish ceremonial houses
at every spirit dance event. The learning experience of the initiation enables the spirit
dancer to reenter an altered state of consciousness; each dancer relives the initial
guardian spirit possession again and displays in personal spirit song and dance performance the spirit power originally acquired in the guardian spirit vision through
the initiation treatment. Some dancers have become experienced virtuosi in quickly
entering a trance-like state through loud hyperventilation while still awaiting their
turn, then "singing out their song," and jumping up high to dance when the deer hide
drums strike up. The dancer's guardian spirit is dramatically manifested in the individual dance steps, movements, and tempo, and it is expressed in the dancer's gestures and miens. Hundreds of spectators watch a sadly trotting "bear mother"
bemoan her lost cubs, a ferociously yelling "warrior" making flying leaps, or a mighty
"killer whale" grabbing smaller fish.

Through its combination with cathartic abreaction in a culture-congenial group setting, the choreographic drama of the spirit dance becomes a therapeutic psychodrama
that also affects the audience. We can say that Coast Salish spirit dancing affords
catharsis for the actors according to Moreno's criteria of the psychodrama, and also
for the spectators according to Aristotle's function of the drama.

SPECIAL SHAMANIC CEREMONIES AT COAST SALISH SPIRIT DANCES

Special shamanic ceremonies are still performed at Salish spirit dances. The *skwenileč*
ceremony, which has a primarily therapeutic function, had its origin in the ancient,
now obsolete, spirit canoe ritual of the Coast Salish, as I was able to demonstrate on
the basis of older ethnographic records (Jilek, 1982, 2000). In the *skwenileč* procedures
I observed in the 1970s and 1980s, the shamanic healer called upon the audience to
concentrate their "good thoughts" on the patient. Held by four strong young male
assistants, the paraphernalia—two twisted, scarlet clothed *power sticks* and a *power
board* with a facial design—were publicly displayed while dozens of deer hide drums
beat fast rhythms. The power-laden instruments appeared so forceful that they
dragged their bearers through the ceremonial house hall when pulling together with
irresistible attraction. The quasi-magnetic therapeutic tools could only be severed
from each other and handled by the shamanic healer himself who thus demonstrated
his power. The paraphernalia finally guided him to the person whom they themselves
sought out for treatment, as it were. The healer was then gently stroking the patient's
head and body with the paraphernalia, thereby relieving tension and anxiety.

Most impressive of all rituals performed during the ceremonial season is the
sxwaixwe dance. The sxwaixwe mask is the only traditional Coast Salish mask and
only a limited number of families have hereditary rights to it. This mask is still fash-
ioned according to the pattern depicted in earlier ethnographic illustrations (Barnett,
1955; Curtis, 1913; Stern, 1934): Surrounded by a shield-like disk is a flat face dominated by protruding peg-like eyes, a nose shaped like a bird's beak, and a large fish-
shaped tongue hanging down; on top of the front are two bird heads standing up like
horns. The bird-fish nature of the sxwaixwe mask, combining the realms of sky and
sea, is repeated in the elaborate attire of the dancer, who wears a feather costume and
holds rattles made of seashells. The important place occupied by the sxwaixwe mask
and myth in Coast Salish culture has been conclusively demonstrated by C.

Lévi-Strauss (1975, 1979). On the cosmic level the sxwaixwe mediates between distant elements, joining sky and sea; on the societal level it mediates between distant kin groups, joining male and female in exogamous union, and also joining the Salish tribes over great distances in the sxwaixwe ceremony.

Beyond the important mediator role of the sxwaixwe, the myth of origin attests to its shamanic healing power. It tells of the hero, a young man at the time of his guardian spirit quest, who is sick. Rejected by his people, he becomes desperate, even suicidal. In order to recover, he has to undergo a death-and-rebirth experience comparable to a spirit dance initiation. He eventually obtains the sxwaixwe mask from spirit beings and is completely cured. He returns home with the mask and the shamanic healing power is conveyed to him.

Even today the supernatural power inherent in both the sxwaixwe mask and dance is believed to be so strong that during the sxwaixwe ceremonial, the spiritually vulnerable new spirit dance initiates have to avoid looking at it. This power could be seen as deriving from the tension generated by combining binary oppositions, as symbolized in the mask and the costume (bird-fish/sky-sea) and also gender oppositions in the choreographic drama of the sxwaixwe ritual in which the wild behavior of the young male dancers is tamed by the soothing tune of mature female singers. The healing aspect of the sxwaixwe dance is still manifested today by its performance for the benefit of North American Indians who are ill. If necessary, the dance is performed outside the ceremonial season, as it was for the ailing son of a well-known chief near Chilliwack, British Columbia, in June 1997.

RENAISSANCE OF NORTH AMERICAN INDIAN CEREMONIALS IN NORTH AMERICA

The revival of the Salish guardian spirit ceremonial has to be seen in the context of the revival throughout North America of other indigenous ceremonials such as the Sun Dance, the Gourd Dance, the Sweat Lodge Ceremony, or the Peyote Cult (Jilek, 1978) that also have significant socio- and psychotherapeutic functions. Most importantly, they create an opportunity for North American Indian people to establish a positive sociocultural identification and thus to escape the deleterious consequences of anomic depression. Today, the message at the revived and readapted indigenous ceremonials is that of North American Indian moral superiority in spite of humiliation, as well as North American Indian revitalization in spite of defeat. What is essentially a pan-North American Indian opposition mythology (Jilek, 1988) supersedes tribal and regional folklore in the speeches held at the ceremonial houses and becomes an effective weapon in the struggle for individual and collective self-assertion.

The revival of North American Indian ceremonials occurred in the 1950s and 1960s. This was the era of global decolonization and of the geopolitical retreat of Western powers from the "Third World," a historical process that was reflected in profound changes of the prevailing zeitgeist. The once glorious Western self-image was deflated, the once dominant Eurocentric worldview was abandoned, together with Western superiority claims, and at the same time the Western image of non-Western cultures and spirituality was upgraded. In this context, the Western perception of the shamanic healer also underwent a remarkable metamorphosis from the old image of a diabolic charlatan or madman to that of a model psychotherapist (cf. Jilek, 2003). The "North American Indian Renaissance" came about in such a changing ideological climate.

REFERENCES

Barnett, H. G. (1938). The Coast Salish of Canada. *American Anthropologist, 40*, 118-141.

Barnett, H. G. (1955). *The Coast Salish of British Columbi*a. Eugene, OR: University of Oregon Press.

Benedict, R. F. (1923). The concept of the guardian spirit in North America. *Memoirs of the American Anthropological Association*, No. 29.

Boas, F. (1894). The Indian tribes of the lower Fraser River. *Report of the 64th Meeting of the British Association for the Advancement of Science*, 1894, pp. 454-463.

Curtis, E. S. (1913). *The North American Indian, Vol. 9*. Norwood, MA. Written, illustrated, and published by Edward S. Curtis. (New York: Johnson Reprint Corporation, 1970).

Du Bois, C. (1939). *The 1870 ghost dance*. Anthropological Records, Vol. 3(1). Berkeley, CA: University of California Press.

Duff, W. (1952). *The Upper Stalo Indians of the Fraser Valley, British Columbia. Anthropology in British Columbia Memoir 1*. Victoria, British Columbia: Provincial Museum of British Columbia.

Eells, M. (1889). The Twana, Chemakum, and Klallam Indians of Washington Territory. In *Annual Report of the Board of Regents of the Smithsonian Institution for the Year ending June 30, 1887, Part 2, 605-681*. S. P. langley, Secretary of the Smithsonian Institution. Washington DC: U.S. Government Printing Office.

Eliade, M. (1964). *Shamanism, archaic techniques of ecstasy*. London: Routledge and Kegan Paul.

Elmendorf, W. W. (1960). *The structure of Twana culture*. Washington State University Research Series Monograph Supplement 2. Pullman, Washington: Washington State University Press.

Gunther, E. (1927). *Klallam ethnography. University of Washington Publications in Anthropology 1/4*. Seattle: University of Washington Press.

Haeberlin, H. (1918). SbEtEtda'q, a shamanistic performance of the Coast Salish. *American Anthropologist, 20*, 294-257.

Haeberlin, H., & Gunther, E. (1924). Ethnographische Notizen über die Indianerstaemme des Puget-Sundes [Ethnographic observations about the Indian tribes of the Puget-Sound]. *Zeitschrift für Ethnologie*, 1-74.

Hill-Tout, C. (1902). Ethnological studies of the Mainland Halkomelem, a division of the Salish in British Columbia. *Report of the 72nd Meeting of the British Association for the Advancement of Science*, 355-449.

Hill-Tout, C. (1904). Ethnological report on the Stseelis and Skaulits tribes of the Halkomelem Division of the Salish of British Columbia. *Journal of the Royal Anthropological Institute of Great Britain and Ireland, 34*(3), 11-376.

Hill-Tout, C. (1905). Report on the ethnology of the Stlatlumh of British Columbia. *Journal of the Royal Anthropological Institute of Great Britain and Ireland, 35*, 126-218.

Jenness, D. (1955). *The faith of a Coast Salish Indian. Anthropology in British Columbia Memoir 3*. Victoria, British Columbia: Provincial Museum of British Columbia.

Jilek, W. G. (1974). *Salish Indian mental health and culture change*. Toronto, Ontario: Holt, Rinehart & Winston.

Jilek, W. G. (1978). Native renaissance—The survival and revival of indigenous therapeutic ceremonials among North American Indians. *Transcultural Psychiatric Research Review, 15*, 117-147.

Jilek, W .G. (1981). Anomic Depression, Alcoholism, and a culture-congenial Indian response. *Journal of Studies on Alcohol*, Supplement No. 9, pp. 159-170.

Jilek, W. G. (1982). *Indian healing—Shamanic ceremonialism in the Pacific Northwest today*. Surrey, British Columbia: Hancock House.

Jilek, W. G. (1988). Pan-Indian opposition mythology and Indian renaissance in Canada. *New Observations* (New York), *60*, 16-23.

Jilek, W. G. (1989). Therapeutic use of altered states of consciousness in contemporary North American Indian dance ceremonials. In C. Ward (Ed.), *Altered states of consciousness and mental health—A cross-cultural perspective* (pp. 167-185). Newbury Park, CA: Sage.

Jilek, W. G. (1992). The renaissance of shamanic dance in Indian Populations of North America. *Diogenes* (Quarterly publication of the International Council for Philosophy and Humanistic Studies/UNESCO), *158*, 87-100.

Jilek, W. G. (1996). Ethnopsychiatric aspects of modified states of consciousness. In J. M. Fericgla (Ed.), *Lectures, Second International Congress for the study of the modified states of consciousness*, pp. 122-127. Barcelona, Spain: Institut de Prospectiva Antropologica.

Jilek, W. G. (2003). La métamorphose du chamane dans la perception occidentale [The metamorphosis of the shaman in the occidental perception]. In R. N. Hamayon (Ed.), *Chamanismes* (pp. 209-237). Paris: Presses Universitaires de France.

Jilek, W. G., & Jilek-Aall, L. (2000). Shamanic symbolism in the revived ceremonials of the Salish Indian Nation of the Pacific Northwest Coast. *Shaman—Journal of the International Society for Shamanisitic Research, 8*, 3-34.

Jilek-Aall, L., & Jilek, W. G. (2001). The woman who could not escape her spirit song. In W. S. Tseng & J. Streltzer (Eds.), *Culture and Psychotherapy—A Guide to Clinical Practice*, Chapter 4 (pp. 43-56). Washington, DC: American Psychiatric Press.

Lévi-Strauss, C. (1974). Discussion comments by Professor Claude Lévi-Strauss upon this author's presentation at the Department of Anthropology, University of British Columbia, July 9, 1974.

Lévi-Strauss, C. (1975). *La voie des masques* [*The way of the masks*] Geneva, Switzerland: Editions d'Art Albert Skira.

Lévi-Strauss, C. (1979). *La voie des masques et trois excursions* [*The way of the masks and three excursions*]. Paris: Plon.

Ludwig, A. M. (1966). Altered states of consciousness. *Archives of General Psychiatry, 15*, 25-234.

Mooney, J. (1896). *The Ghost-Dance religion and the Sioux outbreak of 1890.* Bureau of American Ethnology 14th Annual Report, 1892/93. Washington, DC: U.S. Government Printing Office.

Neher, A. (1961). Auditory driving observed with scalp electrodes in normal subjects. *EEG and Clinical Neurophysiology, 13*, 449-451.

Neher, A. (1962). A physiological explanation of unusual behavior in ceremonies involving drums. *Human Biology, 34*, 151-160.

Olson, R. L. (1936). *The Quinault Indians. University of Washington Publications in Anthropology 6/1.* Seattle: University of Washington Press.

Smith, M. W. (1940). *The Puyallup-Nisqually.* New York: Columbia University Press.

Spier, L. (1953). *The prophet dance of the Northwest and its derivatives: The source of the Ghost Dance.* Menasha, WI: Banta.

Stern, B. J. (1934). *The Lummi Indians of Northwest Washington.* New York: Columbia University Press.

Suttles, W. (1955). *Katzie ethnographic notes. Anthropology in British Columbia Memoir 2.* Victoria, British Columbia: Provincial Museum of British Columbia.

Willoughby, C. (1889). Indians of the Quinaielt Agency, Washington Territory. In *Annual Report of the Board of Regents of the Smithsonian Institution for the Year ending June 30, 1886.* Part 2, 267-282. Washington, DC: U.S. Government Printing Office.

Wilson, Captain E. E. (1866). Report on the Indian tribes inhabiting the country in the vicinity of the 49th parallel of northern latitude. *Transactions of the Ethnological Society of London, 4*, 275-332.

Traditional Healers in Mexico:
The Effectiveness of Spiritual Practices

Kaja Finkler
University of North Carolina, Chapel Hill

It was believed that as biomedicine increasingly succeeded in treating the body, alternative healers would disappear. Biomedicine has acquired an exquisite understanding of anatomy and physiology; it has developed spectacular techniques in organ transplantation, in emergency medicine, and in new reproductive technologies. Despite biomedicine's extraordinary achievements, a multitude of alternative healing forms continue to flourish. Interestingly, in present-day United States a significant change in how traditional healers are viewed has occurred. Whereas, until recently, traditional healers have been regarded as charlatans and quacks, at present enormous interest exists in alternative healing systems of all kinds, both sacred and secular. In fact, the Department of Health and Human Services opened a section dedicated to the study of alternative healing systems and, in the January 28, 1993 issue of the *New England Journal of Medicine*, Eisenberg et al. reported with some surprise that 34 percent of all Americans have used what they call "unconventional medicine." More recently, the same authors found that the percentage of individuals resorting to alternative medicine had gone up to 42.1 percent in 1997 (Eisenberg et al., 1998; see also Chapter 12 in this volume).

A wide variety of alternative healers practice around the world. These healers can be classified into at least two broad categories: sacred and secular. Secular healers may include herbalists, bonesetters, naturopaths, acupuncturists, homeopaths, yogi, and chiropractors. In Mexico, for example, where I have done extensive fieldwork (Finkler, 1991, 1994a, 1994b) there are injection specialists and a variety of traditional healers known as *curanderas/curanderos*.

Cross-culturally, sacred healers include many different types of shamans and other specialists who form part of a religious system and whose practices are embedded in a religious ideology. I studied one type of sacred healer in Mexico, known as Spiritual healers, over a span of 25 years. Unlike secular healers, sacred healers have some connection with divinity and are usually legitimated by their contact with the divine. For this reason, sacred healers share many similarities, including the fact that they often, if not universally, resort to altered states of consciousness by entering into a trance. Each healing system is, of course, unique and embedded in the culture of which it forms a part and from which it sprang. Nevertheless, healing systems, such as Mexican Spiritualism that I discuss in this chapter, share similarities with sacred healing everywhere as, for example, in disparate systems such as those of the bushmen (!Kung) of South Africa and Botswana, Native Americans, and even contemporary Americans (Jones, 1972; Katz, 1982; McGuire, 1988).

In this chapter I briefly describe the healing practices of the spiritualist healers, summarize my research findings of their successes and failures, discuss how they heal from our Western and their own perspectives, and lastly, and arguably most importantly, compare the treatment outcome of Spiritualist healers with that of biophysicians. The comparison brings into bold relief the strengths and weaknesses of both healing systems.

HEALING PRACTICES OF SPIRITUALISTS

Mexican Spiritualism is both a religious movement and a healing system. As a religious system, Spiritualism provides its followers with a well-defined cosmology, ethics, and liturgical order transmitted orally to its adherents through a medium in trance during weekly rituals consisting of sermons. Although Spiritualism incorporates an anti-Catholic stance, it is firmly rooted in Judeo-Christian teachings. Mexican Spiritualists believe in a threefold division of human history; the first stage belonged to Moses, the second to Jesus, and the the third, in which we live today, was ushered in by their founder in 1861. During their rituals, the founder known as Father Elias, the Virgin Mary, and Jesus Christ descend to the congregation in the body of a medium in trance, who irradiates, or conveys their teachings, and who, according to Spiritualists, is but a radio transmitter for their messages. During the irradiation, the congregants sit motionless, silent, transformed, and in a mild trance state. Spiritualist healers encourage those who seek their treatments to attend these rituals because, according to their teachings, listening to His word forms part of the cure.

As a healing system, Spiritualism attends to hundreds of patients.[1] The healers, primarily women, minister to the sick through spirit protectors who posses their bodies when they enter a trance. Each healer acquires a spirit protector during training, or what are called "development" sessions that are required for all potential functionaries of the temple, including healers, once the person has been recruited into the movement. The healers are usually recruited as a result of having themselves had an affliction unsuccessfully treated by physicians, a point to which I return shortly. The spirit protector identifies him- or herself in the body of the trainee during a development session, at which time the person is prepared to treat others. At this point, Mexican Spiritualists will tame spirits of the dead that are believed to roam the universe and harness them for the good of humankind, that is, for healing the sick. Healers may be in training as long as 10 years or, less usually, as little as 3 months, with an average of about 1 year.

Spirit protectors, who are referred to as Brother or Sister,[2] manifest themselves on healing days after the practitioner has arrived in the temple, put on a white robe, approached the alter of the temple to listen to a brief prayer recited by the temple

---

[1]Sylvia Echaniz Ortiz (personal communication) reported that in one Mexico City Spiritualist temple where she had studied for more than 20 years, she counted as many as 5,000 patients in 1 day. In the temple where I did my field research that was situated in a rural area, I recorded as many as 125 patients in a day (Finkler 1994a). Moreover, during the 14 years that I have visited this temple, there has been a three-fold increase in the number of healers working in 2 shifts ministering to the sick, reflecting the increase in the number of people seeking Spiritualist treatment from the healers.

[2]Presumably, spirit protectors are often, but not exclusively, of pre-Conquest origins with names of pre-Conquest tribes.

head, and then entered the healing room. At no time is a healer permitted to summon her protector outside the temple. To summon the protector, the healer sits down, closes her eyes, and mildly shakes the upper half of her body. She ceases to shake when the spirit protector temporarily settles in her body, identifies itself by name, and greets everyone present. Following this proceeding, which may take no more than a minute or two, the healer is prepared to receive patients. The healers usually treat patients in a room adjacent to the temple where religious rituals are conducted. On healing days the temple anteroom becomes transformed into a waiting room where men and women sit separately waiting as long as two to four hours to be seen by a healer. The temple head, who usually officiates over the healing procedures, urges people to contemplate the altar and concentrate on it as they wait because the cure begins when the patient sits silently in contemplation.

The healing procedure can be divided into four major phases. The first phase begins when the patient is directed to the healer by the temple head or a temple functionary overseeing patients in the waiting room. Upon approaching the healer, a patient is required to recite a salutation that initiates a customary response from the spirit protector. Once the salutation is given, the healer moves her hands up and down the patient's body and recites a blessing. This phase of the treatment episode is referred to by the Spiritualists as a "dislodgment," whereas patients speak of it as a cleansing. Additionally, some healers move their hands up and down the patient's body, lightly massaging the person throughout various phases of the treatment. The second phase of the treatment consists of the healer inquiring about the purpose of the visit, at which time the patient reports his or her symptoms and the healer touches the affected part of the body. Some healers may even anticipate the patient's symptoms by stroking the patient's body part affected by pain.

During the symptom exploration phase, a healer may suddenly faint away and begin speaking seeming nonsense. Careful attention to the words spoken reveals that the healer maintains a standard repertoire of set sentences that are uttered during a fainting incident, declarations such as "What am I doing here?" or "Take me away from this sacred place." The fainting episode, which may last no more than two to five minutes, suggests that a foreign evil spirit has briefly displaced the spirit protector in the healer's body. When such an episode occurs, the temple head quickly runs over to the healer and with a special prayer chases the evil spirit away. The spirit protector then repossesses the body of the healer.

The fainting episode as a healing technique occurs on infrequent occasions and is practiced only by some healers. More commonly, all Spiritualist healers resort to a wide variety of healing techniques, including the use of extensive pharmacopoeia, ritual cleansings, purgatives, massages, baths, spiritual surgeries, religious rituals, pharmaceuticals, and what I call "passive catharsis," when a patient experiences a sense of release and relief without having said anything. It is important to stress that along with these standard techniques, healers differ in their comprehension of patients' problems. Some exude more personal warmth in their tone of voice than others, some are brusque and angrily scold patients, and others speak in a soothing and reassuring manner. Some question a patient exhaustively and even ask for the patient's name, native town, and other biographical data. Others make few inquiries and even fail to ask the patient's name. I have observed consultations in which the patient never uttered a word during the entire healing episode, at which time the patient experienced a sense of passive catharsis.

In general, Spiritualist healers do not provide a patient with a definitive diagnosis, and when they do, it usually consists of informing the person either that he or she possesses a gift (a *don*) that requires cultivation, or that an evil spirit occupies his or her body and requires extrication. Normally, people whose illnesses are not readily alleviated by standard Spiritualist procedures, such as teas, massages, and baths, are given this type of diagnosis. If a patient is found to possess a gift or an evil spirit, he or she is instructed to enter training to develop the gift for healing so that the evil spirit is expelled during the training process. In this manner the patient is also recruited into the ranks of Spiritualism in a special ceremony when God "marks" the individual for a designated task, either to become a healer or another type of temple functionary. Such persons become what I call regulars, meaning adherents of Spiritualism.

SPIRITUALIST SUCCESSES AND FAILURES

When I began my research on the efficacy of Spiritualist healing in Mexico and mentioned my project to physicians there, they invariably responded by saying that such people were quacks. The doctors usually added that, because of the Spiritualist healers, they [the physicians] could not treat patients successfully because by the time a patient arrived at their door his or her maladies were too advanced for them to treat. Ironically, when I began attending Spiritualist healing sessions, the Spiritualist healers advised me that frequently they could not heal patients successfully because by the time people came to them to seek treatment, they were too sick to be healed.

During the course of my two-year research in the Spiritualist temple, I discovered that, in fact, the claim made by the Spiritualist healers was correct. Of the 400 patients that I studied who came to the temple for the first time, every one of them had sought treatment from more than one physician before seeking treatment from the Spiritualists. Thus, Spiritualist healing was a last rather than a first resort for the patient.

Commonly, people who arrive at Spiritualist temples originate from the poor strata of Mexican society and, with few exceptions, they usually seek treatment for what is generally described as a non-life-threatening chronic illness, the kind of affliction that biomedicine fails to alleviate.

The literature often refers to those seeking alternative healers as an undifferentiated mass of people who employ similar health-seeking strategies and have similar expectations and treatment outcomes. I observed in total 1,200 patients who came to the temple, and I found at least three categories of patients. *First comers* had seen numerous physicians for gastrointestinal, musculoskeletal, and respiratory distress; skin eruptions; gynecological problems; headaches; and personal problems that were usually associated with bodily discomforts. A second category was what I call the *habitual temple users*. These people were usually successfully treated by temple healers after their first visit, but may have had a recurring episode and returned to seek treatment for less severe disorders, such as mild diarrhea, catarrhs, nerves, pain in the throat (usually referred to as *anginas* in Mexico), back pain, and general discomfort.

The third category of patients were the *regulars* that I had mentioned earlier. These were people whose afflictions were not alleviated by routine temple treatments, and they were recruited into the movement. It is especially important to keep in mind these separate categories of patients when we examine the efficacy of traditional healers because each responds differently to temple treatment. I therefore discuss separately the three categories of patients.

Before I turn to my findings pertaining to the efficacy of Spiritualist ministrations, I must emphasize that it is extremely difficult to assess the effectiveness of any treatment. How can we know that a treatment is efficacious? From a biomedical perspective, therapeutic efficacy is defined as the capability of an agent to alter, demonstrably and measurably, the statistically predictable natural history of the disease. Effective medical treatment eliminates the primary cause of the disease and alters its natural course. The fact is that even with present medical knowledge, and with the exception of antimicrobial agents that remove infectious pathogens, few therapeutic agents are capable of removing the causes of most diseases. Even the treatment of heart contractions with digitalis, diuretics-promoting sodium extraction in coronary failure, thyroid hormone replacement in hypothyroidism, insulin in diabetes, or chemotherapy or radiation in cancer, to mention some of the most prominent treatments, fail to eliminate the cause of the disease at which they are targeted; they can but alter its course. Most chronic diseases that cause suffering in developed nations lack a cure, because for the most part the causes are not clearly understood and are of unknown etiology.

If the underlying causes of most pathologies cannot be eliminated, either because the cause is not known, as with most cancers, or because they lack cures, as with AIDS, how then can effective treatment be assessed using objective measures, except to say that a patient's symptoms were alleviated? Any measurement of effective treatment has its pitfalls, not the least of which is the obvious fact that diseases are often self-limiting and that in some measure, the body heals itself with or without ministration.

Because few objective measures of efficacy exist, I used patients' subjective evaluations to establish the outcome of both Spiritualist healing and biomedical treatments in Mexico (Finkler, 1991). The use of subjective measures is important because people usually regard themselves as healed when they subjectively experience alleviation, rather than when they are told that they are well by a doctor or a healer while they continue to feel sick. By objective measures a person may be considered well and his or her condition alleviated, whereas the patient's pains persist. Consequently, the person will go "doctor shopping" until his or her pains are eliminated.

Using systematic techniques,[3] I interviewed patients at the temple and followed them up at home after they had received treatment. During these follow-up interviews, I asked each person whether he or she followed the prescribed treatment, and whether his or her condition was alleviated, remained the same, or got worse. If the person's condition was alleviated, I asked the respondents to what they attributed the removal of the symptoms.

In my sample of 108 nonregulars–first-comers and habitual temple users— Spiritualist healers succeeded in healing 25.9 percent of the patients, they failed to heal 35.3 percent of them, and the remaining 38.8 percent of the case histories were inconclusive, as shown in Table 10.1. The category of inconclusives refers to people who either did not follow the prescribed treatment on my follow-up visit at home or reported that they felt only partially well.

Generally speaking, those that were successfully treated were people who had experienced mild diarrhea, mild gynecological treatments, and chronic disturbances. Consider Esperanza, who was initially carried in on a chair to the temple, visibly in

---

[3]I interviewed every fifth patient seeking treatment at the temple. Each patient was interviewed before seeing the healer and then followed up between seven and 14 days later. For a detailed discussion of the methodology used, see Finkler (1994a).

great pain. Gradually, she regained her ability to walk after she was given several treatments by three to four healers who simultaneously worked on her to dislodge her illness. The healers used several techniques that form part of the Spiritualist healing repertoire, including massages and dislodgments, or cleansings, to remove the evil spirit possessing her body.

Ten percent of the sample population was comprised of regulars. The regulars included patients to whom physicians may have even recommended surgery, or patients who experienced abdominal pain, back pain, headaches, epilepsy, blurred vision, heart palpitations, feelings of asphyxiation, and a general nervous state. Those who became regulars gradually recovered fully with Spiritualist healing and participation in temple rituals. I must emphasize that these recoveries took place very gradually. Improvement could be seen during periods of months rather than days. It is important to stress that the regular's recovery is dependent on their ongoing participation in temple rituals.

HOW SPIRITUALIST HEALERS HEAL FROM A BIOMEDICAL-SCIENTIFIC AND A SUBJECTIVE PERSPECTIVE

Several interrelated processes are at work in the alleviation of patients' sickness from a scientific perspective. Let me mention but four of the several possibilities I discuss elsewhere in great depth (Finkler, 1994a). First, Spiritualists use a large pharmacopoeia and it is quite possible that many of the botanical plants they prescribe are pharmacologically active. In cases such as diarrhea, for example, these plants may be effective in removing the symptoms, if not the cause.

Second, Spiritualists are very dependent on constant touching of the patient during the consultation, especially when they give patients massages and cleansings. The therapeutic touch seems to relax the patient and to produce a calming effect. The skin itself plays a role in inhibitory and excitatory interaction in mitigating pain. In fact, it has been found that direct stimulation of the skin by vibration is an effective method of decreasing pain (Melzack, 1976; Melzack & Wall, 1975). Moreover, pain may be mediated by increasing endorphins resulting from symbolic treatments through the cleansings.

Third, it is quite likely that Spiritualists induce physiological changes by their reliance on trancing during healing and rituals. Altered states of consciousness have their physiological correlates. Studies have shown long ago the therapeutic value of trance and meditation that is linked to their effects on the autonomic nervous system and on electroencephalogram (EEG) patterns (Benson, 1974; Benson, Klotch, Crassweller, & Greenwood, 1976; Lex, 1976, 1978).

Fourth, and this brings me to the patients' subjective experience, alleviation is mediated through the symbolic aspects of Spiritualist healing. When I asked patients which aspect of Spiritualist treatment eased their condition, all cited the cleansings they received at the temple. Some added massages and baths, but the cleansings were regarded as the most salient feature of Spiritualist healing. Symbols, of course, reach us at the deepest level. Symbols develop in a particular culture and speak to people's most profound concerns in that culture. Cleansings symbolically purify by removing evil. Purification represents a form of restoring order to a condition that previously had been a disorder. The disorder and pain that one encounters in one's life is relieved by symbolic manipulation through purification by cleansing. By way of illustrating the ways in which Spiritualist symbols become transmitted during treatment, consider one patient who subsequently became a curer and who had suffered from heart palpitations. The healer linked these heart palpitations to crystalline drops that fall into an empty glass; the palpitations become drops that symbolize God's words transmitted during Spiritualist rituals and the patient represents the empty glass. The patient constantly referred to this metaphor when she spoke about having gradually recovered from her chest pains and headaches.

Moreover, on an existential level, regulars who become healers embody a spirit protector when they enter a trance, and by so doing they experience their bodies in a new and sacred way. Uniformly, all healers and functionaries enter a trance to fulfill their healing roles, and they report that they experience a tingling effect in their bodies, a heightening of the senses, and a vision of extraordinary colors. People regard these new experiences as transformative and healing. As I noted before, from a scientific perspective, being in a trance may alter the physiology of the body, and a trance may possess physiological correlates that influence the healing process.

At this juncture, it is noteworthy that not all patients respond similarly to the symbols supplied by Spiritualist healers. It is evident that Spiritualists do not heal everyone successfully. Not all people with an illness episode are amenable to Spiritualist therapeutic intervention. In fact, I found that people with fewer self-perceived symptoms were more likely to obtain relief from Spiritualist treatment than persons with a greater number of expressed symptoms. But there are those with symptoms who totally fail to respond to temple therapies and Spiritualist symbolic manipulations, such as individuals with psychotic disorders. Symbolic manipulation by healers is crucial for perceived treatment efficacy, and a patient's capacity to respond to these symbols is equally crucial.[4]

COMPARISON OF SPIRITUALIST HEALERS AND BIOPHYSICIANS

Before I turn to a comparison between Spiritualist healers and biophysicians, I must emphasize that the Mexicans I studied did not usually distinguish between types of healers, nor were they concerned with epistemological questions. Their preoccupation is much more pragmatic; they are interested in who gives the best medicine rather than how healers gain their knowledge, whether it be through spirits or through a scientific education.

The strengths and weaknesses of Spiritualist healing come into bold relief when we compare Spiritualism with biophysicians. After having spent two years studying Spiritualist healers, I spent a similar time period studying Mexican physicians because, as I noted earlier, people sought treatment from Spiritualist healers only after they had been unsuccessfully treated by physicians, and therefore I wished to assess people's responses to biomedical treatments. The physicians' patients I studied were of the same social class as the patients in the Spiritualist temple and they presented similar types of disorders as those reported by patients in the temple.

Table 10.1 displays a comparison between the percentage of patients who reported successes, failures, and inconclusive outcomes of the treatment received from Spiritualist healers and physicians.

---

[4]For an in-depth discussion and specific examples of those who do not respond to Spiritualist ministrations, see Finkler (1985/1994a).

TABLE 10.1
Comparison of Patients' Perceived Recovery by Type of Healer (in Percent)

	Failures	Successes	Inconclusives	Total
Spiritualists (N=108)	35.3	25.9	38.8	100
Physicians (N=205)	25.4	17.1	57.5	100

As displayed in Table 10.1, interestingly, using patients' subjective evaluation of whether they were feeling better, worse, or the same from the time they received the treatments, the percentages of Spiritualists' successful treatment outcomes were somewhat better than the physicians, 25.9 percent and 17.1 percent respectively. But whereas the failure rate among Spiritualists was 35 percent, it was only 25.4 percent among physicians. However, among the overwhelming majority of physicians' patients (57.5 percent), the outcome was inconclusive because in this instance patients reported feeling only partially better as compared with 38.8 percent of Spiritualist healers' patients. The comparison between the treatment outcomes of Spiritualist healers and of biophysicians as perceived by patients suggests that Spiritualist healers had a somewhat higher rate of full success, but that they also had a higher percentage of failures. Most interestingly, the majority of patients were neither healed by Spiritualist healing or by biomedicine at the time of the first follow-up home visit. Those that continued to feel sick returned to the healers, went doctor shopping, and then sometimes returned to the healers again.

What about those who have been successfully healed by Spiritualist healers? What does Spiritualist healing achieve for patients that can contribute to and explain even the relatively low success rate?[5] Before I turn to the differences between the two systems of healing that might illuminate the outcomes of Spiritualist healing, it is worth noting certain similarities between Spiritualist healers and biomedicine. Both adhere to a dualist view of the body and its attendant disturbances. Spiritualists clearly and forcefully distinguish between corporeal (or, in their words, "material") and spiritual disturbances in much the same way that physicians distinguish between organic and psychological sickness, though biomedicine is frequently criticized for this distinction.[6]

In both Spiritualist and biomedical encounters, the patient takes on the role of a passive recipient of the practitioner's ministrations, and in both healing systems practitioners insist on patients' compliance. In fact, a healer's spirit may reprimand a patient if the spirit detects that the patient has not followed the prescribed treatment.

Moreover, the Spiritualist healers always remind patients that they can see "inside the body" because the spirits are omniscient, in the same way as biophysicians see inside the body using complex technologies. But unlike patients at a physician's office, patients seeking treatment from Spiritualist healers do not have to say anything precisely because the healing spirits are omniscient. The patients tend to experience, as I noted earlier, a passive catharsis when the healer describes to them the pains he or she is experiencing, eliminating the need for the patient to actively verbalize his or her distress.

---

[5]For a full discussion of the reasons for success and failures among the physicians I studied, see Finkler (1991).
[6]I should stress, however, that the duality of body and mind in both healing systems may be experienced very differently by the patients.

ATTRIBUTION, DIAGNOSIS, AND TREATMENT

The differences between the two healing systems, however, are much more pronounced. First, spiritual healing is a communal experience. Numerous healers sit in the same room ministering to patients, usually accompanied by a relative. There is a cacophony of sounds in Spiritualist healing rooms that imparts a sense of a collective experience, unlike the physician-patient encounter that takes place in isolation in a cubicle.

Second, in Mexico, faith in the power of biomedicine is such that when biomedical treatment fails, many people assume that the infirmity was produced by witchcraft. Patients seeking treatment from Spiritualist healers usually arrive at a Spiritualist temple believing that witchcraft has been perpetrated on them. Nevertheless, the Spiritualist healers I studied categorically deny the existence of witchcraft, that is, that people can do harm to others by magical machinations. In this manner, Spiritualists remove blame for the patient's disorder from a neighbor, relative, or other human being with whom the person interacts; they place the culpability squarely on impersonal spirits for which neither the patient nor his or her social circle can be blamed. By doing so, they restore order in the person's disrupted social relations and thereby possibly avoid future anger and other upsets that Mexicans believe cause sickness. Although biomedicine lacks a belief in witchcraft, it does blame patients for their sickness, a point to which I return shortly.

Third, in day-to-day practice, Spiritualist healers, unlike physicians, are not concerned with etiological explanations, the cause of the sickness. Such etiologies that they do offer are relatively limited and unchanging compared to those of biomedicine. Spiritualist healers confer a coherent system of explanation, which in the final analysis is usually reduced to assaults by evil spirits. As I noted earlier, Spiritualists believe that those afflictions stubbornly resisting both biomedical and Spiritualist ministrations have been caused by the intrusion of a bad spirit that requires removal from the body, as we saw in Esperanza's case.

Physicians' causal explanations are relatively complex, and they usually include the breaking down of the bodily machine by the invasion of a large variety of pathogens, as well as stress, obesity, diet, poor personal health habits (e.g., drinking and smoking) that place the person at risk (Mckeown, 1979), or genetic inheritance (Finkler, 2000a). Whereas biomedical causal explanations stress an individual's personal behavior, placing the blame on the person or his or her family rather than impersonal spirits or witchcraft performed by other people, Spiritualism tends to remove the blame from the person.

Most important, unlike Spiritualists, physicians may provide various causal explanations and also change them, as good biomedical practice requires. In biomedicine, a diagnosis is always provisional. Good medical practice requires physicians to constantly reevaluate their diagnosis. However, from the patient's perspective, diagnostic revisions are distressing. For example, a physician may change the diagnosis if a patient's complaints were not alleviated by the prescribed treatment. A modification of the diagnosis suggests to the patient that the doctor lacked the certainty and knowledge to cure the illness. Frequently, if patients seek treatment from several physicians, they might be offered various diagnoses. Getting several diagnoses for the same pains and symptomatologies is often puzzling and disturbing to patients.

Unlike physicians, Spiritualists draw on a limited diagnostic repertoire and eschew multiple diagnoses. A Spiritualist healer is usually consistent about diagnosis, and that same consistency exists among different healers regarding the cause of the person's affliction, as well as treatment. Thus, Spiritualists tend to provide decisive explanations and one diagnosis, whereas physicians furnish various and multiple diagnoses that become confusing to the patients.

THE PRACTITIONER / PATIENT RELATIONSHIP

It is commonly said that traditional healers, including Spiritualists healers, show great understanding and possess more empathy and compassion for patients than physicians do, an assertion that by now has become commonsense knowledge. Spiritualists are presumably more attentive to patients than physicians, a quality often measured in terms of healers having more eye contact with patients and spending more time with them. In short, traditional healers are often idealized when they are not demonized. My observations of Spiritualist healers reveals that, unlike physicians, they lack eye contact with their patients and do not recognize the individual standing before them. The healers sit in a trance with expressionless faces; their eyes are closed and they hold or stroke the patient who briefly murmurs a description of his or her disorder. Actually, being in a trance state precludes the healers from displaying any kind of affect for their patients. By contrast, the physician sits facing the patient, who is given a physical examination, and physicians often show a great deal of affect during the encounter.

I found that physicians spent about 21 minutes on average with a first-time patient, whereas Spiritualists healers usually spent half that time. But there is an inherent tension and conflict between the patient and the physician that is absent in the Spiritualist healer/patient encounter. I characterize the physician/patient interaction as a drama, a drama that is lacking in the Spiritualist healer/patient encounter. In both Spiritualist healing and biomedical practice, the meeting between the health provider and the patient is not an ordinary encounter between two strangers, since the conditions that bring healer and patient together are extraordinary: One is in pain and under duress, and the other is expected to eliminate or transform the condition. However, in contrast to the Spiritualist healer/patient encounter, in the biomedical consultation the drama is revealed when the two actors stand in opposition to one another. Unlike Spiritualist healing, the encounter, as scripted by the biomedical model, brings two players into conflict. Moved by a crisis, the patient arrives on the stage to seek advice from an expert who presumably knows more about how bodies work than the patient does. The physician claims to have a monopoly on the knowledge of disease. He is the authority on what went wrong. The patient comes laden with personal knowledge encoded by cultural understanding about the working of his or her own body and the authority of experiencing the specific condition. The patient is *certain* of his or her individualized experience of pain, whereas the physician is often *uncertain* of the diagnosis. One of the doctors I studied said, "I must sometimes invent a diagnosis."

The drama that exists in the doctor/patient relationship is minimized in the Spiritualist healer/patient encounter. Whereas a physician's clinical judgment entails uncertainty and is grounded in a process of exclusion, the spirits treat patients with great certainty. Spiritualist healers are as sure of their diagnoses and course of cure as patients are certain of their pain. Spiritualist healers do not doubt that the spirits possessing their bodies "in the service of mankind" are omniscient, or that they know the person's pain and suffering as well as the required cure.

Significantly, too, whereas the physician must cast the patient's sickness in a temporal frame and localize the pain in a specific part of the body, the omniscient spirits transcend time and space in the same way that the patient's sickness transcends temporal and spatial dimensions. The patient cannot confine the onset of the afflictions to a specific time because the patient experiences the pain as timeless. The biomedical diagnostic process incorporates a temporal and topographic dimension, but for the patient the sickness transcends time and body topography. The physician is often frustrated by the patient's inability to compartmentalize symptoms to a particular anatomical region, to conform to the medical history format, or to locate the symptoms within a time frame. I observed numerous instances when physicians would say to a patient "tell me where it hurts" and the patient, to the physician's frustration, would point to many different areas of the body.

The patient's major concern is that the healer or physician knows his or her pain. When the patient confronts a Spiritualist healer, he or she need not tell the healer very much for the healer to know everything, and may experience a passive catharsis, as I mentioned earlier. In fact, the spirit constantly reminds the patient "I know everything." In this way, the healer reassures the patient and also establishes legitimacy in the healing role. The physician, however, must question the patient, anchor the condition, and locate it in chronological time and in a specific part of the body in order to make an accurate diagnosis.

In sum, whereas Spiritualist healers' diagnoses are relatively simple, their treatment repertoires are relatively complex. In contrast, the physicians' diagnoses are complex, but their curing repertoire is limited. Thus, a comparison of treatment techniques reveals that physicians' treatments include chiefly medications, or, in extreme cases, surgery or replacement of body parts. In contrast, the Spiritualist healers' treatment kit contains a large array of treatment options, which also involve patients' participation in various treatment activities. These include the use of pharmaceuticals or herbs and other botanicals (which people are either required to find in the fields, grow at home, or purchase), massages, baths that require preparation by the patient, and other such activities, including participation in Spiritualist rituals. These activities in effect engage patients in their recovery. In keeping with this point, physicians take full responsibility for the patient's successful cure, if not for their failure to heal. On the other hand, Spiritualist healers assign responsibility to patients for their cure by constantly reminding them that they must have unrelenting faith in the Spiritualist God and His benevolence, further involving them in their own therapy.

RECRUITMENT INTO THE HEALING ROLE

Significantly, patients are also assured that the Spiritualist healer knows their pain because they know that Spiritualist healers too have suffered afflictions before becoming healers. This brings me to the important difference between the recruitment of healers and physicians. The different ways in which Spiritualist healers and physicians are recruited into their respective roles have different effects on patients. Whereas those recruited into the medical profession are usually healthy individuals, those recruited into Spiritualist healing usually have experienced an affliction before becoming healers. As formerly sick people who have become health providers, Spiritualist healers serve as examples of the potential for recovery through Spiritualist ministrations. Importantly, they convey to the patient that they have grasped the patient's anguish through their personal experience. They experienced the pain in the past in the same way as the patient is experiencing it in the present. A doctor cannot provide the patient with experiential evidence, as Spiritualist healers proudly do, or that his or her ministrations induce a transformation from having been sick to healing others.[7]

Lastly, when we focus on the regulars who become members of the movement, we find that these are the people who benefit most from Spiritualist healing. The conversion of a patient to health practitioner, or to a functionary serving God and the spirit world, forms part of the Spiritualist therapeutic repertoire, a technique that the biomedical therapeutic kit lacks. By becoming Spiritualists, they become members of a religious community, and their lives take on new rhythms that revolve around communal rituals and activities. Spiritualist healing can gradually transform the person's existence by incorporating him or her, and sometimes the entire family, into a religious community. Over the long term, Spiritualist healing provides new interpersonal networks and also places the person in a new relationship with God and a new experience of transcendence. In the latter instance, relationships with other human beings become subsumed under the person's interaction with God.

Spiritualist healing progressively reorders the regulars' existence in several ways: by incorporating them into a community of sufferers who share a satisfying religious reality and symbolic meanings, by God appointing them to become functionaries in the movement, and by His having chosen them to become healers because they posses a gift. In this manner, the Spiritualists convert the person's sick role into a healing role. In this context, a point I made earlier merits repeating. Spiritualist healers do not produce miraculous cures. All transformations are achieved gradually, and some patients may even experience great pain in the process of recovery, as well as conflict in joining a new religious movement.[8]

Importantly, Spiritualist healing differentially reorders men and women's lives. It reorders men's lives to the ostensible advantage of women. Spiritualists preach against machismo in men, leading them to cease heavy drinking and womanizing if they join the movement. The men tend to spend their leisure time with their wives and families rather than with their former friends or other women. By restructuring men's lives, Spiritualists promote smoother marital relationships, a change women recognize as salutary and healthful.

To summarize, the dissimilarities between Spiritualist healers and biophysicians include the fact that the Spiritualist healers resolve contradictions for patients that physicians cannot because physicians focus on discrete physical pains, while the patient is experiencing a timeless and overbearing pain that is not necessarily localized in chronological time or confined to specific parts of the body. Physicians do not address the contradictions in which patients are enmeshed and that may have contributed to the development of these symptoms. Physicians may blame impersonal pathogens that attack the body or the patient, as well as his or her poor habits. Biomedicine requires patients to alter their behaviors, such as diet, work, or drinking habits, but it does not attempt to transform the circumstances of a patient's life in the way Spiritualists do, especially *for those who become regulars*.

This brings me to my last point. Elsewhere (Finkler, 1991, 1994b), I proposed the concept of life's lesions as a source of people's non-life-threatening chronic sickness.

---

[7]This is analogous to the underlying assumptions of support groups in United States that are based on the notion that people who have themselves experienced a given sickness can best understand another's experience.

[8]Mexican Spiritualism is anti-Catholic and for individuals who are devout Catholics, joining the Spiritualist community may create a conflict.

By life's lesions, I mean a perceived adverse existence, including inimical social relationships and unresolved moral contradictions in which a person is entrenched that gnaw at the person's being and fester through time, thereby producing myriad non-life-threatening symptomatologies. Life's lesions intrude on the body in much the same way as any pathogen or anatomical lesion, but they are not fatal. Life's lesions express through the body deleterious conditions of existence, be they poverty, malnutrition, adverse life events, or unreconcilable contradictions, and, most important, moral indignation at social relations that have gone sour.

An important facet of life's lesions is marital discord and adverse social relations that can be as pathogenic as any virus. Women's health in Mexico, as is true around the world, is greatly influenced by their relations with their mates, especially by domestic violence, which produces a life's lesion not easily alleviated by medical ministrations (Finkler, 1994a, 1997).

To the degree that Spiritualist healers succeed in easing the marital relationship and changing the person's existence, they are also promoting a woman's health. Clearly, the biomedical model is not designed to address existential dilemmas that produce life's lesions, reinterpret these dilemmas, and give them new meanings, or change relationships in which a patient is embedded, especially those between husband and mate.

Spiritualist healing encompasses the lives of those patients whom it succeeds in converting into participants and believers, a minority at that. For regulars, their bodies become extensions of the Spiritualist congregation upon which they become totally dependent, and paradoxically this reliance on the temple also forms part of their cure. Although it may not succeed in eradicating life's lesions, participation in the Spiritualist movement exerts power over the patients' existence because, as many patients readily admit, if they failed to attend to the various rituals and to heal others, they would revert to their morbid states.

In the final analysis, Spiritualist healers, like physicians, fail to fully heal their patients when they fail to attend to their patient's lived world and to the conditions that shaped the life's lesions. Not surprisingly, therefore, the majority of patients reported inconclusive perceived treatment outcomes. To succeed in resolving non-life-threatening subacute disorders, a healing system must address patients' life lesions and concurrently help them transform their existence. Biomedicine fails in these tasks, whereas Spiritualist healing succeeds with a minority of patients, mainly with the regulars, in transforming their lives.

By way of conclusion, I will add that during the course of 25 years of contact with Spiritualist healers in Mexico, I have watched Mexican Spiritualism grow immensely. In the temples where I carried out my research, there were initially 8 healers, but when I visited them in 1997, 24 healers were working in 2 shifts attempting to heal many hundreds of patients a day.

This growth is probably associated with many factors. To cite but two, as globalization comes into full force, and Mexico is certainly involved in the globalization process, people tend to dig in their heels and hang on to their own understanding of healing and other cultural practices, arguably in response to the homogenization that globalization tends to impose (Finkler, 2000b).

But even more important, as modern medicine advances and people's expectations are heightened regarding its success, biomedicine's failures become less explicable and more frustrating. People therefore turn more and more to alternative healing of the secular and sacred kind for conditions that biomedicine fails to heal, including those that are produced by life's lesions. The non-life-threatening symptomatologies produced by life's lesions cannot be healed unless their causes are addressed and the person's life is transformed. Biomedical practitioners do not have anything in their toolkit to transform people's lives, whereas Spiritualism, although it does not address the causes of life's lesions, does transform the lives of those who become regulars. For this reason I anticipate that traditional healing of the Spiritualist kind will continue to grow and thrive.[9]

REFERENCES

Benson, H. (1974). Your innate asset for combating stress. *Harvard Business Review*, July-August, 49-60.
Benson, H., Klotch, J., Crassweller, K., & Greenwood, M. (1976). Historical and clinical considerations of the relaxation response. *American Scientist*, 65, 441-445.
Eisenberg, D., Davis, R., Ettner, S., Appel, S., Wilkey, S., Van Rompay, M., & Kessler, R. (1998). Trends in Alternative Medicine use in the United States, 1990-1997. *Journal of the American Medical Association*, 280, 1569-1575.
Eisenberg, D., Kessler, R. C., Foster, C., Norlock, F., Calkins, D., & Delbanco, T. (1993). Unconventional medicine in the United States. *New England Journal of Medicine*, 28, 246-283.
Finkler, K. (1991). *Physicians at work, patients in pain*. Boulder, CO: Westview.
Finkler, K. (1994a). *Spiritualist healers in Mexico*. Salem, WI: Sheffield. (Originally published in 1985 by Praeger and Bergin and Garvey).
Finkler, K. (1994b). *Women in pain*. Philadelphia: University of Pennsylvania Press.
Finkler, K. (1997). Gender, domestic violence and sickness in Mexico. *Social Science and Medicine*, 45(8), 1147-1160.
Finkler, K. (2000a). *Experiencing the new genetics. Family and kinship on the medical frontier*. Philadelphia: University of Pennsylvania Press.
Finkler, K. (2000b). Diffusion reconsidered: Variation and transformation in biomedical practice: A case study from Mexico. *Medical Anthropology 19*(1),1-39.
Jones, D. (1972). *Sanapia, Comanche medicine woman*. New York: Hold, Rinehart, and Winston.
Katz, R. (1982). *Boiling energy*. Cambridge, MA: Harvard University Press.
Lex, B. (1976). Physiological aspects of ritual trance. *Journal of Altered States of Consciousness*, 2, 109-122.
Lex, B. (1978). Neurological bases of revitalization. *Zygon, 13*, 276-312.
McGuire, M. (1988). *Ritual healing in suburban America*. New Brunswick, NJ: Rutgers University Press.
McKeown, T. (1979). *The role of medicine*. Princeton, NJ: Princeton University Press.
Melzack, R. (1976). Pain: Past, present and future. In M. Weisenberg & B. Tursky (Eds.), *Pain* (pp. 135-146). New York: Plenum Press.
Melzack, R., & Wall, P. (1975). Psychophysiology of pain. In M. Weisenberg (Ed.), *Pain, clinical and experimental perspectives* (pp. 8-23). St. Louis, MO: C.V. Mosby.

---

[9]On my most recent visit in June 2003, I found that the temple was being expanded to accommodate 1500 worshipers and about 30 to 40 healers.

Women as Healers: A "Gendered" Exploration in Puerto Rico and Elsewhere

Joan D. Koss-Chioino
Arizona State University
George Washington University

Why are women more numerous and important as healers in some medical systems and men in others? Do women healers have special attributes that differ from those of male healers? Relatively few accounts address why and how gender may be important to the healing role, and even fewer answer these questions by exploring the experiences of women as healers. Decades ago, I. M. Lewis (1971) offered the now classic thesis that women are healers where there are "cults of affliction," covert protest movements with possession-trance rituals that seek to compensate gender inequalities. Other anthropologists, such as Morsy (1978), suggested that because some men suffer the same types of initiation illness as do women, and also participate in possession cults, an explanation of why more women are healers in these cults can be found in the relationship between the gender system and systems of power and authority. More recently, Lewis's notion has been critically reviewed by Janice Boddy (1989). Based on studies of the Zar cult in northern Sudan, she suggests that although the idea of status and power balancing may be accurate, it is too one-dimensional to adequately explain Sudanese women's behavior. Boddy describes, in beautiful detail, how complementarities in men's and women's roles underlie women's involvement in the cult, expressed in Zar spirit possessions. The aim of the Zar cult is to address the "major issue" of "cultural over determination of women's selfhood" as reproductive beings (Boddy, 1988, p. 4). Finally, in contrast to appealing to sociocultural factors such as gender role constructs, Jeanne Achterberg (1989, p. 197) suggests that certain gender-related, stereotypical personal attributes are found in women who become healers—subjectivity, relatedness, and understanding—which are also the attributes of the "wounded" healer, considered by her to be the ideal healer.

In my book, *Women as Healers, Women as Patients*, I elaborate on a perspective of the cultural construction of the healer role that selects for female gender, partially constrained by culturally defined gender-role attributes and behavior (Koss-Chioino, 1992). To briefly summarize, women's predisposition to affiliate as a lifelong pursuit can manifest as an enlarged capacity to receive. A woman can more easily learn "to receive herself, receive what is other than herself and also be received by others" (Ulanov, 1981, p. 15). She can then learn to grasp previously unattained attributes of her personal reality, such as power, aggression, spirituality, and earthiness, characteristics that may be denied to her in conventional social intercourse but are essential to the healer role in many healing systems, even though denied to women generally.

The goal of this chapter is to offer a perspective on women as healers in which personal characteristics, gender role, and sociocultural context are interrelated (see also Glass-Coffin, 1996). It incorporates aspects of the formulations briefly described earlier but adds an ontogenetic perspective. I suggest that the twin processes of early life and healer-role socialization, as perceived by healers themselves, are central to an understanding of why some women become healers. This exploration is carried out in five phases. The first section, "Traditional Healers in Puerto Rico: The Process of 'Development,'" describes Espiritismo (Spiritism) and how the healers (Spiritist mediums) are initiated into their healing role. The second section, "Generalizing the Healer's Myth," utilizes material from my studies of traditional healers in Puerto Rico. I examine 3 main themes in a life story of a Spiritist medium, a composite of more than 30 life stories of women Spiritist healers collected some 25 years ago in Puerto Rico. In the third section, "Mental Health Professionals and Medical Doctors in Puerto Rico," I assess the life stories of mental health professionals in Puerto Rico for parallels to the prototype themes in the life stories of traditional healers. The fourth section, "Mental Health Professionals and Medical Doctors in the United States," briefly explores evidence for further generalization of the model. In the final phase, I offer the thesis that many healing systems, like life stories (and life itself), are "engendered." To account for why women or men predominate as traditional, psychological, or medical healers in particular medical systems and societies, I propose that we also need to examine the paradigms, beliefs, and practices of the healing systems in which the healers are involved.

TRADITIONAL HEALERS IN PUERTO RICO: THE PROCESS OF "DEVELOPMENT"

How do traditional healers attain and sustain the healer role? The background and experiences of one type of popular healer in Puerto Rico, an *espiritista* (a spirit-medium), are briefly described as characteristics of a prototype. *Espiritismo,* a mixture of popular religious healing practices and a cult that originated in France in the latter part of the nineteenth century, has been a widespread healing cult in Puerto Rico and most Latin and Mediterranean countries (Koss, 1976). Its main ritual consists of a small group of spirit mediums who call spirits to the "table" and into their bodies in order to alleviate the suffering of assembled clients. This takes place in *centros*, usually small buildings or rooms located in or near the homes of the "president" of a group of healers. The healers sometimes offer individual consultations, but they generally practice in small groups. There are also a few larger temples in Puerto Rico, where perhaps 50 to 100 persons come to be healed in a session; however, they are not as large as many in Brazil and other Latin countries. Spiritist healing is well documented among Puerto Ricans in the United States (Harwood, 1977; Garrison, 1977; Koss, 1975), where it has been syncretized with Afro-Caribbean cult practices, particularly Cuban *Santería*.

In Puerto Rico, approximately three-fourths of the healer-mediums who work at the table and call spirits into their bodies on behalf of suffering clients are women. A woman in an emotional crisis with multiple bodily complaints will be brought to the centro. In about one-third of the cases, she will be diagnosed as "in development" to become a healer-medium and enjoined to apprentice herself to an experienced medium in that centro's group of healers. Thus, all Spiritist healers can be said to be "wounded" and "healed" of an initiation-illness, as well as subsequent illnesses they or close family members have suffered or are suffering. This is a cyclical process with the healer continuing to move between a state of being wounded and being self-healed with the aid of the spirits.

An important aspect of the process of "development" as a healer involves entering into a new arena of social relationships within the center's healing circle, and it leads to changes in the pattern of social relationships (and sometimes also social identity). It also can involve changes in self-concept and a restructuring of personal notions and experiences of the body. Among Spiritist healers, the experience of this process is reconstructed as a personal myth that signifies that the healer has undergone the pain and difficulties that accompany entry into the role and the identity. The process of becoming a healer prepares a woman (or man) for the healing work she will learn from her Spiritist mentor and from wise spirit guides. She will learn to envision her client's distress, capture their bodily distress within her own body, and become possessed by the spirit cause of clients' distress.

GENERALIZING THE HEALER'S MYTH

McAdams (1993) asserts that a person's story is his or her identity and we know ourselves through stories we create about ourselves. These stories have two major psychological motivations: power and love. Although story-making goes beyond the healer's myth into other identity arenas, for women as healers (as well as some men), if the prescribed initiation into the role is programmed and experienced as a transformation, it can become the central myth for persons whose identity includes the healer imago. (*Imago* is defined by McAdams as "predominant theme.") The healer combines both "agentic" (purposive, task-oriented) and "communal" (love, intimacy) orientations in the development of her life story. The structure of the healer's myth follows guidelines defined by the culture and differs in special ways from the life stories of other persons. Although the myth takes on patterns related to gender and individual differences, it is qualitatively different from everyday life stories because it has a prescribed task and context, that of the self-presentation of the person as healer, and it emerges from a transformed sense of self (Koss-Chioino, 1992). Women healers' myths are typified by themes not commonly found in other women's life stories because of the importance of the relationship between empowerment attained through agency and self-nurturance attained through caring for others. Moreover, the healer's myth is constructed within the context of a situation in which the healer finds it both advantageous and necessary to both advertise and socially negotiate whom she has become. This need is conditioned by the circumstance that popular healer identities are contested in many societies (Boddy, 1989).

Using the life narratives of Puerto Rican spirit mediums as a prototype, healer life stories can be viewed as composed of three themes: a life-threatening illness crisis and a prolonged, but successful, health-restoring response; the revisioning of childhood experiences and events; and a series of special experiences with nonliving beings (often involving altered states of consciousness) that both pre- and postdate the acquisition of the healer role. Although these elements create a well-defined pattern, they are intertwined with idiosyncratic themes making each narrative partly unique. Traditional and folk healers are widely reported to have an episode of illness and/or extreme suffering as a central feature of their initiation into the healer role (see Koss-Chioino, 1992; Lewis, 1971; Peters, 1981; Wallace, 1966 as only a few examples). This experience marks the beginning of an ongoing series of special events, incorporated into the life story of the emerging novitiate-healer, which become standard features of the stories of mature healers. The initiation illness and subsequent events anchor a continually expanding narrative that highlights both childhood (sometimes even birth) and later life events subsequent to becoming a healer. These events are frequently recalled by the healer when she tells her story in order to justify and project her persona as a "healer." This is "the story the healer lives by" (to paraphrase McAdams's 1993 title). It is not simply a story that tracks change in one's life, but instead a personal myth that speaks to and about a change in the self that now exists largely to serve others. A prominent (perhaps the most prominent) aspect of this myth for women is the documentation and legitimization of the empowerment of someone who formerly lacked power and self-determination. The initiation stories of male healers also include the themes of distress and illness crisis. However, men as healers typically overcome these obstacles by owning and utilizing their innate and socially conferred power, with which they battle evil, world-destroying forces on behalf of humankind and their clients. Women as popular healers are much more focused on personal survival and responsibility, through which they become empowered to assist others to accept distress, acknowledge responsibility, and survive. Glass-Coffin (1996) describes in detail a similar distinction in the work of male and female healers in northern Peru where women healers emphasize responsibility and try to mobilize a sense of agency in the suffering client (particularly in women clients) in contrast to male healers who struggle with and overcome dark, negative forces and harness forces of good on clients' behalf.

The healer's myth can be thought of as an integral part of a continuing process of transformation. It focuses on a set of events that describe and sustain the healer's persona, but it also illustrates obstacles and endangered places in her life. This type of personal myth-making is similar in some ways to the use of life narratives in psychoanalysis. However, it differs from the way life narratives are supposed to work in psychodynamic therapies in that its goal is reconstruction rather than the revelation of early life traumas, even though both kinds of life stories are influenced by the audience. Some views of the psychoanalytic enterprise assert that the stories of analysands are retrospectively installed fictions (Spence, 1982). If we accept this approach, then both healer and analysand life stories could be characterized as intentionally transformative personal myths, and perhaps can be more accurately thought of as "self representations" rather than as "experienced" autobiographical events (Wikan, 1995).

Healers' narratives resemble life-story testimonials by members of Alcoholics Anonymous (AA) and other 12-step programs (Cain, 1991). As a first step, the life stories of AA members are essential to their taking on an identity as an abnormal person when they strive to become healed of the identified "disease" of overdrinking. Members reinterpret their past until it comes to reiterate the prototypic AA life story.

Although sharing many aspects, such as a history of woundedness and overcoming disease, healer life stories differ from those of "recovering" alcoholics in that they are directed toward individual constructions of new identities rather than to achieving an identity prototype required by a particular group. However, the shaping through repetition of key themes is found among AA members as well as among popular healers. It is also found in the testimonials of Pentecostal converts (Saunders, 1995).

The following excerpts from the life story of a Spiritist healer are translated from a recording of her narrative. Shorter excerpts from other healer narratives are provided to illustrate special points. They are representative examples from a data set of 35 written and oral narratives of women Spiritist healers in Puerto Rico (Koss-Chioino, 1992).

One Healer's Story: Overcoming Chaos

Doña Rosa is a woman of more than 60 years who became a healer in her later twenties. She recalled:

> I began to feel weak, I lost weight, my mind was mixed up, I was very irritable, the economic situation was desperate and I began to look for work, but I didn't feel well, and because I had to depend on public welfare the doctor did not really show concern for my problems. At this time I was going to church, where I had made my first Holy Communion when I was small. I took communion, confessed and asked God for my health and also prayed for my dead mother. But every day I felt worse; I felt as if I walked on air. My husband decided to take me to the hospital. Some godparents got me a bed and they left me for 20 days, but nothing happened. I went home in the same condition. I then found that I had a mania to drink water; I was very agitated and couldn't stay still from early morning; I couldn't do anything. I sat. A friend said, "You should go to an *espiritista* because it seems you have something (a bad spell or spirit causing the problem)." I said, "I don't believe in that." But I went and the healers prescribed many baths, at home from well water, and in the sea, and many other remedies, but they didn't help because I had no faith.

At this point in the story, doña Rosa related that one day a man gave her a small boy to raise (he replaced an only child who had died), and she also had to take care of her ailing father during the five years prior to his death. (The mention of these events implied that she had extra responsibilities and concerns.) She related that the same young friend visited her again, saw that she looked "very pale," that she was "deteriorating," and said, "Are you still drinking water?" At that, doña Rosa began to scream and "knew nothing more of the world." She thought she had "died." "They brought me an *espiritista*, but she came in very angry." This healer insisted that doña Rosa's body and spirit had separated and a bad spirit had taken over body and self (a fairly typical explanation). Doña Rosa was diagnosed as having "powers" (*facultades* with which to see into the spirit world) but, she recalled, "they were so hardened, so obdurate, that I had to suffer this bitter experience to loosen them."

Doña Rosa remembered hearing a voice speak to her saying that she had no body; it told her to look down at herself. She could see a gray coffin in which her body lay. The voice repeated many times, "You see, spirits exist; look at your body in the box." She recalled, "I couldn't see anything; my blood circulated and my feet felt the floor, but I couldn't open my eyes. But I did see a tall black woman in a rough, woven dress. She was laughing, but I felt very afraid and surprised. I found I could then open my eyes and saw many people there." Someone in this group commented that she looked like a cadaver and she ran out of the house and leaned against a wall shaking with fear because she thought she had died. However, the people there took her to bed and after two weeks, to another Spiritist healer, who guided her in developing her faculties to deal with the spirit world and set her to work at the table as a healer-medium.

Commentary on Theme 1: "Overcoming Chaos"

A death or resuscitation rescue theme is central to doña Rosa's personal myth. It is repeated in the stories of all of the other healers. In another case, for example, the healer tried to commit suicide with poison, but her spirit guide "stole the container" and confronted her. Sometime later she felt "obsessed" (out of control of her behavior) and in desperation asked what she should do. Soon afterwards, on a special evening, she saw a cloud descend from the sky. It opened and Jesus appeared. Later she dreamed of a very old woman who said, "Either give yourself to dying or conquer the feeling." Although she continued to be "obsessed," she no longer wanted to die. Another healer dreamt that her daughter would die the next day, and then the daughter fell ill and was close to death. She was saved by herbal medicine prepared by a neighbor who appeared unbidden at the bedside.

Although the death/rebirth experience is considered a universal metaphor of transformation, and in this case seems to serve as a strong boundary between the past and current (transformed) life, there is an interesting difference. Rather than rebirth, doña Rosa experiences resuscitation by "stranger-others" who care for her. The implication is that a new consciousness has been awakened through the help of wise spirit beings. When resuscitated, the healer keeps much of her former identity but has been empowered through a crisis of severe illness, involving chaotic experiences of dissociation, extreme fear, and disbelief.

An accompanying theme in doña Rosa's case is the presence of a strong, "primitive," black woman spirit, who later becomes her principal guide-protector. This spirit is a *madama*, an Obeah healer of West Indian origin, who is also a sorceress and witch. (See Comas-Díaz [1994] on the theme of "lati-negras" as special feminine figures.) Doña Rosa is thus further empowered by the addition of a strong, feminine alter ego to her personal identity representations. In the next part of the life narrative, she recalls that she "felt happier, stronger, and gained weight" after beginning to work at the table on behalf of other sufferers. And she continued to improve. She said that she prayed daily; prayer "was like medicine."

The mix of a communal and agentic orientation typical of these healers' stories is especially clear in doña Rosa's story. In addition to facilitating her healing work, the spirit can be seen to add agency to her self-representations because this spirit is the metaphor for a strong powerful woman. The next event that doña Rosa recalled was that additional family responsibilities led her to pray for a job. While working at the centro one day, a city official attended her session on behalf of a suicidal friend. After doña Rosa "worked" the spirit cause of the disturbed friend, the official complemented her on her spirit work and offered her a job as a caretaker at the local school.

Revisioning Childhood

Doña Rosa began her life narrative by saying "I was Catholic, but now I am an *Espiritista*." She gave her birth date, her parents' names, and her *barrio* and then emphasized that they were "very poor," working as farm laborers "like slaves." She remembered that her parents punished their children very harshly; after a good beating the children were made to kneel on a large grater in front of a cross until released from their penance. Because of their poverty, her older siblings could only complete two grades of school. However, her mother told her, "If God helps me, you will become a teacher." Doña Rosa commented, "I continued believing and thinking about my mother's words. I went to school and when I was about to begin the second grade my mother found a woman in the town with whom I could live and she sent me to school." Later, the whole family moved to town and doña Rosa was finally able to complete the eighth grade. She was then 17 years old, but couldn't afford to continue her education. She married a farmer, gave birth to the child who died, and then went through the illness crisis described earlier.

Commentary on Theme 2: "Childhood and Special Experiences"

Doña Rosa describes her childhood in terms of two notions: suffering poverty and being singled out by her mother to achieve a position in life beyond her expected destiny. Her main helpers on this difficult life journey, as she narrates it, are older women who exemplify the orientation of love. Transformation into the healer role reinforces her belief in the power of love but is also empowering, as indicated by her various experiences with the madama and other spirits who come to guide her. Personal power, first to overcome adversity and then to achieve the teaching position she most desires, comes slowly but increases as she works to help others. According to doña Rosa, the most important outcome was that she achieved a relationship with God. "God pays me every day," she stated emphatically.

Theme 3: Post-Initiation Experiences

Special experiences with spirit beings punctuate doña Rosa's life story as a healer and seem to mark decision points with life-changing commitments. One of these decision points was particularly relevant to the theme of agency. She recalled that when she was notified that the job as a school caretaker was official she began to have doubts regarding her ability to carry out this commitment, despite her desperate need for money to care for her family that included her father, an orphaned nephew, and a younger brother. With the letter naming her to the post in her purse, she went to see her espiritista mentor but did not reveal the reason for her visit. She recalled:

> "I entered the house and sat down and she kept looking at me and said, 'I see a *madama* (spirit) with you with a large white letter in her hand and it has to do with some job.' I began to cry; I couldn't explain why (I was so hesitant) because my economic need was so great."

She then told the espiritista about the job offer and her unreasonable doubts. The healer replied, "How can you *not* accept this job when this has been the work of a spirit who has been fighting to get it for you." The next day doña Rosa felt happy and went to the superintendent's office, got all of the official documents together and began to work. She explained that she only worked part of the day and thus had time to continue her spiritual work.

One night while working at the centro, she had a revelation that she was writing on a blackboard and talking to some children who all looked like angels. In her morning prayers the next day she asked God to reveal the meaning of this vision. She then heard a voice from far away which said, "Now that you are a spiritual teacher, helping people who are like children, I assure you that they are helping you prepare to become a material teacher." Shortly after this vision, opportunities for teacher training developed, and her job benefits made further schooling possible. Eventually, doña Rosa finished high school, then two years of normal school at night, and after waiting several years for a teaching post (while continuing to work as a school caretaker), she got a job as a teacher some 16 years later, at the very school where she first worked as a caretaker.

Commentary on Theme 3: Post-Initiation Experiences

The recounting of these experiences illustrates an important aspect of the traditional healer's convictions, the firm belief that she is not in control of her or anyone's life events. Control is ceded to a higher power—God, the Holy Spirit. The Spiritist healer is not empowered to heal anyone, but rather to develop her faculties spiritually, so that she can help others by offering her body and her being. This parallels differences in women's and men's life stories as interpreted by Gergen (1992), who sees women's narratives as clustering around themes of love versus themes of power in men's narratives. It is love that empowers women who become healers.

MENTAL HEALTH PROFESSIONALS AND MEDICAL DOCTORS IN PUERTO RICO

Because publicized self-representations as healer personae (the healer's myth) are not an expected part of the role of the mental health professional, or of the physician, the life stories of 22 women mental health professionals and 7 medical doctors in Puerto Rico (collected at the same time as those of the healers) contain only glimpses of special experiences and personal transformations. This is reflected in the number of studies in the United States that provide aggregated facts about women physicians, but rarely offer an in-depth look at their experiences, or an understanding of the difficulties women health professionals endure, or how they react to personal events (Geis, Jesilow, & Geis, 1991; however, see Bowman & Allen, 1990; Lorber, 1984). A recent book describing the lives and work of women doctors in England and Australia remedies this deficiency for those societies and references a large literature (Pringle, 1998). Sussman (1992) also points to this deficiency in the literature on women psychotherapists and social workers in the United States.

Some themes of the life stories of Puerto Rican women mental health professionals parallel those of Spiritist healers. Most of the 29 women health professionals recalled events of their childhood when close relatives had experienced chronic or terminal illnesses; in one-third of the cases the relative was a mother or sibling. Several remembered mothers as having suffered from persistent *nervios* (a folk term for emotional distress and/or psychiatric illness); other close female relatives also had similar problems. Many of the women mental health professionals had suffered serious illnesses in childhood, including a chronic heart ailment, benign tumors, asthma, severe allergies, and removal of an ovary. Their interest in nurturing others was reported to have stemmed from religious orientations, from which they developed a strong sense of morality. These experiences directly related to concepts of themselves as "good women" who focus their lives on helping others.

Over half of the women professionals recalled the encouragement to study and become a professional person provided by mothers who had few resources themselves. Many mentioned sources of distress in childhood, such as deep and pervasive feelings of abandonment by fathers who left home, or by mothers who had to leave them with maternal relatives because they were too ill or poor to care for their daughters. Some women remembered mothers as emotionally rejecting but as having facilitated scholastic achievement. Only a few mentioned experiences with extraordinary beings (mostly by relatives) that would parallel the spirit intrusions and visions common to Spiritist healers, but they did recall odd or "strange" incidents, such as the miraculous recovery of a very ill younger brother, or the sudden appearance of a relative or friend who helped them get through a desperate situation.

Although the life stories of the mental health professionals are not "healer's myths," their narrative form and content are parallel to many features of traditional healer stories. They are clearly "gendered" narratives and include restrictions on expressive forms imposed by their culture. As Mary Gergen (1992, p. 140) so aptly describes, the "story lines that lead a woman from childhood to maturity (do) not show a path by which strong achievement strivings could be satisfied without great personal sacrifice, [and] women could not become all that they had the potential to be." Unlike the straight-line life stories of men, womens' stories are multiplex, meandering, and relational (Gergen, 1992). I suggested earlier that the healer's myth is different in content from those of most other women in Puerto Rico, not in its recall of suffering, but in its focus on overcoming suffering through a relationship with spirits and God and at the same time expressing high achievement goals. Professional women's narratives echo those of the traditional healers in frequently crediting their mothers for their goals and achievement.

MENTAL HEALTH PROFESSIONALS AND MEDICAL DOCTORS IN THE UNITED STATES

Does the healer's myth fit women as mental health professionals and physicians in the United States? Like professionals in Puerto Rico, their frequent, deep commitment to their work leads them to endure the dilemmas and conflicts engendered in reconciling personal ("feminine") values around home and family with their vocations (Geis, Jesilow, & Geis, 1991; Koss-Chioino, 1992; Lorber, 1984). Although psychotherapy is only one dimension of mental health care, in the past it has been central to the treatment of emotional and cognitive disorders. Phillipson asserts that it represents the "professionalization of motherhood," in part because private practice and employment" are convenient for women raising families, but more importantly because the form and content of psychotherapeutic practice fits with what have been women's more traditional roles in the home" (Philipson, 1993, pp. 50-51).

There are indications that women manage their distress more successfully than men when carrying out therapeutic work. One study of burnout among mental health professionals showed that although males and females reported the same numbers of job stressors, strong associations existed between stressors and burnout only for males; no clear associations were found for the women (Hiscott & Connop, 1989). Perhaps the emotional demands of mental health care are more compatible with women's ideas and self-expectations. The socialization of the traditional Spiritist healer into her healing role aims at protecting her from the "contagion" of malignant spirit-causes of distress through sharing the healing process with a group at the centro and working spiritually to attract spirit-protectors as personal guides. This suggests that enhanced relatedness among women mental health professionals (a professional "sisterhood") may serve as protective support against burnout.

Evidence for gender role-based differences between male and female physicians comes from a study of stress among 72 male and female physicians in the Philadelphia area who were randomly selected from four specialties: psychiatry, pediatrics, obstetrics-gynecology, and family practice (Gross, 1992). Although both genders reported time pressures to about the same extent, women much more often felt deprived of time for themselves given more familial responsibilities. They tended to work part-time more often than did male physicians but still worked 90 percent as much as male physicians. However, in medicine as a profession, long hours of hard work show high dedication and are considered more prestigious. This study also showed that in regard to the second stressor listed, the doctor-patient relationship, significantly more men reported strain with patients. Moreover, male physicians reported much more dissatisfaction both with patients and colleagues. Concerns over malpractice were much greater among male physicians and fewer claims were filed against women physicians. Gross suggests that because male physicians are more attached to the authority and power inherent in the physician's role, they are more affected when that role is attacked. Finally, the study showed that women worried more about responsibility than men (a parallel to the Peruvian popular healers as described by Glass-Coffin [1996].) Gross (1992) notes that several studies indicate that men attribute their successes to ability and their failures to chance, whereas women's attributions are the opposite.

Numerous studies compare men and women physicians regarding differences in provider-patient communication. Seven key studies are reviewed by Hall and Roter (2002). They note that "significant findings" were that "patients spoke more to female physicians, disclosed more psychosocial and biomedical information, and made more positive statements to female physicians" (Hall & Roter, 2002, p. 217). In general, regardless of gender, patients of women physicians expressed greater comfort, were more engaged, disclosed more, and were more assertive. What might also be noted is that when communication between diverse gender dyads was examined in Western Europe, diverse cultural norms and values also influence these patterns (van der Brink-Muinen, van Dulmen, Messerli-Rorback, & Bensing, 2002). This makes generalization of the effect of gender on provider-patient communication more difficult because it is culturally specific.

The theme of overcoming chaos (and distress) in the healer's myth is reflected in the findings of a study that systematically compared large samples of women mental health professionals and women nonmental health professionals (Elliot & Guy, 1993). Female therapists reported significantly higher rates of physical and sexual abuse in childhood, alcoholism and severe mental illness in parents, and death of a parent or sibling. Moreover, they experienced a relatively high prevalence of trauma and family dysfunction during childhood. And like the Puerto Rican mental health professionals, they reported significantly more moral emphasis and achievement orientation in their earlier family lives. The authors note that these facts imply a "wounded healer" syndrome as motivation to enter mental health care careers, but discount the notion that these women professionals entered the field to resolve personal conflicts without really documenting this retrospective evidence. The study shows that the women mental health professionals had significantly less anxiety, depression, dissociation, sleep disturbances, and impaired relationships than other professionals. Perhaps, like traditional healers, mental health professionals experience less distress because they have managed to overcome it (and utilize this capacity in their work). This would explain their relatively good mental health despite difficult childhoods.

A study of Asian American women as psychiatrists offers a tantalizing glimpse of the experiences of ethnic minority women physicians. Fujii, Fukushima, and Chang (1989, p. 637) comment that those who choose psychiatry are often the eldest in their family and have experienced "unusual life circumstances," such as fleeing a native land under siege, facing possibly fatal illness, and dealing with severe emotional stress and mood disturbances. They "rely on family and religion" to get them through difficult times.

In a set of 91 life narratives recorded from women doctors born at the beginning of the twentieth century, 17 were from non-Western countries. Sixteen of these narratives describe experiences parallel to those of popular healers: These physicians were deeply affected by their own childhood illness and/or the serious illness or loss through death of a parent or sibling. They enjoyed the encouragement and support of a mother who, because of strong societal attitudes that women should not have careers, could never have achieved the career she encouraged in her daughter. Several mentioned meeting a woman doctor who became a role model, which may be similar to traditional healers acquiring a healer-teacher and a principal spirit guide (actually two mentors). Moreover, many of the physicians were affected by and overcame conditions of hardship, poverty, or social upheaval. All of the women from non-Western countries, and about half of the others, described how they felt empowered through acts of medical caring; many focused their later careers on helping disadvantaged women and/or their own struggling countries.

Finally, Pringle (1998, p. 220) raises the question: "Do women doctors make a difference in the practice of medicine and to women's health?" She answers with a very firm "yes," and predicts a transformation in medical education and the practice of medicine in the West once women are in the majority as practitioners.

ENGENDERED HEALING SYSTEMS

A number of authors have argued that the mental health and medical professions are undergoing a process of "feminization" (Bowman & Allen, 1990; Philipson, 1993; Pringle, 1998). This view suggests the final piece in understanding the "why" and "how" of women as healers. It seems that a devaluation of psychotherapy and medicine as professional pursuits is occurring, in part due to the policies of managed care systems. This appears related to the entry of growing numbers of women into health care professions, replacing men who find these careers less attractive. In my opinion, however, this reasoning does not fully account for why women find health professional careers more attractive, or why women's participation has recently become more accepted (apart from the effect of the women's movement). Even a cursory examination of medicine as practiced in the United States (including Puerto Rico), during and since the nineteenth century, reveals its basically androcentric disposition. Medicine's dominant principles have objectified body experience and have focused health care on the rational, scientific, prestigious achievement of restoring physical well-being, often to the neglect of including subjectivity, the sharing of meaning, and experience in patient care. Descriptions of medicine's androcentric orientation in the literature are not hard to come by: Traditionally, medicine has "been the preserve of men" (Geis, Jesilow, & Geis, 1991, p. 967). In medical relationships, "men as doctors 'do dominance' while women 'do deference;' female surgeons are sanctioned for displaying the dominant and agonistic behavior exhibited by their male colleagues" (Cassell, 1997, p. 47); and medicine "traditionally has been a male bastion of power" (Geis, Jesilow, & Geis, 1991, p. 967). One of relatively few studies of women physicians in the United States notes that a conflict of values is inherent in the acquisition of the medical role by some women: "Nurturant, emotional and supportive women are tracked into lower prestige work and not considered leadership material, but aggressive women are also heavily penalized because of the implied threat to men's dominant position" (Lorber, 1984, p. 11).

The medical system of the United States is undergoing change in ways other than economic and political; the entry of nonmedical alternatives has begun to take hold. More physicians are utilizing complementary and alternative healing systems. Homeopathy, Chinese medicine, and naturopathy are the most popular second choices (Eisenberg, Kessler, Foster, Nurlock, & Calkins, 1993; see Chapters 12 and 13 in this volume). More psychiatrists are also advocating a role for spirituality in treating patients (Lukoff, Lu, & Turner, 1992).

The situation of nonphysician mental health care professionals is somewhat different. Although men dominate clinical psychology, women are predominant in the alternative routes for practicing psychotherapy, such as counseling psychology, psychiatric nursing, and social work. Despite the large presence of women, most guidelines in the mental health field are set by psychiatry and therefore most often conform to rules of practice in medicine, particularly those that shape practitioner-patient relationships. Clinical psychology has had its own paradigm, largely behavioristic and individualistic (intrapsychic), with the experimental approach as a gold standard. However, feminist paradigms are emerging in both disciplines. For example, the Stone Center's relational approach based on "help[ing] the client reestablish a sense of empathic possibility and movement or growth in relationship" is notably different. It involves the establishment of mutual empathy and empowerment between therapist and client (Jordan, 1995, p. 260). Guidelines for the therapeutic relationship parallel those in Spiritism and other traditional healing systems. For example, Jordan (1995) states that therapists and clients each have a different kind of power; the therapist carries the power of the expert, whereas the client has emotional power that must be taken fully into account. Jordan also describes the incorporation of uncertainty into the therapy, which leads the therapist to be more "real, more vulnerable, and more mutual than many psychodynamic models advocate" (1995, p. 262). Somewhat like the Spiritist healer (who actually practices "radical empathy"), in the relational model traditional boundary-maintaining techniques between therapist and client are set aside in favor of relatedness and the sharing of personal experiences.

The healer's myth, and its expression in female-oriented healing systems, may not be salient for Western mental health professionals because of obstacles to the full integration of the goal of integrating the intermeshed attributes of power and love into their roles. Constraints relate to differences in the basic principles (though not always in practice) of most traditional healing systems and of medicine. Here I suggest only two. First, there is a large gap, yet to be negotiated, between authoritative knowledge predicated upon a scientific/experimental base, and "intuitive" knowledge, or "inner knowing," based on experience, bodily sensations, and emotional connections between healer and client (Davis-Floyd & Sargent, 1996). Most mental health professionals rely on intuition, but are not trained to develop or trust it. (This may be due in part to continually having to confront within themselves emotionally wrenching issues around craziness and disorder.) Second, a related difference is that medicine and psychology have become vigorously secular, which makes recourse to a "higher power," and to spirituality, difficult for both practitioner and patient.

This discussion has suggested that if change toward a female-oriented model of healing is to occur, two conditions must be met: first, that women continue to undergo experiences that deny them power in social and vocational arenas but keep them intimately connected to important others, particularly other women. Some will respond to these circumstances by being transformed through overcoming fortuitously occurring distress, and by attaining inner wisdom and personal power. One could argue that physicians and psychotherapists exercise a great deal of control over their patients, which makes them powerful. However, the healer's myth suggests that the special combination of power and love for others, hypothesized as central to women's revisions of their early and later life experiences (particularly as participants in a female-gender type of healing system), can be self-empowering. Stein aptly remarks, "it is important to recognize that power assertions—whether in the form of brow beating, advice giving, technique teaching or pill pushing—never cured anyone of a deep psychological problem and have often done a lot of harm" (Stein, 1984, p. 75).

The second condition is that a particular healing system provides a "fit," that is, an ideological and practice context that facilitates a female-oriented love/power approach to healing. Although traditional and alternative healing systems are still widely viewed as unorthodox in the United States, both medicine and clinical psychology have recently become more open to them. (Certainly, there is popular support.) We might predict that we are on the threshold of a new medical era in which alternative ways of healing, especially those in which women (and feminine values) assume increased importance, will be more fully appreciated and integrated into medical and psychological healing.

ACKNOWLEDGEMENTS

Data for this paper were collected, in part, in the Therapist-Spiritist Training project in Puerto Rico, funded by the National Institute of Mental Health (MH 14310-03; MH 15210) and sponsored by the Department of Health of Puerto Rico, for which, many years later, I am still grateful. Dr. Hector Rivera Lopez, Ms. Fredeswinda Román, Mr. Edgardo Rivera Saez, and numerous mental health professionals (especially Drs. José Gomez, Juan Moran, and Michael A. Woodbury) and Spiritist healers (especially, Don Jorgé Quevedo, Doña Guané Clara de Millan, and Doña Dominga Vasquez among many others) were wonderfully wise and giving colleagues during the project's tenure. They deserve my deepest appreciation but are in no way responsible for my interpretations.

REFERENCES

Achterberg, J. (1989). Mind and medicine: The role of imagery in healing. *Journal of the American Society for Psychical Research, 83*(2), 93-100.

Boddy, J. (1988). Spirits and selves in the northern Sudan: The cultural therapeutics of possession and trance. *American Ethnologist, 15*, 4-27.

Boddy, J. (1989). *Wombs and alien spirits: Women, men, and the Zar cult in northern Sudan.* Madison, WI: University of Wisconsin Press.

Bowman, M. A., & Allen, D. I. (1990). *Stress and women physicians* (2nd ed.). New York: Springer-Verlag.

Cain, C. (1991). Personal stories: Identity acquisition and self-understanding in Alcoholics Anonymous. *Ethos, 19*(2), 210-253.

Cassell, J. (1997). Doing gender, doing surgery: Women surgeons in a man's profession. *Human Organization, 56*(1), 47-52.

Comas-Díaz, L. (1994). Lati-negras: Mental health Issues of African Latinas. *Journal of Feminist Family Therapy, 5*(3-4), 35.

Davis-Floyd, R., & Sargent, C. (1996). Introduction. *Medical Anthropology Quarterly, 10*(2), 111-120.

Eisenberg, D., Kessler, R. C., Foster, C., Nurlock, F. E., & Calkins, D. R. (1993). Unconventional medicine in the United States. *New England Journal of Medicine, 328*(4), 246-252.

Elliott, D. M., & Guy, J. D. (1993). Mental health professionals versus non-mental health professionals: Childhood trauma and adult functioning. *Professional Psychology: Research and Practice, 24*(1), 83-90.

Fujii, J., Fukushima, S., & Chang, C. (1989). Asian women psychiatrists. *Psychiatric Annals, 19*(12), 633-638.

Garrison, V. (1977). The Puerto Rican syndrome in *espiritismo*. In V. Crapanzano & V. Garrison (Eds.), *Case studies in spirit possession* (pp. 383-450). New York: Wiley.

Geis, R. E., Jesilow, P., & Geis, G. (1991). The Amelia Stern Syndrome: A diagnosis of a condition among female physicians? *Social Science and Medicine, 33*(8), 967-971.

Gergen, M. (1992). Life stories: Pieces of a dream. In G. C. Rosenwald & R. L. Ochberg (Eds.), *Storied lives: The cultural politics of self-understanding* (pp. 127-144). New Haven, CT: Yale University Press.

Glass-Coffin, B. (1996). Male and female healing in northern Peru: Metaphors, models and manifestations of difference. *Journal of Ritual Studies, 10* (1), 63-91.

Gross, E. B. (1992). Gender differences in physician stress. *Journal of the American Medical Women's Association, 47*(4), 107-114.

Hall, J. A., & Roter, D. L. (2002). Do patients talk differently to male and female physicians? A meta-analytic review. *Patient Education and Counseling, 48,* 117-124.

Harwood, A. (1977). *Rx: Spiritist as needed.* New York: Wiley.

Hiscott, R. D., & Connop, P. J. (1989). Job stress and occupational burnout: Gender differences among mental health professionals. *Sociology and Social Research, 74*(1), 10-15.

Jordan, J. V. (1995). Female therapists and the search for a new paradigm. In M. B. Sussman (Ed.), *A perilous calling: The hazards of psychotherapy practice* (pp. 259-272). New York: John Wiley & Sons.

Koss, J. D. (1975). Therapeutic aspects of Puerto Rican cult practices. *Psychiatry, 38*(2), 160-171.

Koss, J. D. (1976). Religion and science divinely related: A case history of spiritism in Puerto Rico. *Caribbean Studies, 16,* 22-43.

Koss-Chioino, J. D. (1992). *Women as healers, women as patients: Mental health care and traditional healing in Puerto Rico.* Boulder, CO: Westview Press.

Lewis, I. M. (1971). *Ecstatic religion.* Harmonsworth, England: Penguin Books.

Lorber, J. (1984). *Women physicians: Careers, status, and power.* New York: Tavistock.

Lukoff, D., Lu, F., & Turner, R. (1992). Toward a more positive DSM-IV: Psychoreligious and psychospiritual problems. *Journal of Nervous and Mental Disease, 180*(11), 673-682.

McAdams, D. P. (1993). *Stories we live by.* New York: William Morrow.

Morsy, S. (1978). Sex roles, power, and illness. *American Ethnologist, 5,* 137-150.

Peters, L. G. (1981). An experiential study of Nepalese shamanism. *Journal of Transpersonal Psychology, 13*(1), 1-26.

Philipson, I. J. (1993). *On the shoulders of women: The feminization of psychotherapy.* New York: Guilford Press.

Pringle, R. (1998). *Sex and medicine: Gender, power and authority in the medical profession.* Cambridge, UK: Cambridge University Press.

Saunders, G. R. (1995). The crisis of presence in Italian Pentecostal conversion. *American Ethnologist, 22*(2), 324-340.

Spence, D. P. (1982). *Narrative truth and historical truth: Meaning and interpretation in psychoanalysis.* New York: Norton.

Stein, M. (1984). Power, shamanism, and maieutics in the countertransference. *Chiron: A Review of Jungian Analysis,* 67-87.

Sussman, M. B. (1992). *A curious calling: Unconscious motivations for practicing psychotherapy.* Northvale, NJ: Jason Aronson.

Ulanov, A. B. (1981). *Receiving woman: Studies in the psychology and theology of the feminine.* Philadelphia, PA: Westminster Press.

Van der Brink-Muinen, A., van Dulmen, S., Messerli-Rohrbach, V., & Bensing, J. (2002). Do gender-dyads have different communication patterns? A comparative study in Western European general practices. *Patient Education and Counseling, 48,* 252-264.

Wallace, A. F. C. (1966). *Religion: An anthropological view.* New York: Random House.

Wikan, U. (1995). The self in a world of urgency and necessity. *Ethos, 23*(3), 259-285.

IV

Asian Approaches to Therapy and Healing

Indigenous Chinese Healing: Theories and Methods

Ting Lei
The City University of New York

Ching-Tse Lee
The City University of New York

Cecilia Askeroth
St. Francis College, New York

The first author wishes to dedicate this chapter to Professor Kuo-shu Yang in honor of his contribution to the indigenization of Chinese social sciences. He also wishes to thank Profs. Bridie Andrews and Ellen LaForge for their valuable help.

Indigenous Chinese healing (ICH) is a time-tested tradition that has endured for 3000 years. It is also a human-honored medical modality that is not based on generalizations from in vitro experimentation as is conventional biomedicine. Instead, as other approaches involved in traditional Chinese medicine (TCM), ICH is derived from one billion people's folk-friendly experiences of in vivo applications (Benson, 1996; Kaptchuk, 2002; Jonas & Levin, 1999).

Generally speaking, ICH includes three major modalities, namely, acupuncture/moxibustion, qigong (vital energy work), and herbal medicine. Acupuncture and qigong are unique to Chinese culture, whereas herbal medicine has been developed in other cultures as well. Although traditional healers in other cultures employ herbs as the major modality, Chinese healers commonly use herbs in conjunction with other modalities in order to complement the treatment effect produced by acupuncture/moxibustion or qigong. This complementary approach reflects Chinese people's dialectical reasoning. This means that medical modalities based on different mechanisms (e.g., the biophysical mechanisms that acupuncture/moxibustion is based on, the electrophysiological mechanisms that qigong is based on, and the biochemical mechanisms that herbal medicine is based on) can be synthesized into a therapeutic approach to certain disorders. Another reflection of Chinese people's dialectical thinking regarding indigenous healing can be seen in the convergence on the same theoretical foundation of these three healing modalities despite their methodological divergence. This theoretical foundation in terms of philosophy of life, premises of health, and purpose of treatment serves as the common thesis for the three antithetical modalities, and it is briefly introduced later.[1] After that introduc-

---

[1]A more comprehensive description can be found in *The web that has no weaver: Understanding Chinese medicine* (Kaptchuk, 1983).

tion, an investigative review of the mechanisms underlying the three healing modalities is presented.

THEORETICAL FOUNDATION

The theoretical foundation of TCM is deeply rooted in Chinese culture, which, however, is not as homogeneous as has been generally portrayed. From the native's point of view (Lei, 1991), the official or *great* tradition is socially presented as Confucian in name, whereas the unofficial or the *little* tradition subtly represented in people's daily life is mostly Taoist in nature. As most indigenous healers would agree, it is the Taoist weltanschauung (worldview) that provides the principal concepts for TCM.

The weltanschauung referred to here is part of the culture's ideational system. It includes a conception of how the human body/mind/spirit function, a premise of health, the assumptions of pathogenesis, and a philosophy of life. Readers should note that these conceptualizations do not merely remain at a metaphysical level that rationalize TCM practices. They also serve as guidelines that are reflected and concretized in the healers' practices. To put it in a slightly different way, mystical-transcendental Taoism is not simply a modus vivendi for Chinese people, but also a modus operandi for TCM.

The Taoist Worldview

Taoists perceive human beings as microcosms of the universe that surrounds them, suffused with the same primeval force that motivates the macrocosm. All the microcosms are viewed as participants in a general system in which they synergistically interact with each other in the context of a larger and continuous process of transformation. The thread that connects all the parts in this continuous process is called qi, which is a type of subtle/vital energy. People and things come and go, while qi remains to be the continuum across time and space that instills itself into different participants, who are the visible manifestation of qi. From this perspective, qi can make and/or break a person. To cultivate and regulate qi is the major concern in the traditional Chinese concept of health and healing.

In a metaphorical sense, the aforementioned general system or macrocosm can be seen as a four-dimensional web of wholeness. Different parts of the macrocosm are organically intertwined with each other just like different layers of a web are interwoven three-dimensionally (mechanical intertwinement can be graphically represented as two-dimensional). The fourth dimension refers to the temporal dimension that runs through the first three (spatial) dimensions. In Chinese cosmology, on that temporal dimension are five phases (coinciding with the five elements on the spatial dimension) that interconnect with each other to form a constantly-moving cycle. The five phases are symbolically represented as metal, wood, water, fire, and earth,[2] which reciprocally relate to each other and vitalistically correspond to other components of

---

[2]It should be noted throughout this chapter that Chinese language is ideographical in nature; thus, sometimes the meaning of words should not be taken literally but metaphorically. Along the same line, as Kaptchuk (1983) noted, the Chinese description of reality does not penetrate to an objective truth; it can only be a poetic description of a truth that cannot be grasped. The semiotic referents of the five phases and yin-yang do not exactly correspond to the physical reality; instead they are metaphors in a natural drama that seem to be sensible in explaining the ongoing process of the universe and the workings of the human being.

the macrocosm.[3] Besides the five phases, microcosms and macrocosm also correspond to *yin* and *yang*.

So far yin and yang have been simplistically characterized as something static on a two-dimensional plane. A more accurate representation is as follows: Yin and yang can be viewed as two intert wisted vortices in visual representations; one can see a white dot here in the center of the dark yang with a gradation of darkness toward the outer rim, and there is a dark dot in the center of the light yin with a gradation of lightness toward the outer rim. To explain it in words, yin and yang mutually generate and transform each other, and also counterbalance each other in an everlasting dialectical interaction.

The Concept of the Person and the Premises of Health in Taoism

Classical Classification of Body Organs   This classification system is based on the functions rather than the structures of body organs. The tendency of TCM is to seek out dynamic functional activity rather than to look for the fixed somatic structures that perform the activities. There are five organs that correspond to the five phases, namely, liver and wood, spleen and earth, kidney and water, heart and fire, and lungs and metal.

The Meridian System   Meridians are channels for qi circulation following a predetermined circadian sequence to maintain the homeostasis of the body's vital energy system. There are 12 regular meridians spreading all over the human body like a complex matrix. To better capture the meaning graphically, perhaps we can coin the term *innernet* to streamline the term "meridian system," which serves as the basis for acupuncture treatment. Nowadays more than two thousand acupoints are identified on the surface of meridians and function as the gates to the human energy system.

Premises of Health: Consonance in a Cosmic Concert

Homeostatic Configuration of Human Beings   As mentioned in the preceding section on Chinese cosmology and the Taoist worldview, the macrocosm and the microcosms, like a symphony, are composed of complex interweaving patterns of form and movement. These patterns are recapitulated in every miniature system within and beyond each human being, which is at a microcosmic level of organization.

Metaphorically, the human body is to the macrocosm as a harp is to an orchestra. The strings are to a harp as the organs are to the human body. Each string synergistically vibrates together with other strings just as the body organs interact with each other. For the orchestra to play a symphony in harmony, all the instruments must be

---

[3]This notion of merging time and space dimensions seems to defy logic, if the logic is derived from the Newtonian model. However, viewed within the context of models of physics such as relativity/quantum theory, this notion does make sense. In addition, as Needham (1956, p. 474) has suggested, the organic process in which microcosms and macrocosm are involved can be factored into successive states in time and envelopes in space in which every part of the universe is related to others. In the organic view of the world, the universe is one that has the property of producing the highest (human) values when the integrative level of organization appropriate to them has arisen in the evolutionary process. Modern science since Leibniz has embraced the organic paradigm and describes the aforementioned level of organization as a temporal succession of spatial envelopes.

tuned to each other, all the strings of each instrument must be played in tune[4] (Beinfield & Korngold, 1991). By the same token, each body organ has to collaborate with other organs in the organism, which must tune itself to the ecological system in which it is embedded. Otherwise, the organism would be in a state of disequilibrium or disturbance, which is the inception of diseases from the Taoists' pathogenetic perspective.

Etiology Readers should note that we use the word "inception" instead of "cause" of disease. In the West, the dominant philosophy of science postulates that events occur in a series, one triggering another in spatio-temporal sequence. Under this influence, Western medicine often emphasizes the single cause that triggers a pathological process. In contrast to the linear continuum of time and space that links cause and effect, Taoism postulates that events occur in association with reciprocal influence and form configurations that persist beyond their moment of genesis.

Following the Taoist presupposition, the pathogenesis in TCM is not linearly organized. In other words, TCM is not concerned with certain pathogens as the cause of certain diseases. Instead, it attends to the factors that affect the equilibrium of the organism's configuration, which refers to the pattern of events. In Chinese configurational thinking, a precipitating factor might at first appear to be the cause or the beginning of the end in a chain of events. Later on it might become the end of the beginning or part of the configuration, indistinguishable and inseparable from the effect. The lines of causality are bent into circles[5] (Kaptchuk, 1983).

Diagnosis

TCM attempts to locate disorder with a holistic perspective on the person's total physical and psychological condition. Therefore, TCM healers try to obtain as many signs as possible and gather comprehensive information concerning the patient's symptoms. Then they place a given sign of the patient's disturbance or disequilibrium into the patient's entire configuration of signs, including the quality/quantity of pulse, tongue color, body movement, and emotional outlook.

A TCM healer should be equipped with humanistic sensitivity as well as medical sensibility. In addition to the analytic logic required to conduct a differential diagnosis, a synthetic logic is also required for the intersubjective (between the healer and the patient) integration of (in)coherent pathological signs and symptoms. A diagno-

---

[4]This illustrates not only an aspect of Taoism known as the thesis of correspondence, but also a fundamental concept underlying the modern general system theory. These two theoretical theses are different in name and terminology though they converge on a similar principle conceptualization. That is, in order for a larger system to be in balance (equilibrium) as a whole, each system within it must itself be balanced (equilibrated). This principle of harmony applies to all levels of complexity, as orthogenetic theory suggests. Furthermore, according to the orthogenetic hypothesis in terms of recapitulation, patterns of harmony in one system both reflect and generate patterns of harmony in other systems, and at greater and lesser orders of complexity.

[5]The four seasons can serve as an example to illustrate this point. A child who experiences the four seasons for the first time probably thinks that spring causes summer, and in turn autumn and winter. In the following year that child will notice that spring comes after the winter and thus reverses the causal link he or she previously assumed. Even adults can be easily (mis)led into believing the causal link is based on the information of chronological order.

sis cannot be deemed complete until the patient's condition reaches homeostasis, which indicates not merely the efficacy of the treatment, but also the accuracy of the diagnosis.[6]

Traditionally, there are four diagnostic methods, briefly presented as follows:

- **Observations**   The first step is to visually inspect the patient's physical appearance and to note any signs of significance from the following categories:
  - **Body parts** and **posture**
  - **Tongue**   According to the recapitulation or correspondence principle, different areas of the tongue reflect the condition of different body parts.
  - **Static electromagnetic**   Aura and other types of qi manifestation can be detected by the healer's eyes.
  - **Dynamic electromagnetic**   A person's kinesthetic movement is an indication of that person's vital energy or qi and how his or her energy field interacts with that of the environment.
- **Listening and smelling**   The second procedure involves listening to the quality of voice, respiration, and other sounds, as well as being aware of the odors of breath, body, and excreta.
- **Questioning**   TCM healers start by querying patients in detail about sensations when responding to hot and cold, perspiration, previous sickness and treatment, and life style in detail. Furthermore, some important but not readily apparent information can be discovered in the interview process. Given the nature of the Chinese language as ideographic/metaphorical and given the common tendency of somatizing psychological symptoms among Chinese patients (Kleinman, 1980), TCM healers should know how to interpret the meaning of patients' words, and how to conduct probing in order to help patients reflect on and reveal their body/mind/soul (Lei, 2002).
- **Touching**   TCM healers temporarily end diagnosis with palpation, which means systematic feeling of the surface of the body in order to detect any external/internal disharmony. The following are four aspects of palpation:
  - **Body temperature**   Feeling the skin to see whether it is warm or cold. Warm skin indicates yin deficiency and an openness of the person's qi or subtle energy field while cold skin suggests yang deficiency and a closure of the person's qi field.
  - **Body moisture**   Dry skin reveals an abundance of the fire element (phase) and a deficiency of body fluids, whereas moist skin shows the dominance of the water element (phase) in that person's configuration.
  - **Pain**   Pain is a symptom of qi stagnation. The area suffering from pain may not be the ailing area. To detect whether it is a direct or referral pain, TCM healers usually palpate along the meridians and look for possible tender spots. These spots may indicate a local meridian problem or may reveal a more deep-seated disequilibrium of the organ network.

---

[6]As can be seen here, TCM is not simply a time-tested medical modality, but to a considerable extent, an empirically verified folk science. A remission of a patient's ailment provides evidence for the efficacy of treatment that presupposes the accuracy of the diagnosis. On the other hand, a relapse may contraindicate a specific treatment, which may or may not demonstrate the inaccuracy of the diagnosis, because an accurate diagnosis is necessary but not sufficient for an effective treatment.

• **Pulse**   There are three positions near the radial artery on each wrist. In accordance with the correspondence principle, the pulse taken at each position on the two wrists reflects the condition of various body organs.

THERAPEUTIC TECHNIQUES

Acupuncture and Moxibustion

In the TCM treatment approach, acupuncture and moxibustion are often used together as a yang type of treatment, with moxibustion serving as an adjunct.

Purpose of Treatment   Both acupuncture and moxibustion are prescribed for the regulation of qi flow in order to reach homeostasis. Deduced from the etiological presupposition that all diseases are due to or related to the disequilibrum of qi, these two techniques are generally beneficial for many disturbed conditions. A TCM practitioner's short-term goal of treatment is to obtain or disperse the qi at the site of selection, whereas the intermediate goal is concerned with the reduction of the patient's symptoms, such as pain. The patient's harmonized configuration, which is based on her or his qi equilibration, is usually held as the ultimate goal.

Right after the initial treatments of acupuncture or other TCM therapies, the patient may experience an adaptation syndrome, including such symptoms as aches, discomfort, dizziness, stiffness, and the exacerbation of preexisting problems. Most likely these are signs showing that the patient's body as an organismic system is trying to adjust itself to the new disequilibrium generated by the treatment. This type of reaction is not a side effect, but a normal by-product of TCM.[7]

Method of Treatment   Nowadays acupuncture is performed with a variety of tools and manipulations. The filament of a fine needle is the typical acupuncture tool and comes with different diameter, length, and other structural features. Before selecting appropriate needles, the acupuncturist needs to locate acupoints for needling based on their correlation correspondence with the qi disharmony identified in the diagnosis procedure. Then, the patient and the practitioner design a treatment protocol together, with the patient's idiosyncratic constellation taken into serious consideration. In TCM, there are as many protocols as there are combinations of practitioners and patients, because protocols are not unilaterally determined by the medical establishment, which universalizes to different patients who receive the same diagnostic label.

Needling   Once an appropriate acupoint has been located, the acupuncturist would seek subjective as well as objective indication of qi reaction after inserting the needle into the acupoint. Qi becomes manifest to the acupuncturist through a gripping sensation by the hands, through observation, and through the patient's own words (tingling, swollen feeling, etc.). When the qi is encountered (Eisenberg, 1987),

---

[7]In the West, the adaptation syndrome is also commonly observed when people just start detoxification or smoking cessation, during which those people's organismic systems are not used to the new, though healthy, condition.

the acupuncturist may choose to manipulate the needle in various ways depending on whether the treatment goal is to accelerate or retard the qi, and to adjust the density and flow of qi in the meridians, which in turn affect the circulation of the blood and the function of the organ network.

There are multiple methods of manipulating needles, involving variables such as the angle and depth of inserting needles, the direction and twisting of needles after insertion, and the length of retaining needles. In terms of how long to retain a needle in the body, the retention ranges from a few seconds in the case of infants to an hour or longer in treating difficult conditions. Usually, needles are retained in acupoints for about 15 to 20 minutes. Regarding the first few variables, the choice is according to accumulated experience of applying specific theoretical concepts to clinical cases, as well as descriptions in classical and contemporary texts. The theoretical concepts include the yin-yang dyad, the five phases/elements, the organ network, and the innernet or meridian system introduced earlier.[8]

Operational Mechanisms in a Western View

Brain   Functional mapping of the human brain during acupuncture with fMRI (functional magnetic resonance imaging) or PET (positron emission tomography) scans has demonstrated that acupuncture produced dynamic effects on widespread areas of the brain (Biella et al., 2001; Hui, Liu, Wu, & Wong, 1996). This was especially true during needle twisting, which activated the contralateral somatic sensory cortex of the patients with a headache, toothache, or abdominal pain. Moreover, many regions in the frontal, temporal, parietal, and occipital cortices, the encephalon, the cingulate gyrus, and the cerebellum exhibited a response. These responses indicate the involvement of acupuncture in the crucial structures for pain perception/modulation in the somatic sensory/motor areas of the cerebral cortex besides the subcortical areas.

Spinal Gating Mechanism   Another possible mechanism of pain perception may reside in the dorsal horns, the substantia gelatinosa, that regulate the amount of information conveyed from the peripheral nerve fibers to spinal cord transmission cells. These cells in turn activate the thalamus, which also serves as a relay station for the expression of pain. According to the gate theory (Melzack, 1993), the spinal mechanism transmits more sensory pain information as the proportion of small diameter fibers (A delta or C) firing exceeds the amount of large diameter fiber (A beta) activity. Acupuncture as a form of hyper-stimulation analgesia inhibits pain by activating the large fibers to supersede the small fibers (Melzack, 1993).

Autonomic Nervous System   A clinical study conducted in Japan has confirmed that electro-acupuncture (EA) was able to modulate immunologic response by regulating the autonomic nervous system. Specifically, EA tended to induce parasympathetic nervous activities, resulting in a decrease of one's heart rate and corticosteroid, and normalize the pattern of leukocytes (Hidetoshi, Kazushi, Hiroki, & Toru, 2002).

---

[8]Once again, as can be seen here, TCM is an empirical system. The theoretical concepts involved in TCM are not merely a metaphysical outlier of clinical practices. Rather, clinical practices are driven by theoretical concepts to a great extent though they may in turn either support or fail to support the validity of those concepts.

Biochemical Mechanisms Some neuropeptides have also been identified as the operating mechanism of acupuncture that is able to raise the pain threshold (Ulett, Han, & Han, 1998). These neuropeptides include endorphins, which are located in the pituitary gland and function like morphine for the reduction of the pain in general. Endorphins can also lead to the release of antidiuretic hormone (ADH), follicle-stimulating hormone (FSH), and adreno-corticotropic hormone (ACTH) from the anterior pituitary. It should be noted that ACTH, as a major neurotransmitter, plays an important role in regulating our neurological functions. The endorphinergic systems can also be stimulated by auriculotherapy (ear acupuncture), which has been used for neuro-rehabilitation (Terry, 2002). In Korea, cDNA microarray analysis of the differential gene expression in the treatment of neuropathic pain with electro-acupuncture has been conducted on animal models (Ko, Na, Lee, Shin, & Min, 2002). Dot-blotting results showed that the opioid receptor sigma was involved both in the neuropathic pain and in the electro-acupuncture treatment.

Moxibustion

The purpose of burning compressed dry herb from the species mugwort is to warm one's qi and blood, or to expel moisture from the body. There are several techniques to burn moxa. The first one refers to direct moxibustion, in which the moxa is formed into small cones and placed on acupoints to be lit. The second one is called indirect moxibustion, in which moxa is burned above the skin with or without another medium between the skin and the moxa. The medium can be either a layer of salt, a slice of ginger, or a slice of garlic, which serve different purposes. The third method is to burn mugworts at the end of needles, and using the heat generated, to invigorate the body. This method is suitable for the yin type of patient who can be characterized as cold and suffers from qi deficiency.

Augmentation To augment the effect of acupuncture on qi stimulation, practitioners can connect needles with microelectric current or a laser. Clinical trials have shown that these modern techniques speed recuperation by facilitating the regeneration of neural fibers (Tanaka, Lebman, & Nishijo, 1998). A more traditional technique of augmentation refers to acupressure massage. By applying pressure on acupoints, a healer can send qi or subtle/vital energy to patients and simultaneously stimulate their own production of qi.

Cupping This is an optional adjunct technique to acupuncture/moxibustion and includes burning a taper for a very short period of time in a glass globe or bamboo jar in order to exhaust all the oxygen in the globe and to create a vacuum. Then the globe must be placed down over the skin area in order to draw the qi, speed up the blood flow, and have the heat and moisture dispersed.

ORAL THERAPY

Definition and Distinct Properties

Oral therapy includes anything that carries nutritive or medicinal properties and is applied through the patient's mouth.[9] In addition to many herbs, some minerals, ani-

---

[9]The term "oral therapy" does not mean the treatment is for the mouth. Rather, the operating site of the treatment is from the mouth and down to the digestive system.

mal parts, and food are also employed by TCM healers for therapeutic purposes. They are often used as supplement to other therapies. Following the theoretical concepts introduced earlier, the distinct properties of these so-called oral medicines can be broadly summarized in the three categories below (Beinfield & Korngold, 1991):

- **Nature**   This refers to the oral medicine's cooling or warming character, which is supposed to complement the cool or warm nature of the patients and their current conditions. For example, a cool herb such as a dried chrysanthemum flower can make an iced tea, which is good for the fire phase and characterized as warm; it is thus considered more appropriate for the water phase and can be fried to serve people of the yin type.
- **Configuration**   According to the principle of correspondence, or the orthogenetic concept in terms of recapitulation, the shape, color, or texture of an oral medicine may mimic certain parts of the body. As an example, walnuts look like human brain hemispheres and thus are deemed an excellent tonic for the brain. By the same token, ginseng is believed to enhance men's sexual performance, because the ginseng root resembles the shape of a penis.
- **Taste**   Each taste matches with one of the five phases/elements and implies certain actions. Bitterness matches with the fire element and has an eliminative function that discharges qi downward; spiciness matches with the metal element and has a stimulating function that accelerates the qi flow; sweetness matches with the earth and has a harmonizing effect that smoothens qi; sourness matches with the wood and has a softening action that dissolves stale qi.

Delimitation

Oral therapy includes two approaches. One refers to herbal healing; the other may be called dietetics or culinary alchemy. Sometimes they are difficult to distinguish from each other, though usually oral medicines have a stronger effect and are more functionally specific than culinary alchemy.

Herbal Healing

According to the *Encyclopedia of Traditional Chinese Medicinal Substances* (1977), the medicinal effects of 5,767 natural substances (including some minerals and animal parts) have been recognized. The functional properties of these substances can be described as follows:

- **Dispersing**   Moving or redistributing qi, blood, and moisture throughout the body, disseminating them from one part of the body to another, relieving patterns of stagnation and overconcentration.
- **Consolidating**   Gathering together and consolidating qi, blood, and moisture, relieving patterns of slackness and leakage. Herbs possessing this type of property do not change the quantity of qi, blood, and moisture; instead, they alter the qualities.
- **Purging**   Expelling or vigorously ridding the body of accumulated qi, blood, and moisture that have become obstructive, as well as evicting noxious substances.
- **Toning up**   Strengthening metabolism and enhancing the organism's adaptability by nourishing the essence of the body, improving qi, and replenishing blood.

The Therapeutic Thinking Underlying Herbal Healing   To pick the most appropriate herb requires matching the medicinal properties with the underlying pattern of
disharmony, so sometimes the same symptom may be treated with different substances, depending upon the person within whom it occurs. In other words, prescriptions are to be comprehensive, addressing not merely the complaints patients
have, but also their constitutional dynamics.

Furthermore, substances with complementary properties are combined to create
balanced formulae so that side effects of different substances can cancel or counteract
each other. In a similar vein, ingredients that mutually enhance each other's medicinal effects can be mixed together. For instance, herbs or other substances that have
tonic properties are usually complemented by those that disperse. This means that
while the nutrients of the tonic herbs are being assimilated into the blood circulation,
the nutrients' tonic effect can be augmented by dispersing herbs that mobilize or
accommodate the blood circulation.

Dietetics (Culinary Alchemy)

Given the basic principles in TCM, such as self-cultivation, self-healing, and prevention, nutrition plays an important role in Chinese people's health maintenance and
enhancement. Many of the foods prescribed by healers for therapeutic purposes are
also routinely used by common folks for nourishment, coping with seasonal change,
and invigorating women for reproduction, lactation, postpartum recovery, and
longevity. For example, during the first month of the postpartum period a woman is
supposed to eat one steamed, dark-boned chicken a day, while eggs are recommended
for women before giving birth.

Food Factors   As discussed earlier, there is no universal standard concerning what
constitutes a good food. "One man's meat can be another man's poison" is the commonly held food ideology. Foods are selected on the basis of their compatibility and
complementarity with individual configurations, both of which are comprehended
within the language of yin-yang and five phases/elements and are explained in the
classic prescriptive text, the *Yellow Emperor's Inner Classic* (issued around 200 B.C.,
according to Ergil, 1996).

As an example of these principles of food selection, a person who has too much
yang (nowadays manifested in the Type A personality) should not have hot food, such
as red meat. Similarly, a person who has too much fire element may be allergic to spicy
food and had better absorb more of the water element that can be found in asparagus
or some other green vegetables. Another factor that guides food selection is a person's
particular condition at a given time. As a case in point, when a person suffers from
high fever with parched throat, which is a symptom corresponding to the fire phase,
foods that contain the water element seem to be beneficial. Moreover, climate needs
to be taken into account too. To illustrate, in the damp, windy winter, an enriching
diet can produce a wood element and generates internal fire that protects people from
the cold.

QIGONG

Definition and Background

In Chinese, *qigong* can be separated into qi and gong. Qi is a polysemic word, which may denote the vital/subtle energy, whereas gong means work or function. Thus, qigong literally means to work on vital/subtle energy in order to capitalize on its healing function.[10] The theoretical rationale underlying qigong practice is deeply rooted in the classical Chinese cosmology introduced earlier, which considers each human being as a microcosmic energy system synergistically embedded in the macrocosm, such as the ecological environment. These macro- and microcosms constitute a unified energy field and interchange energy constantly based on the operational principle of homeostasis, or dynamic balance and harmony. Granted that diseases arise in the unbalanced qi (cf. the Theoretical Foundation in this chapter), the ultimate goal of applying qigong is to achieve and maintain homeostasis and to eliminate and prevent disease (Lee & Lei, 1999).

Approaches to Healing/Health and Their Underlying Mechanisms

To achieve and retain qi homeostasis, there are several approaches. The first approach is to rely on the extrinsic qi, which is emitted by the qigong practitioner, and apply it to the patient so that the patient's vital energy state can be brought back to balance immediately. Although this approach can produce an instant effect, this effect cannot last long without the restoration of the patient's intrinsic qi, which is the major concern of the second approach. To that end, both the practitioner and the patient engage in the mutual endeavor of learning how to equilibrate the qi toward greater integration with the Tao (the harmonious configuration). The second approach includes (at least) two steps. One is to let the practitioner demonstrate how to perform movement-oriented qigong for accelerating and channeling the intrinsic qi from meridians to the qi-blocked areas. The other is to teach patients how to practice meditation-oriented qigong in order to cultivate qi and regulate their energy state for health. Moreover, during meditation, patients can also learn how to elicit the power of their mind and spirit/soul[11] that mobilizes healthy qi to ailing areas. As can be seen here, in contrast to other TCM modalities, qigong operates on mind, spirit, and body. In fact, without engaging mind and spirit in the production and preservation of qi, either the movement-oriented or the meditation-oriented qigong (including tai chi) exercise would be downgraded to a level of ballet or snooze respectively. In support of this argument, electroencephalogram (EEG) studies have shown that the brainwave patterns (indicating the functional states of the brain) of meditation-oriented qigong and sleep or snoozing are different. As Green and Green (1986) observed in conducting biofeedback on experimental participants, altered states of consciousness are not only

---

[10]Qigong is exactly the same thing as chi-kong or chi-gong, which was the English translation before the Communist Chinese took over Mainland China and changed the language system. The translations chi-kong and chi-gong are still used by many Chinese people around the world except in Mainland China.
[11]The power of mind and spirit can be generated by guided imagery, visualization, and other special techniques.

correlated with the practice of meditation-oriented qigong but may also serve as an intervening variable between qigong and its effects on the human body. In a similar vein, action consciousness (Lei, 1989) is aroused while conducting the movement-oriented qigong.

A recent study conducted at the Harvard Medical School (Kerr, 2002), which included a randomized controlled trial as well as ethnographic research and in-depth interviews, revealed that biomedical researchers viewed qigong as a nonspecific "mind-body" practice that combines relaxation and exercise. On the other hand, qigong masters framed the same practice as a "mind-in-body" intervention that uses specific movements and visualization to direct qi or vital/subtle energy to specific areas of the body. If qigong can be seen as a mind-body intervention, another study conducted at the Harvard Medical School pointed out that mind-body interventions reduce sympathetic nervous system activation, increase parasympathetic nervous system activity, and thereby restore homeostasis (Jacobs, 2001). In terms of homeostasis, the aforementioned two types of consciousness, from the perspective of the general system theory (Laszlo, 1979), can function as feedback for the human homeostatic system's self-regulation, or as a bridge in the mind-body loop.[12] Furthermore, the engagement of the mind and the spiritual dimension together with the body in qigong practice entails a transcendental intuition that enables a person to transform the experience of being an ordinary mortal to that of becoming a human at a higher level (Lei, 1991). This extraordinary experience can help a person to compassionately go over and beyond the secular life stress, and at the same time to tap the parasympathetic nervous system, which in turn boosts the person's immune function.[13]

In the process of qigong intervention, the brain serves as an underlying mechanism or the hardware for the "mind," which functions as the software. The brain's involvement in the qigong intervention has been indicated by the qigong-induced reproducible changes in transcranial Doppler sonography, EEGs, stimulus-induced 40 Hz oscillations, and near-infrared spectroscopy findings (Litscher, Wenzel, Niederwieser, & Schwartz, 2001).

Exogenous-healing Qigong

Following the previous distinction, the first approach that relies on the extrinsic qi can be called exogenous-healing qigong, because the qi that works on the patient is emitted by the healer rather than being elicited from the patient. The physical basis of the energy transmission between the healer and the patient has been demonstrated by the Chinese Academy of Science. One property of that physical basis is low-frequency infrared radiation (Guo, 1989), which indicates the energetic as well as electromagnetic nature of qi.[14]

---

[12]Perhaps the German word Geist fits better here in depicting the intermingling relationship of spirit, mind, and consciousness. Although Geist denotes spirit, such as zeitgeist, which means the spirit of the time, it also carries the connotations of mind and consciousness. Interested readers can refer to Lei (1989, 1990) for details.

[13]Though this kind of experience does not sound as if it were scientific in the Western sense, it has been documented in some best-sellers written by Yale and Harvard medical professors, such as *Love, medicine and miracles* (Siegel, 1990), *Timeless healing* (Benson, 1996), and *Power healing* (Galland, 1998).

[14]In a case as such, quantum physics instead of the traditional Newtonian physics may be a better frame of reference for the study of qi.

Clinical evidence of the exogenous-healing qigong's efficacy has also been documented, especially in the cases of hypertension, stomach cancer, and spinal disc dislocation (Lee & Lei, 1999). Usually, the extrinsic qi is emitted from the healer's hands and transmitted to the patient in two ways. The first way works as does the Western therapeutic touch[15] (Krieger, 1979), in which there is a close distance between the healer and the patient. For that fact, we may call this healing technique distant-healing qigong. The second way is like acupressure massage, during which the healer instills her or his qi into the patient's meridian system through the system's gates, namely, acupoints on the skin. This type of qigong may be termed as meridian-massage qigong, given that the healer performs massage on the patient's meridian system.

Granted the fast relief contributed by exogenous-healing qigong, it cannot be used as a panacea due to the following constraints. First, a healer's energy reservoir has its own limit. While utilizing his or her qi (vital energy) to heal another person, the healer also taxes his or her energy system tremendously. That is the reason why qigong healers can only treat a certain number of patients a day, for the healer needs time to recuperate herself, and to do some qigong to regenerate energy for her own system. Otherwise, not only will the qigong healer suffer from qi depletion, but the quality of the qi she delivers will tend to be low.

The other constraint of using the extrinsic qi can be derived from the Taoist concept of people discussed earlier. Each person's organismic system has his or her idiosyncratic constellation, in which the whole is greater than the sum of all parts. When one pivotal part of the system is dysfunctional, the entire constellation may become disequilibrated.

Introducing extrinsic qi into the disturbed person's system may functionally compensate for that broken part and thus eliminate the disturbance of qi or the symptoms. In so doing, the patient may be healed. However, he may not become holistically healthy and armored with his immune strength. This is because, although extrinsic qi can fix the patient's problem, it cannot fit into his constellation. To change the constellation or configuration is the ultimate therapeutic goal, and the injection of extrinsic qi is merely a temporary solution to a permanent problem. As one old saying points out, "Health cannot be purchased. It has to be earned." To reach that ultimate goal, endogenous-healing qigong seems to be the royal road.

Endogenous-healing Qigong

Several forms of qigong that operate on different subsystems of the human organism can contribute intrinsic qi to equilibrate the organism's general system and consolidate its constellation. These forms of qigong can thereby help heal a person, who is able to ameliorate his illness and at the same time enhance his wellness. For that reason, we call those forms of qigong "endogenous-healing" qigong, which is briefly discussed in this section.

---

[15]In some sense, therapeutic touch or healing touch is a misnomer, since the healer does not necessarily touch the patient. On the other hand, touch may not have to be in a physical sense, provided that the healer's energy is in contact with the patient's.

Movement-oriented Qigong   This is a series of elegant, slow movements, and in some way like a solo dance. There are many styles of movement-oriented qigong that differ not only in choreography, but also in functional purpose. That means they are designed for different parts of the organ network, and for people with different combinations of yin-yang and the five phases/elements. Among them, the most popular one is called *tai chi chuan*, which is good for strengthening the heart and for various configurations of yin-yang and the five phases/elements. However, tai chi chuan is not good for patients who already have cardiovascular problems, because it demands too much of the heart as empirically demonstrated in Ganlante's (1981) longitudinal study.

Wild Swan Gong   This another popular movement-oriented qigong that is especially suited for women. This style is tailored for producing the qi that protects females' reproductive system. Underlying the various styles of qigong, there is a common concern, that is, that the qi has to be cultivated and carried by apparently gentle and supple movements.

Meditation-oriented Qigong   This form can be practiced in a sitting, squatting, standing, or sleeping position. No matter what position is taken, the important thing is to let the mind float with the flow of consciousness or swim in the stream of serenity. While doing this, a person can feel that his or her microcosmic energy system is in touch with the macrocosmic energy system,[16] and he or she should keep body movement to a minimum since it may disrupt the flow of qi or consciousness in the mind.

Basically, there are two types of meditation-oriented qigong. One is mindless meditation, which means thinking nothing while meditating and letting the qi circulation unfold its natural course in the meridian system. This qi circulation starts from the midline of the front to the back of the body and is called microcosmic orbit circulation. While mindless meditation is useful for regulating qi in the whole organismic system, mindful meditation, which resembles guided imagery techniques, is required to direct qi to specific parts of the body for particular functional purposes.[17]

Breathing Qigong   In the Chinese language, the most frequently used denotation of qi refers to air. In fact, fresh air has long been considered as one of the sources of vital energy by Chinese, and breathing qigong was developed to extract high-quality air from the outside and exhale stale air from the inside of the body. In order to inhale as much fresh air as possible, it is best to practice breathing qigong in the morning, especially under pine trees, which are believed to release the best air. During the daily breathing exercise, a person deliberately breathes out the overnight stagnated qi, and then wholeheartedly takes in the good air.

If the immediate goal of practicing qigong is to heal rather than to become healthy, then the person should expel the sick qi by prolonged exhalation before he inhales the fresh air. This exercise should be done several times a day and for as long as it takes to store sufficient qi in the body. Only after the patient accumulates enough sound qi can he or she directly use his or her intention to channel that stored qi to counteract pathogens.

---

[16]Another way to put it is that one's soul/spirit or individual consciousness is transacting with the collective consciousness, including the spirit of the cultural-ethnic group (volkgeist), of the time (zeitgeist), and of the place (ortgeist).

[17]By intentionally moving qi to or out of certain ailing areas of the body through the operation of the mind, about 3000 years ago mindfulness-meditation earned a recognition as the precursor of mind/body medicine (Brigham, 1994).

The traditional Chinese vocal therapy can be employed as an adjunct to breathing qigong. In short, the patient is instructed to vocalize the following Chinese words: *she, shu, su, tzua, kir,* and *fou.* According to TCM theory, these six sounds auditorily represent six body organs in the organ network, namely, triple burner (refers to the three body cavities—pelvis, adomen, and chest), liver, lung, spleen, kidney, and heart. Their pronunciation is believed to ameliorate the disorders involved in each of those organs.

Therapeutic Process

The therapeutic process starts with the typical TCM diagnostic procedure mentioned earlier, of which the information gathered will serve as the backdrop for further diagnosis of the qi state. There is a unique diagnostic tool employed in detecting the patient's qi state, namely, the practitioner's expanded consciousness. A practitioner can apply his or her expanded consciousness in the following ways:

- **Hand scanning**   To perform this type of scanning, the diagnostician brings her hands close to the patient's and moves around in an attempt to feel the patient's qi (subtle energy and/or electromagnetic field). The healer's qi in the form of expanded consciousness (cf. Note 12) emitted from her hands can interact with the patient's qi and thereby create special sensations, such as tingling. Actually, these kinds of sensations are rather subjective and subtle. In that sense qigong diagnosis is more like an art than a technique, and it requires talent as well as training and toil.
- **Visual/mental scanning**   In the qigong diagnostician's eyes, a patient's qi manifests itself in the aura surrounding him or her. The color, brightness, and thickness of the aura indicates a patient's general condition. To detect any variation of the patient's qi distribution, activity level, and other qi characteristics, the diagnostician needs to visually scan every part of the patient's body. Even without conducting any scanning, a gifted healer can sometimes "feel" something went wrong with the patient by mentally projecting herself into the patient's qi field. An anecdotal episode is provided here for illustration:

Once we were in a meeting with a qigong master in our lab, when a woman walked in and took a seat behind the master. To our amazement the master told us a few minutes later that the person sitting behind him was suffering from hypothyroidism, which was probably due to an overdone surgical removal of her thyroid. When we asked this master how he could know the pathological condition of a person he had never seen, he simply said, "Because I feel." Conventional medical experts may argue that perhaps the woman's lethargic movement, slow mental process, and sensitivity provided hints of hypothyroidism to the master. Although all of these could be true, such signs could also indicate other disorders and might not necessarily indicate hypothyroidism. (Lab meeting/personal communication, October 12, 1994)

Diagnostic Criteria   The healer assesses a patient's qi according to the following criteria:

- The evenness of the qi distribution, which reflects the degree of equilibration.
- Leakage of energy. Although the openness of the qi field (which will be discussed in the next section shortly) indicates the two-way transaction between the person's qi system and the outside environment, leakage is only from the inside out and shows that the person's qi system is not well contained.

- Scattered quality of qi, which discloses the irregularity of patient's qi flow in the meridian system.
- Directionality of the qi flow, or whether the qi smoothly follows the microcosmic orbit.
- Stagnation or blockage of the qi circulation, which indicates that the qi may be stuck in some ailing areas.

Diagnostic Results The following conditions may be directly detected from the qigong diagnosis. First, in terms of the quality of qi, the yin-yang quality of the qi as passive or active can be detected via the sensation of the qi's vibration frequency; the hot-cold quality can be detected via thermal sensation, and the wet-dry quality can be detected via moist and dry sensation. So far as the quantity is concerned, the abundance of qi detected by the practitioner may reveal the openness of the patient's electromagnetic energy field, whereas the thin layer of qi may be attributed to either the deficiency of qi or the closure of the patient's qi field.

The previous specific results of qi diagnosis should be evaluated in conjunction with the general diagnostic report, and be referred to the TCM framework for interpretation and the allopathic theory for explaining the operational mechanisms.[18] The specific and general results put together can be categorized into four dialectical patterns that combine four pairs of bipolar factors, namely, yin/yang, hot/cold, interior/exterior, and fullness/emptiness.

Healing Procedure

The guidelines for qigong healing can be summarized as follows: (a) correcting the direction of misled qi flow, (b) homogenizing unevenly distributed qi, (c) balancing the unbalanced qi in terms of yin/yang, hot/cold, and wet/dry, (d) replenishing the leaked or depleting qi system with better qi, (e) mobilizing stagnated qi circulation, (f) releasing the sick qi, and (g) organizing scattered or dispersed qi.

Induction Phase Several sequentially organized phases are involved in the healing process. The initial treatments are conducted by the qigong practitioner during the Induction Phase, which utilizes exogenous-healing qigong. Following the guiding principles aforementioned, to correct the direction of misled qi flow, a practitioner can apply the first method of exogenous-healing qigong: the therapeutic touch. This technique is performed at a distance near enough to manipulate the patient's electromagnetic energy field, especially its bipolar (positive and negative) resistance, but not so close as to lose that resistance. This method can also be used to organize scattered or dispersed qi.

On the other hand, to remove the qi blockage, or to facilitate the stagnated qi flow, it would be more effective to use meridian-massage qigong. In so doing, a practitioner can exert pressure on acupoints and along the meridians, and chop and knead affected areas. Both distant-healing qigong and meridian-massage qigong can be employed to homogenize unevenly distributed qi by means of rotative movement

---

[18]For instance, at the level of physiological structure, yin/yang is homologous to the parasympathetic/sympathetic dyad, and at the neural activity level, yin/yang is functionally analogous to inhibition/excitation.

from the center of the affected area toward the peripheral region. To release the sick qi from a patient, meridian-massage qigong seems to be particularly useful.

While conducting qigong healing, the healer should pay close attention to the patient's reaction. At the beginning, the pressure applied on the patient's acupoints and meridians should be light. Later on, the pressure can be increased gradually to achieve greater effect should the patient adjust him- or herself to a higher level of extrinsic qi. No matter what type of healing qigong is used and whatever the disorder is, at this initial phase patients may experience the adaptation syndrome discussed earlier. This includes some discomfort signs and/or symptoms, which may not be contraindications of qigong treatment. Most likely, they indicate that the patient is going through a process of adapting his system to the incoming foreign substance, which refers to the extrinsic qi in this case (Lee & Lei, 1996).

Remedial/Recovery Phase   Right after the Induction Phase, the second phase of healing process commences, the Remedial/Recovery Phase. During this phase, in a step-by-step process the patient learns how to master the endogenous-healing qigong in order to utilize his own intrinsic qi to help himself from a long-term perspective. This is a life-long learning process and requires patience during which the patient constantly consults the healer concerning the following matters:

- Among those three endogenous-healing qigong methods, namely, movement-, meditation-, and breathing-oriented qigong, which one(s) should be prescribed to the patient? For example, the movement-oriented qigong is necessary to correct the direction of qi flow and to mobilize stagnated qi circulation, whereas the breathing-oriented qigong may be needed for the release of sick qi and for the repletion of a depleted qi system. To generate qi and to homogenize qi distribution, the mindless-meditation qigong is most appropriate, whereas mindful meditation is required to channel qi to certain blocked areas.
- Which style(s) of each qigong method fit(s) the patient best? Each individual has his idiosyncratic condition, including the configuration of his organismic system, his existing energy level, his personality, available time, and contra-indications. For instance, the Young Clan Chuan demands a lot of energy to perform, and a person with a Type A personality or someone who has a tight schedule may experience difficulties when practicing the mindless-meditation qigong.

Maintenance Phase   To remedy and to recover are necessary steps in completing the healing process, though they are not sufficient. The healing comes to a full circle at the third or last phase: maintenance. After a person is fully recovered from the disorder, he or she still needs to practice endogenous qigong in order to maintain the healing effect, and to better regulate his or her system for preventive purposes. To that end, a person may also need some TCM adjunctive therapies besides qigong, such as culinary alchemy, or herb medicine.

THE PAST IS IN THE PRESENT, AND THE PRESENT PROCEEDS INTO THE FUTURE

Paradigm Continuity

In contrast to the Western medical mainstream, which shifts with the natural science paradigm, indigenous Chinese healing relatively maintains its continuity. To be sure, indigenous Chinese healing is traditional but not traditionalistic. Being traditional is about the living faith of the dead, whereas being traditionalistic is related to the dead faith of the living (Bellah, Madsen, Sullivan, Swidler, & Tipton, 1985). Unlike the scientific revolution or the paradigm shifts observed in the West, science (including medical theory) in China witnessed an evolution that did not pass through sequential stages.

In fact, the structure or syntax of science in China has stood the test of time and has remained the same since its inception, even though changes have occurred in the content of which the vocabularies have been enriched and the applications have been expanded. To use the layer cake as an analogy, the old ingredients are never discarded but only recycled into the new layers. No matter how many new ingredients are added in or how many layers are added on, the design or the structure of the layer cake is still identical or homologous with the previous ones.

The structural stability of Chinese science and medical theory should be attributed to the paradigm it is based on, of which the sine qua non is of a human science (*Geisteswissenschaft*) nature. As such, no matter how medical technology advances itself, the fundamental principles underlying indigenous Chinese healing always honor human beings first and never use them as means to test novel medical technology. To recapitulate, these principles include viewing the patient as a whole person with spiritual, psychological, and physiological dimensions, rather than as a bag of diseases; treating the person from a long-term and a proactive/preventive perspective, rather than passively reacting to disorders; and respecting the patient as an active participant in the healing process, who is encouraged to listen to his or her body and tune into intuitive feelings.

Present: Old Wine in a New Bottle (Lee & Lei, 1995)

ICH has attempted to apply the recent developments in biochemistry and analytic techniques in the West by exploring them in at least a few of the following areas. First, as Kaptchuk and Croucher (1986) observe, current research on ICH attempts to isolate the effective components of particular Chinese medical treatments in dealing with diseases recognized by the West. Second, research also attempts to evaluate the efficacy of ICH with contemporary (Western) scientific research designs and with reference to the allopathic taxonomy of disease. Due to the topics and page limit of this chapter, a microanalysis of each ICH method and a meta-analysis of empirical and clinical outcome studies on ICH's efficacy will be presented in another chapter.

Forecasting the Future of ICH: A Promised Land?

Theory-(meta)physics From the perspective of contemporary mainstream science, the theoretical paradigm of ICH does not make sense. Be that as it may, marginal streams led by intellectual prophets in the Western science have pointed out that some of those exotic theoretical aspects may actually promise a brave new direction for science to take (Eisenberg, 2002; Kaptchuk & Eisenberg, 1998, 2001). As an example, the application of the Taoist correspondence or correlative principle to psychology has been made by Heinz Werner (1948) in delineating the recapitulation principle in ontogenetic theory. Along the same line, Carl Jung (1950) resorted to the Taoist *Book of Change* (*I Ching*) to reconstruct the correspondence principle into the synchronicity principle in his grand theory.

More important, ICH concepts of the nature of man and his environment have been echoed in emerging quantum physics and ecological theory (Lei, 1988, 1994), which may shift the paradigm that underlies conventional Western medicine. In terms of quantum physics, it echoes the logic of the Taoist treatise, which suggests that we live in a relatively process-oriented universe, in which no sharp line of distinction can be drawn between mass and energy[19], time and space, or mind and matter. The affinity between quantum physics and the Eastern philosophy that originated from the Taoist tradition has been described by physicist Werner Heisenberg in this way:

> For instance, the great scientific contribution in theoretical physics that has come from Japan [of which the philosophical tradition has been heavily influenced by Chinese heritage, such as Taoism and Confucianism—authors' note] since the last war may be an indication for a certain relationship between philosophical ideas in the tradition of the Far East and the philosophical substance of quantum theory. It may be easier to adapt oneself to the quantum-theoretical concept of reality when one has not gone through the naïve materialistic way of thinking that still prevailed in Europe in the first decades of this century. (1962, p. 202)

More than 60 years have passed since the quantum revolution in modern physics, and Western medicine just began to take advantage of this insight in natural science. Considering that it took 200 years for allopathic medicine to adopt the standards of classical or Newtonian physics, perhaps we still have a long way to go before we reach the new promised land of medicine.

Technique-method: A Web with Worldwide Weavers? Indeed, the indigenous Chinese healing system was originally a unique cultural construction, and it can be considered part of the whole web of reality, which is interwoven with so many other parts of Chinese culture. In the development of this healing system, the Taoist tradition of epistemology has played a facilitative role by providing a common theoretical ground that integrates different ICH modalities. In spite of its positive contribution, the Taoist theory may not be required for the application of each specific ICH technique, and it does not set constraints on the mastery of each method either. This statement is supported by the booming practice of acupuncture since the 1970s in the West, where qigong (including tai chi chuan) is also enjoying an emerging popularity despite the fact that Taoism is still far from being well received. In such a case, can we take a pill without its sugar coating? Meaning, can we just employ the techniques of ICH without adopting its theoretical basis (Yuen, 2001)?

The present authors recommend the inclusion of the sugar-coating for the following reasons: First, ICH theory has its own intrinsic interest and provides us with a different window or vantage point to view the world. Second, sometimes it seems difficult to swallow a pill without its sugar coating, which is to say that although the theory is not the essential component of the ICH system, the belief it supplies to the patient's mind can produce some placebo effects, which are said to account for 50 to 60 percent of the efficacy in allopathic medicine (Benson & Epstein, 1975; Benson & Friedman, 1996), and which may contribute to at least the same degree of the efficacy

---

[19]This is supported by Albert Einstein's famous formula, $E=MC^2$.

of alternative medicine. Indeed, results of clinical and empirical studies generally show that ICH works best when left in the context of Chinese logic. In most cases, an open-minded adoption of the theoretical underpinnings has led to better clinical outcomes than the mechanical application of Chinese remedies within a Western context (Kaptchuk & Croucher, 1986).

To foster rigorous research and still preserve the essence of acupuncture and other ICH modalities, recently Chinese, British, American, and German researchers have jointly proposed novel research methodology (Lao, Ezzo, Berman, & Hammerschlag, 2001). In essence, four steps are recommended to systematically and logically examine particular acupuncture/ICH research questions, as summarized in the following:

1. Use clinical observation to identify a condition that may respond to acupuncture/ICH.
2. Set up a preliminary study for exploration purposes. This preliminary or pilot study should provide the data needed to do the statistical power calculation for a larger clinical trial. It should also assess the feasibility of the research setting, including staffing availability and ability. In addition, it should contribute to a forum in which unforeseeable problems arise and can be addressed so that a solid study protocol can be developed for the later randomized and placebo-controlled trial.
3. Conduct a randomized and placebo-controlled blind study to determine whether the effectiveness is due to placebo effect. Using acupuncture as an example, in the past sham acupuncture referred to the insertion of a needle into nonacupoints or inappropriate manipulations of a needle that should not have any treatment effect. However, these types of sham acupuncture have serendipitously shown some treatment effect, especially for pain management. Now non-needle insertion sham acupuncture is available, and guidance for how to optimize this control has been presented (cf. Kaptchuk, 2003).
4. Carry out a randomized, sham-controlled, double-blind study, in which the healer follows a given protocol without knowing the patient's diagnosis while the treatment effect is measured by a nonhealer researcher. This type of study can rule out the researchers' expectation effect and other experimenter-related effects.

Process Versus Product Approaches   Importing ICH techniques without their theoretical foundations is like planting trees without their roots. Some of those trees may be grafted to the trees with roots and some may soon fade away after a shining start. To us visitors sightseeing in botanic gardens, we couldn't care less about where the trees came from and what they are going to become as long as they look nice.

On the other hand, if we consider ourselves as gardeners, we would want the trees to grow nicely in our soil; they are not merely objects to be seen but also subjects to interact with and whose growth process involves our own. Without engaging ourselves in the developmental process of a product, it is probably infeasible for us to control or change the quality of the product. By the same token, to get involved in the developmental process of a tree right from the beginning is to adopt a bottom-up approach with initial attention being paid to laying down the foundation. With this notion in mind, to design a long-term strategy of adopting ICH in the West and to adapt it to the new host culture, we need to take into account the theoretical foundation and how it unfolds its course in a foreign land. We believe that interweaving the Eastern and Western webs (metaphors of medical modalities) will strengthen both of them, and the uniqueness of each web will shine through the other web by contrast.

REFERENCES

Beinfield, H., & Korngold, E. (1991). *Between heaven and earth: A guide to Chinese medicine.* New York: Ballantine Books.

Bellah, R. N., Madsen, R., Sullivan, W. M., Swidler, A., & Tipton, S. M. (1985). *Habits of the heart: Individualism and commitment in American life.* Berkeley, CA: University of California Press.

Benson, H. (1996). *Timeless healing.* New York, NY: Scribner.

Benson, H., & Epstein, M. (1975). The placebo effect. *Journal of the American Medical Association, 232*(12), 1225-1227.

Benson, H., & Friedman, R. (1996). Harness the power of the placebo effect and renaming it "remembered wellness." *Annual Review of Medicine, 47,* 193-199.

Biella, G., Sotgiu, M., Pellegata, G., Paulesu, E., Castiglioni, I., & Fazio, F. (2001). Acupuncture produces central activations in pain regions. *Neuroimage, 14*(1), 60-66.

Brigham, D. D. (1994). *Imagery for getting well: Clinical applications of behavioral medicine.* New York: W. W. Norton.

Eisenberg, D. (1987). *Encounters with qi: Exploring Chinese medicine.* New York: Penguin Books.

Eisenberg, D. (2002). Complementary and integrative medical therapies: Current status and future trends. In D. Eisenberg (Ed.), *Complementary and alternative medicine: State of the science and clinical application* (pp. 3-32). Boston, MA: Harvard Medical School.

Ergil, K. V. (1996). China's traditional medicine. In M. S. Micozzi (Ed.), *Fundamentals of complementary and alternative medicine* (pp. 183-224). New York: Churchill Livingstone.

Galland, L. (1998). *Power healing.* New York: Random House.

Ganlante, L. (1981). *Tai Chi: The supreme ultimate.* York Beach, MA: Samuel Weiser.

Green, E. E., & Green, A. M. (1986). Biofeedback and states of consciousness. In B. B. Wolman & M. Ullman (Eds.), *Handbook of states of consciousness* (pp. 553-589). New York: Van Nostrand Reinhold.

Guo, L. (1989). *New qigong method for cancer treatment.* Beijing, China: Doun Xing.

Heisenberg, W. (1962). *Physics and philosophy.* New York: Harper & Row.

Hidetoshi, M., Kazushi, N., Hiroki, K., & Toru, A. (2002). Unique immunomodulation by electro-acupuncture in humans possibly via the stimulation of the autonomic nervous system. *Neuroscience Letter, 320*(1-2), 21-24.

Hui, K. K. S., Liu, J., Wu, M. T., & Wong, K. K. K. (1996, September). *Functional mapping of the human brain during acupuncture with magnetic resonance imaging.* Paper presented at the Fourth World Congress on Acupuncture, New York.

Jacobs, G. D. (2001). Clinical applications of the relaxation response and mind-body interventions. *Journal of Alternative Complementary Medicine, 7* (Supplement), 93-101.

Jiangsu College of New Medicine (1977). *Encyclopedia of traditional Chinese medicinal substances.* Jiangsu, China: Jiangsu College Press. (In Chinese).

Jonas, W. B., & Levin, J. S. (1999). Models of medicine and healing. In W. B. Jonas & J. S. Levin (Eds.), *Essentials of complementary and alternative medicine* (pp. 1-15). Baltimore, MD: Williams & Wilkins.

Jung, C. G. (1950/1977). Foreword to the I Ching. In *The collected works of C. G. Jung, Vol. 11,* 589-608. London: Routledge & Kegan Paul.

Kaptchuk, T. (2002). Traditional Chinese medicine: State of the science. In D. Eisenberg (Ed.), *Complementary and alternative medicine: State of the science and clinical application* (pp. 121-131). Boston, MA: Harvard Medical School.

Kaptchuk, T., & Eisenberg, D. (1998). The persuasive appeal of alternative medicine. *Annals of Internal Medicine, 129,* 1061-1065.

Kaptchuk, T., & Eisenberg, D. (2001). Varieties of healing. 1. Medical pluralism in the United States. *Annals of Internal Medicine, 135,* 189-195.

Kaptchuk, T. J. (1983). *The web that has no weaver: Understanding Chinese medicine.* New York: Congdon & Weed.

Kaptchuk, T. J. (2003, March). *The wonder pill: Placebo effect.* A special PBS presentation. Boston: WGBH.

Kaptchuk, T. J., & Croucher, M. (1986). *The healing arts.* London, UK: British Broadcasting Corporation.

Kerr, C. (2002). Translating "mind-in-body:" Two models of patient experience underlying a randomized controlled trial of qigong. *Culture, Medicine, and Psychiatry, 26*(4), 419-447.

Krieger, D. (1979). *The therapeutic touch: How to use your hands to help or to heal.* New York: Prentice-Hall.

Kleinman, A. (1980). *Patients and healers in the context of culture: An exploration of the borderland between anthropology, medicine, and psychiatry.* Berkeley, CA: University of California Press.

Ko, J., Na, D. S., Lee, Y. H., Shin, S. Y., Kim, J. H., Hweng, B. G., et al. (2002). CDNA microarray analysis of gene expression in neuropathic pain and electro-acupuncture. *Journal of Biomedical Molecular Biology, 35*(4), 420-427.

Lao, L., Ezzo, B., Berman, B., & Hammerschlag, R. (2001). Future directions for clinical trials in acupuncture research. In G. Stux & R. Hammerschlag (Eds.), *Scientific basis of clinical acupuncture* (pp. 187-210). Berlin, Germany: Springer-Verlag.

Laszlo, E. (1979). *System, structure, and experience: Toward a scientific theory of mind.* New York: Gordon and Breach.

Lee, C. T., & Lei, T. (1995, April). Effects of vital energy exercise on physiological and psychological changes. In U. P. Gielen (Chair), *Cross-cultural psychology.* Symposium conducted at the 66th Annual Meeting of the Eastern Psychological Association, Boston, MA.

Lee, C. T., & Lei, T. (1996, September). All rivers flow to the sea: Encountering energy through qigong without acupuncture. Paper presented at the Fourth World Congress on Acupuncture, New York.

Lee, C. T., & Lei, T. (1999). Qigong. In W. B. Jonas & J. S. Levin (Eds.), *Essentials of complementary and alternative medicine* (pp. 392-409). Baltimore, MD: Lippincott, Williams & Wilkins.

Lei, T. (1988, February). From a drop of water to see the sea: Universality and Chinese moral reasoning. Paper presented at the 18th Annual Philosophy Symposium, Fullerton, CA: State University of California.

Lei, T. (1989). The physical and metaphysical bases of the mind, self (consciousness), and society. In H. Kao & C. F. Yang (Eds.), *The Chinese and the Chinese mind* (pp. 147-197). Taipei, Taiwan: Long Stream Press. (In Chinese).

Lei, T. (1990). Geisteswissenschaften of Sittlichkeit and political Umwelt: Sinnverstehen in the East. *Pacific Focus, 5*(1), 19-59.

Lei, T. (1991). Ethnogenesis of person and ontogenesis of self: Experience of being and becoming moral in Taiwan. In Y. G. Hwang (Ed.), *The concept of the person, meaning, and society* (pp. 305-361). Taipei, Taiwan: Academia Sinica.

Lei, T. (1994. July). Preventing paradise from perishing: Chinese culture's contribution to eco-ethics. In L. Eckensberger (Chair), *International Conference on Ecological Ethics.* Saarbrücken, Germany: University of Saarbrücken.

Lei, T. (2002, July). *Applications of alternative health/healing models: Freedom of choice, personal responsibility, and just community.* Paper presented at the 2nd Biannual International Conference on Personal Meaning: Freedom, Responsibility, and Justice. Vancouver, BC, Canada.

Litscher, G., Wenzel, G., Niederwieser, G., & Schwartz, G. (2001). Effects of qigong on brain functions. *Neurological Research, 23*(5), 501-505.

Melzack, R. (1993). Pain: Past, present, and future. *Canadian Journal of Experimental Psychology, 47,* 615-629.

Needham, J. (1956). *Science and civilization in China.* Cambridge, UK: Cambridge University Press.

Siegel, B. S. (1990). *Love, medicine, and miracles.* New York: Harper & Row.

Tanaka, T. H., Leisman, G., & Nishijo, K. (1998). Dynamic electromyographic response: Possible influence on synergistic coordination. *International Journal of Neuroscience, 95*(1-2): 51-61.

Terry, O. (2002). Auriculotherapy stimulation for neuro-rehabilitation. *NeuroRehabilitation, 17*(1), 49-62.

Ulett, G. A., Han, S., & Han, J. S. (1998). Electroacupuncture: Mechanisms and clinical application. *Biological Psychiatry, 44*(2), 129-138.

Werner, H. (1948). *Comparative psychology of mental development.* New York: International University Press.

Yuen, C. F. (2001). Oriental medicine. *Alternative Therapy, Health, & Medicine, 7*(4), 71-82.

Indigenous Chinese Healing: A Criteria-based Meta-analysis of Outcomes Research

Ting Lei
The City University of New York

Ching-Tse Lee
The City University of New York

Cecilia Askeroth
St. Francis College

Dmitry Burshteyn
Siena College

Andrea Einhorn
White Plains, New York

The first author wishes to dedicate this chapter to the Shining Star in the dark sky and Alison Aplin. He would also like to express his gratitude to Ronald Doviak, Sadie Bragg, Antonio Perez, Manuel Matinez-Pons, Ellen Ciporen, Emily Anderson, Nora Eisenberg, Barbara Tacinelli, and Tracy November, for their valuable support.

In 1990, David Eisenberg from the Harvard Medical School conducted a large-scale national survey ($N = 1,539$) on the use of alternative medicine in this country and published the results in the *New England Journal of Medicine* in 1993 (Eisenberg, Kessler, Foster, Norlock, Calkins, & Delbanco, 1993). This survey, which has been well received in the fields of both conventional and complementary medicine, revealed that 33.8 percent of Americans used alternative medicine in 1990, and the total visits to alternative medicine practitioners were about 427 million. In 1997, Eisenberg conducted another national representative survey ($N = 1,720$) and published the findings in the *Journal of the American Medical Association (JAMA)* in 1998 (Eisenberg et al., 1998). The later finding indicated a significant increase in the use of alternative medicine in the past 7 years (from 33.8 percent to 42.1 percent, $p < .001$). Extrapolations to the U.S. population suggest a striking 47.3 percent increase in total visits to alternative medicine practitioners during the past 7 years, thereby exceeding total visits to all U.S. primary care physicians (628,825,000 visits to alternative medicine practitioners versus 385,919,000 to all primary care physicians). Data also show a 65 percent increase in the total number of alternative therapies used, from 577 therapies per 1,000 people in 1990 to 953 per 1,000 in 1997. At the same time, estimated expenditures for alternative medicine professional services increased 45.2 percent and were conservatively estimated at $21.2 billion in 1997, with at least $12.2 billion paid out-of-pocket. This is more than the 1997 out-of-pocket expenditures for all U.S. hospitalizations.

Furthermore, according to that *JAMA* report, use of alternative or complementary therapies in 1997 was not confined to any narrow segment of this society, although use was higher among those who had some college education (50.6 percent) than those without college education (34.6 percent) ($p < .001$). Among the 16 modalities of alternative therapies included in the surveys, the percentage of those using non-Western alternative therapies increased significantly. For example, acupuncture increased from 0.4 percent in 1990 to 1.0 percent in 1997 ($p < .05$), whereas energy healing and folk remedies increased even more dramatically (from 1.3 percent in 1990 to 3.8 percent in 1997, with $p < .001$ for energy healing; from 0.2 percent in 1990 to 4.2 percent in 1997, with $p < .001$ for folk remedies). On the other hand, Western modalities of alternative therapies, such as biofeedback, retained their usage (1.0 percent in 1990 and 1997), while chiropractic, hypnosis, and dietary therapies increased insignificantly (10.1 percent in 1990 to 11.0 percent in 1997 for chiropractic; 0.9 percent in 1990 to 1.2 percent in 1997 for hypnosis; 3.6 percent in 1990 to 4.0 percent in 1997 for lifestyle diet, and 3.9 percent in 1990 to 4.4 percent in 1997 for commercial diet). Consistent with this finding, an independent national survey ($N = 1,035$) conducted by Dr. Astin at the Stanford Medical School, and also published in the 1998 *JAMA*, demonstrates that the percentage of people in the United States using alternative therapies rose to 69 percent in 1998, and education emerged as the sociodemographic variable that predicted its use. That is, individuals with a higher educational background were more likely to use alternative therapies (as an example, 31 percent of the respondents with a high school education or less reported use, compared with 50 percent of the respondents with graduate degrees) (Astin, 1998).

As can be seen from the above-mentioned Harvard and Stanford studies, alternative medicine has been enjoying more and more popularity in this country, and this popularity is not capitalizing on less-educated people's ignorance of health care. On the contrary, the multivariate regression conducted in the Stanford study revealed that "cultural creatives" were significantly more likely to use alternative forms of health care. Among this subcultural group, 55 percent adopted alternative health care, versus 35 percent of the respondents not in this group. "Cultural creatives" are individuals who tend to be on the leading edge of cultural change and innovation, coming up with the most new ideas in the society and/or manifesting a commitment to environmentalism as well as involvement with esoteric forms of spirituality and personal growth psychology. The value orientations that characterize cultural creatives have been operationally defined and empirically verified with factor analysis and multiple dimensional scaling (Ray, 1998; Ray & Anderson, 2001). According to Ray's demographic studies, this cultural creative group has been steadily growing since the late 1960s. According to the recent Stanford survey, the dominant reason for this group's adoption of alternative medicine was neither a dissatisfaction with conventional treatment nor a need for personal control, as some scholars pointed out (e.g., Ruggie, 2002). Rather, it was due to "philosophical congruence," meaning that, cultural creatives were more likely to subscribe to a holistic philosophy of health. They might be attracted, therefore, to alternative healing, because they see in these healing systems a greater acknowledgment of vitalistic/organic/quantum (nonmechanic physical) components in creating health and illness.

To be sure, it was also possible that individuals who had tried alternative healing had their belief systems influenced or reinforced by the philosophical rationales underlying these healing modalities. Indeed, users of alternative health care in the Stanford study were more likely to report having had a transformational experience, which might be related to the involvement with alternative healing, or other aspects of life, that changed their worldview. This transformational experience factor emerged as a significant ($p < .005$) predictor of alternative health care usage in the multiple logistic regression. In any case, these survey data suggest that the engagement in alternative health care may be reflective of shifting cultural paradigms regarding assumptions of how things are, including beliefs about the nature of life, humanity, and the world in general. In line with this empirical finding, another important piece of evidence from the Stanford study also lends support to the elite cultural theory of alternative medicine usage. The most influential factor in individuals' decision to use alternative medicine was its perceived efficacy. The response, "The treatment promotes health rather than just focusing on illness" was the third most frequently reported benefit. As such, users of alternative medicine in the United States were not misled due to their insufficient training in scientific research (especially in evidence-based medicine), as some editorials of leading medical journals have implied (cf. Jonas, 1998).

Against this backdrop of a cultural paradigm shift and the rising rival popularity of alternative medicine, the November 1998 theme issue of *JAMA*, and the annual coordinated theme issues of the nine American Medical Association Archives journals published in the same month, were specifically on alternative medicine. They included more than 80 articles, editorials, and systematic reviews on 30 different alternative medicine topics. On the basis of these documents, the *JAMA* editorial arrived at the following conclusion, which should be heeded by every consumer and practitioner of alternative medicine: "Until solid evidence is available that demonstrates the safety, efficacy, and effectiveness of specific alternative medicine interventions, uncritical acceptance of untested and unproven alternative medicine therapies must stop" (Fontanarosa & Lundberg, 1998, p. 1619). To that end, the editorial suggested, "Alternative medicine therapies and interventions can and should be evaluated using explicit, focused research questions along with established and accepted rigorous research methods (e.g., appropriate control, effective blinding procedures, adequate power, state-of-the-art techniques for systematic reviews); incorporating measurable, objectively assessed end-points (e.g., blinded assessment); and reporting meaningful patient-centered outcomes" (p. 1619).

The objective of this chapter is to take the *JAMA*'s suggestion into account in reviewing the research on acupuncture and on energy healing (also called *qigong*), which are two representative forms of indigenous Chinese healing (ICH). The theories and methods of these two ICH treatment modalities are presented in Chapter 12 "Indigenous Chinese Healing: Theories and Methods" (Lei, Lee, & Askeroth, in this volume). Specifically about qigong's rationale, interested readers can refer to Lee's and Lei's chapters on qigong, which appeared in the *Essentials of Complementary and Alternative Medicine* (Jonas & Levin, 1999). In this chapter, we focus on the systematic review of the outcomes research of the two representative ICH modalities.

METHODS

Two types of research documents were reviewed. The first were papers presented at the Fourth World Conference on Acupuncture, which was held in New York City in 1996, and was cosponsored by the World Health Organization. Two of the present authors (Lei and Lee) served on the academic committee of that conference and evaluated 586 abstracts from more than 40 countries. Each of the seven members on the committee had doctorates. Together they worked out general inclusion/exclusion criteria before the evaluation, in which expert opinion played an important role. Full-length papers of the abstracts were requested when the need for more information or detail arose. Only papers with good research quality (rather than those that demonstrated good clinical outcomes) that were approved by at least two reviewers were selected for the conference presentation. Consensus meetings were held regularly to resolve any disagreements among reviewers.

The justification for including these unpublished or prepublished materials in systematic review or meta-analysis has been provided in clinical journals. For example, authors in *JAMA* (Cook et al., 1993) and *Journal of Clinical Psychology* (Eppley, Abrams, & Shear, 1989) have argued that studies with results that reached a conventional level of statistical significance were considerably more likely to be published (odds ratio: 2.54).

As such, it would be difficult to get a complete picture of the results of the clinical trials conducted on certain interventions using only published reports, which tend to be biased toward statistically significant results and do not reflect the whole truth of the clinical trials. Consumers may thus be misled to believe the near-perfect efficacy of the medical intervention and may not know that they only see the stars without the sky of the clinical trials. This publication bias seems to be particularly salient in some countries, especially those that dominate the research on alternative/complementary medicine. As the international Cochrane Collaboration found,

> studies published in Russia and China had a disproportionately high number of statistically significant results (97 percent and 99 percent, respectively) when compared with England (75 percent). It is not yet evident whether these high proportions are due to extreme forms of publication bias or low study quality, which overestimated treatment effects (Ezzo, Berman, Vickers, & Linde, 1998; Lei, Lee, Burshteyn, & Schnoll, 2002).

In a similar vein, another article appearing in *JAMA* (Jadad & Rennie, 1998) maintained that clinical trials with positive results were published years faster than those with negative results. Thus, new interventions have been accepted as effective in the absence of evidence to the contrary, even though such evidence may already have been gathered. In relating to indigenous Chinese healing, an article entitled "Do certain countries produce only positive results?" (Vickers, Goyal, Harland, & Rees, 1998) specifically identified that researchers in some countries may publish only positive results, such as those from randomized controlled trials (RCTs) evaluating acupuncture conducted in China, Japan, and Taiwan, which are the home base of ICH research. Given these publication biases, the inclusion of unpublished materials is not only recommended but also required.

The second type of research documents were articles selected from peer-reviewed journals (e.g., *JAMA, New England Journal of Medicine, Lancet, Stroke, Pain*, etc.), as well as searches on CD-ROMs (e.g., LEXIS-NEXIS). The inclusion criteria for the second type of documents are the common criteria for publication in peer-reviewed journals, while the exclusion criteria refer to the languages other than English, Chinese, German, and Japanese.

Design

Systematic review, including criteria-based meta-analysis, was employed in this research. Usually, the main purpose of meta-analysis is to pool data from existing studies of a certain intervention in order to come up with a better overall estimate of the efficacy achieved by that particular intervention. In so doing, meta-analysis may resolve the conflicts that arise when reports of primary studies disagree, or it may increase the likelihood of detecting small but clinically important effects with the help of larger sample sizes and greater statistical power. Before conducting this quantitatively oriented pooled analysis, a qualitatively oriented methodological analysis seems to be necessary, in which the quality of the research concerning the intervention is scored according to predetermined criteria.

Given the two types of documents (unpublished and published) reviewed in this chapter, two sets of evaluation criteria were set up in accordance with the nature of each set of documents. Most of the unpublished documents reviewed here follow a paradigm that is different from the predominant Western model and are concerned with the nitty-gritty of ICH theory and clinical procedure, rather than logical deduction and the analytic procedure involved in the research process. Furthermore, these documents were based on observational or quasi-experimental studies, which attempted to identify the association between the intervention used and the outcome observed. In contrast, a majority of the published documents analyzed here included randomized controlled trials (of which the sine qua non is an experimental design) that were aimed at testing the causal relation between intervention and outcome. Although all criteria employed in our systematic review relied to a large extent on well-accepted principles of intervention research, the criteria for the unpublished documents were derived from the consensus committee. Committee members took into special consideration the congruence between the documents and their own understanding of ICH theory, as well as clinical practice.

In comparison with the aforementioned cut-and-try or (inter-) subjective expert opinion approach, a more cut-and-dry or objective approach was applied to establish the criteria for the published materials. These criteria and the weight of each criterion are listed and briefly described in Table 13.1. The selection of criteria and the decision of weightings are based on theoretical rationales as well as recent research results in this field. Inter-rater reliability was assessed by means of an intraclass correlation between two authors' (Lei's and Einhorn's) ratings of 20 studies.

RESULTS

Acupuncture

Gray Literature (Abstract Presentations and Unpublished Data) Key data from the previously unpublished but presented studies are summarized in Table 13.2, which is concerned with the efficacy of acupuncture with the data being presented according to disease categories. Most of these studies were conducted in China, in which the data analysis is quite different from the Western approach. Instead of employing statistical analysis, percentages are used to represent the cure rate, improvement rate, and total effectiveness (which is the sum of cure rate and improvement rate). The first category examined refers to the pain that had been managed by acupuncture. Usually acupuncture should be applied to treat specific types of pain by manipulating relevant acupoints. Nevertheless, four studies have been carried out to evaluate the treatment effect of acupuncture on general (various or cancerous) pain.

Pain management. The cure rate for general pain ranged from 58 to 73 percent, and the total effectiveness was from 85 to 98 percent. These numbers seem to be better than the placebo effect, which may be estimated at about 30 to 60 percent (David,

TABLE 13.1
Methodological Criteria (and Weight)

Comparability of Prognosis

(A) Homogeneity (3) Homogeneity should be high within each group in order for parametric statistical analysis.
(B) Randomization (12) Research participants should be randomly assigned to treatment or control groups in order to avoid selection bias (or rule out confounding factors). This procedure also takes intention to treat into consideration.
(C) Comparability of relevant baseline characteristics shown (2) Baseline characteristics of each group and their intergroup differences can intervene in the IV-DV relation and should be documented.
(D) ≧ 50 participants per group (5) Sample size should be derived from an appropriate formula with alpha and beta errors taken into account. Small sample size may reduce statistical power.
(E) ≦ 20 percent loss to follow-up (3) Attrition of participants can be selective and thus may affect the variation on DV.

Adequate Intervention

(F) Avoidance of the nonspecific effect produced by active placebo (2) Inappropriate selection of acupoints for sham intervention (for control purpose) can turn the sham into an active placebo and produce a nonspecific effect.
(G) Acupuncturist's qualification (9) The quality of the acupuncturist plays an important role in determining the variation on the IV.
(H) Sufficient treatment sessions and adequate (individualized) protocols or regimen (15) This is another major determinant of IV variation.
(I) Existing treatment modality in reference group (3) To see whether the new intervention is better than the existing one.
(J) Participants blinded (10) This is to control for the participants' expectation effect.
(K) Evaluator blinded (5) This is to eliminate some potential biases from the evaluator.
(L) Follow-up after treatment ≧ 3 months (10) Placebo effect wears out with time, but real treatment effect is less likely to wear out.
(M) Remark on side effects (2) Side effects should be taken into serious consideration in making clinical decisions about (contra)indication.
(N) Major outcomes measure (10) The reliability, validity, and other characteristics of the outcome measure are an important concern in evaluation.
(O) Data analysis (9) Whether the qualitative/quantitative (including statistical) analyses employed serve the research purpose.

TABLE 13.2
Acupuncture Efficacy: Gray Materials

Treatment Categories	Sample Size	Cure Rate	Improvement	Total Effectiveness	Sources (1996)
Pain management:					
Anesthesia	50			98%	Bao
Pain (various)	**696**	**68%**	**28%**	**96%**	**Wang et al.**
Pain (various)	361	58%		93%	Borisova et al.
Pain (cancerous)	56	73%	12%	85%	Lai
Musculoskeletal	**90**	**84%**	**14%**	**98%**	**Lynn**
Muscle sprain	125	67%	30%	97%	Xia
Knee joint	30			93%	Tan
Lower back	100	43%	53%	96%	Makiyama & Wu
Lower back	148	70%	20%	90%	Liu & Zhou
Lower back	210	70%	24%	94%	Wang & Wang
Spinal cord	61			75%	Rapson & Bieman
Arthritic	30/30 (control)			$p < .05$	Schiantarelli
Lumbar	120	73%	22%	95%	Li

Treatment Categories	Sample Size	Cure Rate	Improvement	Total Effectiveness	Sources (1996)
Dysmenorrhea	144/120 (med)	88/32%	9/43%	97/75%	Dai
Dysmenorrhea	106	70%	26%	96%	Sun
Abdominal	160/140			95/95%	Yu
	(medicated as the control)				
Headache	**383**	**97%**	**2%**	**99%**	**Huang et al.**
	110	62%	35%	97%	Bao
	85/45 (med)	93/56%	6/33%	99/89%	Yu
Migraine	68/20			94/55%	Niu et al.
	(medicated as the control)				
	72	37%	56%	93%	Zeng
Osterotraumatology					
Osteophyte formation	**86**	**2%**	**88%**	**90%**	**Gui et al.**
Osteoarthritis	95			76%	Cai et al.
Osteoarthritis	19/19 (control)			$p < .001$	Lao et al.
Rheumatoid arthritis	42	20%	67%	87%	Yu
Rheumatoid arthritis	378	23%	75%	98%	Sun
Rheumatoid arthritis	56	26%	64%	90%	Sun
Periarthritis	60	93%	7%	100%	Lu
Periarthritis	268	84%	15%	99%	Cong
Sciatica	38	66%	32%	98%	Jin & Wang
Sciatica	60	55%	33%	98%	Zhang et al.
Sciatica	34	64%	32%	96%	Wu
Sciatica	250	68%	28%	96%	Wang
Arthritic hip	30	90%		90%	Tsai et al.
Lumbago	85	82%	18%	100%	Liu & Dong
Lumbago	50	90%	10%	100%	Zhang
Lumbosciatagia	150			92%	Marino et al.
Lumbar hernia	418	65%	33%	98%	Guan
Lumbar hernia	26	38%	39%	77%	Hu & Hu
Lumbar hernia	26	60%	23%	83%	Hu & Hu
Lumbar hernia	108	56%	41%	97%	Yang
Lumbar hernia	144			94%	Zhou
Lumbar hernia	245	57%	37%	97%	Hao
Paralysis cerebral:					
Hemorrhage	30/30 (med)	53/27%	4/26%	57/53%	Zhu
Hemorrhage	30/32 (medicated as the control)			90/69%	Wang
Infarction	188/188 (medicated as the control)			90/44%	Niu
Injury	37/36	3/?%	50/47%	83/47%	Wu et al.
Stroke	**5798**	**61%**	**38%**	**99%**	**Pagon et al.**
Stroke	214	83%	7%	90%	Chen
Stroke	85	45%	49%	94%	Cheu
Facial paralysis	200			98%	Zhao & Yang
Facial paralysis	20	25%	70%	95%	Liau-Hing
Lumbar paralysis	58			78%	Yang
Vertebral fracture	67	35%	63%	98%	D'Acunzo
Nervous system					
Autonomic	**51**			**85%**	**Imai**
Dementia	38	43%	43%	86%	Chen
Multiple sclerosis	332	2%	40%	41%	Tsuchiya
Vertigo	70			93%	Xue
Addiction					
Neonatal					
Abstinence	35/26 (medicated as the control)			$p > .05$	Schwartz
Alcoholism	**20**	**80%**	**20%**	**100%**	**Bayer**

TABLE 13.2 (continued)

Treatment Categories	Sample Size	Cure Rate	Improvement	Total Effectiveness	Sources (1996)
Smoking	127	65%	28%	93%	Xu
Chronic fatigue syndrome (CFS)					
CFS	**155**			**91%**	**He & Zeng**
CFS	111	77%	18%	96%	Ma & Wang
Opthalmology					
Myopia prevention	22/22 (control)			*p* < .01	Eory & Senyi
Glaucoma	68	75%	7%	82%	Pippa et al.
Infection diseases					
Hepatitis B	**44/44 (control)**			*p* < .05	Yuan
Internal organ disorders					
Coronary heart	**30**			65–78%	Yio et al.
Angina	**16**			87%	Jin & Zhou
Hypertension	138			83%	Chen
Hypertension	100	68%	25%	93%	Guan
Hypertension	69			96%	Zhao
Irritable bowel syndrome	39			75%	Lu
Gall stone	58			91%	Su
Ulcer	80			38%	Jin
Obesity	58			94%	Xial
Obesity	146			100%	Xia
Dermatology; surgery					
Facial correction	**120/56 (control)**			81/41%	**Guan**
Burns	**285**	91%		91%	**Jiang**
Dermatitis	16/12 (control)	50/?%	37%	87/?%	Cantoni et al.
Hair loss	**76**			89%	**Tjandra**
Gynecology; obstetrics; pediatrics					
Uterine					
Fiberomyoma	**18**			66%	**Spitali et al.**
Hysteromyoma	**32**	34%	63%	97%	
Infertility	**35**			34%	**Zheng**
Infertility	20			20%	Katai et al.
Child digestion					
Functional disturbance	140			92%	Wu & Han
Infantile cerebral paralysis	87	36%	30%	66%	Ye
Urologic disorders					
Urinary incontinence	76			97%	Zhang
Prostatitis	60	47%	38%	85%	Ma
Impotence	**48**	62%	32%	94%	**Lam**
Others					
Allergic rhinitis	**50**	76%	4%	80%	**Kim**
Endolymphatic edema	30	79%	14%	93%	Wu
Leukopenia	113	62%	33%	95%	Gong & Wang

Friedman, Siegel, Jacobs & Benson, 1992; Weil, 1995), even though these studies were not controlled for the placebo effect. Along the same line, studies conducted on specific types of pain that were managed by acupuncture also showed similar efficacy. Of these types, some can be categorized into musculoskeletal, spinal cord, lower back, lumbar, knee joint, and arthritic pain, whereas others are grouped into dysmenorrhea and abdominal pain by taking into account both traditional Chinese medicine (TCM) and allopathic taxonomic systems. Ten of the 12 studies reviewed here were completed in East Asia and appear to be efficacious (total effectiveness ranges from 90 to 98 percent). One study (Rapson & Biemann, 1996) conducted in the United States reported a total effectiveness of 75 percent. The other study, which was carried out in Italy (Schiantarelli, Pippa, Bernini, & Terza, 1996), included a control group and reports a statistically significant difference ($p < .05$). There was also a study (Yu, 1996) done in China using medicated participants as control, but it revealed no difference between the medicated group and the control group (total effectiveness is 95 percent for both groups).

Consistently high total effectiveness also appeared in the treatment of headaches and migraines, even though the cure rate is not consistent across different studies. Acupuncture seemed to result in a better cure rate in treating headaches than in treating migraines. Medicated participants served as the control group in one headache study (Yu, 1996) and in one migraine study (Niu & Yang, 1996). The first study demonstrates that acupuncture had a much higher cure rate (93 percent) than medication had (56 percent), whereas the second study shows a better total effectiveness for acupuncture (94 versus 55 percent).

Osterotraumatology. This is a common treatment category of acupuncture under which the first subcategory includes a variety of arthritis. The data presented in Table 13.2 indicate that acupuncture had a better result in treating periarthritis than in treating other types of arthritis. Of the eight studies reported here, only one included a control group and this controlled study showed a statistically significant difference ($p < .001$) in treating osteroarthritis. Under osterotraumatology, sciatica is another subcategory of acupuncture treatment in which the results in terms of cure rate as well as total effectiveness were convergently impressive from different studies. The results in the lumbago subcategory were even more impressive, of which the cure rates were 82 percent and 90 percent, while the total effectiveness achieved 100 percent. Although the cure rates (ranging from 38 to 65 percent) were not so excellent in the lumbar hernia subcategory, the total effectiveness was still pretty high (from 77 to 98 percent).

Paralysis. This is the third treatment category evaluated here, under which the first subcategory was concerned with the cerebral etiology, including hemorrhage, infarction, and injury. Medicated control groups were included in all of the four studies reviewed here. Among these four studies, one (Zhu, 1996) reported similar total effectiveness between acupuncture and control groups (57 versus 53 percent), but a better cure rate for the acupuncture group (53 versus 27 percent). The other three studies revealed a much better total effectiveness for the acupuncture groups (ranging from 83 to 90 percent) than the control groups (44 to 69 percent). Among the three studies in the stroke subcategory, one (Pagon et al., 1996) involved 5,798 participants and indicated a 99 percent total effectiveness for acupuncture treatment. Partial (such as facial, lumbar, etc.) paralysis seemed to be a difficult-to-cure disorder for acupuncture, which registered 25 to 35 percent cure rates in this subcategory.

Nervous system. Disorders related to the autonomic nervous system (ANS), dementia, multiple sclerosis (MS), and vertigo are investigated under the treatment category of nervous system here. The data in Table 13.2 indicate that acupuncture can improve ANS disorders, dementia, and vertigo to a great extent (as indicated by 85 to 93 percent total effectiveness). Nevertheless, acupuncture had a very low cure rate (2 percent) and an unimpressive improvement rate (40 percent) in treating MS. In the treatment category of addiction, one controlled study on neonatal abstinence reported a statistically nonsignificant difference ($p > .05$) between acupuncture and medication (control) groups (Schwartz et al., 1996). In contrast, acupuncture registered a 65 percent cure rate and a 93 percent total effectiveness rate for smoking cessation, as well as 80 and 100 percent rates respectively in treating alcoholism (Bayer, 1996).

Internal organs. In the treatment category of internal organ disorders, including cardiovascular and gastric-intestinal diseases, overall the studies are not so fine-grained as the ones reviewed earlier. None of the studies to be discussed here included a control group, and only one study used the cure rate as an indicator, whereas all the others relied on the total effectiveness (TE) as the sole indicator. In any case, acupuncture appeared to be a rather effective treatment for coronary heart diseases (TE: 65 to 78 percent), angina (TE: 87 percent), hypertension (TE: 83 to 96 percent), irritable bowel syndrome (TE: 75 percent), gall stone (TE: 91 percent), and obesity (94 to 100 percent). However, acupuncture was not so effective in treating ulcers (38 percent).

Dermatology; cosmetic surgery. The total effectiveness of acupuncture in this category is in the 81 to 91 percent range. In the subcategory of facial correction, one study involved 176 participants and reported the total effectiveness for the control group as 41 percent, in contrast to the 81 percent for the treatment group (Guan, 1996). Overall, acupuncture could be indicated for dermatological disorders (including hair loss) and/or cosmetic surgery.

Gynecology; obstetrics; pediatrics. The total effectiveness for this category is not impressive, especially for infertility purposes (20 percent and 34 percent respectively for two different studies). Among all the subcategories, acupuncture seems to be most effective for hysteromyoma, in which the cure rate is 34 percent, the improvement rate is 63 percent, and the total effectiveness is 97 percent.

Urologic disorders; infection diseases, etc. Acupuncture seems to be effective in treating urologic disorders, with total effectiveness ranging from 85 to 97 percent. The cure rate for impotence is 62 percent, and the total effectiveness is 94 percent (Lam, 1996). One controlled study involving 88 participants (randomly assigned into two groups) revealed a statistically significant total effectiveness ($p < .05$). Acupuncture can also cure allergic rhinitis (75 percent) (Kim, 1996), endolymphatic edema (79 percent), leukopenia (62 percent) (Gong & Wong, 1996), and glaucoma (75 percent) (Pippa et al., 1996). One controlled study (N=44, randomly assigned into two groups) indicated a significant total effectiveness ($p < .01$) in preventing myopia (Eory & Senyi, 1996).

Published Documents The published data of acupuncture efficacy are presented in Table 13.3, which are arranged by treatment categories.

Psychological disorders. Acupuncture has not been commonly used to treat psychological disorders, of which anxiety and/or depression are reviewed here. The results generated by three studies are not consistent. In the first study (Ulett, Han, & Han, 1998), electrical acupuncture (EA) appeared to be more effective than manual in producing analgesic effects. Both low- and high-frequency EA induces the release of enkephalins and dynorphines. The second study on depression compared the efficacy

TABLE 13.3
Acupuncture Efficacy: Published Data

Treatment Categories	# of Participants	Comments	Primary Author
Psychological disorders			
Review: Ac. for anxiety, depression, and pain	38	Ac. produces analgesic effect. Electrical Ac. (EA) is more effective than manual Low- and high-frequency Ac. induces the release of enkephalines and dynorphines.	Ulett, G.A. 1998.
Depression		64% in full remission. Ac. group significantly more improved than other two control groups.	Allen, J.J. 1998.
Depression		No difference between placebo and adjuvant whole body acupuncture therapy.	Roschke, J. 1998.
Stress management	19	Ac. significantly attenuates the increase in blood pressure during mental stress.	Middlekauff, H. 2001.
Addiction			
Nicotine	78	12.5% of Ac. group completely stopped smoking after six months. 0% in the control group.	Waite, N. 1998.
Cocaine	236	No difference between three levels of Ac, sham Ac, or placebo.	Nielson, O. 1999.
Dermatology			
Progressive systemic sclerosis (PSS)	11	EA decreases plasma ET-1, which is thought to induce vasodilation and elevates the surface temperature in patients with PSS.	Maeda, M. 1998.
Urologic disorders			
Sperm count	32 men	Ac. increased the fertility index ($p < 0.05$). The total functional sperm fraction, the percentage of viability, total motile spermatozoa per ejaculation, and the integrity of the axonema improved ($p < 0.05$).	Siterman, S. 1997.
Prostatic cacinoma	7 men	70 percent showed a substantial decrease in the number of hot flashes.	Hammer, M. 1999.
Cystitis in women	67 women with UTI	85 percent of Ac. group free of cystitis during the six months of treatment. 58 percent of the sham group free of cystitis ($p < 0.05$). 36 percent of the control group free of cystitis ($p < 0.01$).	Johnstone, P. 2003.
Pain management			
Analgesia in tempero-mandibular dysfunction	15 studies	In 4 studies, Ac. had no effect; in 11 it was effective, suggesting Ac. to be a valuable alternative treatment.	Rosted, P. 1998.
Dental analgesia	6 studies	In most Ac. groups, it was effective.	Ernst, E. 1998.
Sympathetic nerve activity	14	Ac. increases heart rate, arterial pressure, and muscle sympathetic nerve activity, and produces hypoalgesia.	Knardahl, S. 1998.
Post-traumatic pain	38	Ac. and sham Ac. improved the patients' condition.	Fialka, V. 1998.

TABLE 13.3 *(continued)*
Acupuncture Efficacy: Published Data

Treatment Categories	# of Participants	Comments	Primary Author
Gouty polyarthritis	44	Ac. enhances the efficacy of the prescribed treatment.	Zhererbrin, V. 1998.
Cancer pain	12	Ac. is not effective.	Sellik, S. M. 1998.
Postoperative patient controlled analgesia (PCA)		Ac. (high-intensity transcutaneous acupoint electrical stimulation [TAESl] decreases PCA significantly and thus decreases opioid-related side effects.	Wang, B. 1997.
Analgesia in rats		Monoamine contents (5-HT and 5-HIAA) in rat brains, after droperidol-enhanced acupuncture is increased.	Sheng, L. 1997.
Peripheral diabetes neuropathy	44	77 percent significantly improved in primary and/or secondary symptoms (p < 0.01).	Abuaisha, B. 1998.
Chronic pain (back pain, arthritis, and fibromyalgia)	74 63 65	Only preliminary data was presented.	Berman, B. 1997.
Chronic pain (skin temperature)	12	The skin temperature at the beginning of the EA sessions was significantly lower than three months after the EA sessions were completed.	Dyrehag, L. 1997.
Migraine	32 children	Ac. significantly reduced the frequency and intensity of the pain, and the beta-endorphin levels. It also gradually increased the panopioid activity in plasma that correlated with the clinical improvement. After 10 sessions the treated group resembled the healthy group.	Pintov, S. 1997.
Paralysis			
Stroke	45	Significant improvement in the Ac. group during six weeks of treatment period, even more during follow-up.	Kjendahl, A. 1998.
Stroke	41	Significant improvement in the Ac. group during six weeks of treatment period, even more during one-year follow-up. Ac. has a positive effect.	Kjendahl, A. 1997.
Nervous system **Dizziness during migraine:**			
Episodic vertigo	74	92% effective	Johnson, G. D. 1998.
Positional vertigo	63	89% effective	
Non-vertiginous dizziness	65	86% effective	
Aural fullness	40	85% effective	
Ear pain	16	63% effctive	
Phonophobia	19	89% effective	
Tinnitus	54	No significant difference between Ac. and placebo.	Vilhom, O. J. 1998.

Treatment Categories	# of Participants	Comments	Primary Author
Multiple sclerosis	624	No significant relationship between the frequency of using Ac. and the reported efficacy ($r = 0.17$, $p > 0.10$)	Nayak, S. 2000.
Gynecology, obstetrics, pediatrics			
Maternal serum levels	180	Prenatal Ac. significantly reduces the duration of the first and second stages of labor. Since serum levels of interleukin-8 and prostaglandin F2, alpha, and beta endorphins are not significantly influenced by Ac., they are not likely to mediate the acupuncture effects.	Tempfer, C. 1998.
Pain relief during child birth	120	58 percent of the women in the Ac. group and 14 percent of the women in the control group managed their delivery without further pain treatment, $p = 0.01$.	Ternov, K. 1998.
Labor duration		Women in the Ac. group endured 196 min. of labor; women in the control group endured 321 min. of labor, $p = 0.0001$. Women in the control group received significantly more oxytocin in their first stage of labor compared with the Ac. group (85 percent and and 15 percent respectively, $p = 0.001$) as well as during the second stage of labor (72 percent and 28 percent, $p = 0.03$). Thus, Ac. is recommended during labor.	Britt-Ingjerd, N. 2003.
Internal organ disorders			
Hypertension	50	30 min. of Ac. decreased plasma renin, heart rate, systolic, and diastolic pressure. Systolic pressure went from $169+/-2$ to $151+/-2$ mm; diastolic from $107+/-1$ to $96+/-1$ mm; heart rate from $77+/-2$ to $72+/-2$ bpm, $p = 0.01$; and plasma renin from $1.7+/-0.4$ to $1.1+/-0.2$ ng/ml, $p = 0.01$. The author concludes that Ac. lowers blood pressure due to the decrease in renin secretion.	Chui, Y. 1997.
Hypertension		Ac. and dieting are recommended in the treatment of hypertension.	Darwin, L. 2002.
Others			
Asthma	23	Review of present literature: Ac. is beneficial in the treatment of asthma.	Davies, P. 1998.
Asthma	32	Some improvement—reduced need for bronchodilators.	Biernacki, W. 1998.
Nonallergic rhinitis	24	No significant difference between Ac., sham, and control group.	Davis, A. 1998.
Allergen-provoked rhinitis	21	Ac. group showed some improvement, but not statistically significant.	Wolkenstein, E. 1998.
Functional muscular distortion	8	Ac. beneficial for decreasing muscular distortions.	Tanaka, T. 1998.
Sjogren's syndrome		No significant difference.	List, T. 1998.
Release of neuropeptides in saliva		Improvement of salivary flow rates in xerostomic patients, and CGRP, NYP, and VIP (immunoreactivity) increase due to Ac.	Dawidson, I. 1998.
Dystonia syndrome	30	Ac. enhances the efficacy of the medicamentosus treatment.	Murashko, N. 2001.
Disability after stroke	1,213 from 14 trials	Ac. has no additional effect on motor recovery but has a small positive effect on disability	Sze, F. K. 2002.

of acupuncture with that of medication and/or no treatment. The acupuncture group improved significantly more than the other two groups in which 64 percent of the patients were in full remission (Allen, Schnyer, & Hitt, 1998). The third study on depression, however, revealed no difference between placebo and adjuvant whole-body acupuncture therapy (Roschke, Wolf, Kogel, Wagner, & Bech, 1998). An empirical study of 19 healthy volunteers, who underwent mental stress testing pre- and postacupuncture, shows that acupuncture significantly attenuates the increase in blood pressure during mental stress (pre- vs. postacupuncture 4.5 versus 1.7 mmHg, $p < 0.001$) but does not modulate baseline muscle sympathetic nerve activity (Middlekauff, Yu, & Hui, 2001).

Pain management. Two meta-analyses are reviewed here. The first one investigated acupuncture as an analgesia in treating tempero-mandibular dysfunction and includes 15 studies (Rosted, 1998). Of these 15 studies, acupuncture was effective in 11 studies and had no effect in the other four studies, suggesting acupuncture to be a valuable alternative treatment for this special purpose. The second meta-analysis includes six studies, in most of which acupuncture was effective as a dental analgesia (Ernst & Pittler, 1998).

As to individual studies, one study on sympathetic nerve activity indicated that acupuncture can produce hypoalgesia, in addition to increasing heart rate and arterial pressure (Knardahl, Elam, Olausson, & Wallin, 1998). Another study included sham acupuncture (puncturing needles into other spots of the body instead of the indicated acupoints) as a control, and revealed that both acupuncture and sham acupuncture can relieve post-traumatic pain (Fialka et al., 1998). In a similar vein, a study on postoperative patient-controlled analgesia (PCA) showed that transcutaneous acupoint electrical stimulation acupuncture decreases PCA significantly and thus decreases opioid-related effects (Wang et al., 1997). Electrical acupuncture was also used to reduce chronic pain (Dyrehag, Widerstrom-Noga, Carlsson, & Andersson, 1997). In this study, skin temperature was employed as an objective index of pain reduction and was significantly lower three months after the EA sessions was completed. This demonstrates that the acupuncture's analgesic effect was not a placebo.

In the case of peripheral diabetes neuropathy, 77 percent of the patients treated by acupuncture significantly ($p < .01$) improved with respect to primary and/or secondary symptoms (Abuaisha, Costanzi, & Boulton, 1998). For patients who suffered from gouty polyarthritis, acupuncture can be used as an adjunct therapy to enhance the efficacy of the prescribed treatment for pain relief (Zherebrin, 1998). However, acupuncture is not effective in reducing cancer pain (Sellik & Zaza, 1998). To relieve the pain involved in the rheumatic conditions, a review study has found positive evidence in relation to acupuncture (Ernst, 2002).

For pediatric pain, 67 percent of 30 patients (including 7 migraine headache cases, 6 endometriosis cases, and 5 sympathetic dystrophy cases) reported a positive or pleasant experience, whereas 13 percent had a negative or unpleasant experience and 6 percent reported a neutral or strange experience. Of the same sample, 70 percent deemed the acupuncture treatment helpful and consequently their symptoms improved, whereas 27 percent considered themselves not harmed by or benefited from the treatment, and only 3 percent thought his/her condition got worse due to the side effect (Perrin et al., 2000).

Some biochemical mechanisms underlying acupuncture's analgesic effect have been identified in experimental studies. For example, in a study on 32 children's migraines, acupuncture significantly reduced the frequency and intensity of the pain, and after 10 sessions the treated group resembled the healthy one. At the same time, the beta-endorphin levels were reduced too, while acupuncture gradually increased the panopioid activity in plasma, which correlated with the clinical improvement (Pintov, Lahat, Alstein, Vogel, & Barg, 1997). Another experimental study was conducted on rats in which droperidol was enhanced, whereas acupuncture increased the monoamine contents (5-HT and 5-HIAA) in the rats' brains (Wei, 2003).

Paralysis, musculoskeletal system, and nervous system disorders. Paralysis caused by stroke can be effectively treated by acupuncture. In prospective controlled studies, acupuncture significantly improved the symptoms during six weeks of treatment, and even more during the one-year follow-up (Kjendahl, Sallstrom, Osten, Stanghelle, & Borchgrevink, 1997). Acupuncture appeared to be effective in treating dizziness during migraines (Johnson, 1998). The symptoms and effective rate of acupuncture treatment can be summarized as follows: non-vertiginous dizziness (86 percent), episodic vertigo (92 percent), positional vertigo (89 percent), aural fullness (85 percent), phonophobia (89 percent), and ear pain (63 percent). On the other hand, the outcome was either unclear in treating severe tinnitus (Vilhom, Moller, & Jorgensen, 1998), or there was an insignificant difference between acupuncture and placebo (Nielsen, Moller, & Jorgensen, 1999). In a recent survey conducted on a southern Arizona convenience sample of 430 enrolled children, 66 cases of cerebral palsy, 37 cases of spina bifida, 24 cases of other musculoskeletal problems, and 27 cases of other nervous system problems reported that they infrequently used acupuncture to treat their problems (Sanders et al., 2003).

Gynecology and obstetrics. Acupuncture can be used to facilitate the delivery process in a variety of ways. For example, prenatal acupuncture can significantly reduce the duration of the first and second stage of labor, and this facilitative effect was not mediated by the biochemical mechanisms (Tempfer et al., 1998). As Tempfer et al. pointed out, the serum levels of interleukin-8 and prostaglandin F2, alpha-endorphin, and beta-endorphin are not significantly influenced by acupuncture. Another study on labor duration included 120 women, in which women in the acupuncture group endured 196 minutes of labor, whereas women in the control group endured 321 minutes of labor ($p < .0001$, Zeisler, Tempfer, Mayerhofer, Barrada, & Husslein, 1998). Furthermore, women in the control group received significantly more oxytocin, which is used for the induction and stimulation of labor, compared with the acupuncture group (85 percent and 15 percent respectively, $p < .001$), and they also received more during their second stage of labor (72 percent and 28 percent, $p < .03$). In addition, acupuncture can also relieve pain during child birth, as demonstrated in a study on 180 women. In that study, 58 percent of the women in the acupuncture group and 14 percent of the women in the control group managed their delivery without further pain treatment (Ternov, Nilsson, Lofberg, Algotsson, & Akesson, 1998).

Other disorders. In treating hypertension, acupuncture reduced the renin secretion first, and in turn lowered systolic and diastolic pressure, as well as heart rate. In other words, the acupuncture effect in this case can be attributed to the biochemical mechanism (Chiu, Chi, & Reid, 1997). Acupuncture was also recommended in conjunction with diet changes in treating hypertension (Guo & Ni, 2003; Sutherland, 2001; Townsend, 2002). Given the lack of effective conventional treatments, auricular (ear) acupuncture has been widely used for cocaine addiction. In spite of its popularity,

clinical trials so far have been inclusive due to the difficulty of selecting an appropriate control group. In one of the few rigorous trials, 82 patients who received auricular acupuncture were compared with a group of patients who received "sham"
acupuncture and another group who received relaxation. At the end of the eight-week
treatment, 53.8 percent of the auricular acupuncture group tested free of cocaine compared with 23.5 percent of the sham acupuncture group, and 9.1 percent of the relaxation control (Morris & Margolin, 2000).

Qigong

Inceptive Research (cf. Lee & Lei, 1995a, 1995b, 1995c, 1996, 1997, 1999; Lei, 1997;
Lei & Lee, 1997a, 1997b) The efficacy of qigong at the inceptive stage is presented in
Table 13.4, which is organized in accordance with disease categories. Different types
of study are included in documenting qigong's efficacy. They are expert opinion,
experimental studies, and clinical studies. The efficacy is not quantitatively presented;
instead, it is categorized into "useful as a primary therapy," "useful as adjunct therapy," "not useful as adjunct therapy," and "contraindicated." Adjunct therapy means
it can be used in addition to another therapy, which is primary. "Contraindicated"
means the therapy may produce adverse effects.

TABLE 13.4
Qigong Efficacy: Gray Material

Treatment categories	Types of study	Source	Comments
Abdominal distension	expert's opinion	Xu, '94	contraindicated
Anxiety	clinical data	Xu, '94	experiment is needed to tease out the causation
Asthma	clinical data	Zhang, '88	
	experiment	Lim, '93	useful as adjunct therapy
	clinical	Yang, '90	useful as adjunct therapy
Bursitis	clinical	Wang, '91	useful as adjunct therapy
Cancer	experiment	Fu, '93; Xie, '88	*
	clinical	Zhao, '82	*
	clinical	Chen, '89; Lo, '90; Sum, '88; Yu, '93	useful as adjunct therapy
		Wang, '93; Hong & Lu, '93	with herb
Congestive heart failure	clinical	Zhang, '88	*
Constipation	experimental	Hu, '92	*
Diabetes	clinical	Du & Chan, '88	useful as adjunct therapy
Mellitis		Jing et al., '93	useful as adjunct therapy
Diarrhea	clinical	Zhang, '88	useful as adjunct therapy
		Mou et al., '91	contraindicated
Emphysema	experiment	Zhang, '88	*
Formication	expert's opinion	Xu, '94	contraindicated
Gastroenteritis	clinical	McGee et al., '88	useful as adjunct therapy
Headache	expert opinion	Cohen, '92	useful as adjunct therapy

Treatment categories	Types of study	Source	Comments
Heart disease	clinical	Wang, '88; Wang, 91	useful as adjunct therapy
	experiment	Jin, '92	not useful as a therapy
	expert opinion	Galante, '81	contraindicated
Hepatitis	clinical	Hong et al., '88	*
Hypertension	experiment	Li, '93; Li et al., '88	useful as adjunct therapy
	clinical	Bian, '90; Bornorni, '93	
		Jing, '88; Kuang et al. '91;	
		Mou, '91; Wu & Liu, '93	
		Xu & Wang, '94	
	clinical	Wang, '95	not useful as therapy
Immuno-deficiencies	expert's opinion	Huang, '88	useful as adjunct therapy
		Hong et al., '88	useful as adjunct therapy
Immune function enhancement	experimental	Chen, 2003	prophylactic
Micro-circulation	experimental	Mou et al., '92, '93, '94;	*
		Zhang, '88;	*
	expert's opinion	Xiu, '88	useful as adjunct therapy
Myopia	clinical data	Wang et al., 92	*
Nephritis	clinical data	Tsai, 1995	useful as adjunct therapy
Migraine	**clinical**	**Lee, 92; Liang, '92**	*
Otitis media	clinical	Zhang, '88	*
musculoskeletal rehabilitation	clinical	Ives, 2000	useful as physical therapy
Pain	clinical	Eisenberg, '85	useful as adjunct therapy
Peptic ulcer	clinical	Chau, '90	*
	clinical	Zhang, '88	useful as adjunct therapy
Pharyngitis	**clinical data**	**Chan, Sung, & Chan, '94**	**useful as adjunct therapy**
Pneumonia	clinical	Zhang, '88	useful as adjunct therapy
Chronic obstructive pulmonary disease	clinical	Gigliotti, Romagnoli, & Scano, 2003	inconsistent results
Rheumatoid arthritis	clinical	Gou, '94	*
Sinusitis, acute/chronic	clinical	Chang, '86	*
Stroke	experiment	Mou et al., 95	*
	clinical	Huang, '88	
		Liu, He, & Xie, '93	useful as adjunct therapy
Tuberculosis	clinical	Zhang, '99	
Upper respiratory infection	clinical	Zhang, '88	useful as adjunct therapy

*Means it is useful as a primary therapy

Pain, migraine, headache. As Table 13.4 shows, much less pain research has been done in the field of qigong than in the field of acupuncture. Clinical studies have demonstrated that qigong can be used as an adjunct therapy to treat general pain (Eisenberg, 1985) and as a primary therapy to treat migraines (Lee, 1992; Liang, 1992). In some experts' opinion, qigong is useful as an adjunct therapy in treating headaches (Cohen, 1992).

Cancer, emphysema, and immno-deficiency.   Qigong is useful as a primary therapy for cancer, as demonstrated in experimental studies (Fu, 1993; Xie, 1988) and in a clinical trial (Zhao, 1982). In treating cancer, qigong can also be useful as an adjunct therapy without (Chen, 1989) or with herbal treatment in clinical trials (Huang, personal communication, September 20, 1996). In treating emphysema, an experimental study showed that qigong can be used as a primary therapy (Zhang, 1988). In some experts' opinion, qigong is useful as adjunct therapy for patients with immunodeficiencies (Hwang, 1988).

Hypertension, microcirculation, and stroke.   Qigong is useful as adjunct therapy for hypertension as revealed in experimental studies (Li, 1993; Li, 1988) and clinical trials (Bornorni, 1993; Jing, Li, & Wang, 1988; Kuang, Wang, Xu, Quian, & Kwang, 1991; Mou, Yen, Li, & Chao, 1991; Xu & Wang, 1994). However, one clinical trial (Wang, Hsu, Chang, & Chang, 1995) showed that qigong is not useful as therapy in treating hypertension. Qigong is useful as a primary therapy for microcirculation problems as well, as documented in experimental studies (Mou, Shi, Hsu, & Chao, 1994; Mou, Wang, & Chao, 1992; Zhang, 1988), although it is useful as an adjunct therapy in one expert's opinion (Xiu, 1988). In treating stroke, qigong can be used as a primary therapy as indicated by experimental data (Mou, Yen, Li, & Chao, 1991) and a clinical trial (Hwang, 1988). In addition, one clinical trial (Wong & Nahin, 2003) showed that qigong can be useful as an adjunct therapy.

Cardiac disorders.   Qigong has not demonstrated consistent effects in this disorder category. For instance, a clinical study reported that qigong can be employed as a primary therapy in treating congestive heart failure (Zhang, 1988), and other clinical studies maintained that qigong is useful as adjunct therapy in treating heart disease (Wang, Xu, Quian, & Kuang, 1988; Wang et al., 1995). However, an experimental study revealed that qigong is not useful in treating heart diseases (Jin, 1992), and some experts even assert that qigong is contraindicated in treating heart disease (Galante, 1981). From Galante's point of view, qigong can be applied to strengthen the cardiopulmonary system before the disease starts, but not afterwards.

Respiratory disorders.   Both clinical data (Zhang, 1988) and experimental results (Lim, Boone, Flarrity, & Thompson, 1993) indicated that qigong is useful as adjunct therapy in treating asthma. Clinical data also show that qigong can be useful as adjunct therapy for pneumonia (Zhang, 1988), tuberculosis (Zhang, 1988), and upper respiratory infection (Zhang, 1988), and as primary therapy for acute/chronic sinusitis (Chang, 1986). For chronic pulmonary disease (COPD), qigong and other types of breathing-retraining strategies have been applied to reduce dyspnea, but have not yet produced consistent results (Gigliotti, Romagnoli, & Scano, 2003).

Digestive system.   Qigong's efficacy seems to be controversial in this category. It is contraindicated for diarrhea as revealed in clinical data (Mou, Yen, Li, & Chao, 1991), and also contraindicated for abdominal distension according to an expert's opinion (Xu & Wang, 1994). On the other hand, some clinical data demonstrated that qigong can be useful as adjunct therapy for diarrhea (Zhang, 1988) and gastroenteritis (McGee & Chow, 1988). Qigong can even serve as a primary therapy for constipation, as discovered in an experimental study (Cohen, 1992), and for hepatitis, as indicated in a clinical study (Fang, Zu, & Zhu, 1992). Along the same line, clinical studies reported that qigong can be successfully used either as primary therapy (Chau, 1990) or as adjunct therapy in treating peptic ulcers, or pharyngitis (Chan, Sung, & Chan, 1994).

Circulatory, metabolic, and urinary diseases. Experimental studies have confirmed that qigong is useful as a primary therapy to improve microcirculation. In an expert's opinion, qigong can be useful as an adjunct therapy for the same purpose (Xiu, 1988). In treating metabolic disorders, clinical studies reported that qigong can be useful as adjunct therapy for diabetes mellitus (Du & Chan, 1988; Jing, Li, Wang, et al., 1993). Qigong is also useful as adjunct therapy for nephritis, as indicated in a pioneering clinical study (Tsai & Rothenberg, 1996).

Other disorders. Qigong's efficacy in the treatment of psychological disorders is not clear. Qigong seemed to be effective to reduce anxiety, but further experiments are required to tease out the causation (Xu & Wang, 1994). For formication, qigong is contraindicated (Xu, 1994). On the other hand, qigong is useful as primary therapy for eye or ear disorders. For instance, clinical data have shown qigong's efficacy in treating myopia (Wang et al., 1992) and otitis media (Zhang, 1988). For inflammation of joints or sacs, qigong appears to be useful. In the case of rheumatoid arthritis, for example, clinical data indicated that qigong can be used as a primary therapy. For bursitis, clinical data also confirm that qigong is useful as adjunct therapy.

Recent Research The key points of recent research are summarized in Table 13.5 by treatment categories.

Pain management. In terms of pain management, qigong appeared to be an effective adjunct therapy for fibromyalgia (Singh, 1988, cited in Xie, 1988). In a well-designed controlled study on complex regional pain syndrome, 82 percent of patients being trained in qigong reported less pain after their first session, and 91 percent after their last session. This effect is not merely a placebo effect, because only 45 percent of the controls reported less pain at the onset, and 36 percent after the last session. Moreover, significantly less transient pain and less long-term anxiety was reported by the treated group (Wu et al., 1999). In a comparative study on muscular pain, all three treatment groups (external qigong, needling to an acupoint, and needling to the pain muscle) showed pain reduction.

Internal organs. Qigong appeared to coordinate heart and brain functions. Empirical data indicate that EEG synchronicity was increased in the anterior and midline regions during the heart-focused attention. Reliable and different topographic patterns of the EEG emerged, as indicated by differences in the shape of peaks in spectra, which is mediated by increased vagal activity (Litscher, Wenzel, Niederwieser, & Schwartz, 2001). Qigong was also able to improve the perfusion of the coronary artery and the cardiac dysfunction produced by myocardial ischemia (Jin, 1992). Along the same line, qigong led to significantly lower blood pressure after two and half years of training. No stroke, congestive heart failure, or acute myocardial infarction occurred during that time (Xing, Li, & Pi, 1993). For chronic gastritis, the total effective rate of qigong was 97.1 percent, according to the conventional Chinese diagnostic criteria. At the same time, gastroscopy revealed that qigong therapy's total effective rate was 64.5 percent, and pathology also showed that the total effective rate was 87.1 percent. In addition, 92.2 percent of the qigong participants gained weight.

TABLE 13.5
Qigong Efficacy: Published Data

Treatment Categories	# of Participants	Comments	Primary Author
Pain management Complex regional pain syndrome	26	82% of patients being trained in qigong reported less pain after their first session, 91% after their last session. 45% of the controls reported less pain at the onset, and 36% after the last session. Also significantly less transient pain and less long-term anxiety was reported by the treated group.	Wu, W. 1999.
Muscular pain		All three groups (external qigong, needling to the pain muscle, and needling to an acupuncture point) reduced pain.	Takeshige, C. 1995.
Fibromyalgia **Disorders of the internal organs** **Chronic gastritis**	28 103	Qigong appears to be (no control group) an effective adjunctive therapy. Qigong was markedly effective in 69.9%; effective in 27.2%. The total effective rate was 97.1%. 92.2% gained weight (110 +/- 70g per day). Gastroscopy revealed that the therapy had a marked effectiveness in 35.5 percent of the participants, and was effective in 29 percent. The total effective rate was 64.5 percent. Pathology showed that there was a marked effectiveness of 48.4 percent, and it was effective in 38.7 percent. The total effective rate was 87.1 percent.	Singh, B. 1998. Feng, Y. 1989.
Heart brain organization	22	EEG was recorded from 19 sites (P, Q, R, S, and T waves) during baseline-focused attention, and during enhanced awareness. Results indicate that the EEG synchronicity is increased in the anterior and midline regions during the heart-focused attention, and during the enhanced awareness condition. Reliable and different topographic patterns of the EEG were observed as a function of the ECG cycle.	Song, L. 1998.
Heart rate	26	Different qigong breathing exercises correlate with differences in the shape of peaks in spectra. Certain breathing exercises can increase the amplitude of peaks in the high-frequency area, and the ratio of low frequency 2/high frequency (LF2/HF) is reduced. This is an indication of increased vagal activity.	Sun, F. 1992.
Heart rate	17	Heart rate was evaluated with an electrocardiographic autopower function (EASF) before and after a qigong exercise. The positive rate of EASF of lead V5 ($Gxx_{1/2}$) decreased from 59% (10/17) to 0% (0/17), and the lead 2($Gvy_{1/2}$) from 82% (14/17) to 41% (7/17) $p < 0.01$ and 0.05. Qigong can improve the perfusion of the coronary artery and the cardiac dysfunction produced by myocardial ischemia.	Jin, K. 1992.

Treatment Categories	# of Participants	Comments	Primary Author
Blood pressure	56	Significantly lower blood pressure after 2.5 years of qigong training. No stroke, congestive heart failure, or acute myocardial infarction occurred during that time.	Xing, Z. 1993.
Brain function **Evoked potentials**		Qigong generated significant changes in cerebral evoked potential (EP) components of the cortex. It seems that qigong has inhibiting and facilitating effects. There were no significant changes in the subcortex, or in EEG power percent. Acupuncture had the same effect as qigong.	Xu, M. 1998.
EEG		After six months of training there was no change; however, after one year the alpha index of the right frontal lobe and of the right temporal lobe decreased significantly ($p < 0.05$). The EEG gradually synchronized.	Xu, S. 1994.
Stimulus-induced 40 Hz oscillations	2	22.2 percent increase in mean blood flow velocity (vm) in the posterior cerebral artery, and a simultaneous 23.1 percent decrease in vm in the posterior cerebral artery.	Litscher, 2001.
Psycho-physiological systems		EEG, EMG, respiratory movement, heart rate, skin potential, skin temperature, finger tip volume, sympathetic nerve function, stomach, intestine, metabolism, endocrine system, immune system, motor movements, and perception were affected by qigong exercises.	Xu, S. 1994.
Electrical conductivity		Robert Becker found that meridian lines transmit current more efficiently than nonmeridian lines.	Roach, M. 1997.
Blood level of monoamine neuro-transmitters	30	Qigong exercises reduced 5-HT from 0.43+/-0.21 to 0.21+/-0.13 microgram/ml ($p < 0.01$). NE and DA showed a tendency to increase.	Liu, B. 1990.
Stress hormones		Qigong significantly increased beta-endorphin, and significantly decreased ACTH.	Ryu, H. 1996.
Psychoses		Inappropriately practiced qigong induces psychoses.	Ng, B. 1999.
Immune system Tumor growth control	Tumor-bearing mice (TBM)	Emitted external Qi (QEQ) has inhibitory effects on tumor growth of TBM. It has enhancing effects on antitumor immunologic functions of the tumor host. QEQ and cyclophosphamide (a chemotherapeutic agent) improves the antitumor immunologic function of the tumor host and significantly increases the antitumor efficacy.	Lei, X. 1991.
Neuromuscular disorder Myotonic dystrophy	7	Qigong and other types of breathing exercise elicit an improvement in respiratory function (2.2 to 2.6 percent increase of arterial oxygen saturation).	Nitz & Burke. 2002.

Treatment Categories	# of Participants	Comments	Primary Author
Respiratory Disorder			
Chronic obstructive pulmonary disease	9	Practice three times a week for eight weeks resulted in significant improvements in respiratory muscle strength and endurance.	Sturdy et al. 2003.
Asthma	30	17 exercisers improved; none of the 13 nonexercisers improved.	Reuther, I. 1998.
Asthma	22 men, 22 women	Baseline maximal inspiratory mouth pressure was significantly lower ($p < 0.01$) while perception of dyspnea and mean daily beta (2)-agonist consumption were significantly higher in the female subjects.	Weiner, P. 2002.
Ventilation weaning	10	9 out of 10 medically complex patients were weaned from mechanical ventilation after 44 days of training.	Martin, A. 2002.
Other disorders			
Biochemical cell function of a human fibroblast FS-4 and of boar sperm	86	In the fibroblast facilitating qi increases 1.8% of the cell growth in 24 hrs., 10-15% of DNA synthesis in 2 hrs., and 3-5% of the protein synthesis of the cell in 2 hrs. Inhibiting qi decreases 6% of the cell growth in 24 hrs., 20-23% of the DNA synthesis in 2 hrs., and 35-48% of the protein synthesis in 2 hrs. In boar sperm facilitating qi increases 12.5-13% the respiration rate in 5 min., inhibiting qi decreases it 45-48% after 2 min.	Chien, C. 1991.
Heroin addiction	Ex = 34 Rx = 26 Ctr = 26	Reduction of withdrawal symptoms in the qigong group occurred more rapidly than in the other groups.	Li, M. 2002.
Diabetes		Qigong walking reduced plasma glucose (from 223 to 216 mg/dL) after lunch without inducing a large increase in the pulse rate.	Iwao, M. 2001.

Psychophysiological responses. Several experimental studies revealed that qigong can affect brain functioning. For instance, qigong generated significant changes in cerebral evoked potential (EP) components of the cortex, on which qigong has both inhibitory and facilitative effects. However, the subcortex function was not affected by qigong (Xu, Tomotake, Ikuta, Ishimoto, & Okura, 1998). Another brain study using electroencephalogram (EEG) data as indicators showed no change after six months of qigong training. Yet after one year the alpha index of the right frontal lobe and of the right temporal lobe decreased significantly ($p < .05$), and the EEG gradually synchronized (Xu, 1994). In addition to the EEG, electromyogram (EMG), skin potential, skin temperature, fingertip volume, heart rate, respiratory movement, motor movement, stomach, intestine, endocrine system, sympathetic nerve function, the immune system, and perception were also affected by qigong exercise.

Moreover, an experimental study on neurotransmitters demonstrated that qigong exercise reduced 5-HT (hydroxytryptamine or serotonin), while norepineprine and dopamine showed a tendency to increase (Liu, Jiao, & Li, 1990). Another experimental study on stress hormones reported that qigong exercise significantly increased beta-endorphin, and significantly decreased andrenocorticotropic hormone or ACTH (Ryu et al., 1996). Given the various effects of qigong on neurotransmitters, it is reasonable to hypothesize that inappropriate practice of qigong could induce psychosis-like symptoms (Ng, 1999). It should be noted that qigong comes with many forms, which match with the needs and types of the patients. If a patient already has too much dopamine which leads to schizophrenia–like symptons, placticing dopamine–enhancing qigong could aggavate his condition.

Respiratory disorders. Qigong has been commonly applied as a form of respiratory muscle training to treat chronic obstructive pulmonary disease. In a randomized, sham-controlled study that involved 14 male patients, the training group showed significant improvement. This improvement was associated with increases in the proportion of type I fibers (38 percent, $p < 0.05$) and in the size of type II muscles (21 percent, $p < 0.05$) in the external intercostal muscles (Ramirez-Sarmiento et al., 2002). A meta-analysis has been performed on the studies of the effects of qigong and other inspiratory muscle training (IMT) methods on chronic obstructive pulmonary disease. Significant training effects were found for dyspnoea at rest and during exercise, and on inspiratory muscle strength and endurance, thereby indicating that qigong along with other IMTs can be an important addition to a pulmonary rehabilitation program (Lotters, van Tol, Kwakkel, & Gosselink, 2002).

Immune/reproductive systems and others. An experimental study conducted on tumor-bearing mice revealed that the extrinsic qi from the qigong master had inhibitory effects on tumor growth by enhancing the tumor host's antitumor immunologic function (Lei, Bi, Zhang, & Cheng, 1991). On the other hand, the intrinsic qi produced from qigong exercise can enhance women's reproductive functions by increasing women's sex hormones, as indicated in their serum/saliva and the ratio of E2/P, and by improving their ovarian function (Kuang, Chen, & Lu, 1989). For male reproductivity, an experimental study conducted on boars' sperm found that the "facilitative qi" emitted from qigong masters increased the respiration rate by 12.5 percent to 13 percent in 5 minutes, while the "inhibitory qi" emitted from qigong masters decreased it 45 to 48 percent after 2 minutes (Chien, Tsuei, Lee, Huang, & Wei, 1991). The extrinsic "facilitative qi" and "inhibitory qi" can manipulate other physiological functions as well, such as DNA and protein syntheses (Chien, et al., 1991).

Intrinsic qigong can reduce the glucose levels in diabetics, the frequency and severity of angina pectoris, coronary heart disease, and blood pressure. A randomized controlled clinical trial that includes three groups, namely, treatment group ($n = 34$), medication group ($n = 26$), and no-treatment control group ($n = 26$), indicates a rapid reduction of withdrawal symptoms in the qigong group in comparison with other groups. Specifically, 50 percent of the qigong group had negative urine tests on day 3, and 100 percent on day 5, compared to day 9 for the medication group and day 11 for the control group (Li, Chen, & Mo, 2002).

Methodological assessment In spite of the overall positive findings presented, the interpretation of these outcomes should be cautious. The methodological quality of the research needs to be taken into account, which could affect the results—most likely a bias toward the false positive direction. In Table 13.6, we select representative studies from different treatment categories in order to evaluate their methodological quality. Hopefully, the data presented here will reflect the field to a considerable extent. In addition, the U.S. Department of Health and Human Services recently also published the evaluation criteria offered by the leading researchers in the field of complementary and alternative medicine (CAM). In short, each CAM therapy is graded by "level of evidence," a system used by the U.S. Preventive Services Task Force in assessing evidence for diagnostic and preventive interventions (Reynolds, 2003).

As can be seen in Table 13.6, 10 studies were evaluated against the 15 predetermined methodological criteria. Out of the total 100 points, assessed studies scored from 18 to 86 points, with an average of 43 points. The second category reviewed is related to hypertension. The four studies evaluated here are not so heterogeneous in terms of methodological quality as those in the pain management. Hypertension studies scored from 40 to 55 points, with a mean of 47 points. The third category is about cardiovascular/pulmonary functions, in which five studies were assessed. They scored from 28 to 53 points, with an average of 41 points. Within the homogeneous category in terms of stroke, the methodological quality of the four studies assessed was not so homogeneous. The scores ranged from 28 to 78, with a mean of 44 points. The fifth category included gastric-intestinal and urinary disorders, in which four studies were evaluated, and they showed poor methodological quality. The mean of their methodological score is merely 38, which would have been even lower if the outstanding study of Tsai, Lai, Lee et al. (1995) had not been included in this category. The sixth category refers to the eye/ear/nose/respiratory category. The methodological quality of the five studies assessed in this category seemed to be on a similar level. The scores ranged from 43 to 68, with a mean of 51 points. The last category included everything else, such as electroencephalogram (EEG), electromyogram (EMG), sympathetic nervous system's operations, and so on. Given the diversity of this category, the methodological quality of studies included in it also varied tremendously. The seven studies assessed scored from 24 to 92 points, with an average of 55 points.

From the mainstream medical point of view, the methodological quality across various treatment categories of the indigenous Chinese healing research scored below 60, and therefore cast the clinical outcomes into doubt. This was one of the reasons why we abandoned the statistical pooling of data using meta-analysis. In other words, the methodological quality of the studies reviewed does not warrant further quantitative analysis. The other reason for omitting a quantitative analysis was the level of heterogeneity of the studies reviewed in this chapter—especially because there was no common measure across different studies for meta-analytic techniques to be applied.

TABLE 13.6
Methodological Assessment of Sample Studies

Studies

1. Pain management — Methodological criteria	Neck pain British 1999	Neck pain #54	Myofacial Birch, 1998	Regional pain Wu et al., 1999	Fibromyalgia Sign et al., 1998	Diabetic pain Abuaisha, 1998	Cocaine addiction Morris & Margolin, 2000
Homogeneity—3	2	3	3	2	3	3	3
Randomization—12	8	9	12	9	3	2	12
Comparability—2	2	2	2	1	2	2	2
>= 50 Ss per group—5	4	3	2	3		3	5
<+ 20% attrition—3	0	0	2	1		2	2
Active placebo—2	0	0	2	2		1	2
Expertise—9		1	9	9		4	8
Protocol—5			10	5	12	12	15
Existing treatment—3	3	1	2	1		3	3
Participant blind—10		10	10	10		3	3
Evaluator blind—5		0	1	3		2	2
Follow-up—10		0	10	8	15	6	5
Side effect—2		0	2			2	1
Outcome measure—10		9	10	10	10	10	10
Data analysis—9		0	9	5		6	9
Subtotal	19	38	86	69	44	61	86

Methodological criteria	Dental pain Ernst et al., 1998	Dental pain Rosted, 1998	Post-surgery pain Fialka et al., 1998	Back pain Ernst, 1998	2. Hypertension(HP)	Heart-brain Sung, 1992	HP/CHD Wang, 1988
Homogeneity—3		2	3	3			2
Randomization—12	8	10		3			8
Comparability—2		2				1	2
>= 50 Ss per group—5		2		4			5
<+ 20% attrition—3		2				6	

TABLE 13.6 (continued)
Methodological Assessment of Sample Studies

| | Dental pain | Dental pain | Post-surgery pain | Back pain | 2. Hypertension(HP) | |
					Heart-brain	HP/CHD
Active placebo—2	1	1	2	1	2	
Expertise—9		5	2	1	3	
Protocol—5		2		1		9
Existing treatment—3		2		1	9	
Participant blind—10	4	3	10	3	15	
Evaluator blind—5	2	4	5	1		
Follow-up—10		5				10
Side effect—2	1	1		3		
Outcome measure—10	2	7	6	1	10	10
Data analysis—9		6		7	9	9
Subtotal	18	54	28	39	55	55

| | HP/LDL | HP 3. Cardiac | Cardio-respiratory | CHD | Micro-circulation | Cardiovascular |
	Wang, 1995	Sun, 1995	Lim, 1993	Chiu, 1992	Wang, 1995	Hwang, 1995
Methodological criteria						
Homogeneity—3		2	1	2	2	2
Randomization—12	3	4		2	3	3
Comparability—2	2				3	
>= 50 Ss per group—5						
<+ 20% attrition—3			2	3		
Active placebo—2				2		
Expertise—9	9				9	9
Protocol—15	10	13	13	2	1	15
Existing treatment—3	2	2	2			
Participant blind—10	9					
Evaluator blind—5						
Follow-up—10	10	10			10	
Side effect—2						
Outcome measure—10	8	9	10	10	10	7
Subtotal		40				

						5. Gastric, Intestinal,urinary
Data analysis—9	9	9	9	8	3	
Subtotal	43	35	28	46	39	

	Vasomotor	4. Stroke	Stroke	Stroke	Paresis	Stroke	
	Hammar, 1999		Gosman, 1998	#34	Johansson, 1993	Kjendahl, 1997	
Methodological criteria							
Homogeneity—3	3						
Randomization—12	1		2		3	2	
Comparability—2	1		9		9	9	
>= 50 Ss per group—5	1		2		2	2	
<+ 20% attrition—3	2		5		2	2	
Active placebo—2	2		2	3		2	
Expertise—9	4					2	
Protocol—15	15					9	
Existing treatment—3	1						
Participant blind—10	1			7		3	
Evaluator blind—5	1					1	
Follow-up—10	10		8	10	10	10	
Side effect—2	1						
Outcome measure—10	3			10	7	10	
Data analysis—9	7			10	7	10	
Subtotal	53		28	30	40	62	

	Gastritis	Nausea, vomiting	Cystitis	Renal disorder	Myopia	Accomodation
	Cheng, 1967	Sadial, 1997	Aune, 1998	Tsai, 1996	Wang, 1992	Shih, 1995
					6. Eye/ear/nose respiratory	
Methodological criteria						
Homogeneity—3	2	2	2	2		
Randomization—12	5	4	9	7		2
Comparability—2			2	1		
>= 50 Ss per group—5	4	4	3	2	4	2
<+ 20% attrition—3					2	3
Active placebo—2			2			
Expertise—9				8		

239

TABLE 13.6 (continued)
Methodological Assessment of Sample Studies

	Gastritis	Nausea, vomiting	Cystitis	Renal disorder	6. Eye/ear/nose respiratory	Myopia	Accomodation
Protocol—15	12			13		9	15
Existing treatment—3				2			
Participant blind—10		10	10				10
Evaluator blind—5		5					
Follow-up—10				6		10	
Side effect—2				2			2
Outcome measure—10	7			10		9	10
Data analysis—9			8	7		9	9
Subtotal	30	25	36	60		43	53

Methodological criteria	Rhinitis Davies et al., 1998	Asthma Biernacki, 1998	7. Others Asthma Reuther, 1998	Migraine Pintov, 1997	EEG Xu, 1998
Homogeneity—3	2	2	1	3	1
Randomization—12	2	10		9	3
Comparability—2	1	2			
>=50 Ss per group—5	1	1	3	2	1
<+20% attrition—3	1	3	2		3
Active placebo—2	1	1			1
Expertise—9	5	7			5
Protocol—15	10	5	15		1
Existing treatment—3		1			1
Participant blind—10	1	10			1
Evaluator blind—5	1	5	9		1
Follow-up—10	1	2			1
Side effect—2	1	2			1
Outcome measure—10	10	10	9	10	10
Data analysis—9	4	7	9		8
Subtotal	41	68	48	24	34

Methodological criteria	EMG	Sympathetic NS Knardahl, 1998	Sclerosis Maeda, 1998	Cocaine Bulluck, 1997	Smoking cessation Waite, 1998
Homogeneity—3	2	2	1	2	3
Randomization—12	10	1	1	10	10
Comparability—2	1	1	1	2	2
>=50 Ss per group—5	1	1		5	5
<+20% attrition—3	3	3	3	1	3
Active placebo—2	2	2	2	1	1
Expertise—9	5	2	2	9	9
Protocol—15	5	15	3	12	15
Existing treatment—3	2	2	1	2	1
Participant blind—10	4	10	1	1	10
Evaluator blind—5	2	1	1	4	1
Follow-up—10	1	1	1		10
Side effect—2	1	1	2	1	1
Outcome measure—10	10	9	9	8	8
Data analysis—9	9	9	9	9	8
Subtotal	58	70	38	67	92

It should be noted that the problem of heterogeneity is not only unique to the present meta-analysis of complementary/alternative medical research, but appears in other meta-analyses of CAM research (e.g., Astin, Harkness, & Ernst, 2000; Ernst & Pittler, 1998) as well. Because of the aforementioned methodological limitations, a criteria-based meta-analysis or systematic review that was employed in the current study is more appropriate than an effect-size-oriented meta-analysis.

Methodological Relativity

Most ICH research does not apply the medical mainstream's "gold standard," that is, randomized controlled trials, and thus is downgraded in terms of methodological quality. Methodological considerations, such as sample size, statistical power, control for placebo and experimenter's expectation, intention to treat, and comparability of relevant baseline characteristics are not of primary concerns to ICH researchers, although they are indispensable criteria in conventional (Western) medical research. Whether ICH research should be universally evaluated by the same gold standard is not just a medical or methodological issue, but also an issue related to the philosophy of science.

Philosophically speaking, Western science is based on empiricism and dominated by logical positivism, which emphasizes "seeing is believing" and hypothesis-testing. On the other hand, from the traditional Chinese point of view, "feeling is believing," and to operationalize complex human phenomena into variables to be tested constitutes a kind of reductionistic fallacy. As an example of "feeling is believing," one major sign of acupuncture's effect is called "de qi," which translates into whether the healer and the patient feel the qi travel through the needle into the patient's meridian. Nobody can see qi, and yet its existence is indicated by electromagnetic measures, and its effect manifests itself through clinical outcomes. With regard to the reductionistic fallacy, ICH researchers would argue that the fact that Western critics do not accept ICH's efficacy is due to their own methodological limitation, rather than to the shortcomings of ICH itself. As an analogy, this relationship appears to be like a blind baby blaming God for creating a dark world without taking into account that the darkness is due to his or her own vision problem. A well-trained ICH practitioner can feel the patient's pulse, scan the patient's energy field against the backdrop of the environment's electromagnetic field, smell the patient's body odor, sense the patient's mood, and check the patient's tongue for clinical signs. All of these (inter-) subjective evaluations are by no means objective and would be considered esoteric, if not occult by Western scientists.

The way ICH practitioners evaluate their treatment effects is deeply rooted in their worldview, which includes the concept of a person, as well as the way in which the world operates. They attend more to the healing process than to the clinical outcomes, take a long-term perspective rather than focus on immediate consequences, treat the person as a whole rather than as a bag of specific disorders, take into consideration the social-emotional milieu outside as well as inside of the person rather than the symptoms alone, validate the patient's subjective feedback rather than rely on objective measurement per se, and emphasize prevention or promoting well-being in general rather than reacting to a specific disease.

INTEGRATING INDIGENOUS HEALING WITH MAINSTREAM MEDICINE

Even though evidence-based mainstream (conventional, Western, or allopathic) medicine is the royal road to relieving human suffering, it is not the only road to that destination. If the intriguing human organism can be viewed as the dark sky, perhaps the variety of healing modalities (including medical) should be seen as stars in the sky. Each of the stars sheds its specific light on the darkness, and at the same time the stars mutually highlight each other, and thus the illumination they contribute together is greater than the sum of each specific light alone. In that sense, it would be better to have more than less different healing modalities, which should synergistically coexist in an amicable rather than antagonistic way.

Whether each specific healing modality works for a person or not depends on what kind of a person you are, and how you use a therapy. If you happen to grow up in a certain culture, in which some healing modalities come to you naturally as an indigenous method to alleviate illness, you are more likely to enjoy its efficacy, because your belief in the modality itself could contribute to the placebo effect (in addition to the method's specific effect), regardless of whether it really manipulates your system in the way the healer expects it to. In China, acupuncture and qigong (in addition to herbal medicine) are not merely popular therapies, but also time-tested traditions in which therapeutic techniques are derived from 3,000 years of in vivo application of folk wisdom rather than based on the generalization from in vitro experimentation on animals only. In fact, these healing modalities are not merely modus operandi in treating a disease, but also ingrained in life as a modus vivendi (e.g., tai chi or qigong exercise, acupressure massage, or herbal diets, which have become part of the daily-life routines of many Chinese). Thus, faith in these therapies is deep-rooted, and through a mind-body connection it could result in the activation of the parasympathetic nervous system, enhancement of the immune function, and the reduction of physical symptoms.

To a certain extent, the psychosomatic effect just mentioned might explain why China has generated more outstanding therapeutic outcomes than any other country. For instance, the total effectiveness of acupuncture documented in China is about 99 percent, which is significantly greater than that attained in England (75 percent) and the United States (70 percent). However, belief or faith is not the only explanation for the differential effect, because Russia has also produced a 97 percent effectiveness rate. To give the benefit of the doubt, the "file-drawer effect" mentioned in the Methods section on pages 215 and 216 (viz., the selective reporting and publishing of only positive results) may play some role when presenting the too-good-to-be-true data. On the other hand, acupuncture and qigong therapists may be better trained in China and Russia, and thus are more likely to bring about better clinical efficacy. Or perhaps the cultural context in Russia is more congruent with the philosophical rationale underlying ICH and is thereby facilitating the psychosomatic healing effect.

Concerning the United States, which represents Western mainstream medicine, "cultural creatives" have brought in non-Western worldviews, led New Age and other movements, and have aroused awareness of complementary/alternative medicine (CAM), including ICH. Many Americans have welcomed CAM, as pointed out in the beginning part of this chapter and as can be seen in recent surveys. According to the *Nutrition Business Journal*, February 2001, American's expenses on herbal remedy have steadily increased from about $8 billion in 1995 to $16 billion in 2000; and, as reported in the cover story of *U.S. News & World Report*, February 12, 2001, about 123.5 million Americans try "natural" products to treat a variety of ills. Yet whether they are going to embrace CAM as part of the medical establishment or just as a fad will be determined by the perspective they take. If they expect immediate outcomes, they will most likely be disappointed. As this chapter has presented, ICH research (along with other CAM as reviewed elsewhere) does not have the methodological rigor as does mainstream medical research; consequently, ICH has only rarely been exposed to the rigorous tests provided by conventional medicine. However, if Americans can take a broader and more long-term perspective, they could realize that the well-being of both body and mind should be the central concern of the health care industry, which should have taken a much more proactive approach in the first place.

To that end, ICH may serve a better purpose. Indeed, every star shines in the sky. Whether you are able to appreciate the illumination of the shining star depends on how close you are to the star, where you are positioned, and how bright the sky happens to be. Given all these variables, it would be better to have an open mind in search of the star that suits you best, rather than to follow the convention and ignore some rising stars.

REFERENCES

Abuaisha, B. B., Costanzi, J. B., & Boulton, A. J. (1998). Acupuncture for the treatment of chronic painful peripheral diabetic neuropathy: A long-term study. *Diabetes Research and Clinical Practice, 39*(2), 115-121.

Allen, J. J. B., Schnyer, R. N., & Hitt, S. K. (1998). Research report: The efficacy of acupuncture in the treatment of major depression in women. *Psychological Science, 9*(5), 397-401.

Astin, J. A. (1998). Why patients use alternative medicine: Results of a national study. *Journal of American Medical Association, 279*, 1548-1553.

Astin, J. A., Harkness, E., & Ernst, E. (2000). The efficacy of "distant healing:" A systematic review of randomized trials. *Annals of Internal Medicine, 132*(1), 903-910.

Bao, S. (1996). The application of acupunctural anesthesia on thyroid operation. *Proceedings of the Fourth World Conference on Acupuncture, 83.* New York: World Federation on Acupuncture & Moxibustion.

Bayer, A. H. (1996). A treatment of chronic alcoholism by combining acupuncture and supervision. *Proceedings of The Fourth World Conference on Acupuncture, 173.*

Biernacki, W., & Peake, M. (1998). Acupuncture treatment of stable asthma. *Respiratory Medicine, 92*, 1143-1145.

Birch, S., & Jamison, R. (1998). Controlled trial of Japanese acupuncture for chronic myofascial neck pain: Assessment of specific and nonspecific effects of treatment. *The Clinical Journal of Pain, 14*, 248-255.

Borisova, N. (1996). The efficiency of the Su Jok acupuncture in treating pain syndromes of different etiologies. *Proceedings of the Fourth World Conference on Acupuncture, 128.*

Britt-Ingjerd, N., Ragnhild, K., Bertha, B., Birgitta, A., Eibjorg, A., Gry, H., et al. (2003). Acupuncture during labor can reduce the use of meperidine: A controlled clinical study. *Clinical Journal of Pain, 19*(3): 187-91.

Bulluck, M., Kiresuk, T., Pheley, A., Culliton, P., & Lenz, S. (1997). Auricular acupuncture in the treatment of cocaine abuse: A study of efficacy and dosing. *Journal of Substance Abuse Treatment, 16*, 31-38.

Cai, S. (1996). Proliferative arthritis of knee joint treated by sensation propagated along channels (SPAC) induced by tranquilization: A report of 95 cases. *Proceedings of the Fourth World Conference on Acupuncture. 96.*

Cantoni, G. (1996). A clinical study on uremic itching of dialyzed patients treated by acupuncture. *Proceedings of the Fourth World Conference on Acupuncture, 210.*

Ceniceros, S., & Brown, G. (1998). Acupuncture: A review of its history, theories, and indications. *Southern Medical Journal, 91*, 1121-1125.

Chang, H. M. (1986). *Pharmacology and applications of Chinese material medica.* Singapore: World Scientific Publishing Co.

Chen, Y. C. (1989). A study of medical qigong's efficacy. *Chinese Journal of Integrative Medicine, 9*(2), 76.

Chen, Y. R. (2003). Aerobic exercise (including qigong) helps in warding off cancer: An experimental study. *China Post,* February 17, 1-2.

Cheu, Y. (1996). A clinical observation on the acupuncture treatment of 85 cases with apolexy sequela. *Proceedings of the Fourth World Conference on Acupuncture, 147.*

Chien, C. H., Tsuei, J. J., Lee, S. C., Huang, Y. C., & Wei, Y. H. (1991). The effect of emitted bioenergy on the biochemical function of the cell. *American Journal of Chinese Medicine, 19*(3-4), 285-292.

Chiu, G. F., Chou, S. F., Gin, Y., Li, H. T., Li, T., & Yu, M. S. (1992). Qigong effect on patients with coronary heart disorder. *Chinese Journal of Sports Medicine, 11*(2), 79-84.

Chiu, Y. I., Chi, A., & Reid, I. A. (1997). Cardiovascular and endocrine effects of acupuncture in hypertensive patients. *Clinical Experiments on Hypertension, 19*(7), 1047-1063.

Cohen, K. S. (1992). *External qi healing: Chinese therapeutic touch*. International Society for the Study of Subtle Energies and Energy Medicine, Second Annual Conference, June 26-30, Boulder, CO.

Cong, Y. (1996). An accupuncture treatment for 268 patients with shoulder joint disease. *Proceedings of the Fourth World Conference on Acupuncture*. 94.

Cook, D. J., Guyatt, G. H., Ryan, G., Clifton, J., Buckingham, L., Willan, A., et al. (1993). Should unpublished data be included in meta-analyses? Current convictions and controversies. *JAMA, 269*(21), 2749-2753.

D'Acunzo, G. (1996). The treatment of vertebral fractures in 67 cases by specific traditional Chinese exercises combined with acupuncture. *Proceedings of the Fourth World Conference on Acupuncture*. 150.

Dai, X. (1996). An analysis of 120 cases with dysmenorrhea after acupuncture at the sanyinjiao point. *Proceedings of the Fourth World Conference on Acupuncture*. 136.

Darwin, L., & Carma, A. (2002). Nondrug interventions in hypertension prevention and control. *Cardiologic Clinicians, 20*(2), 249-63.

David, D. S., Friedman, R., Siegel, W. C., Jacobs, S. C. O., & Benson, H. (1992). Distress over the noneffect of stress. *JAMA, 268*(2), 198

Davies, A., Lewith, G., Goddard, J., & Howarth, P. (1998). The effect of acupuncture on nonallergic rhinitis: A controlled pilot study. *Alternative Therapies, 4*, 70-74.

Davies, P., Chang, C., Hackman, R., Stern, J., & Gershwin, M. (1998). Acupuncture in the treatment of asthma: A critical review. *Allergol et Immunopathologie, 26*, 263-271.

Dawidson, I., Angmar-Mansson, B., Blom, M., Theodorsson, E., & Lundeberg, T. (1998). Sensory stimulation (acupuncture) increases the release of vasoactive intestinal polypeptide in the saliva of xerostomia sufferers. *Neuropeptides, 32*(6), 543-548.

Dyrehag, L. E., Widerstrom-Noga, E. G., Carlsson, S. G., & Andersson, S. A. (1997). Effects of repeated sensory stimulation sessions on skin temperature in chronic pain patients. *Scandinavian Journal of Rehabilitative Medicine, 29*(4), 243-250.

Eisenberg, D. (1985). *Encounter with qi: Exploring Chinese medicine*. New York: Penguin Books.

Eisenberg, D. M., Davis, R. B., Ettner, S. L., Appel, S., Wilkey, S., Van Rompay, M., et al. (1998). Trends in alternative medicine use in the United States, 1990-1997: Results of a follow-up national survey. *JAMA, 280*, 1569-75.

Eisenberg, D. M., Kessler, R. C., Foster, C., Norlock, F. E., Calkins, D. R., & Delbanco, T. L. (1993). Unconventional medicine in the United States. Prevalence, costs, and patterns of use. *New England Journal of Medicine, 328*(4), 246-52.

Eory, A., & Senyi, K. (1996). The efficacy of Chinese massage in the prevention of juvenile onset myopia. *Proceedings of the Fourth World Conference on Acupuncture*, 253.

Eppley, K. R., Abrams, A. I., & Shear, J. (1989). Differential effects of relaxation techniques on trait anxiety: A meta-analysis. *Journal of Clinical Psychology, 45*(6), 957-974.

Ernst, E. (2002). Complementary and alternative medicine for pain management in rheumatic disease. *Current Opinion of Rheumatology, 14*(1), 58-62.

Ernst, E., & Pittler, M. H. (1998). The effectiveness of acupuncture in treating acute dental pain: A systematic review. *British Dental Journal, 184*(9), 442-447.

Ernst, E., & White, A. (1998). Acupuncture for back pain. *Archives of Internal Medicine, 158*, 2235-2241.

Ezzo, J., Berman, B. M., Vickers, A. J., & Linde, K. (1998). Complementary medicine and the Cochrane Collaboration. *JAMA, 280*(18), 1628-1630.

Fialka, V., Korpan, M. I., Nikoliakis, P., Dezu, I., Schneider, I., & Leita, T. (1998). Acupuncture in the treatment of a posttraumatic pain syndrome. *Lik Sprava, 7*, 152-154.

Fontanarosa, P. B., & Lunberg, G. D. (1998). Alternative medicine meets science. *JAMA, 280*(18), 1618-1619.

Ganlante, L. (1981). *Tai chi: The supreme ultimate*. York Beach, MA: Samuel Weiser.

Gigliotti, F., Romagnoli, I., & Scano, G. (2003). Breathing retraining and exercise conditioning in patients with chronic obstructive pulmonary disease. *Respirator Medicine, 97*(3), 197-204.

Gong, Y., & Wang, Z. (1996). Acupuncture and moxibustion for 113 cases of leukopenia caused by chemotherapy. *Proceedings of the Fourth World Conference on Acupuncture*, 225.

Gosman-Hedstrom, G., Claesson, L., Klingenstierna, U., Carlsson, J., Olausson, B., Frizell, M., et al. (1998). Effects of acupuncture treatment on daily life activities and quality of life: A controlled, prospective, and randomized study of acute stroke patients. *Stroke, 29*, 2100-2108.

Greenwald, J. (2001). Herbal healing. In D. Eisenberg (2002), *Complementary and integrative medical therapies* (pp. 3–27). Boston, MA: Harvard Medical School.

Guan, F. P. (1996). A clinical study on making facial correction by needling. *Proceedings of the Fourth World Conference on Acupuncture*. 228.

Guan, Z. (1996). A clinical observation of 418 cases of lumbar intervertebral disk hernia treated with hot needles. *Proceedings of the Fourth World Conference on Acupuncture*, 117.

Guo, W., & Ni, G. (2003). The effects of acupuncture on blood pressure in different patients. *Journal of Traditional Chinese Medicine, 23*(1), 49-50.

Hammar, M., Frisk, J., Grimas, O., Hook, M., Spetz, A., & Wyon, Y. (1999). Acupuncture treatment of vasomotor symptoms in men with prostatic carcinoma: A pilot study. *The Journal of Urology, 161,* 853-856.

Hao, J. (1996). Needle-edge and cupping therapy in the treatment of periarthritis of shoulder joint. *Proceedings of the Fourth World Conference on Acupuncture, 95.*

He, J., & Zeng, Y. (1996). A clinical strategy and method to treat chronic fatigue syndrome by acupuncture. *Proceedings of the Fourth World Conference on Acupuncture, 177.*

Hu, Y., & Hu, K. (1996). A clinical observation on 52 cases of herniated lumbar disk treated with acupuncture. *Proceedings of the Fourth World Conference on Acupuncture, 114.*

Huang, X. M. (1996). Personal communication at the Fourth World conference on Acupuncture, September 20–22, New York.

Huang, Y., & Huang, M. (1996). A special acupuncture treatment for headache (383) cases. *Proceedings of the Fourth World Conference on Acupuncture, 85.*

Hwang, M. G. (1988). Qigong therapy on neurological system. In C. P. Lin (Ed.), *Chinese Qigongology* (pp. 66-89). Bejing, China: Bejing College of Athletic Education (in Chinese).

Imai, T. (1996). The experience in the combination of acupuncture and chiropractic therapy for autonomic nerve dysfunction. *Proceedings of the Fourth World Conference on Acupuncture. 156.*

Ives, J. C. (2000). Beyond the mind-body exercise hype. *Physician and Sportsmedicine, 28*(3), 67-74.

Iwao, M., Kajiyama, S., Mori, H., & Oogaki, K. (2001). Effects of qigong walking on diabetics patients. *Neurological Research, 23*(5), 501-505.

Jadad, A. R., & Rennie, D. (1998). The randomized controlled trial gets a middle-aged checkup. *JAMA, 279*(4), 319-320.

Jiang, K. (1996). A clinical study on slight burns and scalds of skin treated by needling methods. *Proceedings of the Fourth World Conference on Acupuncture. 212.*

Jin, K. Q. (1992). The effect of qigong on electrocardiographic autopower spectrum function. *Chung Kuo Chung His I Chieh Ho Tsa Chih, 12*(7), 412-413, 389.

Jin, Y., & Zhou, J. (1996). A clinical observation on the treatment of angina pectoris by acupoint plastering. *Proceedings of the Fourth World Conference on Acupuncture. 187.*

Jing, Y., & Wang, J. (1996). An observation on therapeutic effect of sciatica treated by acu-moxibustion. *Proceedings of the Fourth World Conference on Acupuncture. 109.*

Jing, Y., Li, X., & Wang, Z. (1988). *Observations on the treatment effects of emitted qi.* Research report presented at the Qigong Institute, Beijing, China.

Johnson, G. D. (1998). Medical management of migraine-related dizziness and vertigo. *Laryngoscope, 108*(1, Pt. 2).

Johnstone, P., Bloom, T., Niemtzow, R., Crain, D., Riffenburg, R., & Amling, C. (2003). A prospective, randomized pilot trial of acupuncture of the kidney-bladder distinct meridian for lower urinary tract symptoms. *Journal of Urology, 169*(3), 1037-1039.

Jonas, W. B. (1998). Alternative medicine—learning from the past, examining the present, advancing to the future. *JAMA, 280*(18), 1616-1617.

Katai, S. (1996). Acupuncture and moxibustion treatment for infertility. *Proceedings of the Fourth World Conference on Acupuncture, 248.*

Kim, N. S. (1996). *A treatment of allergic rhinitis with sneezing nasal discharge and congestion by acupuncture.* Paper presented at the Fourth World Conference on Acupuncture, September 20-22, New York.

Kjendahl, A., Sallstrom, S., Osten, P. E., Stanghelle, J. K., & Borchgrevink, C. E. (1997). A one-year follow-up study on the effects of acupuncture in the treatment of stroke patients in the subacute stage: A randomized controlled study. *Clinical Rehabilitation, 11*(3), 192-200.

Kjendahl, A., Sallstrom, S., Osten, P. E., Stanghelle, J. K., & Borchgrevink, C. F. (1998). Acupuncture in stroke. *Tidskrift Norge Laegeforen, 118*(9), 1362-1366.

Knardahl, S., Elam, M., Olausson, B., & Wallin, B. G. (1998). Sympathetic nerve activity after acupuncture in humans. *Pain, 75*(1), 19-25.

Kuang, A. K., Chen, J. L., & Lu, Y. R. (1989). Changes of the sex hormones in female type II diabetics, coronary heart disease, essential hypertension and its relations with kidney deficiency, cardiovascular complications and efficacy of traditional Chinese medicine or qigong treatment. *Chung His I Chieh Ho Tsa Chih, 9*(6), 331-334, 323.

Kuang, A., Wang, C., Xu, D., Qian, Y., & Kwang, D. (1991). Research on the anti-aging effect of qigong. *Journal of Traditional Chinese Medicine, 11*(2), 153-158.

Lai, S. S. (1996). *Clinical observations: A Chinese herbal formula for the treatment of pain and associated symptoms for cancer.* Paper presented at the Fourth World conference on Acupuncture, September 20-22, New York.

Lam, C. L. (1996). *A clinical observation on the effects of acupuncture and moxibustion on the treatment of impotence in 48 cases.* Paper presented at the Fourth World conference on Acupuncture, September 20-22, New York.

Lao, L. (1996). A controlled acupuncture clinical trial on osteoarthritis of the knee. *Proceedings of the Fourth World Conference on Acupuncture.* 97.

Lee, C. T., & Lei, T. (1995a). *Effects of vital energy exercise on physiological and psychological changes.* Paper presented at the 66th Annual Meeting of Eastern Psychological Association, March 31-April 2, Boston.

Lee, C. T., & Lei, T. (1995b). *Taoist's vital energy exercise as an integration of art and science.* Paper presented at the Fifth Annual Conference of the International Society for the Study of Subtle and Energy Medicine, June 23-26, Boulder, CO.

Lee, C. T., & Lei, T. (1995c). *Eastern art encounters with western sciences: Empirical studies of Taoists' martial art.* Paper presented at the 53rd Annual Convention, International Council of Psychologists, August 4-8, Taipei, Taiwan.

Lee, C. T., & Lei, T. (1996). All rivers flow to the sea: Encountering energy through qigong without acupuncture. *Proceedings of the Fourth World Conference on Acupuncture,* 390.

Lee, C. T., & Lei, T. (1997). *Indigenous Chinese healing.* New York Academy of Sciences. Workshop on Culture, Therapy, and Healing, November 14.

Lee, C. T., & Lei, T. (1999). Qigong. In W. B. Jonas & L. S. Levin (Eds.), *Essentials of complementary and alternative medicine* (pp. 392-409). Baltimore, MD: Williams & Wilkins.

Lee, C. T., & Lei, T. (1999). Qigong. In W. B. Jonas & L. S. Levin, (Eds.), *Essentials of complementary and alternative medicine* (pp. 392-409). Baltimore, MD: Williams & Wilkins.

Lee, C. T., & Lei, T. (1999). Qigong. In W. B. Jonas & L. S. Levin, (Eds.), *Textbooks of complementary and alternative medicine* (pp. 392-409). Baltimore, MD: Williams & Wilkins.

Lei, T. (1997). *Chi-gong: An indigenous Chinese healing method.* Paper presented at the 25th Annual Convention of Psychology, May 3, New York: Hunter College.

Lei, T., & Lee, C. T. (1997a). *Chi Gong: Beyond the body/mind boundary and cultural context.* Paper presented at the Conference of the International Council of Psychologists, July 21-23, Padua, Italy: University of Padua.

Lei, T., & Lee, C. T. (1997b). *Chi Gong: A pan-cultural approach to mental health.* Paper pressented at the 55th Annual Convention of the International Council of Psychologists, July 14-18, Graz, Austria.

Lei, T., Lee, C.T., Burshteyn, D., & Schnoll, R. (2002). *Do not throw the baby out with the bathwater: Adoption of alternative healing in a diverse world.* Paper presented at the Biannual International Conference on Personal Growth, July 18-21, Vancouver, BC, Trinity University.

Lei, X. F., Bi, A. H., Zhang, Z. X., & Cheng, Z. Y. (1991). The antitumor effects of qigong—emitted external qi and its influence on the immunologic functions of tumor-bearing mice. *Journal of the Tongji Medical University,* 11(4), 253-256.

Li, G. C. (Ed.). (1988). *Qigong treatment of commonly seen diseases.* Hong Kong: Su Tun Co., Ltd. (in Chinese).

Li, J. P. (1993). Qigong's effect on hypertension patients' NE and 5-HT. *Chinese Journal of Sports Medicine,* 12(3), 152-156.

Li, M., Chen, K., & Mo, Z. (2002). Use of qigong in the detoxification of heroin addicts. *Alternative Therapy, Health, & Medicine,* 8(1), 50-54, 56-59.

Li, Y. (1996). A clinical obsevation on the selection of abdominal acupoints to relieve lower lumbar pain. *Proceedings of the Fourth World Conference on Acupuncture,* 103.

Liau-Hing, C. (1996). Facial paralysis treated by traditional Chinese medicine and neural therapy. *Proceedings of the Fourth World Conference on Acupuncture.* 152.

Lim, Y. A., Boone, T. F., Flarrity, J. R., & Thompson, W. R. (1993). Effects of qigong on cardiorespiratory changes: A preliminary study. *American Journal of Chinese Medicine,* 21(1), 1-6.

Litscher, G., Wenzel, G., Niederwieser, G., & Schwartz, G. (2001). Effects of qigong on brain functions. *Neurological Research,* 23(5), 501-505.

Liu, B., & Dong, Y. (1996). A clinical study on syndrome of the third lumbar vertebra transverse process treated by the round-sharp needle. *Proceedings of the Fourth World Conference on Acupuncture,* 108

Liu, B., Jiao, J., & Li, Y. (1990). The effect of qigong exercise on the blood level of monoamine neuro-transmitters in patients with chronic disease. *Chung His I Chieh Ho Tsa Chih,* 10(4), 203-205.

Liu,Y., & Zhou, X. (1996). The effect of the acupuncture with TDP on low back pain. *Proceedings of the Fourth World Conference on Acupuncture,* 123.

Lotters, F., van Tol, B., Kwakkel, G., & Gosselink, R. (2002). Effects of controlled inspiratory muscle training in patients with chronic obstructive pulmonary disease: A meta-analysis. *European Respiratory Journal,* 20(3), 570-576.

Lu, J. (1996). The preliminary exploration of applying the biotic holographic acupuncture treatment to cure scapulohumeral periarthritis. *Proceedings of the Fourth World Conference on Acupuncture,* 93.

Lynn, S. (1996). The treatment of musculoskeletal pain—a comparative clinical study of acupuncture versus acupuncture-cupping therapy. *Proceedings of the Fourth World Conference on Acupuncture*, 126.

Lu, A. (1996). Ginger partition moxibustion with acupuncture point injection curing irritable bowel syndrome. *Proceedings of the Fourth World Conference on Acupuncture*, 199.

Ma, W., & Wang, B. (1996). Acupuncture and Chinese drugs (DA-LI-TANG) therapy to chronic fatigue syndrome. *Proceedings of the Fourth World Conference on Acupuncture*, 179.

Maeda, M., Kachi, H., Ichihashi, N., Oyama, Z., & Kitajima, Y. (1998). The effect of electrical acupuncture-stimulation therapy using thermography and plasma endothelin (ET-1) levels in patients with progressive systemic sclerosis (PSS). *Journal of Dermatological Science, 17*, 151-155.

Marino, F. (1996). A comparison of Zhongtiao, Huangzhong and Huantiao; A clinical experience on 150 cases of lumbosciatalgia. *Proceedings of the Fourth World Conference on Acupuncture*, 105.

Martin, A., Davenport, P., McCaffrey, R., & Fowler, N. (2003). Qigong practice: A pathway to health and healing. *Holistic Nursing Practice, 17*(2), 110-116.

McGee, C. T., & Chow, E. P. Y. (1988). *Miracle healing from China*. Coeur d'Alener, Idaho. Thunder Bay Press.

Middlekauff, H., Yu, J., & Hui, K. (2001). Acupuncture effects on reflex responses to mental stress in humans. *American Journal of Physiological Regulation, 280*(5), R1462-R1468.

Makiyama, K., & Wu, B. (1996). The clinical treatment by acupuncture and qigong. *Proceedings of the Fourth World Conference on Acupuncture*. 122.

Morris, K., & Margolin, A. (2000). Needling cocaine addicts helps abstinence. *Lancet, 356*(9230), 658.

Morse, P. (2001). Expenses on herbal remedy. In D. Eisenberg (2002), *Complementary and integrative medical therapies: Current status and future trends* (pp. 3-27). Cambridge, MA: Harvard Medical School.

Mou, F. F., Yen, Z. F., Li, C. Y., & Chao, G. L. (1991). Study of qigong's bi-directional regulation and its mechanism. *Chinese Journal of Modern Deviation in Traditional Medicine, 10*(6), 353-356.

Mou, F. F., Wang, L. J., & Chao, G. L. (1992). An empirical study of qigong's effect on human microcirculation. *Chinese Journal of Physiopathology, 5*, 558-559.

Mou, F. F., Shi, Z., Hsu, G., & Chao, G. L. (1994). Study of qigong on bulbar conjunctiva microcirculation disorder of persons entering highland. *Journal of Microcirculation, 4*(4), 18-20.

Murashko, N. (2001). Variability of cardiac rhythm and treatment modalities for the vegetative state dystonia syndrome. *Lik Sprava, 4*, 81-84.

Ng, B. Y. (1999). Qigong-induced mental disorders: A review. *Australian New Zealand Journal of Psychiatry, 33*(2), 197-206.

Nielsen, O. J., Moller, K., & Jorgensen, K. E. (1999). The effect of traditional Chinese acupuncture on severe tinnitus: A double-blind, placebo-controlled clinical study with an open therapeutic surveillance. *Ugeskrift Laeger, 161*(4), 424-429.

Niu, Y., & Yang, T. (1996). A clinical observation of oxygen-medicine acupuncture therapy for migraine. *Proceedings of the Fourth World Conference on Acupuncture, 87*.

Pagon, A. T., Zhai, N., Chen, H., Li, J., Zhang, C., Lu, S., et al. (1996). The special effect of "Xing-Nao-Kai-Qiao" acupuncture method in the treatment of acute cardio-cerebrovascular diseases: A review of clinical experience and experimental research in the past twenty years. *Proceedings of the Fourth World Conference on Acupuncture*. 139.

Perrin, J., Kemper, K., Sarah, R., Highfield, E. S., Xiarhos, E., & Barnes, L. (2000). On pins and needles? Pediatric pain and patients' experience with acupuncture. *Pediatrics, 105* [Supplement], 941-947.

Pintov, S., Lahat, E., Alstein, M., Vogel, Z., & Barg, J. (1997). Acupuncture and the opioid system: Implications in management of migraine. *Pediatric Neurology, 17*(2), 129-133.

Pippa, L. (1996). A therapy of glaucoma by acupuncture and Chinese herbs. Paper presented at the Fourth World Conference on Acupuncture, September 20-22, New York.

Ramirez-Sarmiento, A., Orozco-Levi, M., Guell, R., Barreiro, E., Hernandez, N., Mota, S., et al. (2002). Inspiratory muscle training in patients with chronic obstructive pulmonary disease: Structural adaptations and physiologic outcomes. *American Journal of Respiratory and Critical Care Medicine, 166*(11), 1491-1497.

Rapson, L. M., & Biemann, I. M. (1996). Acupuncture treatment of pain in spinal cord injuries. *Proceedings of the Fourth World Conference on Acupuncture, 131*.

Ray, P. H. (1998). The emerging culture. *American Demographics*. Retrieved April 10, 1998 from www.demographics.com.

Ray, P. H., & Anderson, S. R. (2001). *The cultural creatives: How 50 million people are changing the world*. New York: Three Rivers Press.

Reynolds, T. (2003). Keeping up with alternative medicine: Researchers offer evaluation criteria. *Journal of National Cancer Institute, 95*, 96-98.

Roschke, J., Wolf, C., Kogel, P., Wagner, P., & Bech, S. (1998). Adjuvant whole body acupuncture in depression: A placebo-controlled study with standardized mianserin therapy. *Der Nervenarzt, 69*(11), 961-967.

Rosted, P. (1998). The use of acupuncture in dentistry. *Oral Diseases, 4*(2), 100-104.

Ruggie, M. (2002). Diversity and healing. In D. Eisenberg (Ed.), *Complementary and alternative medicine: State of the science and clinical application* (pp. 321-332). Boston: Harvard Medical School.

Ryu, H., Lee, H. S., Shin, Y. S., Chung, S. M., Lee, M. S., Kim, H. M., et al. (1996). Acute effects of qigong training on stress hormonal levels in man. *American Journal of Chinese Medicine, 24*(2), 193-198.

Sancier, K. M. (1996). Medical application of qigong. *Alternative Therapies, 2*(1), 40-46, adapted from a database of Chinese qigong proceedings.

Sanders, H., Davis, M., Ducan, B., Meaney, J., Haynes, J., & Buron, L. (2003). Use of complementary and alternative medical therapies among children with special health care needs in Southern Arizona. *Pediatrics, 111*, 584-587.

Schiantarelli, C., Pippa, L., Bernini, A., & Terza, I. (1996). The treatment of osteoarthritic pain using acupuncture and relationship with intake of NSAID. *Proceedings of the Fourth World Conference on Acupuncture,* 91.

Schwartz, L., Sommers, E., Parker, S., Brown, E.R., Winters, M., & Bauchner, H. (1996). Acupressure augmentation of standard medical therapy in the management of the neonatal abstinence syndrome. *Proceedings of the Fourth World Conference on Acupuncture,* 171.

Sellik, S. M., & Zaza, C. (1998). Critical review of five nonpharmocologic strategies for managing cancer pain. *Cancer Prevention and Control, 2*(1), 7-14.

Shih, Y. F., Lin, L. L. K., Hwang, C. Y., Huang, J. K., Hung, & Hou, P. K. (1995). The effects of qigong ocular exercise on accommodation. *Chinese Journal of Physiology, 38*(1), 35-42.

Song, L. Z., Schwartz, G. E., & Russek, L. G. (1998). Heart-focused attention and heart- brain synchronization: Energetic and physiological mechanisms. *Alternative Therapies in Health and Medicine, 4*(5), 44-52, 54-60, 62.

Spitali, R. (1996). Acupuncture treatment of uterine fibromyomas trial of 18 cases. *Proceedings of the Fourth World Conference on Acupuncture,* 240.

Sturdy, G., Hillman, D., Green, D., Jenkins, S., Cecins, N., & Eastwood, P. (2003). Feasibility of high-intensity, interval-based respiratory muscle training in chronic obstructive pulmonary disease. *Chest, 123*(1), 142-150.

Su, J. (1996). A clinical study on the liver and gallstone treated by needling method with the massotherapy of the ear points. *Proceedings of the Fourth World Conference on Acupuncture.* 201.

Sun, F., & Li, S. T. (1995). The efficacy and mechanism in the treatment of 49 cases of hypertension. *Shanghai Journal of Traditional Chinese Medicine, 15*, 22-24.

Sung, F. L., & Yan, Y. A. (1992). Effects of various qigong breathing patterns on variability of heart rate. *Chung Kuo Chung His I Chieh Ho Tsa Chih, 12*(9), 527-30, 516.

Sutherland, J. A. (2001). Selected complementary methods and nursing care of the hypertensive client. *Holistic Nurse Practitioner, 15*(4), 4-11.

Sze, F., Wong, E., Or, K.K., Lau, J., & Woo, J. (2002). Does acupuncture improve motor recovery after stroke? A meta-analysis of randomized controlled trials. *Stroke, 33*(11), 2604-2619.

Tan, C. The clinical use of the 2nd metacarpal radius side micro-acupuncture system of diagnostic and therapeutic method. *Proceedings of the Fourth World Conference on Acupuncture.* 257.

Tempfer, C., Zeisler, H., Heinzl, H., Hefler, L., Husslein, P., & Kainz, C. (1998). Influence of acupuncture on maternal serum levels of interleukin-8, prostaglandin F2alpha, and beta-endorphin: A matched pair study. *Obstetric Gynecology, 92*(2), 245-248.

Ternov, K., Nilsson, M., Lofberg, L., Algotsson, L., & Akesson, J. (1998). Acupuncture for pain relief during child birth. *Acupuncture and Electrotherapeutic Research, 23*(1), 19-26.

Tjandra, J. (1996). The prevention of hair loss and gray hair with acupuncture. *Proceedings of the Fourth World Conference on Acupuncture.* 213.

Townsend, R. R. (2002). Acupuncture in hypertension. *Journal of Clinical Hypertension, 4*(3), 229.

Tsuchiya, M. (1996) The treatment of multiple sclerosis by electric acupuncture: Investigation of 332 cases. *Proceedings of the Fourth World Conference on Acupuncture.* 163.

Tsai, J. R., & Rothenberg, C. (1996). Invasive rectification of arthritic hip, bursitis and tendonitis by five needle deep tissue stimulation (DYS). *Proceedings of the Fourth World Conference on Acupuncture.*

Tsai, T. J., Lai, J. S., & Lee, S. H., et al. (1995). Breathing-coordinated exercise improves the quality of life in hemodialysis patients. *Journal of the American Society of Nephrology, 6*(5), 1392-1400.

Ulett, G. A., Han, S., & Han, J. S. (1998). Electroacupuncture: Mechanisms and clinical application. *Biological Psychiatry, 44*(2), 129-138.

Vickers, A., Goyal, N., Harland, R., & Rees, R. (1998). Do certain countries produce only positive results? A systematic review of controlled trials. *Controlled Clinical Trials, 19*(2), 159-166.

Vilholm, O. J., Moller, K., & Jorgensen, K. (1998). Effect of traditional Chinese acupuncture on severe tinnitus: A double-blind, placebo-controlled, clinical investigation with open therapeutic control. *British Journal of Audiology, 32*(3), 197-204.

Waite, N., & Clough, J. (1998). A single-blinded, placebo-controlled trial of a simple acupuncture treatment in the cessation of smoking. *British Journal of General Practice, 48*, 1487-1490.

Wang, T. (1996). Acupuncture and manipulation massage for 250 sciatica cases. *Proceedings of the Fourth World Conference on Acupuncture.* 119.

Wang, B., Tang, J., White, P. F., Naruse, R., Sloninsky, A., Kariger, R., et al. (1997). Effect of the intensity of transcutaneous acupoint electrical stimulation of the postoperative analgesic requirement. *Anesthetic Analgesia, 85*(2), 406-413.

Wang, C. C., Chang, G. S., Liu, S. C., Geng, G, Y., Chu, M. L., Din, F. D., et al. (1992). An observational study of qigong therapy on 175 college students' myopia. *Journal of Henan Medical University, 27*(1), 20-24.

Wang, C. X., Xu, D. H., Quian, Y. H., & Kuang, A. K. (1988). The beneficial effect of qigong on the hypertension incorporated with coronary heart disease. *Journal of Gerontology, 8*(2), 83.

Wang, C. X., Hsu, D. H., Chang, T. Y., & Shih, W. (1993). An observational study of qigong's effect on hypertensive patients' lipoprotein. *Shanghai Journal of Chinese Medicine, 5*, 22-23.

Wang, C. X., Hsu, D. H., Chang, D. H., & Chang, Y. C. (1995). Effects of qigong on heart-qi deficiency and blood stasis type of hypertension and its mechanism. *Chinese Journal of Modern Development in Traditional Medicine, 15*(8), 454-458.

Wang, S., & Wang, B. (1996). Through needling of the ear point buttock in treating acute low back pain. *Proceedings of the Fourth World Conference on Acupuncture,* 112.

Wang, F., Xu, L., & Bai, G. (1996). A clinical study on the strong stimulation of acupuncture therapy for pain relief. *Proceedings of the Fourth World Conference on Acupuncture,* 124.

Wei, Q., & Liu, Z. (2003). Effects of acupuncture on monoamine neurotransmitters in raphe nuclei in obese rats. *Journal of Traditional Chinese Medicine, 23*(2), 147-50

Weil, A. (1995). *Spontaneous healing.* New York: Alfred A. Knopf.

Weiner, P., Magadle, R., Massarwa, F., Beckerman, M., & Beray-Yanay, N. (2002). Influence of gender and inspiratory muscle training on the perception of dyspnea in patients with asthma. *Chest, 122*(1), 197-201.

White, A., & Ernst, E. (1998). A trial method for assessing the adequacy of acupuncture treatments. *Alternative Therapies, 4*, 66-71.

Wirth, D., Cram, J., & Chang, R. (1997). Multisite electromyographic analysis of touch and qigong therapy. *Journal of Alternative and Complementary Medicine, 3*, 109-118.

Wong, S. S., & Nahin, R. L. (2003). National Center for Complementary and Alternative Medicine perspectives for complementary and alternative medicine research in cardiovascular diseases. *Cardiological Review, 11*(2), 94-98.

Wu, W. H., Bandilla, E., Ciccone, D. S., Yang, J., Cheng, S. C., Carner, N., et al. (1999). Effects of qigong on late-stage complex regional pain syndrome. *Alternative Therapies in Health and Medicine, 5*(1), 45-54.

Xia, X. (1996). The treatment of 125 acute lumbar muscle sprain cases by eye needling. *Proceedings of the Fourth World Conference on Acupuncture,* 104.

Xial, F. A clinical survey of ER YA and Chinese herb for treatment of obesity. *Proceedings of the Fourth World Conference on Acupuncture,* 202.

Xie, H. Z. (1988). *The scientific basis of chi qong.* Beijing, China: Institute of Technology.

Xing, Z. H., Li, W., & Pi, D. R. (1993). Effects of qigong on blood pressure and life quality of essential hypertension patients. *Chung Kuo Chung His I Chieh Ho Tsa Chih, 13*(7), 388-389, 413-414.

Xiu, R. J. (1988). Microcirculation and traditional Chinese medicine. *Journal of the American Medical Association, 260*(12), 1755-1757.

Xu, W. (1996). A clinal observation of ear acupuncture's therapeutic effects on 127 cases of smoking cessation. *Proceedings of the Fourth World Conference on Acupuncture,* 175.

Xu, D., & Wang, C. (1994). Clinical study of delaying effect on senility of hypertensive patients by practicing "Yang Jing Yi Shen Gong." *Proceedings from the Fifth International Symposium on Qigong.* Shanghai, China, 109.

Xu, M., Tomotake, M., Ikuta, T., Ishimoto, Y., & Okura, M. (1998). The effects of qigong and acupuncture on human cerebral evoked potentials and electroencephalogram. *Journal of Medical Investigation, 44*(3-4), 163-171.

Xu, S. H. (1994). Psychophysiological reactions associated with qigong therapy. *Chinese Medical Journal, 107*(3), 230-233.

Xue, A. (1996). An analysis of the treatment of 70 inner-ear vertigo cases. *Proceedings of the Fourth World Conference on Acupuncture,* 159.

Yang, M. J. (1990). *Dayan Gong.* Beijing, China: Renmin Weisheng.

Yang, H. (1996). Observations on 108 cases of lumbar disc herniation treated with traditional chinese medicine. *Proceedings of the Fourth World Conference on Acupuncture* 115.

Ye, C. (1996). A clinical observation on 87 cases of infantile cerebral paralysis treated with acupuncture. *Proceedings of the Fourth World Conference on Acupuncture,* 245.

Yio, X. (1996). An observation of the curative effect on coronary heart disease by acupuncturing neiguan. *Proceedings of the Fourth World Conference on Acupuncture, 182.*

Yu, Y. M. (1996). The clinical and research principle on alleviating upper abdominal pain of 160 patients by needling bilateral zusanili. *Proceedings of the Fourth World Conference on Acupuncture, 135.*

Yuan, Z. (1996). An observation on therapeutic effects of acupuncture in the treatment of chronic active hepatitis B. *Proceedings of the Fourth World Conference on Acupuncture, 231.*

Zhang, H. M. (1988). *Chinese qigong method: Pulling out specific therapeutic abilities.* Tokyo, Japan: Japan Qigong Association (in Japanese).

Zhang, W. B., Zheng, R. G., Zhang, B. K., Yu, W. L., & Shen, X. Y. (1993). An observation on flash evoked cortical potentials and qigong meditation. *American Journal of Chinese Medicine, 11*(3-4), 243-249.

Zhao, X., & Yang, B. (1996). A clinical study on 200 cases of peripheral facial paralysis treated by electroacupuncture combined with indirect moxibustion. *Proceedings of the Fourth World Conference on Acupuncture, 151.*

Zeisler, H., Tempfer, C., Mayerhofer, K., Barrada, M., & Husslein, P. (1998*).* Acupuncture for pain relief during child birth. *Gynecological Obstet Investigation, 46*(1), 22-25.

Zeng, P. (1996). The evidence of angiotensin II involved in the central modulation of electroacupuncture analgesia. *Proceedings of the Fourth World Conference on Acupuncture,* 291

Zheng, G. (1996). The effectiveness of combined Chinese herbs with acupuncture treatment in infertility. *Proceedings of the Fourth World Conference on Acupuncture, 241.*

Zherebrin, V. V. (1998). The use of acupuncture reflexotherapy in the combined treatment of patients with chronic gouty polyarthritis. *Lik Sprava, 2,* 151-153.

Zhou, B. (1996). Treating lumbar disc protrusion with horizontal extension tracting bed. *Proceedings of the Fourth World Conference on Acupuncture,* 107.

Zhu, R. B. (1996). A clinical study on cerebral hemorrhage-yangbi palsy symptom treated by the needling method. *Proceedings of the Fourth World Conference on Acupuncture, 141.*

Psychoanalysis and Buddhism

Jeffrey B. Rubin
Harlem Family Institute, New York City
Visiting Lecturer—Union Theological Seminary, New York City

The relationship between psychoanalysis and Eastern meditative disciplines has intrigued me for many years. I have immersed myself in both traditions since the late 1970s in the hope of ascertaining what light they might shed on the art of living. Judiciously integrating them can open up new vistas that might ultimately enrich our lives and the lives of the people in pain with whom we work.

Imagine the following scenario. A person is in a room with a minimum of sensory stimulations and distractions. She is still, alert, and relaxed. Her eyes are closed. She pays careful attention to whatever she experiences moment after moment . . . I could be describing an analysand in psychoanalytic treatment. In this particular instance, I am actually depicting a person meditating. What I hope to do in this paper is interest you in the possibility that one's experience on the meditative cushion might enrich one's experience in the psychoanalytic consulting room, and one's experience in the psychoanalytic consulting room might aid one's experience on the meditative cushion.

An increasing number of people that I know both in and outside of therapy complain of being too burdened and distracted. They feel oversaturated with e-mails, faxes, and pagers. They frenetically juggle multiple and conflicting roles and responsibilities—parent, therapist, spouse, lover, friend. They often feel a hollowness in their lives. Those of you who feel more grounded and less depleted may still long for a life of greater inner peace and equanimity.

Imagine that you could find a sanctuary in your daily experience from the cognitive overstimulation and the frenetic pace that all too often consumes us. Imagine that within this safe haven you might quiet the inner maelstrom and gain a measure of clarity and focus about what you feel and who you are. Imagine further that you could see and work through restrictive psychological identifications and conditioning. You could then have a less insulated and egocentric view of self and reality. There might be a profound sense of connectedness with yourself and other people. Imagine even further that if this happens, then something sacred will be revealed. Your daily life might be infused with greater meaning and purpose. You might then live with greater compassion and wisdom. This is part of the promise of Buddhism.

WHOSE BUDDHISM IS IT, ANYWAY?

Buddhism, like psychoanalysis, is not one thing. Meaning, as the Russian thinker Bakhtin (1986) knew, is the product of an interaction or dialogue between reader and text, rather than a singular essence waiting to be revealed in a neutral, fixed,

manuscript. There is thus no singular, settled, or definitive Buddhism (or psychoanalysis). "Buddhism" and "psychoanalysis" are heterogeneous and evolving from
a plenitude of beliefs, theories, and practices, cocreated and transformed by readers
and seekers from different historical, psychological, sociocultural, and gendered
perspectives (Rubin, 1996, p. 3). There is thus no such thing as "Buddhism." Given
the diversity in theories and practices within Buddhism, it is more accurate to speak
of Buddhisms rather than Buddhism (Rubin, 1996).

There have been several major schools of Buddhist thought (e.g., Theravadin, Zen,
Ch'an, Tibetan, and Korean) developing in different historical ages and cultures that
have adopted different theories and practices. To cite two examples among many possible ones, anyone familiar with classical Buddhist texts knows that Buddha was not
averse to profound philosophical exploration. After all, he offered profound examinations of the nature of mind, self, suffering, and the path to inner peace. But in
answer to cosmological and metaphysical questions—the existence of a divinity,
divine realms, afterlife, and so forth—he is said to have likened the questioner to a
man who was shot by an arrow and would not pull the arrow out of his body until he
had been told where the arrow was made, what it was made of, and who shot it. The
man was suffering and his time could best be spent, asserted Buddha, in the pragmatic and therapeutic task of pulling out the arrow and relieving his suffering rather
than engaging in endless intellectual speculation about the nature of the universe.

And yet, despite the avowedly pragmatic and nonmetaphysical orientation of
Buddha, subsequent schools of Buddhist thought, such as Tibetan Buddhism, posit
the existence of various deities and adopt a cosmology with magical dimensions that
seems quite foreign to the nontheistic worldview of classical Buddhism (as well as the
contemporary West).

The methods, no less than the worldviews, of the various schools of Buddhism can
also differ greatly. Classical Buddhism placed great emphasis on individual practitioners awakening from their own slumber through concentrated meditative practice
focused on a clear and direct apprehension of reality, living a life based on Buddhist
ethical principles of nonviolence and nonharming, and attention to compassionate
action, livelihood, and speech. As he was dying, Buddha was reported to have said to
his attendant, Ananda: "Be a lamp unto thyself; pursue your deliverance with dili-
gence" (Burtt, 1955, p. 49). No one was selected to teach or govern the Buddhist community that outlived him. The Dharma, that is, the teachings of Buddhism, would be
the teacher not a person or an institution (Kornfield, 1977). In Tibetan Buddhism, sur-
render to the guru as well as various imaginal and visualization practices are an essential facet of the path to awakening. In Pure Land Buddhism from China, faith is
absolutely central to one's salvation.

In the face of these and other differences in worldview and practices, Buddhists
offer an interesting spin to the culture wars that conservatives and multiculturalists
engage in academia in the United States. Members of every school of Buddhist
thought universally idealize Buddha as the founder and most enlightened exemplar
of Buddhism, even as they then proceed to present their particular brand of Buddhism
as the best and most enlightened version. But to have assimilated the crucial currents
in the social sciences and humanities in recent years is to be profoundly skeptical
about any such claims to objectivity or truth. For we are now infinitely more attuned
to the way that such claims are illusory and are based, as Foucault (1980) repeatedly
asserted, on power and a will to dominate. The interesting question then becomes not
"Whose Buddhism is the correct one?" but rather, "What becomes evaded and suppressed by such claims to cultural hegemony?"

The implications of Foucault's reflections on knowledge and power for my own discourse are at least twofold. First, there is no single or superior Buddhism. Second, the Buddhism one chooses to practice or utilize in a study such as this one needs to be justified in terms of its usefulness or pragmatic yield rather than spurious claims to some putative objectivity or authority.

In this chapter I focus on classical Theravadin Buddhism arising in India in the sixth century B.C.E. My reflections will also be informed, sometimes only implicitly, by the iconoclastic spirit of Zen Buddhism of China and Japan, with its eschewing of metaphysical speculation and its attention to the truth of one's experience, rather than conventional or received knowledge. Let me give one example of how the spirit of Zen has shaped my conception of Buddhism. Buddhism is conventionally treated as a world religion with sacred doctrines, ancestor worship, a community of believers, "houses of worship," religious icons, ritualistic practices, and so forth. Believing in Buddhist doctrines such as rebirth and reincarnation, from this perspective, would seem to be central to being a Buddhist. But the answer to the Zen koan "Where did Nansen go after death?" for example, is "Excuse me, I've got to make dinner" (Hoffman, 1975, pp. 129-132). This raises provocative questions about such a conception of Buddhism. Immersion in the antimetaphysical world of Zen—with its emphasis on actuality as opposed to religious doctrines or theories about human beings and the cosmos—can widen our view of it. Might Buddhism be more fertile than the traditional conception implies?

What is most radical and interesting about Buddhism from my perspective (which I realize may be a minority one outside Zen Buddhism) are the meditative methods of self-investigation (by which I mean the operationalizable techniques for studying human thought and emotions) and the Buddhist ethics, not its conventional religious features. I see no evidence that a Buddhism without rebirth or reincarnation would lose its emancipatory possibilities. From my perspective, rebirth and reincarnation are experience-distant constructs far removed from the actual experience of many if not most practitioners. In the spirit of Zen I focus on meditative methods of self-investigation and Buddhist ethics, rather than Buddhist doctrines and speculations such as reincarnation and rebirth.

From the perspective I take, Buddhism can be considered an ethical psychology with a highly developed method for self-investigation. Buddhism is most potentially liberatory and transformative, according to this vision, when it is shorn of some of its doctrinal elements such as reincarnation, magical cosmologies, and so forth. When its experience-near method and its ethics are juxtaposed with psychoanalytic methods of self-inquiry and psychoanalytic perspectives on human development, the dynamics of interpersonal relationships, and the process of change, new and evocative insights and approaches to human beings in the world emerge.

My choice of focusing on one tradition, namely Theravadin Buddhism and occasionally on Zen, is not meant to cast aspersions on other Buddhist schools of thought such as Tibetan Buddhism or the Pure Land sects of Buddhism in China. Different schools of thought are different vehicles. I have chosen Theravadin Buddhism because in my experience it offers a highly sophisticated phenomenology of mind, a nontheistic worldview, and ethics grounded in various facets of everyday life. It is thus very amenable to dialogue and integration with Western psychological thought. Buddha's reflections bear repeating.

> Would he be a clever man if out of gratitude for the raft that has carried him across the stream to the other shore, he should cling to it, take it on his back, and walk about with the weight of it? Would not the clever man be the one who left the raft (of no use to him

any longer) to the current stream, and walked ahead without turning back to look at it? Is it simply a tool to be cast away and forsaken once it has served the purpose for which it was made? In the same way the vehicle of the doctrine is to be cast away and forsaken once the shore of enlightenment has been attained. (Smith, 1986, pp. 209-210)

Before presenting a brief overview of Theravadin Buddhist thought in order to contextualize my subsequent discussion, let me delineate the perspective I adopt in this study. Broadly speaking, there have been three stages in the drama of psychoanalysis and Buddhism. The work of psychoanalyst Franz Alexander (1931) represents the first stage of the encounter of psychoanalysis and Buddhism. Alexander falsely equates meditation with regression and pathology. In his blanket dismissal of Buddhism as training in an artificial catatonia, Alexander illustrates the Eurocentrism that has plagued psychoanalysis. Eurocentrism refers to the intellectually imperialistic tendency in much Western scholarship to assume that European and North American standards and values are the center of the moral and intellectual universe. From a Eurocentric perspective, Eastern thought is pathologized and marginalized. Eurocentrism has played a central role in the literature of psychoanalysis and Buddhism from Freud to the present.

The more sympathetic non-Eurocentric work of psychoanalysts such as Jung (1958); Horney (1945, 1987); Kelman (1960); Fromm, Suzuki, and Dematino (1960); Engler (1984); Rubin (1985, 1991, 1992, 1996); Roland (1988); Finn (1992); Suler (1993); Eigen (1998); Magid (2002); Segal (2003); and Safran (2003) represents the second major trend in the literature on psychoanalysis and Buddhism: an attempt to take Buddhism more seriously. Although they have pointed to various aspects of Buddhism's salutary dimensions, including its ability to sensitize us to the inner life (Jung, 1958), enrich psychoanalytic listening (Rubin, 1985), improve affect demarcation and tolerance (Rubin, 1992, 1996), promote "well-being" (being fully awake and alive [Fromm, 1960]), and expand psychoanalytic conceptions of subjectivity (Roland, 1988; Rubin, 1992, 1993, 1996; Suler, 1993), they tend, with the exception of the work of Roland (1988), Rubin (1991, 1992, 1993, 1996), Engler (1984), Eigen (1998), Magid (2002), and Safran (2003), to neglect clinical issues and case material. There are thus few extant precedents for integrating psychoanalysis and Buddhism.

The two most compelling attempts to integrate Asian and Western psychology are Jack Engler's (1984) "developmental" model and transpersonal theorist Ken Wilber's (1979; 1986) "spectrum psychology." Both thinkers exhibit an exemplary mastery of both traditional psychological theory and spiritual disciplines, as well as an integration of theory and practice.

Engler attempts to integrate conventional psychotherapeutic and contemplative spiritual disciplines by seeing them as complementary facets of a developmental continuum with the former representing "lower" stages of development and the latter representing "higher" stages. Developing a strong, cohesive sense of self is the precondition of the contemplative task of disidentifying from the illusion of substantial selfhood. (Wilber, Engler, & Brown 1986) conclude: "You have to be somebody before you can be nobody" (p. 124). Engler's work makes a highly important contribution to the field of East-West studies by including a greater range of development than either psychotherapeutic or spiritual perspectives alone offer. Both psychoanalysis and Buddhism lack a full-spectrum psychology. The former has little to say about psychological maturity and health. The latter neglects "earlier stages of personality organization and the types of suffering that result from a failure to negotiate them" (Wilber, Engler, & Brown, 1986, p. 49).

There is a tension in the developmental stage model between a complementary view of human development (one is first somebody and then nobody) and a complex, noncomplementary conception. In terms of the former:

> Meditation and psychotherapy cannot be positioned on a continuum in any mutually exclusive way as though both simply pointed to a different range of human development. Not only do post-enlightenment stages of meditation apparently affect the manifestation and management of neurotic conditions, but this type of conflict continues to be experienced after enlightenment. (Brown & Engler, 1986, p. 212)

In terms of the latter view, Brown and Engler conclude that "psychological maturity and the path to enlightenment are perhaps two complementary but not entirely unrelated lines of growth; or . . . they do represent different levels or ranges of health/growth along a continuum, but with much more complex relationships between them than have previously been imagined (p. 212).

Although Engler acknowledges that there are very complex interactions between conventional and contemplative stages and a "rigidly linear and unidirectional model is not at all what we have in mind" (Wilber, Engler, & Brown, 1986, p. 7), the complexity of interaction between "psychological" and "spiritual" perspectives is not addressed or spelled out. The limitations of contemplative perspectives and the value of conventional psychological viewpoints are also neglected—especially the way the latter might enrich the former.

Transpersonal psychology was developed in the late 1960s by thinkers who felt that existing psychologies neglected the full range of human possibilities, including transcendent states. Transpersonal psychology focuses on such things as altered states of consciousness and well-being, meditation, optimal psychological health, and the integration of therapeutic and spiritual disciplines. Ken Wilber (1986), Roger Walsh (1980), Frances Vaughan (1980), Stan Grof (1985), and Charles Tart (1975) are some of its esteemed practitioners.

Wilber's spectrum psychology (1979, 1986) attempts to create a marriage between Western psychological perspectives on human development and psychopathology, and Eastern contemplative understandings of consciousness and optimal states of health. His work exhibits encyclopedic scholarship, an exemplary groundedness in contemplative practices as well as theory, and an openness to diverse psychotherapeutic and spiritual traditions. In Wilber's work the quest to integrate Eastern contemplative and Western psychotherapeutic thought receives its most comprehensive and sophisticated expression.

Central to the spectrum of psychology is what Aldous Huxley (1970) has termed the *philosophia perennis*, the "perennial philosophy," a doctrine about the nature of humankind and reality underlying every major metaphysical tradition. It represents a "reality untouched by time or place, true everywhere and everywhen" (Wilber, 1979, p. 7). According to Wilber, corresponding to the perennial philosophy there exists a *psychologia perennis*, a perennial psychology—a "universal view as to the nature of human consciousness, which expresses the very same insights as the perennial philosophy but in more decidedly psychological language" (1979, p. 7).

For Wilber, the crucial insight of the perennial psychology is that our "innermost consciousness is identical to the absolute and ultimate reality of the universe," which he terms "mind," which "is what there is and all there is, spaceless and therefore infinite, timeless and therefore eternal, outside of which nothing exists. On this level . . . (one) is identified with the universe, the All—or rather . . . is the All" (1979, p. 9).

According to the perennial psychology this is "the only real state of consciousness, all others being essentially illusions" (p. 9).

The perennial psychology is the foundation of Wilber's "spectrum of consciousness" model. The central underlying assumption of Wilber's model is that "human personality is a multileveled manifestation or expression of a single consciousness, just as in physics the electromagnetic spectrum is viewed as a multibanded expression of a single, characteristic electromagnetic wave" (1979, p. 8). Consciousness, like light, exists on and is composed of various bands or spectrums, which develop through a series of stages and which can be correlated with corresponding states of self-organization and self-blindness. Different psychological and spiritual traditions address these different levels.

Wilber (1986) has proposed 10 levels to the spectrum. In ascending order, they are the following: sensoriphysical, phantasmic-emotional, representational mind, rule/role mind, formal-reflexive mind, vision-logic, psychic, subtle, causal, and ultimate. It would distract from the central argument to define Wilber's terms. For our purposes, it is sufficient to note that each stage of development has it own particular type of self-experience, cognitive development, moral sensibilities, potential distortions, and pathologies. Each level is characterized by a different sense of personal identity, ranging from the narrow and circumscribed sense of identity associated with the sensoriphysical level in which one identifies only with the realms of matter, sensation, and perception, to the ultimate level in which one is identified with the totality of the universe. According to Wilber, the great religious sages such as Buddha and the esteemed twentieth-century Hindu saint Ramana Maharshi are exemplars of the highest level of the spectrum.

On this level, one is identified with the universe, the "All," or rather, one *is* the All. This level is not an altered or abnormal state of consciousness but is "the only real state of consciousness, all others being essentially illusions" (Wilber, 1979, p. 9). One's "innermost consciousness is identical to the absolute and ultimate reality of the universe" (pp. 8–9).

Each higher stage is less "selfcentric" than its predecessors (Wilber, 1986). Each level can be correlated with corresponding ways of perceiving and misperceiving reality. Wilber maintains that different psychotherapeutic and spiritual traditions address and are best suited for different levels of the spectrum. Western psychotherapies, such as psychoanalysis, Gestalt therapy, and transactional analysis, address pathology and lower levels of the spectrum, whereas contemplative disciplines such as Buddhism are recommended for higher stages of the spectrum and the deepest kinds of transformation and liberation. For Wilber, psychoanalysis and Buddhism are complementary.

The value of Wilber's work, like Engler's (e.g., Wilber, Engler, & Brown, 1984), is at least twofold: First, it disentangles meditative states of heightened clarity, health, and freedom from psychotherapeutic reductionism. Wilber and Engler (Wilber, Engler, & Brown, 1984) maintain that contemplative practices constitute a higher and advanced level of personality development "beyond ego" or the separate, autonomous, self-centered self that is the acme of mental health in most psychotherapies. Their second contribution is to offer guidance for meditators with psychological disturbances who are failing to make important discriminations in their meditation practice. Meditative practices, according to Wilber and Engler (Wilber, Engler, & Brown, 1986), may attract individuals with self-disorders, by which I mean, people who experience themselves as brittle, fragile, worthless, vulnerable, and prone to self-esteem fluctuations. Meditators who experience self-issues of this sort, obviously not all meditators, may confuse their experiences of identity diffusion and depersonalization with genuine spiritual realization. For such individuals, Engler and Wilber recommend traditional therapy to shore up the self prior to pursuing meditation practice.

* * * *

Psychoanalysis and Buddhism offer fertile possibilities for cross-pollination. Mutual enrichment, however, has been impeded by the restrictive perspective of previous studies, which have adopted one of three monolithic viewpoints in characterizing their multifaceted relationship. These are what I would term the shotgun wedding, bridesmaid, and pseudocomplementary/token egalitarian models. I will briefly discuss each view before presenting my own alternative perspective.

Until relatively recently, much of the literature on Eastern and Western psychology has assumed, either explicitly or implicitly, that Buddhism and psychoanalysis are antithetical and incompatible. It is claimed that they occupy positions of unavoidable disagreement, from which there can be no escape, except by embracing one and abandoning the other (Rinzler & Gordan, 1980). Since psychoanalysis and Buddhism have very "different visions" of the mind and human existence, any attempt to join them is a "shotgun wedding" which "does justice to neither." A synthesis is thus "almost impossible" (Rinzler & Gordon, p. 52).

The most prevalent view of psychoanalysis and Buddhism is what I would term the bridesmaid stance, in which psychoanalysis plays second fiddle to Buddhism. In the earlier Eurocentric literature, Buddhism was often subordinate to psychoanalysis (e.g., Alexander, 1931). In its more recent Orientocentric guise, writers emphasize Buddhism's value for psychotherapy (Boss, 1965; Chogyam, 1983; Deatherage, 1975) while neglecting the latter's value for Buddhism. Orientocentrism does not refer to the "Orientalism" literary and culture critic Edward Said (1979) critiques when he describes the tendency among Western commentators on the Orient to utilize a imperialistic discourse about Asia, which fashions a distorted and reductionistic picture of "the East" in order to intellectually colonize Asia and psychologically fortify itself. Rather, it refers to the mirror-opposite danger to Eurocentrism: the idealizing and privileging of Asian thought—treating it as sacred—and the neglect, if not the dismissal, of the value of Western psychological perspectives. The potential contribution of psychoanalysis is then neglected.

A student of Zen told a Zen master that psychotherapy and Zen had similar effects in overcoming suffering. The Zen master then said that the psychotherapist is just another patient (Matthiessen, 1987, p. 160). This example illustrates Orientocentrism, as does the absence of exploration concerning what value Western psychotherapies might have for non-Western thought in the preeminent, extant anthologies in the field of East-West studies such as Welwood's (1979) *Meetings of the Ways*, Tart's (1975) *Transpersonal Psychologies*, Boorstein's (1980) *Transpersonal Psychotherapy*, and Walsh and Vaughan's (1980) *Beyond Ego*. Orientocentrism is so unconscious that no one has even remarked on its presence! I discuss Orientocentrism later. When the bridesmaid perspective is operative, commerce between Buddhism and psychoanalysis occurs, but only in one direction.

The third way that psychoanalysis and Buddhism have been approached, arguably the most compelling perspective, is Wilber's "spectrum of consciousness" model and Engler's developmental model. The spectrum model has tremendous theoretical and emotional appeal, as it promises to integrate apparently irreconcilable psychological and spiritual systems. Chaos seems to be reduced and seekers after truth no longer feel like UN delegates without an interpreter.

The spectrum model has several fundamental flaws. Development, according to this model, involves progressing through discrete and stratified stages ranging from disavowing aspects of one's identity to recognizing one's fundamental interconnectedness with everything. This presupposes, without actually demonstrating, that there is a uniformity to one's identity and stage of development, and a separation and division of the psychological and spiritual.

The pathology of certain visionaries (Gordon, 1987; Schneider, 1987) and the prescience of some schizophrenics (Searles, 1972) teaches us that human functioning is much more complex than such schematic accounts suggest. One can experience the highest stage on Wilber's scale—unity consciousness—and perceive the interconnectedness of human existence while also operating at times on "lower" levels, demonstrating myopia about one's body, feelings, or relationships. Some of the spiritual teachers embroiled in enormously egocentric and myopic behavior toward others around power, money, and sex demonstrate less interpersonal sensitivity and morality than people who are apparently operating on "lower" levels. One could also be operating on "lower" levels of the spectrum in certain areas while experiencing "higher" facets in other areas. I have worked with schizophrenics, for example, who struggle with the deepest kinds of self-disorders and have also at times perceived insights associated with "higher" levels of development on Wilber's model. They also have not treated others so capriciously and insensitively as the spiritual teachers who have manipulated others for their own benefit.

Because of the asymmetrical nature of human development, we all operate on different levels depending on which particular area of human experience we are confronting. One could be quite aware of one's mental life and be disconnected from one's body—as some spiritual teachers and analysts are—or one could be attuned to one's body and mind and relatively unaware of one's interpersonal relations and impact on others. The complexity and multidimensionality of human experience and development is obscured by linear, hierarchical, developmental models.

Wilber's model does not achieve genuine integration. The attempted "marriage" of psychological and spiritual perspectives is an asymmetrical affair in which Buddhism (and other contemplative disciplines) is actually viewed as superior to psychological thought, offering a privileged and true description of how humans really are. A tacit inequality is hidden underneath the nominal complementary. There is an illusory rapprochement in which psychoanalysis and Buddhism are discreetly segregated to separate and unequal realms of reality, and one is granted a special status. Whereas psychoanalysis usually pathologizes non-Western thought, transpersonal theorists sometimes romanticize it.

Within the transpersonal ranks, what I have recently termed Orientocentrism (Rubin, 1991, 1993, 1996), not Eurocentrism, tends to predominate. When Orientocentrism reigns, then Buddhism is romanticized and uncritically overvalued, and psychoanalysis is disparaged or neglected (Rubin, 1996, 2004). The partiality of the Buddhist worldview then remains unexplored and unconscious, and the value of psychoanalysis is then neglected.

None of these perspectives on the relationship between the Western psychotherapeutic and Eastern contemplative disciplines—the shotgun wedding, bridesmaid approach, or pseudo-complementary view—are wrong, but they reduce to a single factor or characterization what is a complex relationship with a multitude of dimensions. There are ways in which psychoanalysis and Buddhism are antithetical, complementary, and synergistic, but they are not simply any one of these all the time.

BEYOND EUROCENTRISM AND ORIENTOCENTRISM

"Truth" suggested Anatole France, "lies in the nuances." The nuances are exactly what the standard approaches to Western psychotherapies and Eastern contemplative disciplines neglect and eclipse. The relationship between Buddhism and psychoanalysis is more complex than the existing accounts suggest, forming not a singular pattern of influence, but rather resembling a heterogeneous mosaic composed of elements that are, depending on the specific topic, antithetical, complementary, and synergistic. For example, the goals of psychoanalysis and Buddhism are antithetical; the former focuses on strengthening one's sense of self, while the latter views such an enterprise as the very cause of psychological suffering. Meditative techniques for training attentiveness complement and enrich the psychoanalytic perspective on listening, whereas the psychoanalytic account of defense and resistance enhances the Buddhist understanding of interferences to meditation practice. Psychoanalytic and Buddhist strategies for facilitating transformation are, at least in some ways, synergistic.

The Eurocentrism of traditional Western psychology and the Orientocentrism of more recent writings on psychotherapeutic and contemplative disciplines both inhibit the creation of a contemplative therapeutics or an analytic meditation because they establish an intellectual embargo on commerce between Asian and Western psychology. An alternative perspective is necessary for the genuine insights of each tradition to emerge. In contrast to the Eurocentrism of psychoanalysis and the Orientocentrism of much recent discourse on psychoanalysis and Buddhism, I will be recommending a more egalitarian relationship in which there is mutual respect; the absence of denigration, deification, submission, or superiority; and a genuine interest in what they could teach each other.

The egalitarian relationship I am pointing toward is not meant to be a complementarity that erases differences or subsumes either psychoanalysis into Buddhism or Buddhism into psychoanalysis in the act of detecting similarities. Since the advent of deconstructionism, the limitations of searching only for commonalities between two systems of thought appear more problematic. The search misses what is most interesting, which is how the systems are different, what the common denominators eclipse, and how both systems are incompatible and mutually enriching.

The relationship between psychoanalysis and Buddhism is not without disagreements, points of contention, and conflict. But such turmoil can be healthy insofar as it impedes orthodoxy, dogmatism, and premature closure, and can promote cross-pollination and growth.

What I have discovered since approaching psychoanalysis and Buddhism in this way is that both traditions have a great deal of merit, but neither provides a complete picture of human nature, transformation, and liberation. Each offers a valuable and incomplete perspective, neglecting indispensable elements included in the other. For example, Buddhist models of health could teach psychoanalysis that there are possibilities for emotional well-being that far exceed the limits described by psychoanalytic models, whereas psychoanalytic accounts of defensive processes and resistance enhance the Buddhist understanding of the interferences to the meditation practice and the growth process. Since neither tradition has the last word on these issues, both traditions could be enriched if their respective insights were integrated into a more inclusive and encompassing perspective—which currently does not exist—that takes into account their respective contributions and elucidates their blindspots while attempting to bolster their limitations.

Once it is recognized that both traditions are valuable and incomplete, two questions emerge: What does each tradition illuminate? What does each tradition omit?

With these two questions in mind, I shall examine psychoanalysis and Buddhism along three dimensions common to any psychological, religious, or philosophical system: their view of reality and model of ideal health, their view of self, and their conception of the process designed to reach its stated goals, which includes a theory of the obstacles to the process (e.g., Shapiro, 1989). Before addressing these questions, let me give a brief overview of Buddhism. This provides a context for the subsequent discussion.

Buddhism is the codification of the insights about human psychology developed by Gotama Buddha in the sixth century B.C.E. in India in the course of his meditative investigations of his own mind. The Sanskrit translation of the word Budh is "awakened." Whereas his contemporaries were "asleep" in a kind of socially sanctioned trance, unaware of the actual texture of their experience, Buddha was awakened to the realities of birth and death. Classical Buddhism could be considered an ethical psychology of optimal health and wellness, rather than a theistic religion. The primary emphasis is placed on one's learning about and transforming the mind and body through one's own direct experience as opposed to faith in or devotion to a deity.

I briefly describe some essential facets of Buddhist psychology and practice as a reference point for the subsequent discussion. The central teaching of Buddhism is the four Noble Truths. This doctrine delineates the symptoms, diagnosis, and treatment plan for alleviating human suffering. The First Noble Truth of Buddhism presents the salient characteristic of human life, *Dukkha*, a Sanskrit word for a bone out of its socket and a wheel off its axle. *Awryness* and unsatisfactoriness are inherent features of the universe. Life is dislocated and out of joint. No human being, according to Buddhism, escapes some sort of suffering and discontent. The Second Noble Truth presents the cause of suffering: desire, attachment, and craving, that is, the tendency of the mind to grasp or cling. Suffering, from a Buddhist perspective, derives from our difficulty acknowledging a fundamental aspect of life: that everything is impermanent and transitory. We fall in love and anticipate an everlasting joy and ecstasy, and then the honeymoon phase ends. We believe that our favorite psychoanalytic theory is the capital T Truth and then clinical experience demonstrates that something else is more motivationally important for a particular patient. Suffering arises when we resist the flow of life and cling to people, events, and ideas as permanent. The doctrine of impermanence also includes the notion that there is no single self that is the subject of our changing experience. The Third Noble Truth is that suffering can be completely eradicated. The Fourth Noble Truth provides a treatment plan, the Noble Eightfold Path, to address suffering and achieve ideal health. The Eightfold Path includes such things as right understanding, or accurate awareness of the nature of reality; right speech, or speaking truthfully and compassionately; right livelihood, or engaging in work that promotes rather than harms life; and right mindfulness, or seeing things as they are.

The central investigative method of Buddhism is meditation: the careful, nonjudgmental attentiveness to whatever is occurring in the present moment. Meditation often conjures up a host of distorting associations from otherworldly asceticism to narcissistic navel-gazing. Meditation is not religious dogma, self-hypnosis, regression, or pathology (Alexander, 1931).[1] Rather, it is an incisive technique for what I have recently come to think of as *experience-near self-investigation*.

---

[1]This is, of course, not true of analysts such as Jung (1958), Horney (1987), Kelman (1960), Fromm (1960), Roland (1988), Coltart (1996), Eigen (1998; 2001), Grotstein (2000), Magid (2002), Safran (2003), Finn (1992), Cooper (1999), Segal (2003), and myself, among others, who discerned value in Eastern contemplative practices.

There are two main types of meditation, *concentrative* and *insight*. (The analytic meditation found in Tibetan Buddhism could be viewed as a form of insight meditation.) In concentrative meditation, one focuses on a single object, such as the breath, with wholehearted attentiveness. It is an exclusive state of mind. One excludes everything but the object of concentration. When one notices that his or her attention has wandered, one returns attention to the breath. Concentrative meditation cultivates a high degree of mental focus. In the traditional Buddhist practice developed by Buddha, one often begins with concentrative meditation.

When the attentiveness is developed and stabilized, then one practices insight meditation. In insight meditation, one attends without attachment or aversion to whatever thoughts, feelings, fantasies, or somatic sensations one is experiencing. The purpose of such a practice, contrary to popular misconception, is not to make anything happen such as silencing or emptying the chattering mind, but to relate to whatever is happening in one's experience (no matter how painful) in a very different way than we ordinarily do—with tolerance and a sense of inner spaciousness. To those of you who have never meditated, being present to what we are experiencing without aversion or clinging might sound like the simplest task. Given our normal state of distractedness, it is actually enormously difficult. It requires discipline and practice to train the mind to be really present. One can practice meditation either in a retreat-like setting or in one's daily life. An analyst could, for example, meditate between patients, and an analysand could meditate at home or before a therapy session.

In order to meditate, one sits physically still in an upright position and pays attention to the immediate flow of one's moment-to-moment experience, attending to the breathing process and silently noting the experience of inhalation and exhalation at the nostrils or abdomen. The effort is not to control the breathing, but to be attentive to it. Meditation proceeds in stages. At the beginning it is difficult to even pay attention for five consecutive seconds. As meditators know all too well, as we attempt to pay attention to our breathing, we become distracted. Memories, daydreams, anxieties, and insights arise. We replay old experiences or plan new ventures. There is an apparently endless flood of thoughts, feelings, and fantasies. One of these usually catches our attention and before we know it we have traveled down a path toward something far removed from the present moment. We have, for example, constructed a scenario that has never actually happened or we have replayed something that happened many years ago. We are oblivious to the present moment.

As soon as one notices that his or her attention has wandered, one resumes attending to the breath. After a few seconds our attention wanders again. Like a child who reaches for one toy, becomes bored, and reaches for another, and then another, the mind keeps jumping from one thought, feeling, or fantasy to another. Noticing that we have been inattentive slowly cultivates increased attentiveness and focus.

As attentiveness increases and becomes more refined, we can use the developing capacity to focus the mind to observe the nature of our consciousness. Like a movie that is slowed down, we can see how one frame of our consciousness leads into another—how particular feelings condition specific reactions. One might become aware, for example, that he or she is making expansive plans after feeling diminished. Or a person might realize that he or she gets angry at a child when feeling scared about the child's safety.

As our awareness becomes clearer and more focused, we experience a sense of psychological spaciousness: We do not become as entangled in reactive patterns of feeling and thinking. When praised, one might allow oneself to bask in its warm glow instead of automatically devaluing it. Psychological resilience is cultivated; when we are unsettled or distracted, we regain clarity more quickly. We can begin to notice within the first few seconds that we are unthinkingly attacking ourselves, thus avoiding getting emotionally hijacked and caught in a downward spiral of self-contempt and self-destructive behavior.

Meditation lessens distractedness, quiets the inner pandemonium, and concentrates the mind. Fostering what Horney (1987) termed, "wholehearted attention" (p. 18), meditation cultivates precisely the quality that Freud (1912) recognized was essential to psychoanalytic listening, namely "evenly-hovering attention." Unfortunately, Freud identified this state of mind but never offered positive recommendations for how to cultivate it. His writings focused on the interferences to this sort of listening, not what to do to actually facilitate it (Rubin, 1985). Meditation can also reduce self-criticism, aid psychoanalysts and patients in tolerating a greater range of affect without the need to deny or decomplexify it, and foster the capacity to relate to self and others with greater openness and fluidity (Rubin, 1998).

At first glance it might seem that speaking of psychoanalysis and Buddhism in tandem is advocating a forced and unproductive association. After all, several fundamental disparities between them exist. Buddhism is a spiritual system developed 2,500 years ago in India for attaining enlightenment; psychoanalysis is a psychotherapeutic system arising in Europe in the late nineteenth century addressing psychopathology and mental illness. To attain enlightenment, Buddhism recommends recognizing the illusoriness of our taken-for-granted sense of self as a unified, static, unchanging, autonomous entity. Most analysts, with the exception of Lacanians, claim that strengthening the self is crucial to the psychoanalytic process. Buddhism emphasizes the necessity of letting go of all desires and self-centeredness, while psychoanalytic self-psychology maintains that ideals and goals play a crucial role in psychological well-being.

Similarities between both traditions, however, make a comparison between them intriguing. Both are concerned with the nature and alleviation of human suffering and each has both a diagnosis and "treatment plan" for alleviating human misery. The three other important things they share make a comparison between them possible and potentially productive. First, they are pursued within the crucible of an emotionally intimate relationship between either an analyst/analysand or a teacher/student. Second, they emphasize some similar experiential processes—evenly hovering attention and free association in psychoanalysis, and meditation in Buddhism. Third, they recognize that obstacles impede the attempt to facilitate change, such as the self-protective strategies analysts have termed resistance and defensive processes in psychoanalysis, and the "hindrances," "fetters," and "impediments" in Buddhism. In the next section I examine their respective worldviews and visions of ideal mental health.

PSYCHOANALYTIC AND BUDDHIST WORLDVIEWS AND VISIONS OF IDEAL HEALTH

Psychoanalysis and Buddhism are *stories* about and *strategies* for addressing human life. Treating Buddhism and psychoanalysis as *narratives* rather than as sacred *tradition*, by which I mean sources of absolute wisdom that provide a blueprint for how to live in the present, may shift the way we think about tradition in general and each tradition in particular. Instead of viewing either of them as received truths, universally valid for all times and places, we might conceive of them as human creations arising in particular historical and sociocultural contexts. The value of psychoanalysis and

Buddhism thus resides in how well they help people in the present age live with greater awareness, tolerance, and care.

Tradition has two meanings: It means to pass on and it means to betray. Tradition can be enslaving as well as enabling. It may give one an identity and an orientation in the world, even as it limits one's horizon of vision and stifles one's development. It is inhibiting because it assimilates the present into the past and predisposes us to look toward the past to solve dilemmas in the present. "Tradition is important just as history is important, not as a vise to squeeze the present into but as a steppingstone to grow from" (Kramer & Alstad, 1993).

Once tradition is no longer viewed as sacred, its essential revisability becomes more crucial. Buddhism, as well as psychoanalysis, needs to be open to feedback about its limits, and to change, evolve, and grow so that it can respond to the living moment.

Let's return to the stories psychoanalysis and Buddhism tell about human existence. Stories are made, as the historian and cultural critic Hayden White (1973) notes, "by including some events and excluding others, by stressing some and subordinating others" (p. 6, note 5). "Emplotment" is what White terms this process of exclusion, emphasis, and subordination in the interest of creating a particular kind of story. Literary theorist Northrop Frye (1957) has identified four archetypal genres or types of plot structures—tragedy, irony, romance, and comedy. Each genre offers a conception of the world that is particular and partial, highlighting and omitting certain facets of the world.

Psychoanalysis is underwritten by a "tragic" view of the universe, by which I mean, it recognizes the inescapable mysteries, dilemmas, conflicts, and afflictions pervading human existence (Schafer, 1976). Tragic implies an acknowledgment that time is irreversible and unredeemable; that is, humans are beings moving toward death, not rebirth, choices entail conflict and compromise, and suffering and loss are inevitable. Religious consolations are quixotic in the tragic vision. A Buddhist's claims about enlightenment, that is, achieving permanent and irreversible cessation of egoism, vanity, self-deception, and suffering, would seem illusory in a tragic vision.

Psychoanalytic views of health emerge directly from this tragic view of the world. Psychoanalysis is essentially a psychology of illness that focuses on what is wrong with people. It is no accident that health does not appear in the *Standard Edition* of Freud. Freud (Breuer & Freud, 1895) claimed that the best humans can do is transform "neurotic misery" into "common human unhappiness" (p. 304). Psychoanalysis neglects wellness or exceptional states of health and functioning. Health, in the less arid and less depressogenic mood of contemporary psychoanalysis, involves self-integration and self-enrichment—the development of a cohesive, integrated, and multidimensional self and the cultivation of more complex and enriching modes of relatedness. But states of health, wellness, compassion, and wisdom that are central to Buddhism are neglected in even this view of health in contemporary psychoanalysis, except in the writings of such analysts as Grotstein (2000), Eigen (2001), and Rubin (2004).

Buddhism adopts a "romantic" view of the world. "Romance" refers not to romantic involvement, infatuation with another, or idealized love, but rather to a view of the world that personal and familial conditioning can be transcended and that ultimate meaning on a grand design can be achieved. In the romantic vision, life is viewed as a quest involving the hero's or heroine's "transcendence of the world of experience, his [or her] victory over it, and his [or her] final liberation" (Frye, 1957, p. 8). Given the emphasis on the pervasiveness of suffering in Buddhism, it may seem odd to claim that Buddhism is emplotted in a romantic narrative. Buddhism's diagnosis of the human condition is tragic, but its prognosis is romantic. That Buddhism is a romantic narrative about human existence is demonstrated by its belief in the possibility of getting beyond one's psychological conditioning and experiencing transcendence and unqualified fulfillment.

The Buddhist view of health is enlightenment, which is defined differently in each of the three main Buddhist traditions. To Zen master Dogen, the founder of Soto Zen, enlightenment meant "intimacy with all things" (e.g., Rubin, 1996, p. 83; Dogen, 1976). An esteemed Tibetan Buddhist monk-psychiatrist has described enlightenment as "no unconsciousness" (Lobsang Rapgay, personal communication, 1995). In classical Indian Buddhism, enlightenment is described as completely purifying the mind of "defilements," such as greed, hatred, and delusion, the removal of which is said to result in the transcendence of psychological conditioning, the total cessation of suffering, and the presence of profound love and compassion. An enlightened meditator in that tradition is said to be without any trace of egoism and self-deceit, in a permanent and irreversible state of clarity, equanimity, loving kindness, and wisdom (Rubin, 1996).

The times we live in demand both a sobering recognition of the fragility and tenuousness of our condition and a decisive and a progressive or visionary response to the enormous challenges that we collectively face. Optimism is a better strategy for change than pessimism (Joel Kramer, personal communication, 1995). Pessimism often breeds paralysis, which inhibits the motivation to change. But ungrounded optimism can result in an illusory and disabling conception of reality.

With his notion of "pessimism of the intellect, optimism of the will," the Italian Marxist Antonio Gramsci (1971, p. 175, note 75) provides one possible way of theoretically integrating the stories psychoanalysis and Buddhism tell about reality and ideal health so that they might speak to the concerns of citizens confronting meaninglessness, disconnection, self-alienation, and so forth.

Psychoanalysis is a "hermeneutics of suspicion" (Ricoeur, 1970), by which I mean it questions and often demystifies (or attempts to demystify) conventional and unquestioned assumptions about motives and meanings. Psychoanalysis can help Buddhists detect where they neglect unconsciousness and are being self-deceptive—where, for example, self-abasement in a Buddhist meditator can masquerade as spiritual asceticism. Psychoanalysis can temper Buddhism's unqualified belief in self-transcendence. Buddhist teachers are often presented as being beyond self-deceit. For those spiritual seekers who are experiencing an idealizing transference, such a possibility is enormously reassuring. The claim that a Buddhist teacher is without unconsciousness is about as likely as an analyst never experiencing countertransference again. Psychoanalysis teaches Buddhism that psychological conditioning and emotional strife cannot be transcended or eliminated. Psychoanalysis can enlighten Buddhists about where unconsciousness, transference, and countertransference live in Buddhism's theories, institutions, and practices. That Buddhism has pockets of unconsciousness is suggested by three things: the residues of pathology found in enlightened meditators (e.g., Brown & Engler, 1986), the plethora of scandals in Buddhist communities, and the nature of consciousness. Rorschach studies of enlightened meditators at Harvard suggested that these meditators had intrapsychic conflict, struggles with dependency and needs for nurturance, fear and doubt regarding relationships, and fear of destructiveness (pp. 188–189). In recent years, there has been a plethora of scandals in Buddhist communities involving Buddhist teachers from both Asia and the United States (those supposedly self-realized beings who are paragons of self-awareness, health, and virtue) illegally expropriating funds from the community, succumbing to substance abuse, and sexually exploiting nonconsenting female students (Boucher, 1988). Few people have confronted these scandals directly. Typically, they are denied or rationalized. One way of attempting to sidestep and ignore the disturbing implications of this plethora of immoral behavior is to assert that Western Buddhists have insufficiently internalized Buddhism and its ethics because they have grown up in a non-Buddhist culture. But the fact that these scandals involve indigenous Buddhists from Buddhist countries, as well as "homegrown" American Buddhist teachers, casts doubt on this defense. These scandals among Buddhist teachers suggest that these teachers have areas of self-blindness and egocentricity. The nature of mental life also casts doubt on Buddhist claims about the permanent and irreversible transformation of consciousness and the eradication of conflict. Because mental life is fluid and partially unconscious, there is no final resting place of complete self-awareness and inner peace. Conflict and suffering cannot be eliminated from mental life.

Buddhism's romanticism, its belief in radical possibilities of self-transformation, can temper the excessive pessimism in psychoanalysis' psychology of illness. The trace of the tragic psychology of illness in psychoanalysis emerges implicitly in its neglect of such topics as creativity, spirituality, and optimal mental and physical health.[2] The psychoanalytic view of health is, according to Buddhism, a suboptimal state of being, an arrested state of development.

Buddhism can challenge the limitations of a psychoanalytic view of self that is excessively self-centered and restrictive (Rubin, 1996, 1998). This egocentricity emerges when we consider relationships and morality in psychoanalysis. Although a successful psychoanalytic treatment obviously fosters greater empathy for and attunement toward others, there is a tendency in psychoanalysis to cultivate an egocentric sense of self, in which one views the other as an *object* that does (or does not) fulfill the needs of the self, rather than a *subject* with its own separate values and needs. Analysts within the relational fold usefully highlight the relational nature of human development and treatment. But the legacy of a one-person, nonrelational view of patients emerges when moral issues arise in treatment. At such times the questions analysts ask often predispose patients to adopt a self-centered way of thinking about morality. If a patient is struggling, for example, with whether to take in his or her aging mother-in-law, many analysts would, I suspect, tend to ask not, "How would your decision impact the network of relationships you are embedded in?" but rather, "What do you think and feel and need to do?" The question assumes and pulls for an egocentric stance toward morality rather than a relational one (Rubin, 1998). Buddhism can encourage psychoanalysts to think about morality in a less self-centered way so that the needs and claims of the other, as well as the self, are given more weight. Buddhism can also teach psychoanalysis that the integrated self can foster a constricted way of living. The experience of meditation practice points toward a more uncongealed and unfettered sense of self and way of living.

---

[2]There are exceptions to this claim. Winnicott (1971), Milner (1987), Gedo (1996), McDougall (1995), Phillips (1993), Oremland (1997), and Roland (2002), among others, have been interested in the nature of creativity. But there is a pervasive tendency in psychoanalysis to view this topic pathologically and reductionistically. Freud's study of Leonardo Da Vinci was termed, for example, a pathography. In recent years there has also been a greater interest in spirituality in psychoanalysis among such analysts as Grotstein (2000), Eigen (1998, 2001), Ulanov (1985), and Corbett (1999). But again this is an exception rather than the rule.

Buddhism points toward possibilities for self-awareness, freedom, wisdom, and compassion that Western psychology in general and psychoanalysis in particular has never mapped. In other words, the Buddhist vision of health goes beyond the love and work Freud felt were essential to health or the authenticity and creativity that were central to Winnicott's vision (1971). It also goes beyond the humor, creativity, awareness of mortality, and wisdom that Kohut (1985) espoused, or the relational sensitivity and competence that interpersonally oriented clinicians value.

PSYCHOANALYTIC AND BUDDHIST APPROACHES TO THE MIND AND VIEWS OF THE SELF

Psychoanalysts and Buddhists examine self-experience from radically different vantagepoints that lead to very different conceptions of it. The meditative method involves a solitary individual paying careful, detailed attention to whatever she or he experiences in the present moment. I would like to stress three facets of the meditative method: the meditative process is a private, noncommunal[3] examination of one's consciousness, one utilizes a microscopic lens in examining one's experience and the meditative method, to borrow the language of linguistic theory, is synchronic; that is, one studies one's mind cross-sectionally—one examines oneself in the present moment rather than historically.

Examining one's immediate experience with the microscopic, "zoom lens" attentiveness cultivated by meditation lessens inner distractedness, quiets the inner pandemonium, and concentrates and focuses the mind. "Wholehearted attention" (Horney, 1987, p. 19) promotes greater receptivity and attunement to internal and interpersonal experiences. This fosters a clearer and more spacious perspective on one's experience. It can aid one in reducing self-criticism and tolerating a greater range of feelings without fleeing from them or getting lost in them. This is obviously of great benefit to both the spiritual seeker and the person in therapy. Psychoanalysts who meditate would have greater affect tolerance and would listen more attentively and empathetically to their patients. They might also have a less narcissistic relationship to their own favored theories, committing to particular ways of organizing the multidimensionality of the patient's material without being attached to the ultimate truth of their conceptions. Analysts who meditate might thus hold their theories more lightly rather than tightly (Rubin, 1998). Patients who meditate would reduce self-criticism, tolerate a greater range of feelings, and relate to self and others with greater flexibility and openness.

The non- or antiself that Buddhism "discovers" is directly related to its way of investigating self-experience. When self-experience is examined microscopically, one is predisposed to see the discontinuities in one's experience, an apparently unrelated flow of separate states of consciousness rather than a solidified self.

Meditative approaches to the mind are myopic as well as illuminating. They have blind spots that eclipse certain facets of self-experience. In exploring humans with a microscopic perspective, meditation promotes "near-sightedness," by which I mean,

---

[3]Sangha, the community of like-spirited spiritual seekers, is central to Buddhism. Nonetheless, meditation practice, even done in a Buddhist community (or with a group of Buddhists outside a community or retreat context), involves paying attention to one's own inner experience, which is an essentially isolative process and practice.

meditation neglects historical influences on the person arising from the distant past, including the shaping role of unconsciousness, transference, and character. The essentially isolative and noncommunal aspect of the meditative experience insures that there is a neglect of the kind of public dialogue, feedback, and validation that characterizes disciplines such as Western science and psychoanalysis. I say neglect because certain schools of Buddhism such as Zen offer a slight corrective for this with the emphasis on working with a meditation teacher. But the isolated nature of the meditative process still exists. And the Buddhist teacher does not systematically examine or work through transferences, relational enactments, and countertransference. These phenomena remain relatively unconscious in Buddhism.

There are several problems with the meditative method. First, Buddhism has an ambivalent relationship to emotional life. The meditative method counsels nonjudgmental attentiveness to whatever one experiences. This fosters greater openness to experience and helps the meditator access formerly unconscious thoughts, feelings, and fantasies. On the other hand, afflictive emotions, such as greed and hatred, are viewed in some meditative traditions such as classical Buddhism, as "defilements." The goal of meditation, from this Theravadin perspective, is to "purify" the mind of "defilements." (In Tibetan Buddhism the goal is transformation.) Trying to purify the mind establishes an aversive relationship to experience. Thought and emotions are viewed as obstacles that interfere with experiencing a deeper reality. Then we are unconsciously predisposed to devalue our experience, to wish to transcend or get rid of it rather than determine its shaping power and learn what it might teach us. During the first meditative retreat I ever participated in, a wealth of formerly unconscious thoughts and feelings arose during my meditations. I asked one of the Buddhist teachers how to handle this material. "Don't do anything," he counseled me. "Just let go of it."[4]

Letting go has its value when one is hypervigilant and overcontrolled, or caught in obsessive thinking or excessive worrying. But when we let go without investigating the meaning of our experience, like the Buddhist teacher recommended to me, then the unconscious ways that we conceive of and relate to ourselves and others can remain hidden. For patients who have experienced severe trauma, such as sexual abuse or physical torture, and who have "survived" by not registering or disconnecting from and segregating their experience, integrating formerly disavowed experiences seems crucial to the healing process. Prematurely detaching from such experiences makes it more difficult to understand some of the forces that motivate us in the present. Our lives are then restricted.

Psychoanalysis examines the self diachronically and "telescopically," that is, it investigates self-experience historically. It utilizes a wider-angle lens, a more generalized and unfocused mode of introspection, to examine the way the distant past influences the present. When one studies the self in this way, one is predisposed to

---

[4]This may be less true of Zen, in which there seems to be a greater emphasis on experiencing rather than transcending experience. If one cannot let go of an aversive experience such as physical pain in Zen practice, then one is encouraged to be the pain. Many meditators have experienced the way pain shifts or evaporates when one does this. But this strategy may not work as well with certain experiences that our patients struggle with, such as intense self-criticism or severe trauma. The Dalai Lama was shocked to hear that Americans suffered from "self-directed contempt" (Goleman, 1997, p. 196). He told a group of American scientists and mental health professionals that this experience was absent from Tibetan culture (Goleman, 1997).

"see" a substantial agent shaped by his or her past. Understanding our past gives us a powerful tool to transform the self in the present. Although Western psychotherapy goes deep into the roots of mental conditioning, exploring the past can become a way of evading responsibility for living in the present. The psychoanalytic approach to the mind can be "far-sighted," by which I mean that it may eclipse certain near-at-hand aspects of the self. In seeking the historical roots of our difficulties in living, psychoanalysis tends to neglect the shaping role of conditioning that arises in the present moment (e.g., Kramer & Alstad, 1993). This is, of course, less true of analysts who place more emphasis on the intersubjective nature of the analytic process and the "here-and-now" facets of the patient's material or the analytic relationship.

Eastern meditative disciplines teach us that psychological conditioning is caused by experiences in the present as well as the past. Meditative traditions alert us to what I would very provisionally term the *contemporaneous* unconscious, by which I mean, the unconsciousness that we experience in the present. When we speak of the unconscious, we ordinarily refer to formative experiences from the past that we are unaware of in the present. But the unconscious is not only the repository of early traumas and forgotten memories. It is also being continually created in the present by selective processes of perception and attention that filter the way information is taken in and kept out. All perception involves a selective process. One of the most powerful unconscious selective filters involves keeping out of our awareness that which causes discomfort to us. An area of extreme discomfort for most of us is anything that clashes with our ideals and self-images (Kramer & Alstad, 1993). The contemporaneous unconscious, unlike Freud's dynamic unconscious derived from our distant, familial past, is created in the present moment. It is composed of whatever thought or conduct, such as our self-centeredness, laxity, or competitiveness, that does not match our cherished views of ourselves. These phenomena are not registered by us in the present because they would make us feel bad about ourselves. Not seeing how we sometimes think and act in ways that contradict our values and ideals ensures that we do not feel badly about ourselves. It also insures that these facets of our experience tend to be sequestered from our sense of ourselves and thus remain unconscious.

Buddhism teaches psychoanalysis that it also neglects what I have termed non-self-centered aspects of self-experience. Non-self-centered subjectivity is implicated in a wide range of adaptive behaviors ranging from art to psychoanalytic listening to intimacy. It is an unconstricted state of being, a non-self-preoccupied, non-self-annulling immersion in whatever one is presently doing. There is heightened attentiveness, focus, and clarity. Action/response is unconstrained by self-concern, thought, or conscious effort, and restrictive self-identifications and boundaries are eroded. This facilitates a greater sense of freedom and an inclusiveness of self-structure. When excessive self-preoccupation wanes—as may occur, for example, while one is deeply immersed in playing a musical instrument, watching an engrossing cultural event, playing with a child, or making love—one may experience a heightened sense of living.

Neither psychoanalysis nor Buddhism recognizes that there is no immaculate perception. The self (or anti/no-self) that they "discover" is intimately related to how they investigate it. The telescopic approach to self-experience employed by many psychoanalysts yields a substantial self shaped by a particular history. Examining self-experience microscopically, as Buddhist meditation does, reveals the fluid and unfolding nature of identity, the way we are shaped anew, moment by moment.

We need a bifocal conception of self that realizes that the self is both a substantial, embodied, historical agent, as psychoanalysis suggests, that perceives, chooses, and acts, and a fluid, uncongealed process that is created afresh by changing states of consciousness in the present. Each conception of self is useful in particular circumstances. At certain times of the day when we have to evaluate among conflicting values and choose a particular moral course, we need to fixate the self and see it as a substantial agent with a history and a hierarchy of values. When listening to a patient in therapy, observing art, or appreciating nature, we sometimes need to unconstrict our sense of self and see it as an open and unfolding process.

PSYCHOANALYTIC AND BUDDHIST PATHS

In this final section of my paper I discuss the relationship of the psychoanalytic and Buddhist approaches to change. The process of change in psychoanalysis involves the illumination, transformation, and expansion of the patient's subjective world (Stolorow, Brandchaft, & Atwood, 1987). Psychoanalysis has identified three dimensions that are central to change, namely, cognitive insight, the affective bond to the analyst, and the integration of formerly dissociated experience (e.g., Friedman, 1978). I use this model as a point of reference in organizing the vast yet important topic of how psychoanalysis and Buddhism conceive of change and how each discipline might help or hinder people in their quest for self-transformation.

Because most of us may be more familiar with the psychoanalytic process than the Buddhist one, I shall devote more attention here to Buddhism. Buddhism helps and hinders one in the process of change. Meditation, as I suggested earlier, can foster the cultivation of self-introspective abilities. Meditation practice helped a woman I shall call Maureen, a long-term practitioner of Buddhist meditation, cultivate enhanced self-observational capacities; it increased her attentiveness and self-awareness. Meditation practice also aided Maureen in becoming unusually attentive to the nuances of her inner life such as latent motives, formerly disavowed intentions, and subtleties in the way she related to me. When she discussed relationships, for example, she demonstrated great insight into the possible patterns of interaction and the hidden motives and meanings that might be operative. This enabled her to track her reactions to me and others and often detect inchoate perceptions and fantasies. While meditating, for example, she became aware of formerly disavowed feelings of betrayal at the way her parents "gaslighted" or betrayed her and covered it up.

Not only did her receptivity to inner and interpersonal life increase, her attitude to her experience changed. The meditative spirit of attending to experience without judgment or aversion gradually replaced the self-critical stance exemplified by her characterologically contemptuous father. This led to greater affect tolerance. She had a highly developed capacity for tolerating and living in and through a range of affects without having to foreclose or simplify either the confusion or the complexity. She was able, for example, to examine such things as ambivalence and anger without criticizing herself, reducing the complexity of these experiences, or clamoring after premature understanding. As she accepted herself more, emotional warts and all, she developed deeper acceptance of others.

Cognitive insight can develop as a result of meditation. Maureen gained greater insight into the formerly unconscious disappointment, deprivation, and rage that she felt toward her critical and emotionally unavailable parents. Her cognitive insight about the way she had subverted what she called her "voice" so as to remain connected to and not threaten the fragile emotional tie to her parents emerged more clearly for her because of her refined capacity in meditation to attend to her experience with nonjudgmental awareness. As patients who meditate develop the capacity to view their own experience—even troubling facets such as deprivation and shame—with understanding and acceptance, they can more easily integrate formerly disavowed experience.

Meditation also aids the analyst in a variety of ways. Listening to ourselves and our analysands is both the essential tool of psychoanalytic inquiry and the foundation of psychoanalytic technique. And meditation deeply aids analytic listening. The analyst who meditates develops greater self-introspective abilities. Meditation fosters greater access to formerly unconscious material as well as greater receptivity to subtle mental and physical phenomena. The analyst notices thoughts, feelings, fantasies, images, and bodily sensations that he or she is ordinarily unaware of (Rubin, 1996). To cite one example among many, while involved in intensive meditation practice, I have much greater access to and clarity about my own dream life, including frequent occurrences of lucid dreaming.

Meditation practice also promotes greater tolerance for whatever we experience, including affects. By developing the ability to open to the texture of experience with less attachment and aversion, meditation aids the therapist in more skillfully handling affects. The analyst can literally sit with and through a greater range of affect without the need to shield him- or herself by premature certainty or intellectualized formulations. There is then a greater tolerance for complexity, ambiguity, and uncertainty. There is less pressure to know and to do. Not knowing is then a more comfortable state of being for the analyst. The analyst experiences more "beginner's mind." "In the beginner's mind there are many possibilities," notes Shunryu Suzuki (1970), and "in the expert's mind there are few" (p. 21). The analyst who has a beginner's mind takes less for granted, is more receptive to the unknown, and is more capable of being surprised.

The analyst's creativity is then enhanced. She is less filled with preconceptions about treatment, the therapeutic relationship, or life in general. She is freer to question, wonder, and doubt. She relates to analysands less habitually, repetitively, and self-centeredly. Such an analyst also has a deeper respect for differences. She is more tolerant of a wider range of internal and interpersonal phenomena. This creates an analytic environment that decreases the patient's vulnerability and shame.

By aiding the therapist in tolerating a wider range of experiences and reactions without fear or judgment, these experiences can be utilized as grist for the self-investigative mill. This opens up unexpected possibilities for learning and growth.

Meditation also fosters what Buddhists term *nonattachment*, a nongrasping state of mind in which one hold one's viewpoints less tightly. The nonattachment that meditation practice develops also cultivates greater freedom in the analyst. Meditation practice has personally helped me adopt a more fluid relationship to the theories I utilize to organize and make sense of the complex and overdetermined clinical actualities. It has helped me employ theoretical and clinical maps that I find illuminating, while simultaneously recognizing their ultimate provisionality and the inevitability of continually revising them. In cultivating perceptual acuity, attentiveness, and nonattachment, meditation fosters an awareness of, and deautomatization from, previously habitual patterns (Deikman, 1982), including some of the unresolved issues from one's own analysis that create difficulty or conflict for the clinician in conducting therapy.

Buddhism fosters the process of change in another way. It widens the field of psychoanalytic practice to include our lives outside the session. The Buddhist Eightfold Path, which includes right speech, or the effort to speak in a way that is truthful and useful (eschewing gossip, backbiting and so forth) and right livelihood, work that enriches rather than detracts from human life, emphasizes that the stage of our practice is, to borrow from Shakespeare, all the world, including and beyond the therapist's office. Buddhism emphasizes that everything in daily life, from the way we speak to our family and colleagues to the work that we do and the values we live by, is grist for the meditative mill. And Buddhism encourages us to give morality and values a more central role in our lives.

Buddhism hinders as well as facilitates the change process. It interferes with it in several ways. Whereas meditative methods make thoughts, feelings, and fantasies more available to us for scrutiny, the Buddhist stance of detaching from experience rather than exploring its meaning discourages us from using what we have discovered during our meditations to study ourselves. We feel more when we meditate, but we do not do enough with it. Buddhism, to cite one possible example from many, can foster lucid dreaming even as it encourages the dreamer to detach or let go of the dream, rather than exploring and elucidating its meaning and significance in one's life. Psychoanalysis can aid us in getting more mileage from the inner experience that meditation so wonderfully makes available to us. So after becoming aware of our inner experience through meditation, we then need to utilize psychoanalytic methods to investigate what we have become aware of. And psychoanalysis teaches Buddhism that it is crucial for self-transformation that one explore areas in one's life that meditation neglects, such as the shaping role of one's past, unconsciousness and character, our views of self and others, our strategies of self-protection, and the nature and quality of our relationships.

Buddhism occurs in the context of an emotionally intense relationship between a teacher and student. But neither the student nor the teacher reflect upon interpersonal dynamics, transference and countertransference, or relational enactments. And it is not a relationship that is designed to illuminate and transform the patient's characteristic ways of relating to self and other. The Buddhist teacher might relate to the student in such a way as to challenge the student's internalized and limiting beliefs about herself and others. But the absence of a relationship designed to investigate and illuminate the patient's recurrent ways of relating to self and the world makes it impossible to understand and transform the patient's transference or work through archaic self-defects.

By systematically analyzing transference phenomena and relational reenactments, psychoanalysis can illuminate ways of being that may either go unnoticed or be submerged in Buddhism, such as a student's idealization of his teachers and his concomitant self-submissiveness (e.g., Tart & Deikman, 1991). In Buddhism, this dynamic may remain unexamined and the student's self-devaluation and deferentiality may never get resolved and may play itself out in various other relationships.

As the crucible for the reemergence of archaic transferences, the psychoanalytic relationship can aid in the process of aborted development being recognized, reinstated, and worked through. Because it omits the crucial task of self-construction, Buddhism's model of working with self-experience is a necessary but incomplete way of healing the fault line that some of the people we work with struggle with. Such people need self-creation and self-amplification as well as self-deconstruction. When one's life is haunted by absence, emptiness, and virtuality rather than misplaced desires and attachments, one needs to built a *new* life based on one's relational and avocational values and ideals, not simply detach from a bad one—one based on attachments to illusory notions of self and reality. Working through a self-void and building a meaningful life is very different from letting go of illusory conceptions of self. Such a person would thus need psychoanalysis as well as meditation in order to work through their directionlessness and build a meaningful life.

Rudyard Kipling believed, perhaps like many of us, that "East is East and West is West and never the twain shall meet." In *East, West,* a recent collection of stories, Salman Rushdie (1994) offered an opposite perspective: "I too have ropes around my neck, I have them to this day pulling me this way and that, East and West, the nooses tightening, commanding choose, choose . . . Ropes I do not choose between you . . . I choose neither of you and both. Do you hear? I refuse to choose" (p. 211). "East" may be East and "West" may be West, but in my experience, if we are open to what psychoanalysis and meditation might teach us and allow the twain to meet, then our lives and the lives of those we work with might well be transformed and greatly enriched.[5]

REFERENCES

Alexander, F. (1931). Buddhistic training as an artificial catatonia: The biological meaning of psychological occurrences. *Psychoanalytic Review, 18,* 129-145.

Bakhtin, M. (1986). *Speech genres and other late essays.* Austin: University of Texas Press.

Boorstein, S. (Ed.). (1980). *Transpersonal psychotherapy.* Palo Alto, CA: Science and Behavior Books.

Boss, M. (1965). *A psychiatrist discovers India.* London: Oswald Wolff.

Boucher, S. (1988). *Turning the wheel: American women creating the new Buddhism.* San Francisco, CA: Harper and Row.

Breuer, J., & Freud, S. (1895). Studies on hysteria. In *Standard Edition* (Vol. 2, pp. 255-305). London: Hogarth Press.

Brown, D., & Engler, J. (1986). The stages of mindfulness meditation: A validation study. Part II: Discussion. In K. Wilber, J. Engler, & D. Brown (Eds.), *Transformation of consciousness: Conventional and contemplative perspectives on development* (pp. 17-51). Boston: Shambhala.

Burtt, E. (1955). *The teachings of the compassionate Buddha.* New York: New American Library.

Chogyam, T. (1983). Introductory essay. In N. Katz (Ed.), *Buddhist and Western psychotherapy* (pp. 1-7). Boulder, CO: Prajna Press.

Coltart, N. (1996). Buddhism and psychoanalysis revisited. In *The baby and the bathwater* (pp. 125-140). New York: International Universities Press.

Cooper, P. (1999). Buddhist meditation and countertransference: A case study. *The American Journal of Psychoanalysis, 59*(1), 71-85.

Corbett, L. (1996). *The religious function of the psyche.* New York: Routledge.

Deatherage, G. (1975). The clinical use of "mindfulness" meditation in short-term psychotherapy. *Journal of Transpersonal Psychology, 7*(2), 133-144.

Deikman, A. (1982). *The observing self: Mysticism and psychotherapy.* Boston: Beacon Press.

Dogen. (1976). *Zen master Dogen.* New York: Weatherhill.

Eigen, M. (1998). *The psychoanalytic mystic.* London and New York: Free Association Books.

Eigen, M. (2001). *Ecstasy.* Middletown, CT: Wesleyan University Press.

Engler, J. (1984). Therapeutic aims in psychotherapy and meditation: Developmental stages in the representation of self. *Journal of Transpersonal Psychology, 16*(1), 25-61.

Finn, M. (1992). Transitional space and Tibetan Buddhism: The object relations of meditation. In M. Finn & J. Gartner (Eds.), *Object relations theory and religion* (pp. 87-107). Westport, CT: Praeger.

Foucault, M. (1980). *Power/knowledge.* New York: Pantheon Books.

Freud, S. (1912). Recommendations to physicians practicing psychoanalysis. In *Standard Edition* (Vol.12, pp. 218-226). London: Hogarth Press.

Friedman, L. (1978). Trends in the psychoanalytic theory of treatment. *Psychoanalytic Quarterly, 47,* 524-567.

Fromm, E., Suzuki, D.T., & DeMartino, R. (Eds.). (1960). *Zen Buddhism and psychoanalysis.* New York: Harper and Row.

---

[5]This is adapted from an earlier work (Rubin, 1996, 1998). The first and final section introduces new material and extends this previous work. This chapter was enriched by the thoughtful feedback of Barry Magid, Uwe Gielen, Susan Rudnick, and Andrea Koehler.

Frye, N. (1957). *Anatomy of criticism: Four essays*. Princeton, NJ: Princeton University Press.

Gedo, J. (1996). *The artist and the emotional world*. New York: Columbia University Press.

Goleman, D. (1997). *Healing emotions: Conversations with the Dalai Lama on mindfulness, emotions, and health*. Boston: Shambhala.

Gordon, J. (1987). *The golden guru: The strange journey of Bhagwan Shree Rajneesh*. Lexington, KY: The Stephen Greene Press.

Gramsci, A. (1971). *Selections from the prison notebooks*. (Q. Hoare & G. Smith, Eds. & Trans.). New York: International Universities Press.

Grof, S. (1985). *Beyond the brain: Birth, death, and transcendence in psychotherapy*. Albany, NY: State University of New York Press.

Grotstein, J. (2000). *Who is the dreamer who dreams the dream: A study of psychic presences*. Hillsdale, NJ: The Analytic Press.

Hoffman, Y. (1975). *The sound of one hand clapping*. New York: Basic Books.

Horney, K. (1945). *Our inner conflicts*. New York: Norton.

Horney, K. (1987). *Final lectures*. New York: Norton.

Huxley, A. (1970). *The perennial philosophy*. New York: Harper.

Jung, C. G. (1958). Psychology and religion: West and East. In *Collected Works, Vol. 11*. Princeton, NJ: Princeton University Press.

Kelman, H. (1960). Psychoanalytic thought and Eastern wisdom. In J. Ehrenwald (Ed.), *The history of psychotherapy* (pp. 328-333). New York: Jason Aronson.

Kohut, H. (1985). *Self psychology and the humanities*. New York: W. W. Norton.

Kornfield, J. (1977). *Living Buddhist masters*. Santa Cruz, CA: Unity Press.

Kramer, J., & Alstad, D. (1993). *The guru papers: Masks of authoritarian power*. Berkeley, CA: Frog Press.

Kramer, J. (1995). Personal communication.

Magid, B. (2002). *Ordinary mind: Exploring the common ground of Zen and psychotherapy*. Boston: Wisdom Publications.

Matthiessen, P. (1987). *Nine-headed dragon river: Zen journals, 1969-1982*. Boston: Shambhala.

McDougall, J. (1995). *The many faces of eros*. London: Free Association Books.

Milner, M. (1987). *The suppressed madness of sane men*. London: Tavistock.

Oremland, J. (1997). *The origins and psychodynamics of creativity*. Madison, CT: International Universities Press.

Phillips, A. (1993). *On kissing, tickling, and being bored*. Cambridge, MA: Harvard University Press.

Rapgay, L. (1995). Personal communication.

Ricoeur, P. (1970). *Freud and philosophy: An essay on interpretation*. New Haven, CT: Yale University Press.

Rinzler, C., & Gordon, B. (1980). Buddhism and psychotherapy. In G. Epstein (Ed.), *Studies in non-deterministic psychology* (pp. 52-69). New York: Human Sciences Press.

Roland, A. (1988). *In search of self in India and Japan: Toward a cross-cultural psychology*. Princeton, NJ: Princeton University Press.

Roland, A. (2002). *Dreams and drama: Psychoanalytic criticism, creativitiy, and the artist*. Middletown, CT: Wesleyan University Press.

Rubin, J. B. (1985). Meditation and psychoanalytic listening. *Psychoanalytic Review, 72*(4), 599-612.

Rubin, J. B. (1991). The clinical integration of Buddhist meditation and psychoanalysis. *Journal of Integrative and Eclectic Psychotherapy, 10*(2),173-181.

Rubin, J. B. (1992). Psychoanalytic treatment with a Buddhist meditator. In M. Finn & J. Gartner (Eds.), *Object relations theory and religion: Clinical applications* (pp. 87-107). Westport, CT: Praeger.

Rubin, J. B. (1993). Psychoanalysis and Buddhism: Toward an integration. In G. Stricker & J. Gold (Eds.), *Comprehensive textbook of psychotherapy integration* (pp. 249-266). New York: Plenum.

Rubin, J. B. (1996). *Psychotherapy and Buddhism: Toward an integration*. New York: Plenum Press.

Rubin, J. B. (1998). Psychoanalysis is self-centered. In *A psychoanalysis for our time. Exploring the blindness of the seeing I* (pp. 126-140). New York: New York University Press.

Rubin, J. B. (2004). *Psychoanalysis and the good life: Reflection on love, ethics, creativity and spirituality*. Albany, NY: SUNY Press.

Rushdie, S. (1994). *East, West*. New York: Pantheon Books.

Safran, J. (Ed.). (2003). *Psychoanalysis and Buddhism. An unfolding dialogue*. Boston: Wisdom Publications.

Said, E. (1979). *Orientalism*. New York: Vintage Books.

Schafer, R. (1976). *A new language for psychoanalysis*. New Haven, CT: Yale University Press.

Schneider, K. (1987). The deified self: A "centaur" response to Ken Wilber and the transpersonal movement. *Journal of Humanistic Psychology, 27*(2), 196-216.

Searles, H. (1972). The function of the analyst's realistic perceptions of the analyst in delusional transference. In *Countertransference and related subjects* (pp. 196-227). New York: International Universities Press.

Segal, S. (Ed.). (2003). *Encountering Buddhism: Western psychology and Buddhist teachings*. Albany, NY: State University of New York Press.

Shapiro, D. (1989). Judaism as a journey of transformation: Consciousness, behavior, and society. *Journal of Transpersonal Psychology, 21*(1), 13-59.

Smith, H. (1986). *The religions of man*. New York: Harper and Row.

Stolorow, R., Brandchaft, B., & Atwood, G. (1987). *Psychoanalytic treatment: An intersubjective approach*. Hillsdale, NJ: The Analytic Press.

Suler, J. (1993). *Contemporary psychoanalysis and Eastern thought*. Albany, NY: State University Press.

Suzuki, S. (1970). *Zen mind, beginner's mind*. New York: Weatherhill.

Tart, C. (Ed.). (1975). *Transpersonal psychologies*. New York: Harper and Row.

Tart, C., & Deikman, A. (1991). Mindfulness, spiritual seeking and psychotherapy. *Journal of Transpersonal Psychology, 23*(1), 29-52.

Ulanov, A. (1985). A shared space. *Quadrant, 18*(1), 65-80.

Walsh, R., & Vaughan, F. (Eds.). (1980). *Beyond ego: Transpersonal dimensions in psychotherapy*. Los Angeles, CA: Jeremy Tarcher.

Welwood, J. (Ed.). (1979). *Meeting of the ways: Explorations in East/West psychology*. New York: Schocken.

White, H. (1973). *Metahistory: Historical imagination in nineteenth-century Europe*. Baltimore: John Hopkins University Press.

Wilber, K. (1979). Psychologia perennis. In J. Welwood (Ed.), *Meeting of the ways: Explorations in East/West psychology* (pp. 7-28). New York: Schocken.

Wilber, K. (1986). The developmental spectrum and psychopathology; Part I, Stages and types of pathology. *Journal of Transpersonal Psychology, 16*(1), 75-118.

Wilber, K., Engler, J., & Brown, D. (Eds.). (1986). *Transformations of consciousness: Conventional and contemplative perspectives on development*. Boston: Shambhala.

Winnicott, D. W. (1971). *Playing and reality*. London: Tavistock.

Japanese Forms of Psychotherapy: Naikan Therapy and Morita Therapy

Junko Tanaka-Matsumi
Kwansei Gakuin University

Studies on healing practices across cultures have revealed the close relationship between basic cultural concepts and specific forms of treatment, and have underscored the importance of shared worldviews held by client and therapist (Draguns, 1975; Frank & Frank, 1991). Prince (1980) broadened the scope of psychotherapy to include all forms of "altered states of consciousness." He stated that Western conceptions of psychotherapy must be drastically expanded if we are to understand the diverse therapeutic procedures of other cultures. According to Frank and Frank (1991), all psychotherapies share at least four effective features: a therapist-client relationship, a special healing setting, a therapy rationale, and a therapeutic ritual or procedure. Accepting these elements as "exogenous mechanisms," Prince (1980) viewed psychotherapy as the mobilization of the person's "endogenous mechanisms" such as sleep, rest, and social isolation in order to relieve personal distress. Endogenous mechanism such as induced social isolation is a basic element in both Naikan and Morita therapies. It is systematically mobilized to increase client's attention to previously avoided anxiety provoking events or to important interpersonal relations. The interpretation of the meaning or cause of distress and the methods of relieving suffering vary according to culture.

The first goal of this chapter is to present two forms of indigenous psychotherapies developed in Japan and to explore their exogenous and endogenous mechanisms. The second goal of the chapter is to examine both universal and culture-specific aspects of two Japanese therapies.

I applied a combined etic-emic perspective (Segall, Dasen, Berry, & Poortinga, 1999) to organize the relevant literature. The etic position examines universalist features of all forms of psychotherapies (Draguns, 2002). The emic, or cultural relativist position, helps accommodate culture at the individual level in psychotherapeutic practice.

CULTURAL ACCOMMODATION IN PSYCHOTHERAPY

Culture has been defined in many different ways. Culture is "the man-made part of the environment" (Herskovits, 1948, p. 17). It encompasses "behavioral products of others who preceded us and it contains values, language, and a way of life" (Segall et al., 1999, p. 2). From a semiotic perspective, culture is "an historically transmitted pattern of meanings embodied in symbols" (Geertz, 1973, p. 89). Cultural psychologists emphasize a dynamic interaction of the context and the person. Effective communication between the therapist and the client in psychotherapy is based on the shared cultural meanings of the concepts and idioms of distress. Pedersen (1997) advocates that all psychotherapies be "culture-centered" and that multiculturalism should be generic to all counseling relationships.

The goal of cultural accommodation in psychotherapy is the integration of the cultural context with the design of clinical services (Higginbotham, West, & Forsyth, 1988). Cultural accommodation can be enhanced by attending to the indigenous or culture-relevant meanings of deviant behaviors, their perceived causes, and the social reactions they provoke (Tanaka-Matsumi, Higginbotham, & Chang, 2002). Implicitly or explicitly, as Kleinman (1978) advocates, therapy is a series of "negotiations" between the therapist and the client within his or her cultural context. Kleinman suggests four procedures for negotiating both the meaning of the client/therapist interaction and the cultural meaning of the client's presenting problem. First, the therapist encourages the client to give his or her own explanations of the presenting problem. Second, the therapist discloses the explanation, or "explanatory model," that he or she uses to interpret the problem. Third, the two frameworks are compared for similarities and discrepancies. Finally, the client and clinician translate each explanatory model into mutually acceptable language so that they may jointly set the content of target behaviors for treatment and outcome criteria. In both Naikan therapy and Morita therapy, negotiations may take place using predominantly nonverbal but also verbal means.

EMIC AND ETIC ASPECTS IN INDIGENOUS THERAPIES

Indigenous therapies are developed from within a culture to meet the needs of its members in a particular sociocultural context, rather than being imported from the outside. A number of psychotherapy researchers have observed that indigenous therapies have both etic, or universal, and emic, or cultural, aspects. Roland (1988), who has practiced psychoanalysis in Japan and India, proposes that the various concepts of psychoanalysis are universal, but that both therapy and therapist training are highly culture-specific. He uses the individualism and collectivism dimensions to describe cultural differences in therapist-patient relationships and communication styles. In addition, he discusses the limitation of applying individual-oriented confrontational therapy to a culture in which interdependence has been reinforced to maintain highly ritualized interpersonal relations and social roles.

Psychotherapy is often construed as a social influence process; both the client and the therapist variables play an important role in treatment selection and outcome. The context of therapy should be consistent with the beliefs and practices of the client's culture. The goal of cultural accommodation can be enhanced by taking into account the forms and content of indigenous therapies, which reveal culture-specific explanatory frameworks for the diagnosis and treatment of abnormal behaviors (Kleinman, 1978; Tanaka-Matsumi, Seiden, & Lam, 2001).

In the Japanese indigenous Morita therapy (Morita, 1928/1998) and Naikan therapy (Murase, 1996; Tanaka-Matsumi, 1979a), an important therapeutic goal is that of social restoration. This is accomplished not by systematic verbal exploration of problems between the therapist and the client, but rather by initial social isolation from the client's troubling interpersonal networks and by providing a highly structured therapeutic setting and daily schedule to facilitate self-reflection and acceptance of fears and anxieties. Reynolds (1980) calls these Japanese indigenous therapies the "quiet therapies" due to their emphasis on acceptance of the current plight, structured self-observation, and highly limited and ritualized verbal exchanges between the therapist and client.

In this chapter, I examine the themes and therapeutic structure of Naikan therapy and Morita therapy. They both deviate drastically in form and explanatory model from Western-derived psychotherapies such as psychoanalysis, client-centered therapy, or behavior therapy. Despite differences among these Western therapies, they encourage development of the independent self as an active agent of change (Bandura, 1982). On the other hand, Naikan therapy aims to increase clients' appreciation that self is but a part of their valued social network that is maintained by the Buddhist worldview of benevolence of mother, father, teachers, and specific others, whereas, similarly, Morita therapy has an ultimate goal of accepting suffering as part of nature, according to the worldview of both Buddhism in general and Zen Buddhism in particular. Morita and Naikan therapies are both means to achieving "self-illumination" within the Japanese cultural context. The therapist in each therapy provides a highly structured healing setting for self-reflection. The disruption of usual activities and relationships is a basic condition of Naikan and Morita therapies. In Naikan therapy, clients are encouraged to focus on their relationships with specific others in order to reduce self-centeredness. In Morita therapy, clients learn to accept anxiety and to keep performing goal-oriented behaviors. Development of a purpose-centered life is Morita's goal. Emotions and moods are regarded as secondary to behaviors.

NAIKAN THERAPY

Naikan is a Japanese word that means concentrated self-reflection. This word is frequently used in the context of the Jodo Shinshu sect of Buddhism (Yoshimoto, 1989). Ishin Yoshimoto (1916-1988) developed Naikan as an intensive method of self-exploration five decades ago (Yoshimoto, 1989, 1996). Yoshimoto was an ardent Buddhist and repeatedly attempted *mishirabe*, a rigorous meditation and self-examination without eating, drinking, or sleeping, with frequent encouragement of those who had experienced mishirabe themselves. Yoshimoto wished to make such self-reflection available to others. After 15 years of preparation, Yoshimoto drastically modified the system and incorporated the warmth and comfort of regular meals and sleep. In 1954, he converted his own home in Nara into the first Naikan center in Japan. Naikan was first used as a means of rehabilitating prison inmates (Reynolds, 1980).

Naikan therapy is a continuous self-observation in which clients are instructed to examine themselves in their relationship with significant others through the recollection of specific life events in their past (Tanaka-Matsumi, 1979a). Clients sit in a physically and socially isolated corner of a room for more than 15 hours each day for as long as one week (Miki, 1976). Clients follow this routine from 6:00 in the morning until 9:00 at night. The therapist gives specific instructions to the client but does not follow the contents of what the client recollected during Naikan. Yoshimoto called this therapy a way of "self-illumination" (Yoshimoto, 1989), which is based on structured learning experiences about one's attitude and behavior toward significant others who influence one's daily activities.

Naikan Clients

Naikan therapy is designed for individuals who wish to improve their interpersonal relationships with significant others and to learn to control their own activities. Historically, the most appropriate candidates for Naikan therapy have been delinquents, alcoholics, and *shinkeishitsusho* patients (Murase, 1996). Shinkeishit-susho is a Japanese idiom of distress applied to people who present problems with "hypersensitivity, introversion, self-consciousness, perfectionism and hypochon-driacal disposition" (Lin, 1989, p. 108).

According to Naikan therapy, within Japanese culture, psychological problems of the individual are rooted in distorted interpersonal relationships. Therefore, in this model, the Japanese self-concept is relative to one's relationships with significant oth-ers (Kimura, 1972). A common Japanese belief is that basic human happiness derives from harmonious interpersonal relationships within the individual's rather rigidly defined social environment. Positive interpersonal bonds are developed and main-tained by the mutual fulfillment of obligations or what the Japanese call *on* within a hierarchical and collectivitistic structure. People who fail to return favors given by specific others are regarded as self-centered. Such people, according to Naikan ther-apy, disturb the closely knit social structure (Miki, 1976). Naikan therapy attempts to resocialize clients through increased awareness of what other people did for them. Becoming aware of unreturned favors induces self-reproach, guilt, and lowered self-esteem in clients during Naikan therapy.

Naikan Therapists

Naikan therapists see their clients only 3 to 5 minutes at a time, but at 90-minute inter-vals while they are in therapy. The primary role of the Naikan therapist is to direct clients' self-examination by giving them sets of instructions individually. Therapists do not analyze the specific reports of clients' self-observations about their past rela-tionships with significant others. In this respect, Naikan therapy is concerned with procedures rather than the content of the therapist-client relationship (Murase & Johnson, 1974).

Naikan therapists assume a very modest and polite manner toward clients. They use honorific expressions and follow ritualistic forms in their interactions with clients. They seldom interact verbally with clients and they do not reinforce clients' emotional reactions to their recollected interpersonal events. At the end of each brief interview, the therapist and the client exchange gratitude bowing to one another. This thera-peutic interaction style is consistent with the Japanese cultural emphasis on nonver-bal rather than direct verbal communication. Thus, although the Naikan therapist does not interact with the client by talking and analyzing his or her verbal report, the therapist's brief interviews and nonverbal behaviors guide the client's self-observa-tion within the residential Naikan center.

Potentially, anyone is qualified to become a Naikan therapist. The only restriction is that Naikan therapists must have experienced Naikan themselves. Therapists come from various backgrounds: psychology, psychiatry, education, religion, counseling, and others.

Physical Setting of Naikan Therapy

Naikan therapy typically takes place in a residential center. Each client is assigned a semi-enclosed area in a Japanese-style room. This small space becomes a private space for the client during the one-week period. Frequently, four or more clients are assigned to the same room in separate corners. Clients are isolated from social con-tact. They are given only a sleeping bag and meals are delivered to them three times a day. Clients are allowed to leave their space to use the bathroom; otherwise, they spend 15 hours a day in rigorous self-examination for a 7-day period, a total of 100 hours.

Under this isolated social and physical condition, clients engage in Naikan continuously according to specific interpersonal themes and instructions. The physical and social isolation from clients' usual environments creates desirable therapeutic conditions under which clients learn to focus their attentions on recollecting specific interpersonal episodes.

Clients are instructed to take any physical posture that is relaxing to them, so long as their activities are limited within the given space. Clients do not receive any systematic relaxation training and they are not taught how to focus their attention on specific themes. Thus, clients must endure the strains of isolation, fears, boredom, and attention wandering for the first two or three days (Murase, 1996).

Instructions and Themes of Naikan

The theme of Naikan is probably its most unique aspect. It reflects Japanese cultural values, demonstrating how Japanese people relate to their social environments via the concept of reciprocity (Lebra, 1969). Murase (1974, p. 10) summarized the following three instructions given by the therapist as crucial to effective Naikan therapy:

1. Recall and examine your memories on care and benevolence you have received from a particular other person.
2. Recollect and examine your memories on what you have returned to that person.
3. Recollect and examine trouble and worries you have given to that person.

Naikan therapy instructions are entirely concerned with specific interpersonal relationships, regardless of clients' particular presenting problems. The first subject of Naikan therapy is usually clients' relationships with their mothers. The Naikan therapist instructs clients to recall and examine specific life events that involved them and their mothers, from when they were in elementary school chronologically to the present. The therapist indicates a specific phase of clients' lives to be recalled. For example, the therapist says, "Please examine what your mother did for you when you were in high school." Clients are to recall details of their relationships with their mothers. This procedure occupies 25 to 30 hours of the total Naikan therapy.

The importance given to the establishment of a strong relationship with one's mother in Japanese culture is well documented and reviewed (e.g., Johnson, 1993; Miyake, Campos, Kagan, & Bradshaw, 1986; Murase, 1996; Naito & Gielen, in press). These studies emphasize the mutual dependency of the Japanese mother and her child. This dependency is carried into many aspects of Japanese social life and is captured by the Japanese concept of *amae* (Doi, 1973). Doi defined amae as the ability to presume or depend upon the benevolence of another. Group-oriented activities are encouraged among Japanese people because such activities strengthen social roles which are dependent on one another (Azuma, 1994). The Japanese ideal self, as illuminated by Naikan therapy, is therefore an interdependent self (Markus & Kitayama, 1991). Taketomo's (1986) proposition that amae is a culturally reinforced metacommunication strategy suggests that Japanese people learn to distinguish carefully to whom they can express amae. Taketomo's (1986, 1999) definition of amae includes the mutual acceptance of the inappropriate expression of needs and behaviors and the suspension of formality in social interaction. Interpersonal transactions and communications based on amae permeate the hierarchically organized Japanese society. It is, therefore, not surprising that the treatment of problems relating to the inability to express or accept amae has been at the forefront of Japanese psychotherapies (Kitayama, 1999). Naikan therapy also helps clients to resolve inappropriate or frustrated amae needs that they still harbor toward their parents. Murase (1996, p. 226) states that the successful Naikan client accepts his or her own responsibility as a person and resolves unsocialized amae.

In Naikan therapy, the three instructions help clients recall continued benevolence given by their mothers. Naikan therapy defines benevolence in terms of specific acts, so that clients are always told to recall specific events. According to Naikan therapy, the accumulation of those recollected events in which the mother has one-sidedly given favor to the client induces guilt or a sense of indebtedness (Murase, 1974). The Western idea of guilt typically indicates violation of an absolute moral code represented by the Judeo-Christian tradition. To the contrary, guilt in Japanese culture is understood in a more social and concrete framework. To Japanese people, guilt means a debt to a specific other for causing them trouble. The Japanese concept of guilt has an obvious interpersonal context (Kimura, 1965; Murase, 1996). Naikan therapy clients experience guilt and/or shame at the same time they feel their mothers' benevolence (Miki, 1976). This is so because the therapist's instructions always emphasize the mother's positive acts and the client's negative acts, that is, the mother's favors unreturned. The therapist instructs clients to consider another's position. The Naikan therapist often asks, "What would your mother do?" This demonstrates the cultural importance of being able to take another's perspective before asserting oneself. The possibility that clients' mothers may have caused them trouble (for example, child abuse) is not taken into account. If clients criticize their mothers' behaviors, the therapist points out that this is not Naikan but *Gaikan. Gai* means looking outward as opposed to *Nai* meaning inward.

Naikan therapy clients sit in an isolated place and actively review their past lives for 100 hours continuously on single themes of interpersonal obligations and exchanges. A person is regarded as weak and guilty, and the realization of one's guilt, defined in terms of the therapist's three specific instructions, is itself an educational experience (Ishida, 1972). There is a strong social factor in the "self-illumination" of the Japanese people.

Because Naikan therapy does not emphasize a verbal elaboration of clients' self-observation, little objectivity is built into the monitoring procedure. In fact, Ishida (1972) comments that clients' descriptions of their mothers are often idealized and are discrepant with their real mothers. This, however, works favorably for therapy because such ideal images of one's mother enhance gratitude felt toward her. Because a person's introspection or self-observation is not subject to another person's observation, the data of Naikan therapy are in clients' verbal or written reports of their active self-recollections. However, the Naikan therapist makes very few attempts to obtain detailed verbal reports of the events recollected by clients. After all, the Naikan therapist typically sees clients for only a few minutes for each 90-minute self-observation by the clients.

Various Naikan therapists have reported clients' intense emotional arousal. Frank and Frank (1991, p. 201) stated that "in psychotherapy, review of the past inevitably mobilizes feelings of guilt or shame." They also stated that the therapist's continued impartial interest in the face of material that arouses guilt or shame implies forgiveness and ultimately enhances the morale of the client. Successful Naikan clients also report achieving a similar state. Tezuka (1999) compared and contrasted her own experience of receiving psychoanalytic therapy in the United States and Naikan therapy in Japan. She described Naikan therapy as structured monologues assisted by the therapist in concentrated self-reflection, which leads to an intense and powerful reexperiencing of the positive aspects of amae between client and mother.

In conclusion, the goal of Naikan therapy meets the value system of the Japanese people. It emphasizes the fulfillment of mutual obligations within a hierarchical social structure. Just as people in different cultures define their own problems as worthy of intervention according to their value judgments (Draguns, 2002), this is also true of Japanese people in their definition of behaviors and attitudes that they consider deviant and how they resocialize clients.

Current Status of Naikan Therapy in Japan

Naikan therapy continues to obtain support from a wide range of professionals and paraprofessionals in Japan. Today, there are more than 40 Naikan centers in Japan. Also, Naikan therapy is practiced in more than half a dozen inpatient medical settings in Japan for the treatment of alcohol dependency, school refusal, depression, and psychosomatic disorders (Murase, 1996). Additionally, Naikan therapy is offered in some temples and juvenile rehabilitation centers in Japan. Internationally, Naikan centers have been established in Austria and Germany.

In 1978, the Japan Society for Naikan Therapy was founded and its first meeting was held in Kyoto. Reviewing the first 10 years of the conference proceedings, Murase (1996) noted one of the most important future items on the agenda is the development of a conceptual explanatory model of Naikan therapy. Although the field lacks controlled empirical research into Naikan therapy's effectiveness and mechanisms of therapeutic change, Murase's (1996) review of published case studies suggests that Naikan therapy is most appropriate for the treatment of delinquency, crimes, alcohol dependency, and smoking.

According to a comprehensive survey on the practice of psychotherapy in Japan (Sugiwaka, Takeshima, Nishimura, Yamamoto, & Agari, 1992), the most dominant approaches are brief therapy, psychodynamic psychotherapy, and client-centered therapy. Of the 189 of 500 surveys returned by the members of three major professional associations, 7.4 percent of them indicated the use of Naikan therapy as a secondary technique in conjunction with other psychotherapies. Three percent of the respondents, on the other hand, stated that they use Morita therapy as a main therapy and 14 percent reported its use in connection with other therapies.

MORITA THERAPY

Consistent with the criteria of indigenous therapies in the use of original concepts and cultural idioms of distress rather than imported or translated concepts, Morita therapy is replete with Japanese idioms and phrases. To reflect this unique feature, I use the original Japanese words with English translations.

Shinkeishitsu: Symptoms and Functional Characteristics

Morita therapy was founded by the Japanese psychiatrist, Shoma Morita (1874-1938) for the treatment of anxiety disorders with hypochondria, which Morita called *shinkeishitsu*, translated as nervous disposition. As noted previously, shinkeishitsu is characterized by hypersensitivity, introversion, self-consciousness, perfectionism, and hypochondriacal disposition (Lin, 1989). Specific symptoms include headaches, dizziness, palpitations, distention of the stomach, fear of contracting disease, feelings of shame in public, anxiety attacks, paralysis, and insomnia, among others. Shinkeishitsu clients tend to regard any of these conditions as abnormal because of their hypochondriacal tendencies. As their fear increases, they develop anticipatory anxiety. This cycle increases their autonomic arousal and their sensitivity and worry through the process of *seishin kogo sayo*, which was defined as "the vicious cycle of the interaction between one's felt sensation and one's focus of attention on the sensation" (Morita, 1928/1998, p. 1). Morita regarded symptoms of shinkeishitsu to be but a reflection of "the desire for life" or *sei no yokubo*. He considered the fear and the desire to be complementary.

Morita defined anxiety disorders as being due to one's hypersensitivity to felt sensations or hypochondria (Morita, 1928/1998, p. 106). Shinkeishitsu symptoms result from mental preoccupation (*toraware*) with his or her own subjective experience though the process of *seishin kogo sayo* (psychic interaction). Morita was concerned with the mechanism of symptom production in clients. Although Morita was versed in nosology-oriented Kraepelinian psychiatry and had a profound knowledge of Western psychotherapy literature, he used the Japanese language and concepts to describe the functional characteristics of shinkeishitsu (Morita, 1953).

Taijin Kyofusho   Within the interpersonally tight Japanese cultural context, people who have an inclination toward shinkeishitsu may easily develop social phobia. Morita (1928/1998) defined taijin kyofusho as a subcategory of shinkeishitsu. He was particularly interested in treating socially phobic individuals with the diagnosis of taijin kyofusho, a symptom complex that includes a number of social fears. These fears include fear of one's gaze giving displeasure to others, fear of blushing, fear of giving off an offensive odor, and fear of unpleasant facial expressions (Takahashi, 1976; Tanaka-Matsumi, 1979b). Common to all the complaints is an intense awareness of people in their social environment due to their hypersensitivity to the perceived "defect" and anxious apprehension. Patients are obsessed with shame. Their complaints are marked by an intense awareness of others, hypersensitivity to the perceived "defect," and anxious apprehension.

In a collectivistic society that reinforces interdependence and social affiliation, taijin kyofusho clients fear that they disturb the interpersonal harmony due to their "defects." An American therapist assessing a Japanese client who reports a fear of displeasing others due to the client's own gaze might be tempted to call this a "delusion" due to the deviancy of this thought from American norms and fear. However, in Japan, fear of eye contact is common even among "normal" people. The Japanese culture reinforces other-oriented concerns such as "I am offending my colleagues at work due to my eye gaze." The client's fear is an exaggeration of cultural rules regarding eye contact and a culturally normative concern for how one's behavior affects others (Kleinknecht, Dinnel, Kleinknecht, Hiruma, & Harada, 1997; Seiden, Lam, & Tanaka-Matsumi, 1996). Taijin kyofusho has been attributed to the Japanese value of extreme interpersonal sensitivity and to the culturally fostered inhibition of expressing negative emotions, even in a nonverbal manner (Russell, 1989). Patients typically avoid or escape from feared social situations and their social anxiety symptoms generalize to a variety of social situations.

Taijin kyofusho has been classified as a culture-bound disorder because "cultural beliefs or rules and patterns of interaction are constitutive of the disorder" (Kirmayer,

1991, p. 26). The complexity of Japanese norms for interpersonal interaction requires that children, from a young age, learn to read subtle cues as to the thoughts and feelings of others and organize their verbal and nonverbal behaviors accordingly. Children are taught from a young age to "stand in" rather than to "stand out" in social situations (Weisz, Rothbaum, & Blackburn, 1984). Hypersensitivity to one's bodily conditions in social situations may explain the cultural prominence of taijin kyofusho in Japan. Morita therapy directly addresses this concern.

Goals of Morita Therapy

The goals of Morita therapy are the following: the recognition of facts, obedience to nature, focus on the present, the increase of spontaneous activities, the decrease of self-focused preoccupation, the elimination of indulgence in moods and emotions (*kibun honi*), the withholding of value judgments, the reduction of intellectualizing, the cessation of escape into a sick role, and the cultivation of a humble (*sunao*) mind (Iwai & Abe, 1975, p. 84).

Morita therapy "constantly pushes clients to obey nature by means of actual proof and experiential understanding" (Morita, 1928/1998, p. 34). *Taitoku* (experiential understanding) is the "knowledge and awareness obtained from direct practice and experience" (Morita, 1928/1998, p. 7). The treatment of shinkeishitsu aims at the elimination of fear associated with seishin-kogo-sayo. Shinkeishitsu clients exhibit "ideational contradictions" (*shiso no mujun*) that reflect the conflict between their rigid ideas and reality. Shinkeishitsu clients hold high standards for themselves and believe they "should" or "must" achieve such goals. They are likely to be contradicted by reality. They attempt to reduce conflicts by cognitively manipulating, distorting, and/or denying what is real or actual according to their desires of how things "ought" to be. Morita was interested in eliminating contradiction by ideas and fostering acceptance of facts in the state of *arugamama*, which means accepting things as they are. Morita postulated that this was made possible by eliminating avoidance and by teaching clients to accept fears until they dissipate naturally. Morita's original procedure had clients in complete social isolation and in bed, resting for the first 10 days of therapy. Clients would ideally become the focal points of subjective fears without opportunities for escape or avoidance.

Morita therapy reflects a strong Zen influence. Morita rejected the mind-body dualism and considered the "mind" to be of a fleeting nature whose "dynamic flow changes between external events and the self" (Morita, 1928/1998, p. 9). Morita therapy aimed for the development of *mushoju shin*, a Zen term used to describe the state of alertness and mindfulness without narrowly self-focused attention to a particular bodily sensation such as heart palpitations.

Stages of Morita Therapy

The prototypical form of Morita therapy is an inpatient treatment involving four stages: (1) isolation-rest therapy, (2) light occupational therapy, (3) heavy occupational therapy, and (4) complicated activity therapy in preparation for actual life. Treatment in the first and second stages is conducted with clients being placed in completely isolated states; they are not allowed to have any social or family contact. Clients are permitted to leave the hospital grounds for the first time in the fourth stage. Morita stated that the essential characteristics of his therapy are the natural treatment of the mind/body and the practice of experiential methods. In short, shinkeishitsu clients learn to observe and obey nature without fighting anxiety symptoms.

The first stage: Isolation and rest   Clients are given detailed explanations of the functions of the symptoms of shinkeishitsu. The therapist instructs that shinkeishitsusho cannot be treated by intellect. It is important that the client adhere to the therapist's instructions. For seven days, clients are placed in complete isolation and told to maintain a resting or prone state except during use of the toilet and bath. They are prohibited from performing any activities that distract them, including talking with other patients, receiving visitors, and reading for pleasure or distraction. Clients are told to observe their fears and anxieties without escaping. Morita stated, "the more intensely the client suffers, the more s/he achieves the aim of treatment. When a client's distress reaches a climax, it naturally and completely disappears within a short time" (Morita, 1928/1998, p. 39). By the fourth day of complete isolation, clients report feeling bored and a natural desire for activities emerges. The therapist sees the client once a day for a few minutes in Morita's case, while contemporary Morita therapists spend more time with clients to establish rapport (Iwai & Abe, 1975).

The second stage: Light occupational work   The client continues to be isolated. "Conversation and amusements are prohibited . . . and the client is instructed to go outdoors into the fresh air and sunlight during the daytime" (Morita, 1928/1998, p. 44) in order to increase spontaneous mental activity. Twice a day, in the morning and before going to bed, clients are told to read aloud from the Japanese classical literature in order to decrease mental ruminations, particularly at night.

The purpose of the second stage, which can last for two to four weeks, is to let clients endure the boredom of isolation, accept the distress of shinkeishitsusho, and to stimulate spontaneous activities and desires for action rather than following a set schedule of activities. Morita observed that the client begins to show signs of perfectionism when engaging in even trivial activity such as looking at a nest of ants. Clients are driven to examine this thoroughly. Morita therapists thus do not impose large tasks on clients to prevent them from being overwhelmed by the desire for success and perfection. The second stage is designed to stimulate clients' small spontaneous activities to get out of boredom. In this way, clients learn to enact behaviors without self-preoccupation.

From the second day of stage two, clients are directed to constant activities for over 15 hours a day (Morita, 1928/1998). Clients are permitted to engage in heavier and increasingly diversified work according to the purpose-oriented method. Therapists do not reinforce clients' complaints of shinkeishitsu symptoms. At the end of the second stage, clients generally stop complaining about their hypochondriacal symptoms. Morita summarized the second stage: "My therapy aims at radical treatment and breaks down clients' self-evaluating attitudes by de-emphasizing a focus on feelings of comfort and discomfort" (Morita, 1928/1998, p. 48). Clients are encouraged to keep a diary. Therapists read clients' diaries to assess their mental states and attitudes toward therapy and they write brief comments to guide clients.

The third stage: Intensive occupational work   The goals of the third stage, which lasts one or two weeks, are to acquire patience and to endure work, to increase self-confidence, and to provide encouragement through repeated experiences of success. Clients engage in various tasks such as mopping the floor or washing dishes. Through the direct experience of successfully executed tasks, clients are expected to learn the value of taking actions before being preoccupied with symptoms of shinkeishitsu.

The fourth stage: Preparation for daily living   The purpose of the fourth and final stage in Morita therapy is to train clients to adjust to changes in the outside world. Purpose-oriented activities are emphasized. At this stage, clients are trained to act free of preoccupations and fixations. Therapists encourage clients to read as much as they can throughout the day. They are permitted to go outside the hospital for errands and experience the demands of the outside world without anticipatory fears and preoccupations with shinkeishitsu symptoms.

Current Status of Morita Therapy

Iwai and Abe (1975) categorized four types of Morita therapy centers in Japan. The first is the inpatient setting practicing Morita's original ideas for the treatment of shinkeishitsusho. Activity therapy and experiential living are emphasized. The second category includes outpatient clinics. The third category is Morita therapy programs for outpatient treatment within university hospitals. The fourth type consists of meetings of *Seikatsu no Hakkenkai* (Hasegawa, 1990), translated as "association for discovery of life." Yozo Hasegawa founded Hakkenkai in 1970 with the support of Dr. Takehisa Kora, Morita's successor. With more than 4,000 members, group study meetings are organized throughout Japan to assist group members in overcoming mutual problems of shinkeishitsu. The study group is not based on therapist-client relationships. Members believe that the principles of Morita therapy can be applied to education and leading a productive life. Hakkenkai is essentially a self-support group and maintains a very close relationship with Morita-oriented treatment centers to refer clients when professional intervention for their members is necessary. Today, there are close to 150 Hakkenkai meetings in Japan (Seikatsu no Hakkenkai, n.d.).

In 1986, the first international seminar on Morita therapy was held under the sponsorship of Hakkenkai and the ToDo Institute of David Reynolds in Los Angeles. The first volume of the *International Bulletin of Morita Therapy* was published in English in 1988. The publication of this journal has contributed to the accelerated international spread of Morita therapy. In the first volume, Ishiyama (1988) reviewed the status of research methods, instruments, and results of Morita therapy, and called for international efforts to conduct controlled studies. This journal has published excerpts from Shoma Morita's collected works as well as Kora's (1990a, 1990b, 1991) introductions of the theory of practice of Morita therapy. These international efforts helped increase the practice of Morita therapy outside of Japan, including countries such as the United States (e.g., Hedstrom, 1994; Reynolds, 1995), Canada (e.g., Ishiyama, 1986), Australia (e.g., LeVine, 1993), and China (e.g., Lee, Zin, Liu, & Tan, 1990).

Constructive Living

David Reynolds (1976, 1980, and 1983) introduced Naikan therapy and Morita therapy to the United States. He studied Naikan and Morita therapies in Japan in the 1960s and conducted fieldwork in these methods for his doctoral dissertation in anthropology. He saw common value in Morita and Naikan therapies and began integrating the two methods and called the integration of the two methods Constructive Living. According to Reynolds (1995), "one of the goals of Constructive Living is to shake the foundations of clinical psychology and psychiatry in the West" (p. 5). Reynolds challenges the assumptions and models that underlie traditional Western psychotherapies. Constructive Living teaches people to focus on purposeful behavior and "let the feelings take care of themselves" (Reynolds, 1995, p. 5). The three elements of Constructive Living are "accept reality, know your purpose, and do what needs to be done" (Reynolds, 1995, p. 21). Today, certified Constructive Living instructors can be found in Canada, England, Germany, Japan, New Zealand, Mexico, and the United States (Reynolds, 1995). The web site www.anamorph. com/todo can be accessed and members can correspond on the electronic mailing list.

POINTS OF CONNECTION WITH WESTERN THERAPIES

Indigenous therapies are designed to respond to cultural formulations of abnormal behaviors and are replete with cultural values and idioms of distress that are familiar to the members of the culture (Tanaka-Matsumi & Draguns, 1997). Indigenous therapies also mobilize therapeutic change mechanisms that seem to be universal.

Various authors have studied similarities between Morita therapy and Western therapies such as rational emotive therapy (LeVine, 1993), cognitive therapy (Ishiyama, 1986), and behavior therapy (Reynolds, 1976). Morita himself practiced various therapies, including hypnosis and Binswanger's life control method, to treat shinkeishitsu clients. He was critical of Freud's structural approach to personality and psychoanalysis and any approach that used only verbal means, such as Dubois' method of "persuasive arguments," which he found ineffective.

Morita therapy's emphases on performing goal-oriented activities and the reduction of mental preoccupation are similar to current emphases by cognitive behavior therapies on the reduction of avoidance behaviors and the acceptance of emotional distress via exposure to various feared stimuli. Morita therapy uses an extreme social stimulus deprivation via the initial bed rest to teach clients to gradually reappraise and appreciate social interchanges.

Morita therapy's international practice demonstrates its universal therapeutic features. For example, we observe a move within cognitive behavior therapy to accommodate Zen philosophies of life. Linehan's (1993) dialectical behavior therapy explicitly states that life is composed of dialectics defined as "the reconciliation of opposites in a continued process of synthesis" (p. 19). Linehan states that the emphasis on "acceptance as a balance to change flows directly from the integration of a perspective drawn from Eastern (Zen) practice with Western psychological practice" (p. 19). Thus, two different Eastern and Western therapeutic systems may share general conceptual frameworks whose specific contents are nevertheless filled with culture-specific themes (independent self versus interdependent self) and procedures (e.g., nonverbal versus verbal transactions) to maximize therapeutic effects.

Furthermore, Morita's analysis of toraware, or mental preoccupation with various anxiety symptoms by shinkeishitsusho patients, has much relevance to Barlow's (1988) model of anxiety disorders. Barlow focused on the assessment of anxious apprehension and somatic conditioning. Panic patients are alarmed by somatic symptoms (e.g., heart palpitations, cold sweat, and dizziness), which serve to signal intense anxieties as well as anticipatory fears in similar situations. Morita focused on the functional analysis of anxieties and attempted to free patients from preoccupying fears and anxieties by encouraging acceptance of them without avoidance, although he accomplished this goal in a highly structured, stimulus-deprived therapeutic environment without verbal explorations of the problems with clients. Barlow's programs also achieve the same goal of anxiety reduction and panic control via somatic exposure without avoidance. Endogenous mechanisms of therapeutic change may be similar, whereas exogenous mechanisms to accomplish the goals differ.

* * * *

Naikan therapy and Morita therapy are two representative Japanese indigenous psychotherapies whose goals are to resocialize clients to their social networks. Both therapies meet criteria for four universal features of psychotherapy with regard to the prescribed therapist-client relationship, a special healing setting, a therapy rationale, and a therapeutic procedure (Frank & Frank, 1991). Therapists do not engage in elaborate dialogues with clients but make sure that clients engage in prescribed self-reflection in Naikan therapy, or regulated physical tasks in Morita therapy. Both therapies accommodate Japanese cultural themes of specific interpersonal transactions rather than themes of individuation of self as frequently seen in Western therapies. Certain commonalities between Naikan and Morita therapies and cognitive-behavior therapies were also reviewed.

REFERENCES

Azuma, H. (1994). *Nipponjin no shitsuke to kyoiku* [Child discipline and education in Japan]. Tokyo: Tokyo Daigaku Shuppankai.

Bandura, A. (1982). *Self-efficacy mechanism in human agency.* New York: Hold, Rinehart and Winston.

Barlow, D. H. (1988). *Anxiety and its disorders: The nature and treatment of anxiety and panic.* New York: Guilford.

Doi, L. T. (1973). *Anatomy of dependence.* Tokyo: Kodansha International.

Draguns, J. G. (1975). Resocialization into culture: The complexities of taking a world-wide view of psychotherapy. In R. Brislin, S. Bochner, & W. Lonner (Eds.), *Cross-cultural perspectives on learning* (pp. 273-289). Beverly Hills, CA: Sage.

Draguns, J. G. (2002). Universal and cultural aspects of counseling and psychotherapy. In P. B. Pedersen, J. G. Draguns, W. J. Lonner, & J. E. Trimble (Eds.), *Counseling across cultures* (5th ed.) (pp. 29-50). Thousand Oaks, CA: Sage.

Frank, J. D., & Frank, J. B. (1991). *Persuasion and healing: A comparative study of psychotherapy* (3rd ed.). Baltimore, MD: The Johns Hopkins University Press.

Geertz, C. (1973). *The interpretation of cultures.* New York: Basic Books.

Hasegawa, Y. (1990). Hakkenkai's method of studying Morita theory: A group learning approach to overcoming neurosis. *International Bulletin of Morita Therapy, 3,* 26-34.

Hedstrom, L. J. (1994). Morita and Naikan therapies: American applications. *Psychotherapy, 31,* 154-160.

Herskovits, M. J. (1948). *Man and his works: The science of cultural anthropology.* New York: Knopf.

Higginbotham, H. N., West, S., & Forsyth, D. (1988). *Psychotherapy and behavior change: Social, cultural and methodological perspectives.* New York: Pergamon.

Ishida, R. (1972). Naikanho no rinsho igaku [Clinical medicine of Naikan therapy]. In K. Sato (Ed.), *Zenteki ryohou naikanho* [Zen therapy and Naikan therapy]. Tokyo: Bunkodo.

Ishiyama, F. I. (1986). Morita therapy: Its basic features and cognitive intervention for anxiety treatment. *Psychotherapy, 23,* 375-381.

Ishiyama, F. I. (1988). Current status of Morita therapy research: An overview of research methods, instruments, and results. *International Bulletin of Morita Therapy, 1,* 58-83.

Iwai, H., & T. Abe (1975). *Morita ryoho no riron to jissai* [Theory and practice of Morita therapy]. Tokyo: Kongo Shuppan.

Johnson, F. A. (1993). *Dependency and Japanese socialization: Psychoanalytic and anthropological investigations into Amae.* New York: New York University Press.

Kimura, B. (1965). Vergleichende Untersuchungen über depressive Erkrankungen in Japan und Deutschland [Comparative investigations of depressive illness in Japan and Germany]. *Fortschritte der Psychiatrie und Neurologie, 33,* 202-215.

Kimura, B. (1972). *Hito to Hito tono Aida* [Interpersonal space]. Tokyo: Kobundo.

Kirmayer, L. J. (1991). The place of culture in psychiatric nosology: Taijin Kyofusho and DSM III-R. *Journal of Nervous and Mental Disorder, 179,* 19-28.

Kitayama, O. (Ed.). (1999). "*Amae" ni tsuite kangaeru* [Thoughts about "amae"]. Tokyo: Seiwa Shoten.

Kleinknecht, R. A., Dinnel, D. L., Kleinknecht, E. E., Hiruma, N., & Harada, N. (1997). Cultural factors in social anxiety: A comparison of social phobia symptoms and Taijin Kyofusho. *Journal of Anxiety Disorders, 11,* 157-177.

Kleinman, A. (1978). Clinical relevance of anthropological and cross-cultural research: Concepts and strategies. *American Journal of Psychiatry, 135,* 427-431.

Kleinman, A. (1980). *Patients and healers in the context of culture.* Berkeley, CA: University of California Press.

Kora, T. (1990a). An overview of the theory and practice of Morita therapy (Part 2). *International Bulletin of Morita Therapy, 3,* 7-13.

Kora, T. (1990b). An overview of the theory and practice of Morita therapy: III. Methods used in residential Morita therapy. *International Bulletin of Morita Therapy, 3,* 71-76.

Kora, T. (1991). An overview of the theory and practice of Morita therapy: IV. Understanding and treating shinkeishitsu symptoms in Morita therapy. *International Bulletin of Morita Therapy, 4,* 42-46.

Lebra, T. S. (1969). Reciprocity and the asymmetric principles and analytical reappraisal of the Japanese concept of On. *Psychologia, 12,* 129-138.

Lee, Z., Zin, T., Liu, J., & Tan, W. (1990). Is Morita therapy for patients with shinkeishitsu symptoms or shinkeishitsu personality characteristics? A clinical study in China. *International Bulletin of Morita Therapy, 3,* 85-91.

LeVine, P. (1993). Morita-based therapy and its use across cultures in the treatment of bulimia nervosa. *Journal of Counseling & Development, 72,* 82-90.

Lin, T. Y. (1989). Neurasthenia revisited: Its place in modern psychiatry. *Culture, Medicine and Psychiatry, 13,* 105-129.

Linehan, M. (1993). *Cognitive behavioral treatment of borderline personality disorder.* New York: Guilford.

Markus, H. R., & Kitayama, S. (1991). Culture and the self: Implications for cognition, emotion and motivation. *Psychological Review, 98,* 224-253.

Miki, Y. (1976). *Naikan Ryoho Nyumon* [Introduction to Naikan therapy]. Tokyo: Sogensha.

Miyake, K., Campos, J. J., Kagan, J., & Bradshaw, D. L. (1986). Issues in socioemotional development. In H. Stevenson, H. Azuma, & K. Hakuta (Eds.), *Child development and education in Japan* (pp. 239-261). New York: W. H. Freeman.

Morita, S. (1928/1998). *Morita therapy and the true nature of anxiety-based disorders (Shinkeishitsu).* (A. Kondo, Trans.). Albany, NY: State University of New York Press.

Morita, S. (1953). *Shinkei suijyaku to kyouhaku kannen no konchihou* [Treatment of shinkeisuijyaku and obsessional ideas]. Tokyo: Hakugeisha.

Murase, T. (1974). Naikan therapy. In T. S. Lebra & W. P. Lebra (Eds.), *Japanese culture and behavior* (pp. 431-443). Honolulu: East-West Center Press.

Murase, T. (1996). *Naikan riron to bunka kanrensei* [Naikan theory and cultural relevance]. Tokyo: Seishin Shobou.

Murase, T., & Johnson, F. A. (1974). Naikan, Morita, and Western psychotherapy: A comparison. *Archives of General Psychiatry, 31,* 121-128.

Naito, T., & Gielen, U. P. (in press). The changing Japanese family: A psychological portrait. In J. L. Roopnarine & U. P. Gielen (Eds.), *Families in global perspectives.* Boston: Allyn & Bacon.

Pedersen, P. B. (1997). *Culture-centered counseling interventions: Striving for accuracy.* Thousand Oaks, CA: Sage.

Prince, R. (1980). Variations in psychotherapeutic procedures. In H. C. Triandis & J. G. Draguns (Eds.), *Handbook of cross-cultural psychology, psychopathology* (Vol. 6, pp. 291-354). Boston: Allyn and Bacon.

Reynolds, D. K. (1976). *Morita psychotherapy.* Berkeley: University of California Press.

Reynolds, D. K. (1980). *The quiet therapies: Japanese pathways to personal growth.* Honolulu: The University Press of Hawaii.

Reynolds, D. K. (1983). *Naikan psychotherapy: Meditation for self-development.* Chicago: University of Chicago Press.

Reynolds, D. K. (1995). *A handbook for constructive living.* Honolulu: The University Press of Hawaii.

Roland, A. (1988). *In search of self in India and Japan: Toward a cross-cultural psychology.* Princeton, NJ: Princeton University Press.

Russell, J. G. (1989). Anxiety disorders in Japan: A review of the Japanese literature on Shinkeishitsu and Taijin Kyofusho. *Culture, Medicine, and Psychiatry, 13,* 391-403.

Segall, M. H., Dasen, P. R., Berry, J. W., & Poortinga, Y. H. (1999). *Human behavior in global perspective: An introduction to cross-cultural psychology* (2nd ed.). Boston: Allyn and Bacon.

Seiden, D. Y., Lam, K., & Tanaka-Matsumi, J. (1996, February). Taijin Kyofusho: Cultural context of social phobias in Japan. In J. G. Draguns (Chair), *Social phobia, Taijin Kyofusho, and anthropophobia: Three disor-*

ders or one? Observations in China, Japan, and the United States. Symposium conducted at the annual meeting of the Society for Cross-Cultural Research, Pittsburgh, PA.

Seikatsu no Hakkenkai (n.d.). *Introduction to Seikatsu no Hakkenkai.* Retrieved September 27, 2003, from http://hakkenkai.gr.jp/introduct.htm

Sugiwaka, H., Takeshima, A., Nishimura, R., Yamamoto, M., & Agari, I. (1992). Waga kuni ni okeru seishin ryoho no genjyo to kousatsu [The status of psychotherapy in Japan]. *Seishin Ryoho, 18,* 248-255.

Takahashi, T. (1976). *Taijin kyofu.* Tokyo: Igaku Shoin.

Taketomo, Y. (1986). AMAE as a meta-language: A critique of Doi's theory of AMAE. *Journal of the American Academy of Psychoanalysis, 14,* 69-84.

Taketomo, Y. (1999). Taijinkoudouteki AMAE to seishinnaiteki AMAE: Nichijyougo *amae* no encho ni aru seishinbunseki jyutsugo *amae* no mondai. [Interactional AMAE and intrapsychic AMAE: A problem of a psychoanalytic term AMAE proposed as the extension of an ordinary Japanese word.]. In O. Kitayama (Ed.), *Amae ni tsuite kangaeru* (pp. 47-64) [Thoughts about *Amae*]. Tokyo: Seiwa Shoten.

Tanaka-Matsumi, J. (1979a). Cultural factors and social influence techniques in Naikan therapy: A Japanese self-observation method. *Psychotherapy: Theory, Research and Practice, 16,* 385-390.

Tanaka-Matsumi, J. (1979b). Taijin Kyofusho: Diagnostic and cultural issues in Japanese psychiatry. *Culture, Medicine, and Psychiatry, 3,* 231-245.

Tanaka-Matsumi, J., Higginbotham, N. H., & Chang, R. (2002). Cognitive-behavioral approaches to counseling across cultures: A functional analytic approach for clinical applications. In P. B. Pedersen, J. G. Draguns, W. L. Lonner, & J. E. Trimble (Eds.), *Counseling across cultures* (5th ed.). (pp. 337-354). Thousand Oaks, CA: Sage.

Tanaka-Matsumi, J., & Draguns, J. G. (1997). Culture and psychopathology. In J. Berry, M. Segall, & C. Kagitcibasi (Eds.), *Handbook of cross-cultural psychology. Vol. 3: Social psychology, personality and psychopathology,* 2nd ed. (pp. 449-491). Boston: Allyn and Bacon.

Tanaka-Matsumi, J., Seiden, D. G., & Lam, K. (2001). Translating cultural observations into psychotherapy: A functional approach. In J. F. Schumaker & T. Ward (Eds.), *Cognition, culture and psychopathology* (pp. 193-212). New York: Praeger.

Tezuka, C. (1999). Therapy ni okeru *"amae"* to kotoba. Aru kojinteki taiken no ichi kousatsu [*Amae* and language in therapy: Consideration of a personal experience]. In O. Kitayama (Ed.), *"Amae" ni tsuite kangaeru* [Thoughts about *amae*] (pp. 67-82). Tokyo: Seiwa Shoten.

Weisz, J. R., Rothbaum, F. M., & Blackburn, T. C. (1984). Standing out and standing in: The psychology of control in American and Japan. *American Psychologist, 39,* 955-969.

Yoshimoto, I. (1989). *Naikanhou-40nen no ayumi* [Forty years of Naikan therapy] (Rev. ed.). Tokyo: Bunshusha.

Yoshimoto, I. (1996). *Naikan eno shoutai* [Invitation to Naikan] (Rev. ed.). Osaka, Japan: Toki Shobou.

Indian Conceptions of Mental Health, Healing, and the Individual

Rashmi Jaipal
Bloomfield College

Many psychological theories and interventions that prevail have originated in the West and are based on particular conceptions of mental health and the individual that have largely evolved within a Western cultural and historical context. This chapter looks at alternative conceptions of health and the individual as developed by Indian psychologists originating in an Indian cultural context. This different understanding of mental health, which is based on a different definition of the individual, has implications for treatment in India, as well as the potential to significantly contribute to and expand Western concepts of health and interventions. The recent growth of indigenous psychologies originating in non-Western cultures such as India presents an opportunity for psychology to be built on a broader range of cultures and human experience.

Indian indigenous psychology cannot be articulated without taking into account the current situation in India regarding not only psychology and treatment strategies, but also the larger social context of rapid modernization within which Indian psychology operates. Therefore, the first part of the chapter is devoted to the current situation in India regarding the psychological effects of modernization and acculturation, followed by a discussion on the current status of psychology in India, both theoretical and applied, and its gradual indigenization. The second half of the chapter is devoted to a review of Indian indigenous psychology, and an attempt is made to synthesize traditional Ayurvedic conceptions of mental health and the individual with the concepts of *dharma* and *swadharma*. The implications of the Ayurvedic concept of the individual as representing a personality type are delineated as a contribution to the development of an Indian psychology. Since the purpose of the chapter is to review, discuss, and add to the formulation of an Indian indigenous psychology, it draws primarily on the work of Indian psychologists and their use of Hindu philosophical concepts, as well as their articulation of some of the underlying attitudes and beliefs of many Indians that derive from the Hindu worldview and seem to permeate Indian society. It does not therefore rely on philosophical, religious, or anthropological sources, because this would be beyond the scope of this chapter.

THE CURRENT CONTEXT OF PSYCHOLOGY IN INDIA

In India, the status of psychology and psychotherapy is fraught with contradiction. It reflects the disparities of a country in transition; of globalizing, Westernizing forces in an uneasy juxtaposition with older, more deeply rooted traditional worldviews and social relations; of huge divisions between class and caste, urban and rural; of a growing middle class and an increasingly Americanized private sector struggling with entrenched government bureaucracies. Conflicts between older traditional structures and newer modernizing influences are reflected in the disparity between the kinds of mental disorders found.

Some of the most frequent mental disorders seen by general health professionals in India, according to recent research, are depression and anxiety disorders (Patel et al., 2003). However, disorders that are more culture specific are also found such as *dhat* (anxiety, impotence, and an enervated state thought to result from sperm loss) and *koro* (an irrational fear of genitals retracting into the abdomen, resulting in death). These are found mainly in rural areas, in male patients of low socioeconomic status (Varma & Chakraborty, 1995). Also found in rural areas are some kinds of hysterical psychosis and possession states (acute psychoses following a stressor where the person behaves as if possessed by a god, demon, or ancestral spirit, etc.) that are particularly common among young women. Urban areas, on the other hand, appear to show an increase in the previously mentioned problems of depression and anxiety states. Community surveys of rural and urban populations have found that mental illness prevalence rates are higher in urban populations. Most studies show that the highest rates of mental disorders are in the 20- to 45-year age range with a sharp decline after 50 years. Mental disorders are higher for married couples, especially married women who are not working outside the home. Studies also show higher rates for middle-class Indians (Varma & Chakraborty, 1995).

These epidemiological patterns seem to reflect some of the dichotomies that have developed due to modernization. Rural areas seem to have a higher prevalence rate of "traditional" illnesses such as dhat or koro, whereas urban areas seem to have illnesses that reflect the stresses of modernization. Because of the increasing breakup of the extended family, particularly in urban areas, more burdens may be placed on married couples in nuclear family situations, especially on women, leading to higher rates of mental disorder (Varma & Chakraborty, 1995). Conversely, at the same time, the extended family ties are very present psychologically. This is reflected in more care for the elderly and a corresponding decline in mental disorders after middle age. In fact, some studies show that the extended family is relatively strong in some areas and serves to cushion the effects of urbanization (Korom, 2001). The urbanization process may be most conflictual for middle-class, married, nonworking women, who are caught between traditional and changing gender roles (Bhui, 1999). Another major factor contributing to stress for women and implicated in prevalence rates of depression is coping with poverty and economic problems. A recent study of postpartum depression among low-income women in a district hospital in Goa found that the most important factors that put these women at risk for depression were economic deprivation and marital problems (Patel, Rodrigues, & DeSouza, 2002).

Another feature of modernization and urbanization is that migration from the rural countryside to the cities continues to grow. Acculturation stress, alcoholism, and drug abuse have increased in tribal groups who have been uprooted and resettled in urban slums, and are facing massive cultural dislocation. They have increased their reliance on their traditions and rituals rather than adopt modern therapies as a way to cope with the strains of acculturation (Mookherjee, 1995). In addition, a higher frequency of mental disorders is found in refugee populations from Pakistan and Bangladesh even years after migration (Varma & Chakraborty, 1995). An interesting effect of changes in urban areas is the rise of mental health and health problems among the New Delhi police. According to an internal review by the police department, due to severe stress and job-related tensions, many policemen have severe sleep disorders, mental problems, and increasing rates of heart attacks. Another study found nearly 40 percent of police personnel had mental disorders (Kumar, 2000).

In general, the different kinds of psychological disorders that exist in India, from dhat and koro to acculturation stress, reflect the traditional-rural, and modern-urban cultural environments that coexist, as well as the deep divisions between them. These divisions are reflected in higher prevalence rates for many psychological problems in areas that are urbanizing. Such problems seem due to the pressures of modernization and acculturation, resulting in increased stress as people try to bridge the gap.

Treatment for these problems is usually based on the Western psychiatric paradigm by psychologists and psychiatrists trained in the Western traditions. India is coming out of a long period of mental colonization, which is of major importance to the discipline of psychology. When faced with the current situation, many aspects of psychology as practiced in the West are not really applicable to most Indians. A recent study by Chadda et al. (2001) on help-seeking behavior among Indians found that prior to their visit to a psychiatric clinic, they had sought the help of a wide range of indigenous therapeutic modalities, including religious faith healers and alternative medicine such as Ayurveda. Although this tendency, due to cultural beliefs in the supernatural causation of illness, as well as the accessibility of the provider, has been diminishing since the expansion of psychiatric facilities in India, multiple treatment modalities, which include traditional medical approaches, are still widely used (Chadda et al., 2001). The New Delhi police department, for example, has instituted a meditation program for their police personnel to help in stress reduction, which has been found to be very effective (Kumar, 2000).

Unfortunately, the effects of colonization die hard, and many Indian psychologists still continue to unthinkingly apply Western psychological theories and methods (Sinha, 1993). Misra states that due to the effects of colonialism, the Indian academic world looked down on its own cultural heritage. Western concepts were unquestioningly accepted and applied, whereas indigenous concepts were dismissed and not even allowed to enter into academic discourse (Gergen, Gulerce, Lock, & Misra, 1996). Adair, Puhan, and Vohra (1993) propose that the process of indigenization goes through stages and that this process has been taking place very slowly in India. However, there has been a growing awareness of the effects of mental colonization. There are more publications about indigenous psychology, and indigenous concepts are being considered seriously as viable alternatives. Sinha (1993) distinguishes between revivalist Indian psychology, superficial indigenization, and true indigenization, which in his view represents the empirical investigation of Indian modes of operating. He feels that indigenization should not lead to cultural relativism but to more universal categories. In general, one could say that psychology in India has gone through stages—from blindly applying Western psychology to discovering that it was problematic and hence modifying Western theories to be more adaptive to an Indian context, to finally articulating local psychological theories and worldviews.

PROBLEMS WITH THE WESTERN PARADIGM

A review of the literature reveals some of the ways in which the application of Western psychology in India has been problematic. This covers three main areas that have to do with the influence of an individualistic value orientation, and with compartmentalization in Western psychology. One problem is that the Western paradigm contains implicit assumptions regarding mental health that are based on an individualistic value system. These values are mostly incongruent with Indian culture. Theorists such as Roland (1988, 1996) have articulated the very different set of implicit assumptions underlying Indian conceptions of psychological health and social relations, based on a more collectivist value system and the Hindu worldview. Roland states that psychoanalysis is the "psychological theory and therapy par excellence of modern Western individualism. If individuals are set upon their own in society in a way never before done, then psychoanalysis is oriented toward enabling them to be on their own (by resolving all kinds of inner conflicts and deficits)" (Roland, 1996, p. 13). He discusses how psychoanalysis based on individualistic norms defines what healthy human nature should be and how it develops in contrast to psychopathology. Outer ego boundaries between the self and others have to be firm so that closeness does not mean merging with others, which is considered pathological. He states that the norms for "the North European and North American individualized self as formulated in current psychoanalytic theory are considered to be universal and superior" (Roland, 1996, p. 13).

In cultures like India and Japan, however, according to Roland, outer ego boundaries are much more permeable, and there are semimerger experiences of greater emotional intensity and closeness with others. Consequently, firm outer ego boundaries are maladaptive and neurotic for Indians and Japanese. The norms for healthy and unhealthy functioning based on ego boundaries vary with culture. This seems supported by Dhawan et al.'s (1995) findings on the cultural construction of the self-concept. They found that an Indian sample placed significantly more emphasis on a social identity component of the self-concept than an American sample. Roland calls for a new paradigm in psychoanalysis that applies the categories of psychoanalysis such as ego boundaries in a way that takes into account the cultural construction of these categories.

The Western paradigm is also problematic in the area of intervention and treatment. The whole social enterprise of psychotherapy, which involves self-reflection, self-analysis, and verbalization of private feelings to a stranger/therapist on a hired, contractual basis is a fairly recent social construction arising in a Western individualistic context. Social categories for psychotherapist and for contractual relations between therapist and patient as separate individuals do not exist in the Indian cultural context.

Rastogi and Wampler (1997) point out the difficulties in being a family therapist in India. The gender and age of the therapist largely determine how the patient and family will relate to him or her. To admit psychological problems to outsiders brings shame on the family. Traditionally, older members of the extended family intervened in relationship problems within the family. A young, unmarried female stranger intervening in a family problem is not taken seriously, and the therapist has little credibility unless he or she carries the social authority of age, gender, or of being from a higher social class. Social class and caste issues are very important factors when attempting to do therapy. Rastogi and Wampler (1997) discuss the treatment of a rural family living in poverty. The therapist had to act in conjunction with the local activist, who was running a support group for rural women, and had to take macrosocial issues into account such as class and gender roles. She also had to combine social action and advocacy with working on relationship problems. The social categories of family elder or activist are more socially acceptable and familiar than the role of "therapist." There have been some attempts therefore to fit psychotherapy into existing social categories, such as the *guru-chela* or teacher-student relationship (Misra, 1993).

The third aspect of the Western paradigm that has proven problematic in the Indian context is the tendency to focus on the microcontext (Sinha, 1993). Macrosocial issues are left to other disciplines such as sociology and anthropology. Sinha found that this leads to psychology being largely irrelevant in a country where rural development and other pressing social issues are of paramount concern. He recommends focusing on more relevant issues on the macrosocial level, such as rural development, as well as collaborating with other fields to make psychological approaches to these problems more interdisciplinary. This approach was demonstrated by Rastogi (1997) in the discussion earlier on family therapy in rural India. Macrosocial issues such as the effects of mass dislocation from the countryside and acculturation to modern urban environments are also beginning to be investigated, as discussed earlier.

INDIAN INDIGENOUS PSYCHOLOGY

Given the aforementioned problems of applying the Western psychological paradigm in India, recent attempts by Indian psychologists to develop a more relevant indigenous psychological framework constitute an important step in the right direction. They draw mainly upon the vast wealth of knowledge pertaining to psychology and healing represented by the Hindu philosophy and scriptures. There are many different approaches to mental illness in the Hindu tradition. The Samkhya Yoga and Vedanta philosophies, scriptures such as the *Bhagavad Gita*, and traditional medicine or Ayurveda all include conceptualizations of mental disturbance. Paranjpe (1988) discusses the philosophy of Advaita Vedanta and its theory that a person is made up of layers of consciousness. According to this view, the source of suffering comes through wrong identification of the self with the body and the mind. Other psychologists take the principle of nonattachment to the fruits of action from the *Bhagavad Gita* and relate it to the alleviation of stress (Sinha, 1993). Sharma (1995) talks about the role of the *samskaras* or memory traces in determining behavior. Misra (1993) emphasizes the holistic nature of the Hindu worldview and articulates its main features, among them coherence and natural order across all life forms, the concept of dharma or a moral code of action that requires staying in tune with the natural order, and a socially constituted, embedded, and relational concept of the person. He finds that "to a large extent the worldview of the people is organized around the notion of dharma and a belief in the inherent order of the universe" (Misra, 1993, p. 233). Not staying in tune with the natural order can result in ill health and psychological disturbances.

Indian psychologists such as Balodhi (1991) and Sinha (1990) have discussed traditional holistic definitions of health and illness according to the Ayurvedic system of medicine. Balodhi (1991) finds Western therapeutic interventions are incongruent with the Ayurvedic holistic worldview. This holistic worldview influences definitions of the individual and of psychological health and illness. Instead of the Western concept of health based on the separate individual, there seems to be a concept of health based on the individual as a personality type (to be discussed later), and as part of the sociocultural and cosmic whole. In the West, as stated earlier, pathology is often associated with symbiosis and a lack of ego boundaries between self and others. For many psychoanalysts, to restore a person to healthy functioning means helping the individual to separate and become an autonomous, self-reliant individual (Roland, 1996). However, as Roland (1996) observes, the Indian experience of health is based on the connected self, which has semipermeable ego boundaries and greater intimacy experiences with others. This connected self is a product of the holistic Hindu world-view. The aim of traditional Indian medicine is to restore health not by helping individuals to separate, but by helping them maintain their connections with others in a more harmonious fashion, thereby restoring a state of balance with the whole. This has implications for modern psychological interventions that are more applicable in the Indian context.

Balodhi (1991) finds that Western medical or psychological treatment is inadequate, especially when dealing with patients in rural areas, because of its dualistic assumptions of the separateness of mental and physical phenomena. He discusses how the Hindu society is a world of sharing. Illness is seen as an integral part of the whole community and is the fault of the whole community. Health is based on a holistic worldview of no separation between mind, body, and society. Holistic Ayurvedic interventions involve diet, massage, herbal medication, and the performance of rituals that often include family members. Therefore, patients expect more from treatment than just Western-style therapy or medication. Balodhi and others recommend that psychiatrists work with local Ayurvedic practitioners and try to familiarize themselves with Ayurvedic and folk concepts of mental ailments (Balodhi, 1991; Varma, 1995).

Kakar (1982), in his excursions into different Indian healing traditions, describes an Ayurvedic doctor at work with severely mentally ill patients in his clinic. Some of the doctor's patients had tried Western-style psychiatric treatment such as electroshock therapy and medication. They were not satisfied and had come to him for traditional treatment. His therapy consisted of herbal medications and dietary prescriptions administered in a live-in therapeutic milieu with the patient's family and clinic staff working together to help the patient.

For the treatment of mental problems in India, coordinating a variety of treatment options such as allopathic as well as Ayurvedic medicine seems appropriate. Psychiatrists working with the local Ayurvedic physician might be able to provide more comprehensive treatment for the patient within a familiar, supportive social and cultural context. To prevent patients from dropping out of treatment, it is necessary to understand and incorporate the local worldview, including beliefs and concepts of the individual into psychological understanding. These initial attempts by Indian psychologists to develop an indigenous psychology focus on articulating commonly held beliefs derived from Hindu philosophy and medicine that need to be utilized by mental health professionals in their therapeutic interpretations and interventions. Their attempts to incorporate Ayurvedic conceptions of health and especially of the individual have some interesting implications for counseling and therapy strategies.

AYURVEDIC CONCEPTIONS OF HEALTH AS BALANCE

Traditional Indian categories of health, illness, and the individual, based on a holistic approach, are complex and need to be more fully articulated. A comprehensive overview of the Ayurvedic system of medicine from an Ayurvedic researcher and practitioner's point of view is provided in a recent article by Mishra et al. (2001). The following section, however, takes a closer look at Indian psychologists' articulation of Ayurvedic concepts of health and illness. Central to the development of appropriate healing strategies are the Hindu concepts of dharma, or right action, and the Ayurvedic view of the individual. This section draws out the implications of the

Ayurvedic view of the individual as representing a unique psychosomatic type, relates this view to the concept of dharma, and discusses how this synthesized approach may lead to more relevant psychotherapeutic interventions in the Indian context. Sinha (1990) describes the traditional Ayurvedic definition of health as maintaining balance. Sinha's account of the Ayurvedic theory of health is expanded upon later and related to the concept of dharma. The notion of dharma is considered by Indian psychologists such as Kakar (1978) and Misra (1993) to be central to an understanding of the Indian psyche.

Ayurveda, which means the science of life, originated from the ancient Indian scriptures called the *Vedas*. Health in Ayurveda is defined as "a state of delight or a feeling of spiritual, physical and mental well-being. The essential feature of a healthy person is that he possesses various bodily constituents in the right quantity, neither too little nor too much" (Sinha, 1990, p. 5). Having various constituents in the right or *natural* quantities is essential for healthy functioning. *Asantulan* or imbalance is the cause of illness, the quantities of the constituents being out of proportion to each other. For health there should be a balance between the three constituents called the three *dhatus* that support the body—*vayu, pitta,* and *kapha* (Dube, Dube, & Kumar, 1982). The main objective is *dhatu-sama-kriya* or the restoration and maintenance of metabolic equilibrium (Sharma, 1975). This is also related to maintaining equilibrium with the environment. If the dhatus or constituent energies of the body become out of balance and increase or decrease disproportionately, they are called *doshas,* which means "faults."

Imbalance affects not just the physical, but the whole mind-body system reflecting a holistic viewpoint. Illness, or *dukha samyogo,* means "contact with dukha," or contact with physical pain and discomfort, as well as mental anguish, including pangs of jealousy, fear, anger, avarice, and hatred, that is, all that is unpleasant to the body and mind. An imbalance of the dhatus can cause an imbalance at the mental level. Conversely, an imbalance at the mental level can push the dhatus out of balance. There is nothing that can be thought of or experienced that does not affect the mind or body according to Ayurveda (Sharma, 1975). The cause of imbalance can therefore be located at any level of the spiritual-mental-physical system, and it will have repercussions on the other levels. The definition of medical treatment also reflects this holistic approach. Interventions can be of many different kinds that address all the levels of the mind-body system—words and thoughts, as well as medicines on the physical plane, can be used to intervene.

The dhatus, or constituents of the mind-body system, are based on the doctrine of the *Panch-Bhutas,* or the five elements (Kakar, 1982) that in a similar form are also found in Chinese traditional medicine. There is conceptual difficulty in describing these terms, as there seem to be no scientific or conceptual categories in modern Western thought that fit their nature. Terms such as *dhatus* or elements refer to subtle, vital energies of consciousness that are neither physical energies nor subtler mental energies but exist between these two levels. Nature, both animate and inanimate, is thought to consist of these energies of consciousness in the form of the five elements —air, fire, water, earth, and ether. This appears naive from the point of view of the physical sciences, which, in the periodic tables, identify the basic elements that constitute physical matter (air, fire, water, etc.). The latter are not thought of as elements because they are made up of much more basic building blocks of matter or energies. However, the Ayurvedic view of the five elements starts from the very different premise that there are subtle energies of consciousness similar in quality to air, fire, water, and others that make up all living things, including the human being. Each dhatu is composed of a combination of elements. (The vayu dhatu is composed of air and ether, pitta of water and fire, and kapha of earth and water.) These lead to different physical and mental qualities. There are also subdivisions of the dhatus or energies that predominate in different parts and organs of the body. The dhatus exist in different, very complex combinations in each person, often with one of the dhatus, vayu, pitta, or kapha, predominating over the others.

Each human being, therefore, has her or his own constitutional makeup of a particular configuration of the dhatus or doshas that lead to different psychosomatic or personality-body types. Body and mind in this view are not separate but intrinsically related. In addition, body and mind are not separate from the environment (Sharma, 1975). These dhatus or subtle vital energies are also present in nature, in plants, and in animals, which also vary in terms of their psychosomatic "types." Each human being, plant, and animal is a part of the whole because it is made up of the same dhatus and qualities of nature, and it has to stay in balance with the whole. The balance of the dhatus is related to seasonal variation and lifestyle. Thus, the notion of psychosomatic type is intrinsically relational to the environment, and its state of balance is constituted through interactions with nature of which it is a part.

Each type has its own definition of healthy versus unhealthy functioning, expressed as psychological qualities. For the vayu type, healthy functioning is associated with the psychological state of enthusiasm, whereas unhealthy functioning is associated with the psychological state of fear. For the pitta type, health is associated with feeling courageous, and illness with anger, and for the kapha type it is cheerful versus dull (Sharma, 1975). Imbalance leads to different "symptoms" for each type—fear and anxiety with an imbalance of vayu, anger and irritability with an imbalance of pitta, sluggishness with unbalanced kapha, and so forth. Health, here, is based on the concept of the individual as a personality type, and the definition of health varies with each type. (The individual is also seen as unique according to Ayurveda. Although each person is a type, each person's type is unique since the combinations of the doshas are very complex. In addition, each person is a product of the *gunas*, qualities of action, and *samskaras*, memory traces from past lives, which influence the configuration of the doshas in this lifetime.)

When treating disease, the Ayurvedic physician, rather than diagnosing the kind of disease the patient has, diagnoses instead the kind of patient he or she is, because this will provide the information about the problem (Sharma, 1975). It is important to treat each person differently depending on their constitutional makeup, and to restore the balance in functioning. Eating the right food for a particular psychosomatic type and particular season of the year is an example of staying in balance. Different types require different lifestyles and different herbal and psychotherapeutic remedies. Therefore, interventions are based on personality types because what promotes health for one personality type may cause illness for another type. For example, psychological problems such as anxiety, tension, and psychosomatic illness are associated with a *vata* constitution and are treated accordingly (Kumar & Shrivastava, 2000). Also, each individual type has to maintain its own relational balance with the natural and social order, and therapy aims at helping to restore or achieve this balance. The pitta type, for instance, needs to practice moderation in its relationships and lifestyle, whereas the kapha type needs to stimulate itself in its relationships and lifestyle. Health means having an appropriate lifestyle for one's particular personality and body type, and responding to its particular needs for harmonious balance with the world.

BALANCE AS DHARMA

Health is related to actions that maintain a balance between all the bodily constituents and between the body-mind system and the environment. This seems to imply the concepts of dharma and swadharma, which involve the performance of right action in the social and individual spheres to maintain connection with the whole. Misra (1993) and Kakar (1978) both emphasize the central role dharma and swadharma play in the Hindu worldview, and how this permeates Indian society in general. Dharma and swadharma are controversial and complicated concepts that have been used to justify oppressive caste systems in the social sphere. However, both these concepts have implications for psychological functioning because they are considered the means to achieve healthy maturity and eventually *moksha* or enlightenment, the final goal of life (Kakar, 1978). Kakar states that dharma originated in the *Vedas* and comes from the root *dhr,* which means to uphold or sustain. It has various translations, among them, "right action," or "conformity with the truth of things," and is the principle underlying social relations. It has two aspects; one is the social aspect, which is right action that upholds and sustains society. Society is seen as part of the natural order, an organic whole in which all members are interdependent and possess complementary roles.

The other aspect is swadharma, or individual dharma. This refers to "staying true to the ground plan of a person's life, the fulfillment of an individual's own particular life task. If a person does this, he is traveling on the path towards moksha or liberation and enlightenment" (Kakar, 1978, p. 37). A person gets to know his or her swadharma, or right action, by considering four factors. Right action depends on *desa,* the culture in which he or she is born; *kala,* the period of historical time in which he or she lives; *srama,* the actions appropriate for different stages of life; and *gunas,* or innate personality characteristics. Right action can only be determined after taking into account all these factors. What may be an appropriate lifestyle for one person depending on his or her age, culture, and so forth may not be for another person from another culture or historical time period. This is a sophisticated, holistic understanding that accommodates the complexity of human life. Understanding one's swadharma is important, because a person's right action in the world has the purpose of preparing him for the final goal of moksha. Actions are valued not so much for the external rewards they bring, as for the internal effects they have in developing the person spiritually, in furthering him or her along the path toward liberation (Kakar, 1978).

Among the factors in determining swadharma or right action for the individual are the person's innate characteristics. They include the person's particular psychosomatic type given by Ayurveda. Right action for the individual involves considering the needs of one's particular psychosomatic type in conjunction with one's present cultural and historical milieu and one's stage of life. Right action relates individuals in a balanced way both to themselves and to their context. Ayurvedic conceptions of health emphasize the needs of the psychosomatic type; if they are not taken into account while performing actions, it can lead to psychological and physical ill health. Swadharma here means the unfolding of the unique individual toward maturity and moksha through his or her particular constitutional needs and relational balance with the environment. This may seem similar to the Western idea of unique individual self-expression, but it is actually quite different in meaning. Here it is the expression of the personality type as a part of and complementary to the whole. Individual identity in the modern West is created through separation from dependence on others and through self-expression. This includes making individual choices and decisions regarding work, relationships, and so forth. Creating an individual identity is seen as a developmental goal. It is seen as separate from and often in opposition to the social and natural world. Not to conform, to triumph over adversity, and to control nature are frequently seen as the hallmarks of a strong individual.

The Ayurvedic concept of the unique individual based on psychosomatic type is different. Here the goal is to express the unique personality, not through separation, but through relationship and participation with the social and natural worlds. The Ayurvedic view sees the individual as already unique owing to his or her constitutional makeup, so that he or she does not have to create a unique identity; he or she already has one. What he or she has to do is keep his or her unique self and its expression in tune with the larger whole, since he or she is an intrinsic part of it. This can be done through right action for the individual or swadharma, actions that take into account personality, bodily, and social needs. Too little emphasis on personality type and its relationship with society can lead to psychological and physical problems. For example, choosing, due to social pressures, an occupation that is ill suited to a particular personality type can lead to a later midlife crisis.

DIAGNOSIS AND THERAPY

Ayurvedic concepts of health, the individual, and dharma are related to one another and have implications for diagnosis. It is interesting that ancient Ayurvedic diagnostic techniques seem based on the concept of swadharma as innate personality characteristics, kala (historical time), desha (culture), and so on. The Ayurvedic physician is supposed to make a comprehensive diagnosis not of the disease, but of the person, based on a thorough examination of a patient's physical, emotional, and social spheres (Kakar, 1982). The doctor has to assess the patient's current mental status, personality-body type, family background, and social, geographical and cultural context, including his caste, lineage, and *bhumi-pariksha* or "land examination." The doctor has to find out about

> the region the patient comes from, the lifestyle of the people there, their inclinations, food habits, physical characteristics and levels of vitality. Also the kind of diseases they most often contract, any special geographical features of the habitat, the general condition of health in that region, and also what is generally considered wholesome or unwholesome in that region. The person is conceived of as living simultaneously in physical, social and spiritual realms, and so a thorough knowledge of all the realms and their inter-relationships is considered essential for the education of a doctor. (Kakar, 1982, p. 228)

The relationship between Ayurveda and dharma also has implications for therapy. The concepts of swadharma and dharma can be divested from encrusted associations with social division and caste duties, and reclaimed in order to apply to conditions in modern India. The effects of modernization associated with increasing individualism can be understood in terms of Indian categories of the individual. Through swadharma, or right action, based on innate personality characteristics, desa (culture), kala (historical time), and so on, confusing transitions between traditional and modern lifestyles can be more clearly understood.

Swadharma, or the necessity of following one's individual path, can take on a new meaning in modern times, which requires actions that previously were not suitable. Society and the individual's role are in the process of redefinition through modernization, and the concepts of dharma and swadharma can encompass this process and guide it. For example, as stated earlier, urban women have higher rates of mental disorders than rural women, possibly reflecting their feelings of conflict between traditional and modern roles. Therapy interventions could utilize the concepts of dharma and swadharma and personality-body type in order to alleviate these conflicts. Modern times require new actions, and new roles for women (such as getting a divorce or pursuing a career) that will express each woman's unique personality-body type and maintain it in a state of balance with her changing environment. Individuality does not need to mean individualism or separation from context as in the West. Individuality can retain its meaning as a unique personality type embedded in a context, and swadharma, or right action to keep the personality type in balance, can change in accordance with the culture and the times.

In the Ayurvedic understanding, health and illness are intrinsically linked to personality, and interventions need to be correspondingly tailored for each type. This has implications not only for interventions, but also for the classification of disease in India, which is currently based on Western categories and diagnostic procedures. The latter is a system of classification that consists of empirically derived categories based on patterns of co-occurring symptoms, whereas the Ayurvedic classification of mental illness is based on psychosomatic categories. Ayurvedic conceptions of personality-body types with different kinds of healthy and unhealthy functioning may contribute to developing a more indigenous classification system, and to developing more appropriate treatment strategies.

The Ayurvedic approach can also contribute to Western psychology. Ayurvedic concepts of health and illness based on the individual as a psychosomatic type have implications for diagnosis. Psychological health and illness in the West are most often thought to be independent of personality type. It is interesting to note that personality factors are making a comeback in Western psychology through trait theory (such as the "Big Five" trait clusters), and in the classification of mental illness in the *Diagnostic and Statistical Manual* published by the American Psychiatric Association (DSM-IV), which now includes a diagnostic axis for personality disorders. The DSM-IV multiaxial classification system's Axis II includes long-standing problems, such as personality disorders, as possible contributing factors to the presenting problem, or the main Axis I diagnosis. However, most disorders, such as major depression or schizophrenia, are not seen to be based on, nor are they seen to vary with, personality traits or type. (Major depression, for instance, is categorized as major depression, regardless of whether the person has a narcissistic, schizoid, or paranoid personality disorder.) Personality disorders themselves present an exception (and a possible anomaly) to the DSM IV categories of mental illness. They are different from other disorders in that they involve exaggerated personality characteristics that have become dysfunctional. Personality traits in extreme cases can themselves become a psychological disorder. However, they are not necessarily seen as causing other mental disorders.

Ayurvedic psychosomatic classification systems, and the Ayurvedic view of the relationship between personality type and health, may be useful to empirical research on the classification of mental disorders. This has not been attempted thus far in a systematic way, but it could lead to a fruitful line of research. Graha Chikitsa, or the Ayurvedic equivalent of psychiatry, is one of the earliest systems of knowledge about mental illness and its treatment (Kumar & Shrivastava, 2000; Mishra et al., 2001). Ayurvedic psychosomatic classification systems could aid in the formulation of research questions on personality trait clusters and whether they are implicated in the development of different disorders, different kinds of healthy functioning, and varying responses to particular types of treatment.

RITUAL AS DHARMA

The previous discussion looks at how the traditional Hindu concepts of right action and individuality can be applied in a modern Indian and Western setting. However, right action, in the form of ritual action, also plays a role in healthy psychological functioning. Various daily and seasonal rituals are prescribed and practiced all over India, with important regional differences. Varma and Chakraborty (1995) discuss the health-promoting aspects of culture, the social norms and cultural rituals that serve to promote psychological health. This is an important idea that has therapeutic, social, and political implications. Varma feels that rituals play a role in maintaining psychological health, because according to him, they function as cultural defense mechanisms to allay anxiety. Rituals surrounding marriage, death, and adolescence, that is, life events that can be stressful, help to ease these transitions. These rituals are culturally prescribed ways to defend against the anxiety, loss, and conflict that occur while moving through the stages of life. Instead of the individual fabricating internal ego defense mechanisms, he or she uses ready-made ones in the form of these rituals provided by society that exist for all members in similar situations, and which allay anxiety and provide partial gratification. These rituals engender states similar to denial, repression, sublimation, projection, and so on, instead of the intrapsychic activities of the ego (Varma & Chakraborty, 1995). This interpretation of the role of rituals is interesting and important, as it does not separate the individual psychologically from his or her social environment. It reflects a more holistic worldview, which emphasizes the effect of social and cultural factors on healthy psychological functioning.

The psychological role of rituals therefore, according to Varma and Chakraborty (1995), seems to serve as defenses against preexisting uncomfortable emotional states. However, they may also function as *preventive* measures that ensure smooth psychological and spiritual functioning, and prevent the onset of anxiety and conflict. Rather than engendering psychological states similar to the ego's defenses such as denial and repression, they may engender anxiety-free psychological states of attunement with the internal and external natural order, thus diminishing the necessity for ego defenses such as denial, repression, and so on. Rituals are usually perceived as religious observances or worship, but within the context of the Hindu worldview they have the added connotation of maintaining a healthy balance and harmony in relationships with the natural and social order.

Common daily and periodic Hindu rituals in many parts of India include *pujas* or worship, *bratas* or vows and fasts, and *havans* or fire ceremonies. Women were, and still are in traditional families, the chief performers of rituals. According to Karlekar (1991) the dharma, or duty of the traditional Indian woman was to perform a variety of rituals in the home. Women were instructed by the older and senior women of the house on how to perform all the pujas, vows, and fasts necessary to ensure the good health and prosperity of the family, and the smooth running of the household. Mitter (1991) finds that for many traditional Hindu women, the performance of their duty or dharma (*streedharma*) as a wife and mother, (which involves the performance of prescribed rituals), brings them spiritual strength, and advances them on the path toward moksha or spiritual emancipation, the highest goal of life according to the Hindu worldview.

Pujas involve offering light and flowers, incense, and other symbolic substances as a means of honoring the deities who represent higher states of consciousness. Among the deities worshipped are usually Ganesh, the remover of obstacles, and Lakshmi, the goddess of abundance. The action of invoking these deities is supposed to ensure the right relationship with the principles of abundance, and the clearing of one's path in life. According to Karlekar (1991), bratas, which involve taking vows and fasting on certain days of the week, are also seen as a way to mold the character.

Fire ceremonies, or *havans*, conducted by the local Brahmin priest are held on special occasions, such as moving into a new home, or for certain healing purposes such as mental afflictions, or bringing peace to a troubled household as in the *shanti havan*. These ceremonies involve making offerings of clarified butter, grains, fragrant woods, and other substances that symbolize the bounty of the earth to the sacred fire (a small indoor fire), accompanied by the chanting of Sanskrit verses. These havans are expected to purify the atmosphere and restore peace and good relationships within the household and with the wider society. Larger-scale *yajnas*, which are rare in modern times but were more common earlier, are large-scale fire ceremonies carried out by the leaders of a community to maintain the cosmos and keep the invisible natural order in good repair and functioning smoothly.

These fire rituals are based on the notion of sacrifice, a central concept in the Vedic understanding (Lannoy, 1971). This ancient worldview, which is still pervasive among Hindus today and from which the concept of dharma is derived, sees the smooth functioning of the cosmos as based on the principle of sacrifice or offering. All life and living things are involved in a cycle of giving. Human beings keep the cycle going by offering back to nature and the gods all the bounty of life they have received. By making offerings back to life, one is performing dharmic actions to maintain one's place in the natural order and do one's bit to ensure its continuance. This prevents the disorder and imbalance that results from forgetting that one is part of a larger whole.

In addition to maintaining connection with the external environment, rituals may also serve an intrapsychic function by helping to maintain an internal sense of balance. According to the Sankhya school of philosophy, the psyche consists of four psychic instruments: *chitta, manas, buddhi,* and *ahamkara* (Paranjpe, 1998). Chitta is the subconscious mind and a repository for all memory traces and sense impressions. Manas, or mind, is the filter through which all sensory information enters the psyche. Buddhi is the intellect or capacity for discrimination, and Ahamkara is the ego or the process of identification, such as "I am a parent," or "I am this body," and so on.

The misuse of these psychic instruments can lead, among other things, to internal imbalance of the Ayurvedic dhatus or bodily constituents, and to imbalance of the whole mind-body system. An example of misuse of a psychic instrument is wrong identification on the part of ahamkara. Overidentification with the impermanent physical body and its social and psychological roles is thought to be at the root of psychological problems. In contrast, right identification is with the eternal soul at the core of the person that lives on after the body has passed away (Paranjpe, 1998).

Right action, or proper use of the psychic instruments, leads to a state of internal balance. Right action includes ritual action, which may have a therapeutic effect on the identification process, the psychic instruments, and on the whole system. Rituals such as havans and pujas help to rebalance the psychic instruments by directing the ego or ahamkara toward identification with higher, unchanging states of consciousness rather than with passing social role identities, the physical body, and so on. These actions thus help restore the proper functioning of the four psychic instruments.

It is interesting to speculate about the relation of ritual action to ego defense mechanisms. The absence of ritual actions on a regular basis may lead to internal imbalance and the necessity of forming defense mechanisms, or to defensive actions being taken by the ego as a way of dealing with the consequences of imbalance.

In sum, ritual action can be a healing as well as a preventative technique that helps to maintain the balance between the individual and his or her social and cosmic environment. Indian psychologists can utilize the Ayurvedic concepts of the individual personality-body type, the concepts of dharma and swadharma, and daily rituals to make therapeutic interpretations and prescriptions for clients. This is illustrated by the recent case of an Indian woman who tried Western psychotherapy and discontinued it after some months. She turned to Hindu philosophy and the performance of rituals in temples instead, as she could more easily relate to this way of interpreting and dealing with her emotional problems. If she had gone to an Indian psychologist who incorporated these elements into the therapy, she may not have dropped out of treatment.

HEALTH AND ALTERED STATES OF CONSCIOUSNESS

The bulk of the discussion so far has been on the Ayurvedic concepts of health and illness as balance and imbalance. However, there are accompanying approaches for the understanding of psychological disturbances, solely in the realm of the metaphysical, that are beyond the scope of this chapter but that are very much a part of the Indian mindset, such as the doctrines of *karma* and reincarnation, and Vedic astrology. The latter is seen as the companion science to Ayurveda, and consultations with an astrologer are frequent, particularly for the pragmatic daily problems of living, such as infertility and the desire to have children, getting a good job, and arranging a marriage. The astrologer will often recommend lucky or healing stones to wear to prevent some misfortune or alleviate a problem such as infertility. Both astrological predictions and prescriptions, and Ayurveda, are supposed to work hand in hand to prevent ill health, prepare the person for future circumstances, and give advice about how to handle their lives.

On the other hand, supernatural explanations for mental illness, found mainly in rural areas, have not been fully integrated into the Ayurvedic medical paradigm according to Kakar (1982). Possession states are believed to account for the more severe psychological disturbances, and temple exorcisms are the method of treatment, as described in detail in his book *Shamans, Mystics and Doctors* (Kakar, 1982). The book investigates the variety of healing paradigms available in India, from mysticism to traditional Ayurvedic medicine. They largely operate outside the scope of Western allopathic medicine, with patients going back and forth between Western-style clinics and treatment therein and traditional methods such as temple exorcisms. Again, however, as in the case of Ayurvedic physicians, psychiatrists working in rural areas would do well to work with the local priests in treating their clients. Combining exorcism rites with a medication regimen might be effective in preventing recurring episodes of the various disturbances, whether they are labeled psychosis or possession state.

Another metaphysical aspect to the Hindu understanding of mental health is the concept of moksha or spiritual liberation and enlightenment. Psychological health is ultimately the same as spiritual health or moksha (Sinha, 1990). This points to an interesting contrast between some Western individualistic conceptions of health, and the traditional Indian conceptions of health that are based on altered states of consciousness. Modern Western conceptions of health are based mainly on states of consciousness that are grounded in everyday sense reality and biological functioning. The spiritual aspects are for the most part seen as separate from the psychological aspects of human life. Within the general framework first articulated by Freud and still influential today, human beings should have biological drives and desires, ambitions and attachments, regulated by healthy ego functioning, and the mind and senses should be outwardly directed and actively engaged. Not having these would be considered dysfunctional. According to traditional Hindu views (which have implications for psychological health), being true to one's psychological type and to one's swadharma, or groundplan of existence, leads to attaining enlightenment or altered states of consciousness. The person is content, desireless, and nonattached, and in the transcognitive state of moksha (Paranjpe, 1988). Here the senses are disengaged from the outer environment, bodily desires have been transcended, and the mind has become still, leading to new experiences of conscious existence beyond the mind and the body. From this standpoint, Western healthy functioning would be seen as partial and leading to pathology if not directed toward transcendence of the mind and the physical senses.

From the modern, Western point of view, the Indian concept of health appears dysfunctional and not grounded in the body and physical reality. Indeed, the existence of an experiential reality beyond the senses, or altered states of consciousness, is not considered seriously by the dominant schools of psychology, with the partial exception of Humanistic, Transpersonal, and Jungian psychologies. In contrast, what is within the realm of normal, possible, and desirable human experience spans a much wider range in the Indian tradition, so much so that the Indian conception of a mentally healthy state is based on experiences whose existence is considered questionable by the dominant psychological paradigms in the West. As stated earlier, Sinha (1993), in discussing the effects of indigenizing psychology, feels that this need not lead inevitably to relativism, but to the development of a more universal psychology. A contribution that Indian psychology could make toward this end would be to expand the concept of healthy psychological functioning to include a wider range of possible experiences and states of consciousness. In addition, it should prove worthwhile to incorporate into the notion of health Ayurvedic categories for mental health such as psychosomatic types, and the balance between individual and society.

In conclusion, the pervasiveness of the Hindu belief system, notions such as dharma and swadharma, health as balance and illness as imbalance, and the embeddedness of the individual within a social context make it important to develop an indigenous psychology and interventions that are applicable in India. This is slowly starting to happen as Indian psychology tries to become more relevant to local issues. At the applied level, therapists are wrestling with the problem of how to define themselves in ways that are socially acceptable. Some psychologists and psychiatrists are trying to work side by side with traditional physicians, and healers and social activists, to bridge the gaps between traditional and modern, urban and rural. This is an important step in the right direction, but much more needs to be done in this area. The contribution of this chapter is to delineate the Ayurvedic concept of the individual as opposed to the Western psychological concept of the individual. Incorporating Ayurvedic concepts of health as balance, the individual as psychosomatic type, and Hindu concepts of dharma into Indian psychology can result in treatment strategies that would be more applicable in an Indian setting. Hopefully, psychologists will develop a cultural sensitivity in working with other groups such as Muslims, Parsis, and tribal groups as well, and incorporate their understanding and worldviews into appropriate treatment strategies. India is a culture in transition, and psychology must be able to utilize and synthesize what is applicable from both Indian and Western approaches to adequately deal with the psychological issues and contradictions of life in modern India.

REFERENCES

Adair, J. G., Puhan, B. N., & Vohra, N. (1993). Indigenization of psychology: Empirical assessment of progress in Indian research. *International Journal of Psychology, 28*(2), 149–169.

Balodhi, J. P. (1991). Holistic approach in psychiatry: Indian view. *NIMHANS Journal, 9*(2), 101–104.

Bhui, K. (1999). Common mental disorders among people with origins in or immigrants from India and Pakistan. *International Review of Psychiatry, 11*, 136–144.

Chadda, R. K., Agarwal, V., Chandra Singh, M., & Raheja, D. (2001). Help seeking behavior of psychiatric patients before seeking care at a mental hospital. *The International Journal of Social Psychiatry, 47*(4), 71–78.

Dhawan, N., Roseman, I., Naidu, R. K., Thapa, K., & Rettek, S. I. (1995). Self-concepts across two cultures: India and the United States. *Journal of Cross-Cultural Psychology, 26*(6), 606–621.

Dube, K. C., Dube, S., & Kumar, A. (1982). Psychiatric syndromes in Ayurveda with description of epilepsy and alcoholism. In A. Kiev & A. Venkoba Rao (Eds.), *Readings in transcultural psychiatry*. Madras, India: Higginbothams.

Gergen, K., Gulerce, A., Lock, A., & Misra, G. (1996). Psychological science in cultural context. *American Psychologist, 51*, 496–503.

Kakar, S. (1978). *The inner world: A psychoanalytic study of childhood and society in India*. Delhi, India: Oxford University Press.

Kakar, S. (1982). *Shamans, mystics and doctors*. Boston: Beacon Press.

Karlekar, M. (1991). *Voices from within: Early personal narratives of Bengali women*. Delhi, India: Oxford University Press.

Korom, F. (2001). Changing patterns of family and kinship in South Asia. *Journal of the American Oriental Society, 121*(1), 120–122.

Kumar, S. (2000). Tension-ridden job causes mental health problems for police in New Delhi. *The Lancet, 355*, 1082.

Kumar, S., & Shrivastava, R. (2000). Diagnosing mental illnesses by pulse examination in ancient India. *The American Journal of Psychiatry, 157*(3), 450.

Lannoy, R. (1971). *The speaking tree*. London: Oxford University Press.

Misra, G. (1993). On the place of culture in psychological science. *International Journal of Psychology, 28*(2), 225–243.

Mishra, L., Singh, B., & Dagenais, S. (2001). Ayurveda: A historical perspective and principles of the traditional healthcare system in India. *Alternative Therapies in Health and Medicine, 7*(2), 36–42.

Mitter, S. (1991). *Dharma's daughters*. New Brunswick, NJ: Rutgers University Press.

Mookherjee, H. N. (1995). Psychoemotional responses to the existing social systems in tribal populations in India. In R. K. Price, B. M. Shea, & H. N. Mookherjee (Eds.), *Social psychiatry across cultures* (pp. 51-60). New York: Plenum Press.

Paranjpe, A. C. (1988). A personality theory according to Vedanta. In A. C. Paranjpe, D. Y. F. Ho, & R. W. Rieber (Eds.), *Asian contributions to psychology* (pp. 185–214). New York: Praeger.

Paranjpe, A. C. (1998). *Self and identity in modern psychology and Indian thought*. New York: Plenum Press.

Patel, V., Chisholm, D., Rabe-Hesketh, S., & Dias-Saxena, F., et al. (2003). Efficacy and cost-effectiveness of drug and psychological treatments for common mental disorder in general health care in Goa, India: A randomised, controlled trial. *The Lancet, 361*, 33–39.

Patel, V., Rodrigues, M., & DeSouza, N. (2002). Gender, poverty and postnatal depression: A study of mothers in Goa, India. *The American Journal of Psychiatry, 159*(1), 43–47.

Rastogi, M., & Wampler, K. S. (1997). Couples and family therapy with Indian families: Some structural and intergenerational considerations. In U. P. Gielen & A. L. Comunian (Eds.), *The family and family therapy in international perspective* (pp. 257–274). Trieste, Italy: Lint.

Roland, A. (1988). *In search of self in India and Japan*. Princeton, NJ: Princeton University Press.

Roland, A. (1996). *Cultural pluralism and psychoanalysis: The Asian and North American experience*. New York: Routledge.

Sharma, P. S. (1975). *Ayurvedic medicine*. India: Dabur.

Sharma, R. (1995). A note on samskara. *Journal of Indian Psychology, 13*(1), 51–53.

Sinha, D. (1990). Concept of psycho-social well-being: Western and Indian perspectives. *NIMHANS Journal, 8*(1), 1–11.

Sinha, D. (1993). Indigenization of psychology in India and its relevance. In U. Kim & J. Berry (Eds.), *Indigenous psychologies: Research and experience in cultural context* (pp. 30–43). Newbury Park, CA: Sage.

Varma, V. K., & Chakraborty, S. (1995). Social correlates and cultural dynamics of mental illness in traditional society: India. In I. Al-Issa, (Ed.), *Handbook of culture and mental illness: An international perspective* (pp. 115–128). Madison, CT: International Universities Press.

Psychotherapy and Healing in Africa and the Arab World

Western Psychotherapy and the Yoruba: Problems of Insight and Nondirective Techniques

Raymond Prince
McGill University
Montreal, Canada

POSTSCRIPT IN THE YEAR 2003

This chapter was originally written in 1962, when transcultural psychiatry was in its infancy. Shortly after completing my psychiatric training, I had the good fortune to work for three years within the Yoruba culture of Nigeria. Between 1957 and 1959, I practiced as government psychiatrist for the British Colonial Service at Aro Hospital, Abeokuta. During this clinical period, I became aware of the expertise of Yoruba traditional healers in treating a wide spectrum of psychiatric disorders, and during 1961 to 1963, I returned to research their treatment methods in detail.

When I first entered psychiatry in the early 1950s, I was trained in psychoanalytically based psychotherapy, which was then regarded as the most effective and highly valued form of treatment for the neuroses. Later, I would learn the advantages of the nondirective interviewing method. During my work as a clinician in Nigeria, however, I rapidly discovered the culture-bound nature of the psychotherapeutic techniques I practiced in Canada. This chapter briefly describes my discovery of the cultural limitations of insight and nondirective techniques—as seen in the year 1962. Today, with flawless hindsight, we may smile at a discovery that nowadays can seem obvious. It was not, however, at all obvious to me, and at the time it would certainly have come as a surprise to my Canadian teachers and colleagues.

Let me begin with an anecdote. I first came to Nigeria in 1957 and worked as a government psychiatrist at Aro Hospital, Abeokuta. One of my first patients was a young schoolteacher with a walking disorder. When she walked forward, her right leg was stiff and she moved with a severe limp; however, if she ran forward, or walked backward, no stiffness occurred and her movements were normal. Her illness was obviously functional (i.e., the pathology was not in muscles or nerves but in feelings and ideas), and I decided that the best treatment would be intensive psychotherapy aimed at exploring and resolving the fears, hostilities, or guilts that were theoretically behind

This study was supported by the Human Ecology Fund, New York. I would also like to thank Mr. Frank Speed of the Medical Illustration Unit, University College Hospital, Ibadan, and Mr. F. Bale of the Phonetics Department, University College, Ibadan for making the film and sound recordings. I am also grateful to Dr. T. A. Lambo for his help in allowing me access to the facilities and patients at Aro Hospital, Abeokuta. Professor E. D. Wittkower made many helpful suggestions about the text.

her trouble. She seemed an appropriate candidate for such treatment; she was young and intelligent, and spoke adequate English. I followed the technique of psychotherapy I had learned and employed in Canada. I found it quite ineffective. In spite of considerable labor and explanation, I could discover no more than that the illness seemed to be related in some way to an illegitimate pregnancy and that the girl herself attributed her affliction to stepping on some bad medicine planted in her path by the relative of her lover. I could elicit no significant picture of her relationship with her mother, father, or lover, or any emotionally charged material. After some 10 or 12 hours, I abandoned psychotherapy and resorted to drugs and electroconvulsive therapy. There was only temporary improvement, and when Dr. Lambo, the Yoruba superintendent of the hospital, returned from leave, I was relieved to turn her over to him, whose patient she had originally been. It was with some amazement that, a short time later, I saw the girl walking quite normally! I asked Dr. Lambo what magic he had used. He said he had simply given her an intravenous sedative and, during the drowsy state, had suggested strongly that she should walk, which she did. Now such a direct-command approach is frowned upon in the school of psychiatry in which I was trained; it is said that the symptoms would be relieved only temporarily or that other symptoms would appear to take their place: "You push it in here and it comes out there" as it were. Whatever one's theories are, the fact remains that she did walk and, from recent reports, is still walking and doing her work effectively. Such an experience is a little hard on one's professional vanity. I soon learned that the much-prized Western techniques of insight therapy are almost inapplicable when doing psychiatric work among the Yoruba.

It is fortunate for the Western-trained psychiatrist that not all his lore is similarly culture-bound. In fact, a good portion of Western psychiatric practice can be transposed to the Yoruba milieu without alteration. This is particularly true of Western modes of physical therapy. Tranquilizing, energizing, and sedative drugs have similar effects upon Yoruba and Western patients. Electroconvulsive therapy is applicable cross-culturally, as is insulin coma therapy.

Turning to diagnosis, most Yoruba illnesses can be categorized according to Western nosology. It is true that occasionally Western names do not seem to fit the Yoruba pattern comfortably. For example, there is an illness that the Yoruba native doctors call "hunter's head" (ori ode), which is characterized by a painful thumping or crawling sensation in the head, dimness of vision, and sometimes impotence and insomnia. They say that if the illness becomes too intense the patient may "run mad." Several causes for this illness are mentioned by native doctors: (a) It may be due to a worm about the size of a tick found on sheep's heads; when the worm breathes or moves, one feels the crawling sensation. (b) It may be due to bad medicine; an enemy may take a little of your hair, apply certain medicines to it, and then place it under the blacksmith's anvil so that every time the anvil is struck, you feel the thump. Faced with this illness, the Western diagnostician might call it an anxiety state or perhaps a masked depression. However, it must be admitted that such a constellation of symptoms is rather uncommon in the West and one is a little uneasy about using such Western names. On the whole, however, Western names can be used with a relatively clear conscience.

A good deal more could be said about these Yoruba/Western differences in illness patterns for they are of great theoretic interest. However, at this time I wish to return to the problem of insight therapy and discuss a little more thoroughly the nature of the problem and some of its implications.

INSIGHT THERAPY

One of the major preoccupations of Western psychiatry during the past 50 years has been with the idea that many psychiatric disturbances are based upon pathological familial relationships during the patient's childhood. Prior to that time, a psychiatric illness was likely to be regarded as hereditary, constitutional, the result of some unknown circulating toxins, or perhaps as the result of "sin" (e.g., excessive masturbation or alcohol intake producing "degeneration" of some kind). Concomitant with this concept of cause, a variety of methods of "insight therapy" have evolved. In varying degrees, these methods involve the exploration through interview of the patient's past and current relationships, including the one with the therapist. During psychoanalysis, the most intensive form of psychotherapy, the patient relives important infant-like experiences, with the therapist being felt by the patient to be taking the role of his mother or father. He is able to resolve emotional conflicts because the therapeutic situation is more favorable than was the original situation. These procedures may extend over a period of years and involve hundreds of hours.

Various interview techniques are used to encourage these explorations and regressions, which are often painful. Nebulous questions are used such as "Tell me more about that" or "How do you mean?" Feeling-charged or other significant words are repeated as though the therapist did not understand their meaning, and silences are used judiciously. The therapist avoids asking leading questions or offering "advice" of any kind. Patients gradually clarify their own problems and determine their own course within the warmth and protection of the relationship.

One of the important aspects of this nondirective type of interview in conducting research, especially in conducting cross-cultural research, is that by avoiding putting ideas into the patient's mind by direct questions, one can be relatively sure that the experiences and views described by the patient do not come from the interviewer. Furthermore, a blunt question about a feeling-laden area of one's life will rarely elicit any significant material. Thus, the question, "Did you feel jealous of your brother when he was born?" would almost certainly elicit a stout denial, whereas if the area were explored in the patient's own time using the nondirective method, significant material would more likely be obtained from the same patient. The use of the nondirective method is relatively unbiased, yet even then the indirect cues of approval or disapproval, such as nods or "hums" of the therapist, may distort the data in the direction of the therapist's expectations.

To demonstrate the Western type of response to the nondirective interview technique, I present the case of a 30-year-old American housewife who for many years has suffered a psychogenic skin condition. In the interview, she related how her first skin reaction lasted only a few hours and seemed to arise from a disturbing situation when she was 13 years old. She had just begun working in a grocery store in a job she considered beneath her and she did not like her boss. After the first day, she decided to quit but instead her boss discharged her. That night her whole body was covered with a burning, itching rash. The next episode occurred at the age of 16 after her parents sent her off to boarding school as a punishment for being "incorrigible." A further episode occurred when she was 20 when she was "thrown over" by a boyfriend. Since that time, the rash has affected many different parts of her body and has persisted almost continually. She points out the self-inflicted nature of the rash in that if she does not scratch the affected areas, they clear up.

The interview with the patient was conducted in a rigorously nondirective manner. "Silences" were not interrupted. Certain recurring themes readily emerged, such
as the rash seemed to occur in situations when she suffered a decline in self-esteem.
Certain hypotheses suggested themselves for future testing. It would appear that
when she attempted to be accepted in a mature way and failed, the patient would fall
back into a self-induced "sickness," perhaps in order to elicit warmth from others.
There was probably a pleasurable component to the itching, and the behavior may
have been akin to thumb-sucking or masturbating, which is frequently seen in children that feel abandoned or lonely. Thus, nondirective techniques enabled the therapist to learn a good deal about how pathological relationships between parents and
children may produce a disfiguring skin condition.

THE YORUBA AND THE NONDIRECTIVE INTERVIEW

The nondirective technique employed with a Yoruba patient does not produce similar results. After describing their complaints, generally in as few words as possible,
Yoruba patients fall silent. Explanations of the interviewer's requirements evoke little response. Although the Yoruba may superficially agree that their symptoms are
psychological in origin, they do not genuinely seem to believe that their own feelings
or relationships, past or present, could have any causal relationship to their illnesses.
They feel dejected because of their headaches; it is not the dejection that causes the
headache. With further encouragement and some direct questioning perhaps, it may
be possible to unearth beliefs that the illness is due to the ill will of others; further
exploration founders on the bedrock of magic.

To demonstrate Yoruba interview behavior, I present the case of a 30-year-old government clerk who studies in his spare time in preparation for an advanced-level
examination. His ambition is to become a lawyer. He is married and has one daughter.

He suffers from the ubiquitous disease of Nigerian students: pain and burning in
the head aggravated by reading, and reduced ability to grasp and retain what he
reads. In addition, he feels that he has a hard ball in his head that sometimes moves
in a circular fashion; he experiences burning sensations in his limbs; his legs occasionally jerk in an involuntary way, as a kind of spontaneous startle.

His trouble started several years ago when he began to have dreams of being
beaten. These dreams would occur only after he had been reading before going to bed.
He could not see who the people were that were beating him, but there were many of
them and they would beat him with their hands. He had no head trouble at that time,
but he would avoid reading before bed because he was afraid of these dreams. He
considered the dreams to be the result of *asasi*, a kind of bad medicine used against
him by unknown persons who were jealous of his progress as he would often be first
at school. Native doctors prescribed several kinds of protective medicines for these
dreams, including various burnt and powdered herbs mixed with *agidi* (corn) or palm
oil. These cleared up the dreams in about five years, but a few months afterwards the
head trouble described made its appearance. It has become increasingly troublesome
since that time so that now he is scarcely able to read at all.

In the interview, the patient first attributed his head complaints to reading excessively. Later he expressed the idea that they were due to his "ambition" and fear of being
left behind by his colleagues. The nondirective technique was used to attempt to draw
out what specific feelings of jealousy, fear, despair, or hostility lay behind these words
"ambitious" and "left behind." After some 20 unproductive minutes, the trial interpre-

tation was made that he was perhaps afraid mostly of being left behind by his brothers. This elicited a very emphatic denial and resulted in the startle symptom in his legs.

Expressions of feelings, however, were not forthcoming, and a progressively more direct interview approach was attempted. "Did you feel left behind in any other situations, such as at home or as far as girls were concerned?" Finally, he was directly questioned about his feelings when his brother was born at the age of four (based on the hypothesis that his ambitions and fears of being left behind were exaggerated because of earlier painful experiences of this nature). Such direct questions evoked vehement denials and ridicule. "Feeling left out when one's brother was born would be stupid!" This response is what one might expect, of course, with the direct approach, as has already been noted.

Finally, he made it clear that he felt that his head trouble was also due to asasi: "All the other boys are as ambitious as I am, all the other boys read as much as I do, but not all the other boys have this head trouble; that is why I believe this sickness to be not of natural origin." The locus of the problem was then removed from within himself to the outside world and any further discussion of his own feelings was rejected as irrelevant.

During the nondirective part of the interview, the patient seemed to be constantly scanning the situation to find some cue as to what I wanted him to say. Of course, this was exactly what I did not want to communicate. I repeated what he said, expecting an elaboration or clarification, but evidently wishing to please me, he would simply agree by repeating the same words back to me and the interview swallowed its own tail, as it were.

THE IFA SYSTEM AS PSYCHOTHERAPY

In order to illuminate this Yoruba difficulty with the nondirective technique, I will next describe one type of psychotherapy that the Yoruba themselves have elaborated. I do not intend to explain the Yoruba difficulty or attempt to trace its origin, but simply show that it seems to be part of a general cultural attitude toward disease and expectations regarding therapy.

A good deal of the unhappiness, fear, and illness of the Yoruba community finds its way to the ears of the traditional doctor-diviner, the *Babalawo*, father of mysteries, priest of the ancient prophet Orunmila.

I can only deal briefly with the complex system of divination (called *Ifa*) employed by the Babalawo. Essentially, it is a method of summoning and questioning certain invisible agencies who know about the client's sickness or misfortune to learn from them what must be done to alleviate it.

During the divination session, the diviner is seated cross-legged on a grass mat. Before him is the divining board, a bowl of palm nuts, the *irofa* (a horn-shaped carved object with a clapper), a bag containing cowry shells, animal teeth, broken pieces of pottery, and seeds (*sesan*). On the diviner's right hand is his assistant, a Babalawo in training, and on his left the patient. The divination session consists of five sections, as follows:

- *Invocation of ancestor diviners and spirits:* The divining board is covered with a white sawdust (*iyerosun*) and the session commences with the summoning of Orunmila, other ancestor diviners, and the spirit who knows about the patient's problem. A kola nut is split and cast to determine whether everything is favorable for divination. These prayers are accompanied by various ritual acts: the Babalawo beats himself so that Ifa will not beat him, a little water is sipped by all, and some is poured on the ground. Pinches of sawdust are also thrown into the air. The divining board is tapped with the *irofa* to command the attention of the relevant spirits.

- *The patient presents his problem to the palm nuts:* The patient puts a coin into the bowl of palm nuts and then whispers his problem into the bowl. He prays for assistance. The Babalawo does not know the problem during the divination session. The transaction is between the patient and the spirits; the diviner is just the intermediary.

- *The presiding spirit or Odu announces himself:* The diviner commences casting the palm nuts in order to determine which spirit has come to resolve the patient's problem. He places the 16 nuts in his left hand, with his right hand he grasps as many nuts as possible, usually 1 or 2 remain in his left hand because 16 palm nuts are a good-sized handful. If more than two nuts remain, if none remain, or if he fumbles, the cast is repeated. If one nut remains, he makes two marks in the dust on the board. If two remain, he makes one mark. This procedure is repeated eight times. This configuration represents the "call marks" of one of 256 spirits that may be summoned. Each of these configurations of marks has a cluster of verses associated with it, stories and songs which the diviner must memorize. They are like chapters of a book of religio-medical poetry.

- *Ibo, the casting of lots:* The verses have many themes; some refer to people who have good luck, some have bad, some have illnesses, and some want children. All the verses contain sacrifices that must be made to procure their desired ends. The diviner, having determined which chapter of the poem refers to the patient's problem, must next determine which specific verses relate to the problem. Through casting the nuts, the diviner in fact asks the spirit a series of questions of the yes-no type; is it good luck or bad? Good luck, answers the spirit. Is it a matter of children or not? Not of children. Is it a matter of long life and health or not? Yes, of long life and health, and so on. In this way, the spotlight is narrowed to focus on a few relevant verses.

- *Interpretation and recitation:* The specific verses having been revealed to the Babalawo, he commences to tell the patient what the problem is, what is behind his problem in a supernatural sense, and what sacrifices the patient must make to resolve the problem. What seems more to the point from our Western view, he may direct the patient to change his ways—be less arrogant, forgive your wife "because women are always that way," and so on, or he may advise him to change his place of abode, because of the witches in the compound. He promises good luck if the sacrifices are carried out, but gives dire warnings if they are not. Next, he recites the verses, stories, and songs upon which he has based his interpretation. The patient is then given an opportunity to say whether he is satisfied with the interpretation and to ask any further questions he may have. Finally, through further questioning with the palm nuts, the precise sacrifice is determined: a goat, a pig, money, palm oil, a new pot, and so on. The sacrifice session may take place immediately if directed by the oracle, but generally it takes place a week or two afterwards. The sacrifice session may last from two to three hours, but need not concern us here.

The Yoruba patient, on consulting the diviner, is not even required to tell what the problem is. In fact, the specific surface manifestations of the problem are irrelevant;

the important point is to determine the underlying supernatural agencies at work and most of all what these agencies will accept to release their hold on the sufferer. In the worldview of the Babalawo, misfortunes and illnesses are largely determined by agencies outside of the person. There is little rationale for looking inward for the sources of the trouble. Of course, it is clear that if a man mistreats his wives, they will leave him, and the Babalawo frequently points out such surface behavior problems. Still, their cardinal role is in revealing the "hidden" origins of misfortune. There is little traditional awareness of unconscious psychological causes of misfortune.

It is true that many present-day Westernized Yoruba (and probably many laymen in the past) are not at all conversant with this traditional worldview. Yet the worldview, the philosophy as it were, seems to rest on fundamental personality characteristics, so that the basic attitudes persist even when the philosophy is unknown. It is a matter of feeling and not of knowledge, and it cannot be readily explained away. Even if patients do not believe in spirits and sacrifice, they do not regard the causes or remedies of their misfortunes as having origins within themselves. Instead, help rests with the doctor and what he can do for or to the patient. That the doctor should probe into the patient's inner life seems as irrelevant as it would to a Western patient if, when consulting a doctor about a fractured wrist, he or she was questioned about the solar system.

THE IMPLICATIONS OF THE FAILURE OF THE NONDIRECTIVE METHOD

Practically speaking, in the day-to-day treatment of Yoruba psychiatric disturbances, the failure of the techniques of insight therapy is of little importance. Most illnesses can be adequately treated with drugs and electroconvulsive therapy. The psychotherapy that does take place is of the suggestion type—not grossly different from the "divination and command" therapy of the Babalawo's. Indeed, the doctor seems automatically to be invested with the numinous quality that adheres to the Babalawo in the consciousness of the people.

It does, however, have important implications for research. It is largely through this procedure that Western psychotherapists have charted the relation between pathological childhood relationships and adult neuroses. The nondirective interview is at once a therapeutic and a research tool.

This research channel being closed with Yoruba patients, it is very difficult to determine what particular childhood experiences are significant in producing adult neuroses and adult personality characteristics. For instance, what are the effects of the indulgent relation between mother and child, the protracted period of breast-feeding, and the child's apparently sudden dethronement after the birth of the next child? Does this series of events have any bearing on the difficulty the Yoruba schoolboy experiences when he finds himself in the highly competitive school situation? Why is impotence such a common symptom in the Yoruba male? These and a host of similar questions can most satisfactorily be answered through analytic-type explorations.

It is true that much important work has been done in the culture-personality area without the use of the nondirective analytic interview. These studies generally apply Western psychodynamic thinking to field data collected by anthropologists on adult behavior, child-rearing practices, dreams, myths, rituals, and folk beliefs. Various personality tests have been administered and interpreted according to criteria validated for the West. From such studies it would often appear that psychoanalytic personality concepts are applicable in non-Western cultures. Yet such studies often seem to presuppose the mechanisms whose existence they propose to demonstrate. These methods lack the immediacy and, as it seems to me, the validity of the interview approach, on the basis of which personality dynamics were originally formulated in the West.

Consider, for example, the problem of Yoruba impotence. We may marshall the following facts:

- The first three years of the Yoruba mother-son relationship are very close physical ones. During this period the mother is required (at least theoretically) to remain sexually continent.
- There is a Yoruba myth about an ancient queen, Yemaja, whose son fell in love with her. He had sexual relations with her and as a result of which she disappeared into the earth. From her breasts sprang two rivers and from her body emerged several Yoruba deities, including Shopono, the malevolent smallpox god who is implicated very commonly as a cause of mental illness.
- One of the most common explanations for impotence is that it is the result of witchcraft. With the Yoruba the witch is a female entity, a separate name and separate activities being attributed to her male counterpart. It is believed that during the night the witch takes the man's penis, uses it to have intercourse with another woman, and then returns it in the morning. However, it will not function after that.
- Finally, I quote from one of the ritual songs associated with the Gelede cult reported by Beier (1958). This cult protects its members from molestation by witches.

> . . . Great mother with whom we dare not cohabit
> Great mother whose body we dare not see,
> Mother of secret beauties
> Mother who empties the cup
> Who speaks out with the voice of a man
> Large, very large mother on the top of the Iroko tree
> Mother who climbs high and looks down on the earth
> Mother who kills her husband yet pities him.

Now it may be, as some of this evidence suggests, that impotence is related to the early close relationship between mother and child—the arousal of incestuous wishes and the fear of retaliation and castration by the mother. It is plausible to think that these anxieties would be reactivated in the adult sexual situation. Certainly, this mechanism is not without precedent as a background for impotence in the West. Yet it seems to remain very much an armchair theory until a patient explicitly describes these wishes and feelings. It is much more satisfying to get it straight from the horse's mouth.

Perhaps with the Yoruba, the portal of entry into personality is not through illness. During my interviews with native doctors I have been surprised by the richness of some of the fragments of biography they have presented unasked. Some of the fragments are more emotionally colored and more personal than anything I have been able to elicit in the clinic. With the native doctors the relationship is much more as between equals, and there was no question of wanting to be cured of anything. It is interesting that this was the approach of Sachs (1947) whose book *Black Anger* is the life story of a Manyika (South Africa) native doctor. It is true that this study does not demonstrate the bringing of unconscious elements into consciousness as is the case in a more genuinely psychoanalytic study (cf. Freud's "Case of Anna O," for example). Nonetheless, it is a psychologically rich document. The analytic study of a healthy Yoruba in a relationship of equality might prove a profitable research venture for the future.

REFERENCES

Beier, U. (1958). Gelede masks, *Odu, 6*, 5–23.
Sachs, W. (1947). *Black anger*. New York: Grove Press.
Singer, M. (1961). A survey of cultures and personality theory and resources. In B. Kaplan (Ed.), *Studying personality cross-culturally*. Evanston, IL: Row, Peterson.

Healing the Wounds Following Protracted Conflict in Angola: A Community-Based Approach to Assisting War-affected Children

Michael G. Wessells
Randolph-Macon College & Christian Children's Fund

Carlinda Monteiro
Christian Children's Fund/Angola

In the last several decades, a significant shift has occurred in the global pattern of armed conflict. Since the late 1980s, approximately 25 to 30 intrastate wars have occurred each year, whereas the frequency of interstate wars declined to a level near zero (Eriksson, Sollenberg, & Wallensteen, 2002). Intrastate conflicts take a profound toll on civilians (Wessells, 1998a). As evidenced by the conflicts in the former Yugoslavia, Cambodia, Guatemala, Somalia, and Rwanda, fighting occurs increasingly not on well-defined battlefields, but in and around communities. Often it involves personalized acts of violence, rapes and other atrocities committed by former neighbors, and ethnic cleansing and genocide. As a result, the war-related civilian death rate has risen sharply. In the early part of this century and in previous centuries, it is estimated that civilians comprised approximately 20 percent of war-related deaths. By the 1990s, however, civilians comprised nearly 90 percent of war-related deaths (Garfield & Neugut, 1997; Sivard, 1996; UNICEF, 1996).

Associated with this changed pattern of warfare is sharply increased psychological fallout for civilian populations. Intercommunal fighting shatters social trust, and following the fighting, there remain deeply divided societies in which one's neighbors may be people who had done horrible things during the war. Trauma occurs on a large scale, as many civilians are subjected to attack, loss, uprooting, and human rights violations. The attack on homes and communities disrupts daily routines and ruptures people's sense of normalcy and continuity. Large numbers of landmines may make it impossible to return home or to resume agriculture, which for many people in the developing world is both traditional and necessary for survival. Nearly 40 percent of contemporary conflicts have lasted 10 or more years (Smith, 1997), and these protracted conflicts devastate infrastructure, amplify already severe poverty and social injustice, and create hopelessness. Although any one of these problems could have profound psychological impact, it is the accumulation of multiple, chronic stresses that poses the gravest psychological risk to civilian populations (Garbarino & Kostelny, 1996; Straker, 1987). In many areas, violence becomes normalized and saturates various social levels from family to community and society. Worldwide, approximately 300,000 youth get drawn into soldiering, typically by desperation, victimization, and force (Brett & McCallin, 1996; Cohn & Goodwin-Gill, 1994). These youths are at risk of continuing cycles of violence (Straker, 1992; Wessells, 1997, 1998b, 2002; Wessells & Monteiro, 2001).

In war-torn contexts, great need exists for large-scale, psychosocial intervention both to relieve suffering and to enable processes of development and societal reconstruction for peace. People who live in conflict-torn areas frequently report that the emotional and social wounds of war are as or more painful than physical wounds. In many areas, victimization is so pervasive and communalized that it becomes woven into the fabric of social identity. The collective trauma is heroized, takes on mythic proportions, and gets passed from one generation to the next, continuing selective war memories that plant seeds of future conflict (Volkan, 1997). Trauma, depression, and war-related stresses inflicted on a mass scale may reduce people's ability to make decisions needed to insure the survival of themselves and their families.

In constructing psychosocial interventions, it is vital to address the needs of children, defined as people under 18 years of age, because they are key future resources, are vulnerable, and, during adolescence, are making key choices about how they will live their lives. War-affected children may not be in a position to concentrate and to benefit fully from education, job training, and other activities that promote healthy development. Children exposed to violence through witnessing, victimization, or perpetration are at heightened risk of getting involved in violence, either through soldiering or through community violence.

This chapter describes a large-scale program of psychosocial assistance to war-affected children conducted in Angola by an international nongovernmental organization (NGO), Christian Children's Fund (CCF). Focusing on the period 1995 to 1998, during which there were hopes for peace in the aftermath of the Lusaka Protocol, the program places culture and community participation at the center of psychosocial reconstruction. Having described the Angolan war and its impact on civilians, we outline the local cosmologies and cultural practices that color the interpretation of people's war experiences and provide the foundation for culturally relevant methods of healing and social integration. Against this cultural background, we analyze the implications for psychosocial intervention on a mass scale. In particular, we describe two concurrent community-based projects that focus on healing and on the reintegration of former child soldiers, respectively. Although the results of these projects are discussed, we emphasize the process of integrating Western and traditional methods because this process has implications for the conduct of psychosocial work in other regions.

WAR IN ANGOLA

War in Angola is so long-standing that it has become part of the psychological horizon. Having grown up under war conditions, many people do not remember the good times that antedated the war. Many report that they cannot imagine living in conditions of peace, and to speak of peace in times of tension is to endanger oneself.

War erupted in 1961 as a liberation struggle against the Portuguese colonial regime. Although Angola gained independence in 1975, the country was devastated and lacked functional government and social infrastructure (Lodico, 1996). The three main groups—the Movimento Popular de Libertacao de Angola (MPLA), the Frente Nacional de Libertacao de Angola (FNLA), and Uniao Nacional para a Independencia Total de Angola (UNITA)—that had fought the Portuguese then embarked in a power struggle, plunging Angola into civil war. With the socialist, MPLA-dominated government in Luanda receiving extensive aid from the Soviet Union and Cuba, South

African invaded Angola in support of UNITA. At the same time, the United States began providing extensive aid to UNITA and the FNLA, which joined forces against the MPLA (Human Rights Watch, 1994).

In this manner, the Angolan civil war became a proxy war, one of many waged by the United States and the Soviet Union during the Cold War. By the late 1980s, Cuba had 50,000 troops in Angola. But the defeat of South African forces in the 1988 battle of Cuito Cuanavale, together with the end of the Cold War, sharply reduced the outside support for the warring parties. In late 1988, the Cubans agreed to withdraw their troops under the supervision of a U.N. peacekeeping mission, the United National Angolan Verification Mission (UNAVEM I). By May 1991, Cuban troops had left Angola, and the MPLA and UNITA signed the Bicesse Peace Accords, temporarily stopping a conflict that had killed between 100,000 and 350,000 people in combat (Human Rights Watch, 1994).

The Bicesse Accords called for free elections in 1992, and the U.N. dispatched military observers (UNAVEM II) to support the peace agreement. In the September 1992 elections, the MPLA candidate, President Jose Eduardo dos Santos, received 49.6 percent of the vote, whereas Jonas Savimbi, who had led UNITA since 1966 and who had garnered extensive U.S. support over the years, received 40.1 percent. Because the Angolan constitution stipulated that a majority of 50 percent was needed to achieve victory, a second round of elections was planned. But UNITA denounced the election results as fraudulent and withdrew its forces from the newly established national army. Rising tensions and violent acts on both sides led to another round of war, beginning October 31, 1992 (Lodico, 1996).

This time—late 1992 through May 1994—the fighting was particularly intense and inflicted very heavy civilian casualties. The 21-month siege of the city of Kuito devastated the city, where house-to-house fighting and sniper attacks were common and where civilian populations were systematically starved, resulting in 20,000 to 30,000 deaths. Other cities such as Huambo suffered prolonged attacks as well. On both sides of the conflict during this period, there were indiscriminate shellings and bombings of cities, summary executions and tortures, and recruitment of child soldiers (Human Rights Watch, 1994). The rate of killing rose as high as 1,000 people per day, and fighting led to anarchy and hunger in much of the country (Lodico, 1996). The number of internally displaced people rose from 344,000 in May 1993 to 1.2 million people by September 1994. Many lived in desperate circumstances.

This most recent phase of the war profoundly impacted children, who comprised nearly half the 1.2 million displaced people. It is estimated that approximately 500,000 children died as a direct result of the war and that 15,000 children were "unaccompanied," that is, separated from their families and without adult supervision. Throughout Angola, hunger, disease, and the destruction of health facilities boosted morbidity rates. By 1993, UNICEF estimated that nearly 840,000 children were living in "especially difficult circumstances." UNICEF also estimated that 320 out of 1,000 children died before they had reached the age of five. Large numbers of children were killed or maimed by landmines, which were used widely throughout Angola. Today Angola, which has a population of approximately 11 million people, is estimated to have 6 to 10 million landmines, ranking with Cambodia and Afghanistan as one of the three most heavily mined countries in the world.

A stalemate in the fighting, coupled with international pressures, led to the signing in November 1994 of the Lusaka Protocol, which set the stage for the construction of a new Government of National Unity and Reconciliation in April 1997. Many UNITA officials entered the government amidst recurrent U.N. criticisms of UNITA leader

Jonas Savimbi for failure to comply fully with the terms of the Lusaka Protocol. Between 1995 and 1998, tensions remained high and access to UNITA-controlled areas was sporadic, keeping Angola in the situation of being a country inside a country. Because of the grinding poverty, the anarchic environment in many rural areas, and the involvement of many education-deprived youths in the military, many youths turned to banditry, which remains one of the biggest security problems in Angola today.

The war has had a powerful impact on children, who comprise nearly half the population of Angola and have grown up never having known anything other than war. In 1995, CCF/Angola conducted a study of a nonrandom sample of 200 children between the ages of 8 and 16 years from Bie and Huambo provinces, and children who had come to the capital city, Luanda, from 10 other provinces (UNICEF, 1996). Although it was a worst-case analysis, the results were shocking: 27 percent had lost their parents, 94 percent had been exposed to attacks, 66 percent had witnessed mine explosions, 5 percent had been victims thereof, 36 percent had lived with troops, 33 percent had suffered injuries by shooting or shelling, 65 percent had escaped death, and 7 percent had fired guns. These experiences had a powerful psychological impact on the children, who exhibited trauma symptoms such as fright and insecurity (67 percent), disturbed sleep (61 percent), intrusive images (59 percent), frequent thoughts about war (89 percent), and sensory-motor disturbance (24 percent). Moreover, 91 percent of children in the sample exhibited three or more symptoms of trauma. Similar results have been reported by other researchers (e.g., McIntyre & Ventura, 2002).

It would be misleading, however, to focus on symptomatic behavior. The wider psychosocial effects of the war can be understood only in the context of Angolan culture.

CULTURAL BELIEFS AND RITUALS

Angolan culture is variegated and reflects a mixture of indigenous African groups. The main ethno-linguistic groups of Angola are of Bantu origin, including Kikongos (Bakongo), Kimbundos (Kymbundu), Lunda-Kiokos (Lunda-Tchokwe), Mbundos (Ovimbundos), Ganguelas (Nganguelas), Nhaneca-Humbe (Nyaneca-Nkhumbi), Hereros (Tjiherer or Thielele), and Xindongos (Oshindonga). Of non-Bantu origin are the Bochimanes (Vakwankala or Vasekele), Khoisan (Cazama), Cuissis (Kuisi or Ova-Kwanda), and Vatuas.

Due to its colonial heritage, Angolan culture also reflects the strong influence of Portuguese and other European cultures. During the colonial era, much was done to suppress or eliminate local culture, which was viewed as primitive, and led many local people to internalize a sense of inferiority regarding their own culture. In addition, the turmoil and displacement caused by the war disrupted or altered established social patterns and weakened the force of traditions. Nevertheless, it is possible to identify common themes and centuries-old patterns of belief and practice having much in common with wider patterns of Bantu culture seen in countries throughout sub-Saharan Africa.

COMMUNITY AND SPIRITUALITY

In contrast to the individualistic orientation of many modern Western societies, traditional Bantu societies place a strong emphasis on extended family and on community, which includes both the living and the spirits of the ancestors. Traditional cosmology holds that when someone dies, the life of the person continues in the spirit world. The spirits of the ancestors protect the living community, which is an extension of the ancestral community. If the ancestors are not honored through the teaching of traditions and the practice of appropriate rituals, their spirits cause problems manifested in poor health, misfortune, social disruption, and even war. Life is governed by the principle of unity (Altuna, 1985). The ancestors participate in the daily life of the community, the visible, living portion of which is an extension of the ancestral community. In this sense, the visible and invisible realms are indestructibly fused. Life on earth and life beyond are continuous and interdependent. It is as if the world were a spider's web in which any touch of a single thread reverberates throughout the entire structure (Tempels, 1965).

Although the visible and invisible worlds interact continuously, the invisible world is most fundamental, and all major happenings are attributed to it. The spirit world of the ancestors is made up of a god and the founder of the clan, former heroes, spirits, geniuses, chiefs, hunters, warriors, magicians, and all other ancestors. Ancestors can be good or bad and intervene in the visible world, causing both good fortune and problems. Consequently, the living are constantly afraid of upsetting their ancestors and attempt to please them to win favors. Because of ancestors' powers and the fact that the living are an extension of the same community as the ancestors, Bantu people know that they risk annihilation if they damage their relationship with the ancestors or other parts of their community. In this belief system, the individual is an extension of the collective, has rights derived from participation in a wider community, and is responsible for having offspring and for transmitting traditions to them, thereby continuing the community and maintaining spiritual harmony with the ancestors.

FUNERAL RITES

Rites and rituals surrounding death are of great importance in marking the solidarity between the living and the dead and enabling the successful spiritual passage of a person from the visible world to the next world. If the funeral rites are applied according to tradition and the wishes of ancestors, the dead person will arrive safely at his destination, the life force transformed but continued in the spiritual reality of the ancestors.

As soon as the person dies, the relatives cry, shout, dance, and show their grief over the loss. The person is called by name, thanked, and recognized for positive actions in life, and the dead person is wished well for this phase. At the same time, the person or entity who caused the death is cursed. The whole community participates in gestures, body contortions, and dances. In this way, the community shows the ancestors that the person who died was well behaved and respected. This is intended also to placate the dead person so that he or she does not return to harm the community. Festivals and ceremonies are also thought to encourage the dead person to cope with the situation while awaiting transformation into the world of the ancestors.

In the funeral rite, the body is washed, dressed in good clothes, and perfumed. This preparation is a form of honoring the family, but more important, allows the dead person to maintain his or her dignity alongside the ancestors at the point of transition. Personal objects are placed alongside the dead person to help meet needs during the "journey." All relatives should be informed of the death in the family, even if they live some distance away. It is a time in the life of the community that most demands solidarity of all its members. Only in extreme circumstances can relatives be excused from the funeral. The community eats, drinks, and dances for several days. The food and drink are intended not to help the members of the community to cope with the death but to help the dead person to manage the transition.

Through the funeral rite, the family and community "promote" the deceased to the class of ancestors. Conducted properly, the ritual helps to establish harmony with the spirit world and to guarantee protection of the visible world by the ancestors. Failure to conduct the rite properly, however, would betray community solidarity and place the living community at risk. Without proper burial, it is believed that the dead person's spirit wanders around lost and disgraced and may wreak vengeance on the living. This is viewed as a source of permanent danger, as the living community is secure only if the individual really "dies" through the funeral rites and is received into the community of ancestors.

In rural Angola, where spirituality is at the center of life, the failure to perform the burial rituals is a source of psychological distress, as it is believed that the spirits of the deceased person visit and ask to be buried properly. As an elder in Huambo stated:

> During the war my father was killed. I did not perform a burial because I thought that in times of war there is no need for that. But I dreamed with my father telling me that 'I am dead but I haven't reached the place of the dead, you have to perform my obito [burial rites] because I can see the way to the place where other dead people are but I have no way to get there.' (After this dream) I performed the ritual, and I have never dreamed of my father again. (Honwana, 1998, pp. 25-26)

Similarly, Lohali, a *soba* (traditional chief) in Bie province, reported:

> My mother was killed during the war, and because at that time there was no way of performing the burial, we did not do anything. After sometime my daughter became ill, and ordinary traditional treatment did not cure her illness, later a kimbanda [diviner] told us that the spirit of my mother had possessed my daughter because since she died we did not do anything. After performing the obito the child's illness disappeared. (Honwana, 1998, p. 25)

It is not known how many people, faced with difficult war situations, failed to perform burial rituals for loved ones. Some people fear that the spirits of the unburied people wander around and cause significant damage. Thus, it should be an ongoing priority to enable people to conduct the appropriate burial rites.

CONCEPTS OF HEALTH, ILLNESS, AND HEALING

In Angola, the local concepts of health and illness are holistic and spiritually oriented, and distinctions between mind, body, and spirit do not carry the same weight they do in most Western societies. Health is defined as a harmonious relation between the individual and the environment, which includes one's ancestors and other community members. Any gap in that harmony is attributed to harmful interference of ancestors' spirits, which are dissatisfied as the result of inappropriate behavior of the living. Illness affects the whole person, and its causes are attributed to imbalances in the interaction of natural, social, and spiritual forces. Although many illnesses are viewed as having natural causes such as contact with someone who is ill, illnesses are also attributed to social, moral, and spiritual transgressions or to omissions, all of which anger the ancestors. This intermixing of natural and spiritual causes of illness, found in much of Southern Africa, entails the use of two systems of understanding and healing: Western and traditional (Louw & Pretorius, 1995).

In general, local healing is based on an explanation of why the individual was affected in a particular manner. This explanation, which may appeal to both physical and spiritual influences, identifies the "forces" that were disturbed and with which restitution must be made. Healing, too, may have physical and spiritual components and can take several forms from divination to herbal treatment. Not infrequently, treatment involves ceremonies of social integration or appeal and offers of sacrifices to ancestors in hopes of regaining protection. Local communities typically include healers (*kimbandas*) of various kinds. The healer may be an herbalist whose connection with the spirit world is limited, or the healer may be trained as a "channel" between the living and the ancestors. In some instances, healers believe they have been selected by the ancestors as intermediaries with the living.

It is important to avoid essentializing "traditional healing" (Dawes, 1997), as even very old practices reflect extensive interpenetration between different cultures. In addition, traditions are not fossilized but grow and change over time. As a result of Angola's colonial heritage, European ideas and practices have intermixed extensively with local practices. Traditional healing methods and their evolution remain poorly documented, as the traditions themselves have been transmitted orally.

Many Angolans have ambivalent feelings about traditional healing. The colonial regime sought to weaken or eliminate Angolan culture, leading many Angolans to internalize feelings of inferiority. Particularly in urban areas where Portuguese influence was strong, many Angolans lack knowledge of traditional ways. Lacking a sense of rootedness in their own culture, many Angolans feel alienated. An important step toward psychosocial reconstruction is to document traditions and to support them where it is ethically appropriate to do so as a means of strengthening the sense of continuity and social meaning. As will be described, the documentation of local beliefs and practices became an integral part of the psychosocial intervention.

PSYCHOSOCIAL INTERVENTION

Due to the local culture and history of war, psychosocial intervention in Angola faces significant challenges. Large numbers of people have been affected by war, but there are very few trained psychologists. Extreme poverty, badly damaged infrastructure, the very difficult health situation, and the prevalence of unmet basic human needs have necessitated holistic approaches that provide psychosocial assistance in the context of meeting a wider spectrum of needs. Few roadmaps exist for the construction and implementation of such approaches, and poverty and donor fatigue thwart the long-term approaches that are needed.

Amidst the war-related chaos and dire economic circumstances, it is often international NGOs and U.N. agencies that have the resources and will to provide assistance (Dubrow, Lowski, Palacios, & Gardinier, 1996; Minear & Weiss, 1993). External intervention, however, can cause significant problems (Anderson, 1996; Prendergast, 1996), particularly in a historic context of power asymmetry in which external forces exploited Angola. Reliance on external intervention often creates problems of dependency and program unsustainability. Even well-intentioned intervention by Western NGOs can promote colonialism and undermine local beliefs, values, and processes.

When most external NGOs enter a war zone, they typically bring Eurocentric ideas and Western-trained technical expertise. Aside from issues of culture bias and cultural sensitivity, the imposition of Western methods and modes of analysis is an act of psychological imperialism that marginalizes and undermines local ways of understanding and addressing psychosocial problems (Dawes, 1997; Nasanemang & Dawes, 1998; Wessells, 1999; Wessells & Kostelny, 1996). This imposition seldom occurs directly. More often, it occurs subtly through the deference of local people to the presumed wisdom of Western scientific experts, through the Western experts' disinterest in or lack of enthusiasm for learning about local modes of healing, and through the silence of local people who want to please NGOs in hopes that they may obtain valuable food, water, and shelter as part of whatever programs are constructed. In some areas, it is as if one must "give permission" before local people will discuss traditional healing with outsiders. Although NGOs cannot correct the power and resource asymmetry inherent in their work, they can be conscious of it and can work to share power and decision-making, as discussed below.

TRAUMA AND WAR STRESS—THE LIMITS OF WESTERN APPROACHES

Cultural assumptions and values saturate all intervention efforts. In examining psychosocial needs and structuring interventions in a war-torn context, Western-trained psychologists tend naturally to focus on well-validated concepts such as "trauma" and "post-traumatic stress disorder" (PTSD) (cf. Friedman & Marsella, 1996). Although these concepts have considerable value, excessive focus on trauma can detract attention from the fact that even people who do not meet formal diagnostic criteria for PTSD may nonetheless be war-affected, experiencing difficulties such as hopelessness, helplessness, and fear. In addition, psychologists often speak of "trauma" in the context of punctuated life-threatening experiences, whereas in war zones, people face multiple, chronic stressors, not least of which is poverty (Dawes & Donald, 1994; Straker, 1987). Further, the use of such terms tends to medicalize problems that are profoundly political and social (Punamäki, 1989). Excessive focus on trauma can inadvertently pathologize entire populations, encouraging the treatment of local people as victims when, in fact, local people often exhibit remarkable resilience even in the worst war conditions.

Not everyone is affected in the same manner by war experiences. The psychosocial effects of war on children vary according to the multiplicity and chronicity of stressors, the nature of one's war experiences, the meaning assigned to the experiences, the coping strategies used, and the availability of emotional support by adult caregivers, among others (Arroyo & Eth, 1996; Cairns, 1996; Dawes & Donald, 1994; Garbarino & Kostelny, 1996; Leavitt & Fox, 1993; Macksoud & Aber, 1996; Punamäki, 1996; Straker, 1992; Wessells, 1998b).

Furthermore, spiritual cosmology colors the interpretation of traumatic events in Angola. If, for example, a boy's home had been attacked, his parents had been killed before his eyes, and he had fled his village, he might present symptoms of trauma such as sleep disturbances and concentration problems associated with flashbacks. The deeper problem, however, might be spiritual; if he had been unable to conduct the appropriate burial ritual for his parents, the boy might believe that his parents spirits lingered unavenged and caused problems for him and those around him. This spiritual distress extends well beyond the parameters usually associated with terms such as "trauma." Whereas Western societies view trauma as an individual phenomenon, spiritual discord such as that associated with failure to conduct the appropriate burial ritual is highly communal. For these reasons, terms such as "war stresses" or "violence-related stresses" are preferable to "trauma."

Attempts to use strictly Western interventions to assist the boy described previously would be of limited value. Typically, Western interventions for trauma entail the provision of a safe environment and the encouragement of emotional expression in a supportive context as a means of enabling the client to come to terms with and to reintegrate his or her traumatic experience (Herman, 1992). In Angola, however, talking and emotional expression do not always fit the cultural scripts for healing. As in Southern Mozambique, talking about the past is not a key part of coming to terms with it, and talking is viewed as an invitation for the return of bad spirits (Honwana, 1997). What are indicated are culturally appropriate rituals conducted by traditional healers as a means of restoring spiritual harmony. This is not to deny the value of Western interventions in Angola, but to caution against "off-the-shelf" application without appropriate cultural tailoring and against the single-minded use of Western-based methods in a context that warrants the integration of different methods.

The situation in Angola poses equally formidable obstacles to the use of Western methods, which tend to focus on interventions for individuals and families. The surface problem is the paucity of trained psychologists, which is by far incommensurate with the scale of the need. Even if services were available, however, the widespread poverty would severely limit people's ability to pay for them. The deeper problem with the damage is that the psychological wounds are communal and cannot be addressed effectively at the individual or family levels. The war in Angola badly damaged the fabric of social relations, destroyed communities, created loss and displacement on a massive scale, and produced the deterioration of social and cultural norms. In this context, it is meaningless to think of mental health in individual terms, disconnected from wider social, political, and economic systems (Martin-Baro, 1994; Reichenberg & Friedman, 1996). Communal wounds require communal interventions that focus on rebuilding positive community and reestablishing normal patterns of living and tradition that contribute to people's sense of continuity and meaning (Gibbs, 1997). This is best accomplished through a community-based approach.

A COMMUNITY-BASED APPROACH

Angola offers many opportunities for the construction of community-based approaches. Culturally, there is a strong communal orientation. Despite having endured the ravages of 35 years of war, Angolans exhibit remarkable resilience, the desire to break the yoke of colonialism, and a willingness to address societal problems even while living and working under very difficult conditions.

Although community-based approaches come in different varieties, they have five distinguishing features, outlined here with reference to psychosocial interventions.

Partnership   The community is regarded neither as beneficiaries nor as a locus for intervention but as a partner who brings important cultural and human resources to the table and with whom power should be shared in all phases of program conception, design, implementation, evaluation, and reporting. Local people are viewed not as helpless victims, but as people living under difficult circumstances with whom power is shared and decisions are made jointly. Participatory process, joint dialogue, and collaborative problem-solving are emphasized.

Community Mobilization   Because war disrupts society, a central priority is to support and enable the reestablishment of community, physically and psychologically (Boothby, 1996). This entails work with and through local leaders, networks, and social influence processes, mobilization of the community around pressing needs, and building local capacity. It also entails conscientization for empowerment, because, amidst war, many communities lack the luxury of stepping back, asking how they have been affected by the war, what their historic situation and reality are, and what steps they can take to construct a more positive future (Lederach, 1995).

Cultural Relevance   Local culture is regarded as a set of potentially useful resources for identifying, understanding, and addressing psychosocial needs. The aim is to learn from local culture and to construct culturally relevant interventions, recognizing that local methods evolve and may be enriched by integration with methods derived from other cultural systems.

Holism   Diverse social mediators and pathways influence the effects of exposure to violence. Since war zones create systems of violence, ecological approaches that integrate work at family, community, and societal levels are indicated. To assist children, it is necessary to assist the primary caregivers and families that mediate the effects of stress and play a pivotal role in children's development. Some of the worst stresses are economic, as war leads to losses, hunger, and changes in status. Because psychosocial influences are inextricably interconnected with biological needs and with the political, economic, and social milieu, psychosocial interventions should not be stand-alone but integrated and holistic. Ideally, psychosocial work is coordinated with efforts to meet basic biological needs, to restructure the political and economic system, and to introduce appropriate changes in the policy arena. This approach invites participation and minimizes stigma that might be associated with individual counseling and the use of psychological centers.

Sustainability   The emphasis is on processes that will endure and address long-term needs. The main goal is to build local capacity and to use culturally appropriate methods based on community participation and ownership. In this approach, Western psychologists may provide training and consultation, but their role is supportive and aims to strengthen local psychology and psychological services. These features are integral to the philosophy and implementation of the two interventions described next.

Community-Based Healing

In Angola, two key psychosocial priorities are community healing and the reintegration of former child soldiers. Without social healing and coming to terms with the past, it is difficult for people to construct a bridge between the present and a positive future. As discussed earlier, healing is a communal project that is intimately connected with cultural issues. In a context in which war had disrupted traditional practices and normal patterns of living and where Western NGOs were operating, there was a temptation to impose outsider approaches rather than support and strengthen local cultural practices. This section tells the story of how the program developers learned to incorporate local cultural beliefs, practices, and resources into the program on healing.

The Luanda-based Pilot Project

Initially, the work on healing was constructed within a trauma idiom, as indicated by a pilot project conducted in Luanda in 1994 and 1995 and called the Mobile War Trauma Team project (Wessells, 1996). Its strategy was to train adults who could then organize healing activities for traumatized street children and for orphans who had little social support. To build local capacities for psychosocial assistance, CCF formed a national team of five Angolans led by Carlinda Monteiro. This team received an intensive four-week training on basic principles of child development, the emotional impact of war on children, the methods of assisting war-affected children, and non-violent conflict resolution. The assistance methods initially were expressive activities such as song, dance, drawing, and storytelling, all of which aimed to enable emotional expression and integration.

This pilot project collaborated with local communities and with government agencies such as the Ministry of Rehabilitation and Social Reintegration to select and train adults who had worked with children and were in a position to have a positive impact. Working with groups of 15 to 20 people, the national team provided two-week, participatory seminars that included the curriculum elements described previously including methods for assisting children. Following the seminars, trainees used these methods in the context in which they normally worked with children, with the national team providing follow-up support in solving problems or providing additional training on site. The national team, in turn, received ongoing training, support, and supervision from Carlinda Monteiro and from an outside consultant.

During the pilot project, the Angolan team rapidly learned the importance of local beliefs and resources. On one occasion, the children in an orphanage believed that a spirit haunted the premises and they were unable to sleep, making the orphanage a very difficult environment to live or work in. Recognizing that the solution was not to be found in emotional expression or talking, the team suggested the recruitment of a local healer who visited the orphanage and conducted a ritual to get rid of the bad spirit. Subsequently, the children were able to sleep, enabling life in the orphanage to return to normal. Having learned the value of local practices in assisting children, the team made three important changes. First, they networked with traditional healers and elders, developing good working relations that made it possible to draw upon the knowledge and skills of the healers. Second, they incorporated information about local beliefs and practices into the training seminars. They accomplished this through the use of a highly participatory, elicitive pedagogy (Lederach, 1995) that invited the participants to bring to the table their local beliefs and the practices surrounding them. For instance, the trainers stimulated active discussion by asking questions such as "What do children need for healthy development?" and constructed with the participants a basic ecological model, as shown in Figure 18.1. Third, they reconceptualized the seminars as spaces in which the participants discussed how to integrate the Western-based, expressive methods with the local, ritual-focused methods. In this manner, the participants and the trainers became co-learners who sought to use the best insights from different cultural systems to support war-affected children.

This pilot project was instrumental in building participatory processes with local communities, learning from traditional healers, and testing ways of intermixing traditional and Western methods of healing. Through interventions such as organized dances, drawing sessions, storytelling, drama, and sports and games, this project reached nearly 15,000 children, who exhibited improved child-child and adult-child

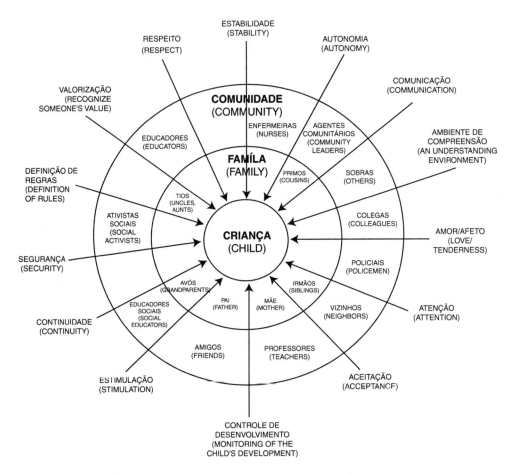

FIG. 18.1. An ecological conception of children's basic psychosocial needs and the key people who influence their development.

relations; decreased sleeping problems; reduced bedwetting, stress reactions, and aggressive behavior; diminished concentration problems and social isolation; and improved future orientation (Wessells, 1996).

A Multiprovince Approach

The next challenge was to apply on a large scale the methodology that had been developed in the pilot project. With the assistance of major funding from the U.S. Agency for International Development, CCF/Angola implemented a program of community-based healing in the eight most severely war-affected provinces: Benguela, Bie, Huambo, Luanda, Malange, Uige, Huila, and Moxico (in the latter two provinces, CCF collaborated with UNICEF). In each province, there was a three-person team of trainers who knew the local language and culture and who were respected by local people. Applying the model that had been used successfully in Luanda, these provincial trainers conducted week-long training seminars aimed to build the local capacity to assist children and to mobilize communities around children's needs. At the national level, most of the work was conducted in Portuguese. Locally, however, the work was conducted in the local languages. The provincial teams spoke both the local language and Portuguese and translated when it was necessary.

The province-based trainers' work included seven steps (Green & Wessells, 1997). First, the team conducted a local situation analysis to identify the geographic areas of greatest need. Second, the team visited local communities, meeting with and demonstrating respect for local sobas (traditional chiefs), elders, influential women, and caregivers. If they expressed having strong material needs, the CCF trainers worked with other NGOs and local agencies to meet the material needs. Third, the trainers conducted sensitization dialogues with community groups. Many local people viewed problems such as children's aggression as signs of disobedience rather than as impacts of war experiences of violence. The sensitization dialogues helped local people understand children's behavior and activated them around assisting children. Fourth, using the community networks identified in the first two stages, the trainers selected well-respected adults such as organizers of youth groups or teachers who were in a good position to assist children. Fifth, the trainers conducted week-long training seminars for groups of approximately 20 adults using the curriculum outlined. Follow-up support was provided through regular site visits.

Sixth, the trainees implemented activities on behalf of children. Following the seminars, trainees applied what they had learned in the venues in which they worked with children in their respective communities. To encourage emotional expression in a supportive group context, trainees arranged group activities such as singing, storytelling, drama, and dancing. Particularly for young or withdrawn children, they often encouraged free drawing, giving children a sheet of paper and crayons and asking them to draw whatever they want. Typically, children drew pictures of their war experiences, enabling discussion and emotional reintegration in a safe environment. Although these activities were accessible to all children, the trainees gave special attention to the children with whom they worked who exhibited the strongest psychosocial impact of war. Activities also included informal educational discussions and noncompetitive athletic activities. These structured activities were designed to encourage prosocial behaviors and to increase the amount of time children spent under the supervision of adults who had a basic understanding of the impacts of war and skills to assist children. Having benefited from discussions of war experiences during the seminars, trainees often talked with others in the community about how they had individually and collectively been impacted by war.

To mobilize communities around the needs of children, the trainees acted as community advocates on behalf of children. They convened community discussions about the status and needs of children, helped to conceptualize projects to assist children, and identified policies that were in children's interests. This work was complemented by trainees' advocacy of policies at the municipal and local levels that serve the needs of children. Recognizing the harmful effects of institutionalizing orphans, for example, they advocated for more intensive work on the tracing and family reunification of orphans. As the project evolved, trainees included more activities such as soccer teams and drama groups for increasing social integration. Because local people needed to see tangible improvements in their circumstances, the teams also began a program of giving small grants for community-planned projects such as school construction or building community huts. These projects were conducted in partnership, with CCF supplying the materials and selected community adults supplying the labor.

The seventh step was to evaluate the work using a mixture of qualitative and quantitative methods and indicators. The results, which have been presented in greater detail elsewhere (Wessells & Monteiro, 2000), are summarized here. Over three years, the project trained 4,894 adults, who in turn assisted nearly 300,000 children. The impacts on children included improved child-child and adult-child relationships; improved behavior and cooperation in the classroom; less evidence of war-related games and toys; diminished isolation behavior; reduced violence and aggressive behavior; fewer concentration problems; decreased hypervigilance; increased hope; and improved school attendance. Adults, too, reported discernible benefits. Many reported that the training seminars had for the first time provided space in which they could begin coming to terms with their own war experiences.

At the communal level, the project had powerful effects. Sobas and elders reported that communities had become more active and hopeful as a result of the project. As schools were built, for example, the physical structures became tangible symbols of communal healing and monuments to people's hope and resilience. There was an intimate connection between physical reconstruction and healing, a topic that has received relatively little attention in the psychological literature. Much of the healing was social as people rebuilt systems of planning, dialogue, and joint activity that normalized life and embodied social trust.

Social healing also occurred through cultural reclamation and the strengthening of traditional social structure and practices. Centuries of colonialism had damaged traditional authority and had led local people to feel inferior about their own culture. People who feel inferior and who doubt their own abilities are not in a good position to plan effectively for the future. Many adults reported that the project, by working in partnership with sobas and healers, had strengthened belief in the value of local culture, helped to restore social traditions and practices, and reinforced belief in the ability of local people to take charge of their own future. In this sense, the project's cultural approach was a key part of the communal empowerment and mobilization process. The project on reintegration of underage soldiers sought to strengthen this process.

THE REINTEGRATION OF UNDERAGE SOLDIERS PROJECT

Approximately 9,000 Angolan children, defined in accord with international law as people under 18 years of age, were drawn into soldiering, mostly on the side of UNITA. Most children were recruited forcibly either through roundups in public places or through imposition of a quota system. In the latter, troops entered a village and demanded that the soba turn over a particular number of young people lest the entire village be attacked and destroyed. Boys usually acted as combatants, porters, cooks, and spies, while girls often assumed roles as concubines or sex slaves.

Brutal tactics were often used to indoctrinate young people into military life. Many young recruits were beaten and threatened with execution if they tried to escape. According to one boy soldier, "escapees who were found were generally killed. They were tied to a post and all the troops would be called to watch. They were killed, and the killer had sometimes to drink the victim's blood. The blood was said to be good for the person not to feel remorse" (Honwana, 1998, p. 40). It was not uncommon to force young people to kill someone who had tried to escape as a means of deterring escape, instilling terror, and normalizing the act of killing. To boost their morale and strengthen their military identities, young soldiers were typically given names such as "Strong" or "Rambo."

When CCF first sought to assist these young people, the term "child soldiers" posed problems. In Angola, as in most Bantu societies, people who have participated in culturally defined rites of passage, typically at 12 or 13 years of age, are considered adults. The term "child soldiers" embodied Western views of childhood and of children's rights that do not fit the local beliefs. Fortunately, the local authorities agreed that it is damaging and undesirable for people under 18 years of age to be soldiers, enabling reference to "underage soldiers."

Concurrently with the community-based healing project, the "Reintegration of Underage Soldiers" (RUS) project was implemented in 1996 through 1998 in partnership with UNICEF in the same provinces and many of the same localities where the work on healing had been conducted. The project strategy was to reintegrate former underage soldiers into families and communities through a holistic approach that combined family preparation and integration, community sensitization, microeconomic development, and traditional healing. This social integration approach contrasts with that of placing returning youth in transitional centers where they receive counseling. Although center-based approaches are valuable in some circumstances, they tend to take on a life of their own. Short-term stays give way to long-term stays, and, too often, insufficient attention is given to reintegration into family and community life, the broader goals to which any rehabilitation program must aspire. In the Angolan context, centers and counseling are unsustainable, as neither has a basis in the local culture.

Preparation, Reentry, and Reintegration

To initiate the project at the grassroots level, the province-based teams identified, trained, and supported a network of approximately 200 *activistas*. Many of the activistas were associated with the local church, had strong networks with the local communities, and were recognized by their communities as being in a good position to assist returning youth. The provincial teams trained the activistas on social mobilization, the psychosocial impacts of child soldiering, and methods of enabling the integration of former soldiers. The activistas conducted their work in three stages: preparation, reentry, and reintegration. These are described briefly since the primary emphasis is on the traditional healing aspects of the project.

While the former soldiers, most of whom had been recruited at 13 to 14 years of age, were in quartering areas, the activistas traced and notified their families. The activistas listened to family members' concerns, educated them about the situation of child soldiers, and advised them on how to aid family and community reintegration. They also worked to increase the understanding that problems such as disobedience might stem not from bad character, but from war experiences. In the community, activistas worked to raise awareness of the needs of former child soldiers, to reduce stereotypes, and to hear concerns about their return. They also worked to gain support of local officials by conducting meetings with sobas, government leaders, and community influentials. These meetings helped to sensitize people to the needs for vocational training, apprenticeships, economic opportunities, and positive roles and life options for returning child soldiers.

The reentry work was very dangerous because Angola remained a divided country, and strong pressures existed in UNITA-controlled areas to continue fighting and to reabduct former soldiers. Recognizing that family reunification is one of the most basic forms of psychosocial assistance to children, the activistas provided extensive logistical and transportation support, accompanying the child soldiers to their rendezvous points and arranging temporary foster care when it was impossible for the families to meet the children. Of the 4,104 youths demobilized into the CCF/UNICEF project areas, over 50 percent were successfully reunited with their families. The activistas also arranged community receptions, which occasioned singing, dancing, and traditional reentry rituals in which adults sprinkled the youths' faces and heads with flour or water.

To promote integration, activistas helped to identify school, job, and vocational training placements. These are vital for building hope for the future and giving young people skills that will enable them to support themselves. In addition, participation in culturally appropriate patterns of activity provides a sense of normalcy, continuity, and social meaning (Gibbs, 1997). Unfortunately, many youths chose not to return to school due to embarrassment over having to take classes with young children in primary school. Since many youth will return to agricultural life, CCF/Angola, with the aid of external funding, provided small grants for quick-impact projects such as starting a small business. Preliminary evidence indicated that youths felt hopeful and were making the transition effectively from military to civilian life as they entered carpentry or agriculture or started small businesses. This approach underscores the importance of linking psychosocial healing with economic reconstruction in an integrated effort.

Among the most important aspects of reintegration is the process of spiritual cleansing of returning soldiers. As will be described, traditional purification is a crucial gateway for social reintegration, and without it, returning former soldiers are viewed as placing the community at risk. Unfortunately, many international NGOs have focused so strongly on trauma and on outsider concepts that they have not put themselves in the positions of students who stand to learn much about local culture. The RUS project sought to study this gateway and to weave it into the fabric of the holistic approach described previously. It assumed that analyzing local beliefs and practices surrounding soldiering and the return home is an important first step in understanding how young people have been affected and in constructing interventions that enable social functionality and integration. The next section describes the gateway and the process through which the Angolan team studied and valorized it.

Traditional Healing and Community Reconciliation

The RUS project sought to document traditional beliefs and rituals that had been transmitted orally across generations and had not, to anyone's knowledge, been described by people who had received appropriate anthropological training. Initiated in a spirit of action research, the documentation effort sought to describe indigenous psychological tools and resources that may be useful in assisting war-affected children. It also aimed to valorize local traditions as part of the process of cultural reclamation and the boosting of collective self-esteem and empowerment. Indeed, the documentation was part of the process of psychosocial healing because it heightened the salience and prestige associated with cultural beliefs and practices that enable social meaning, provided support under difficult circumstances, and built continuity between past, present, and future. The process of documentation was also one of mobilization and strengthening local networks, as many people had become separated from healers or had not been referring with them as frequently as had been the practice before the war.

To prepare for the documentation, Alcinda Honwana, a Mozambiquan social anthropologist, trained the province-based teams in ethnographic methodology. The teams then used this methodology to interview key informants and learn about local beliefs on life and death, illness and health, and ritual purification. A key lesson from this part of the project was the need for ongoing training that contributed not only to technical expertise but also to open-mindedness. The provincial teams consisted of university educated people who had embraced the mindsets of the colonizers and who themselves tended to see traditional practices as being backwards. Accordingly, follow-up trainings used a reflective methodology in which the Angolans discussed why they held such deep prejudices toward their own culture, the value of the local cultural beliefs for people living in the rural areas, and the importance of documenting the beliefs and practices. Although the documentation is still in its early stages, numerous patterns and themes are visible.

One of the main findings is that spiritual contamination rather than trauma is viewed locally as the heart of the problems facing returning underage soldiers. Among the former soldiers and the local communities, the belief is that one who has killed is haunted by the unavenged spirits of the people who had been killed. The spirits are believed to cause mental disturbance. According to one informant, "those who killed unjustly . . . the spirit of the dead person possess [sic] them and they become mentally disturbed. When that happens it is necessary to do traditional treatment—ku thoka—so that the illness goes away" (Honwana, 1998, p. 73).

The local belief is that the spirits of the dead cause injury or harm and that traditional treatment is required to remedy the problem. Speaking of her 19-year-old nephew who had returned following seven years of fighting in the war, a kimbanda from Malanje said the following:

> I could not let him stay without the treatment. He needed it because there he might have done bad things like kill, beat and rob people . . . without the treatment the spirits of the dead would harm him. I do not know what happened there, he said he did not do anything . . . young people sometimes lie . . . I decided to go for full treatment because otherwise he could become crazy or even die. (Honwana, 1998, p. 74)

In the view of local people, the problem is one of spiritual contamination, and it is communal in nature. If a returning soldier who is haunted returns to the village, the haunting spirit causes bad behavior, creating problems such as crime and killing in the community. The members of the living community are obligated to restore spiritual harmony through the conduct of an appropriate purification ritual that avenges the spirits of those who had been killed. The failure to conduct the purification ritual jeopardizes the entire community. This communal distress constitutes a powerful barrier to the reintegration of returning underage soldiers. To open the door for integration, it is necessary to achieve spiritual cleansing or decontamination, which is accomplished through symbolic purification rituals performed by a kimbanda. The performance of these rituals opens the door to reconciliation between the returning young person and the community.

To illustrate the cleansing process, consider the case of M. P., a 20 year old from Huambo who had narrowly escaped death twice while in the military. Speaking of his joyful reunification with his mother, he described the greeting ritual that was performed.

> . . . a chicken was killed and I ate it all. They also scrubbed me fuba (cassava flour) in the face and swept my legs with a broom. I asked why, and she said "It will not do you any harm. We did this because you have been far away for a long time. You didn't die, you returned, that is why." Then we danced batuque [a traditional dance accompanied by drums] with the whole family and the neighbors.

Subsequently, through networks of the CCF trainers, a local healer judged that the cleansing process was incomplete, leading him to conduct a more thorough purification ritual. This and other evidence suggests that there is a two-stage process of cleansing in which more thorough methods are applied if the initial procedures do not achieve the cleansing. The ritual included creation of a safe space, fumigation, offering to the spirits, and a mixture of purgative and preventative elements as described next.

The healer placed several herbs (green leaves, dry leaves, and roots) in a basin containing water, which he put on the threshold of the front door. The healer put dry leaves of the Uvanga plant into a can containing two lighted pieces of charcoal, and he placed the can on the right side of the basin. The burning leaves created a white fume that transformed the atmosphere. Fanning the can to expand the fume all over the room and the back yard, the healer said, "This fume expels the souls of the other world. The souls of the other world, and the spirits, that want to harm you step back when they find in the door Uvanga or its fume." A bunch of dried Jelele branches was then placed in the front part of the basin. The branches were tied as to form a traditional or handmade broom, which was placed in front of the door. The healer said, "This broom is to impede the entrance of the 'filthiness' that was attached to you until now."

M. P.'s mother was allowed to help organize the herbs according to the healer's instructions. When everything was ready, the old man poured some liquor in each of the four corners of the room, around the basin, and finally over it, forming a cross. In the same places, he also poured the Kissangua [a traditional nonalcoholic drink] and small amounts of Kanjika [a local food consisting of corn and beans]. The healer explained that this was a symbolic gesture for offering a banquet or party to the spirits.

Seated on a small bench with the basin of herbs between his feet, M.P. rested his feet on Upu leaves, thereby squashing, stepping on, and killing evils he carried such as spirits of the dead or curses put upon him. M.P. removed his shirt, and the healer then scrubbed his chest with black Jolela root to avoid all evils that might have wanted to attack frontally. The same root was scrubbed on M.P.'s back so that he would have the same protection on both the back and front of his body. The rubbing of front and back was repeated using the rubber stem of the Olunenva plant, thereby blocking evil, removing curses, and adding protection. The bathing continued with Evonguevongue leaves, which the healer explained would block anyone who wants to hinder a person's progress.

Following a full-body bath, the healer covered M.P. with cloths and a bathing towel and turned his face toward the basin. Heated mud stones which had been built by salele (fire ants) were placed in the basin, causing the water to boil and giving off a vapor that caused M.P. to sweat. The healer explained that "Even if somebody wants to harm you, in a short time, he forgets what he wanted to do against you." While M.P. breathed the hot vapor, the old healer began to rotate the chicken around M.P.'s head. He also said, "You didn't make anything. You don't know anything. This already began a long time ago; all the evil that it is in our son, we don't know, the evil that is in our son should leave; if he has done any wrong, it is because he was forced to do, it was not his will; because he did not begin it in the first place." According to the healer, the chicken is important because it serves as payment for the spirit that is causing all evildoing . . . The healer explained that the chicken has to be offered to the spirit to achieve the patient's protection: "If the spirit receives a chicken from somebody wanting him to engage in evildoing, he no longer can do it because he has been paid already. The spirit returns and tells the person who sent the chicken that he cannot do it anymore, so the person who was to have suffered the harm is set free."

The ceremony having ended, the participants and witnesses celebrated by consuming Kanjika, bread, liquor, and Kissangua. Smiling, M.P. dressed himself. The healer observed M.P. and moments later requested that he leave the room by jumping through the door.

M.P. jumped over the basin as requested. The jump signified that starting from that day, all types of wickedness, persecutions by the spirits of the dead, living enemies, envy and diseases, were left behind. Thus began a new life for M.P., who is now seen as having been purified from all evil. "Now he is lighter, all the weight that he carried, all the filthiness came out," the old healer said.

Programmatically, the RUS project did not itself invent or apply traditional treatments. Rather, it played a facilitative role that encouraged local communities to strengthen traditional processes that war, colonialism, and poverty had tended to disrupt. The importance of this facilitative role should not be underestimated, as the entry of humanitarian assistance agencies into war zones brings a host of outsider values and social influences that may subtly contribute to the erosion of local traditions and practices that are valuable sources of psychosocial support. Through documentation processes, local communities may move into a better position to analyze the strengths and weaknesses of their traditions and practices and to make conscious choices about which paths to pursue in community development.

Sadly, the re-eruption of war in Angola in December 1998 disrupted work on the reintegration of underage soldiers. Because additional youths have been recruited since, there will be great need of future work along the lines outlined previously. Although this reintegration work is prevention-oriented in that it seeks to reduce the risks of reabduction and to create positive life options for youths, it is only one element of comprehensive prevention efforts. To strengthen prevention efforts, the CCF teams have consistently supported policies that provide more effective protection for children and that outlaw such objectionable exploitation of children.

TOWARD THE FUTURE

The war in Angola officially ended in April 2002, yet there is great need of additional psychosocial work on healing and the reintegration of underage soldiers as part of the peace-building process. Although the projects described in this chapter have had significant positive impact, they surely raise more questions than they answer. Enormous needs exist for ongoing evaluation research to address questions such as the following. How effective is traditional healing, and to what extent do project effects owe to traditional methods, to Western methods, or to their combination? How long term are the effects of the projects? How will the use of Western-based methods alter traditional beliefs, practices, and values and what are the implications of these changes? What roles does the family play in buffering the effects of stress or, in cases of excessive discipline and child abuse, in spreading and amplifying effects of community-level violence? Much more remains to be learned about the pathways through which violence and healing methods influence stress and behavior. Fortunately, the projects have helped to build a foundation of interest in and expertise for collecting data to address these and related issues. The intent is to refine the interventions through continued evaluation research, enabling the project to serve as a model for conducting culturally relevant interventions in other war-torn countries.

Ultimately, the aim of projects such as these is to contribute to peace. Peace, however, requires political, social, and economic transformations on a large scale. To maximize their impact, psychologists in war zones need to develop more effective means of integrating their work into macro-social programs for transforming cultures of violence into cultures of peace.

REFERENCES

Altuna, P. A. (1985). *Cultura tradicional banto* [Traditional Bantu Culture]. Luanda, Angola.

Anderson, M. B. (1996). Humanitarian NGOs in conflict intervention. In C. A. Crocker, F. Hampson, & P. Aall (Eds.), *Managing global chaos: Sources of and responses to international conflict* (pp. 343–354). Washington, DC: U. S. Institute of Peace Press.

Arroyo, W., & Eth, S. (1996). Post-traumatic stress disorder and other stress reactions. In R. J. Apfel & B. Simon (Eds.), *Minefields in their hearts* (pp. 52–74). New Haven, NJ: Yale University Press.

Boothby, N. (1996). Mobilizing communities to meet the psychosocial needs of children in war and refugee crises. In R. J. Apfel & B. Simon (Eds.), *Minefields in their hearts* (pp. 149–164). New Haven, NJ: Yale University Press.

Brett, R., & McCallin, M. (1996). *Children: The invisible soldiers.* Vaxjo, Sweden: Rädda Barnen.

Cairns, E. (1996). *Children and political violence.* Oxford, England: Blackwell.

Cairns, E., & Dawes, A. (1996). Children: Ethnic and political violence—a commentary. *Child Development, 67,* 129–139.

Cohn, I., & Goodwin-Gill, G. (1994*). Child soldiers: The role of children in armed conflicts.* Oxford, England: Clarendon.

Dawes, A. (1997, July). *Cultural imperialism in the treatment of children following political violence and war: A Southern African perspective.* Paper presented at the Fifth International Symposium on the Contributions of Psychology to Peace, Melbourne, Australia.

Dawes, A., & Donald, D. (1994). *Childhood & adversity: Psychological perspectives from South African research.* Cape Town, South Africa: David Philip.

Dinicola, V. F. (1996). Ethnocultural aspects of PTSD and related disorders among children and adolescents. In A. J. Marsella, M. J. Friedman, E. T. Gerrity, & R. M. Scurfield (Eds.), *Ethnocultural aspects of posttraumatic stress disorder: Issues, research, and clinical applications* (pp. 389–414). Washington, DC: American Psychological Association.

Dubrow, N., Lowski, N. I., Palacios, C., & Gardinier, M. (1996). Traumatized children: Helping child victims of violence. The contribution of non-governmental organizations. In Y. Daniele, N. S. Rodley, & L. Weisaeth (Eds.), *International responses to traumatic stress* (pp. 327–346). Amityville, NY: Baywood.

Eriksson, M., Sollenberg, M., & Wallensteen, P. (2002). Patterns of major armed conflicts, 1990-2001. *SIPRI Yearbook 2002,* pp. 63–76.

Friedman, M. J., & Marsella, A. J. (1996). Posttraumatic stress disorder: An overview of the concept. In A. J. Marsella, M. J. Friedman, E. T. Gerrity, & R. M. Scurfield (Eds.), *Ethnocultural aspects of posttraumatic stress disorder: Issues, research, and clinical applications* (pp. 11–32). Washington, DC: American Psychological Association.

Garbarino, J., & Kostelny, K. (1996). The effects of political violence on Palestinian children's behavioral problems: A risk accumulation model. *Child Development, 67,* 33–45.

Garfield, R. M., & Neugut, A. I. (1997). The human consequences of war. In B. S. Levy & V. W. Sidel (Eds.), *War and public health* (pp. 27–38). New York: Oxford.

Gibbs, S. (1997). Postwar social reconstruction in Mozambique: Reframing children's experiences of trauma and healing. In K. Kumar (Ed.), *Rebuilding war-torn societies: Critical areas for international assistance* (pp. 227–238). Boulder, CO: Lynne Rienner.

Green, E., & Wessells, M. (1997). *Mid-term evaluation of the province-based war trauma team project: Meeting the psychosocial needs of children in Angola.* Richmond, VA: Christian Children's Fund.

Herman, J. (1992). *Trauma and recovery.* New York: BasicBooks.

Honwana, A. M. (1997). Healing for peace: Traditional healers and post-war reconstruction in Southern Mozambique. *Peace and Conflict: Journal of Peace Psychology, 3,* 293–306.

Honwana, A. (1998). *"Okusiakala Ondalo Yokalye": Let us light a new fire.* Luanda, Angola: Christian Children's Fund/Angola.

Human Rights Watch/Africa (1994). *Angola: Arms trade and violations of the laws of war since the 1992 elections.* New York: Human Rights Watch.

Leavitt, L. A., & Fox, N. A. (Eds.). (1993). *The psychological effects of war and violence on children.* Hillsdale, NJ: Erlbaum.

Lederach, J. P. (1995). *Preparing for peace: Conflict transformation across cultures.* Syracuse, NY: Syracuse University Press.

Lodico, Y. C. (1996). A peace that fell apart: The United Nations and the war in Angola. In W. J. Durch (Ed.), *UN peacekeeping, American politics, and the uncivil wars of the 1990s* (pp. 103–133). New York: St. Martin's.

Louw, D. A., & Pretorius, E. (1995). The traditional healer in a multicultural society: The South African experience. In L. L. Adler & B. R. Mukherji (Eds.), *Spirit versus scalpel: Traditional healing and modern psychotherapy* (pp. 41–57). Westport, CT: Bergin & Garvey.

Macksoud, M. S., & Aber, J. L. (1996). The war experiences and psychosocial development of children in Lebanon. *Child Development, 67*, 70–88.

Martin-Baro, I. (1994). War and mental health. In A. Aron & S. Corne (Eds.), *Writings for a liberation psychology* (pp. 108–121). Cambridge, MA: Harvard University Press.

McIntyre, T., & Ventura, M. (2002). Children of war: Psychosocial sequelae of war trauma in Angolan adolescents. In S. Krippner & T. McIntyre (Eds.), *The psychosocial impact of war trauma on civilians* (pp. 39–53). Westport, CT: Praeger.

Minear, L., & Weiss, T. G. (1993). *Humanitarian action in times of war.* Boulder, CO: Lynne Rienner.

Nsamenang, A. B., & Dawes, A. (1998). Developmental psychology as political psychology in sub-Saharan Africa: The challenge of Africanisation. *Applied Psychology: An International Review, 47*, 73–87.

Prendergast, J. (1996). *Frontline diplomacy: Humanitarian aid and conflict in Africa.* Boulder, CO: Lynne Rienner.

Punamäki, R. (1989). Political violence and mental health. *International Journal of Mental Health, 17*, 3–15.

Punamäki, R. (1996). Can ideological commitment protect children's psychosocial well-being in situations of political violence? *Child Development, 67*, 55–69.

Reichenberg, D., & Friedman, S. (1996). Traumatized children. Healing the Invisible wounds of war: A rights approach. In Y. Daniele, N. S. Rodley, & L. Weisaeth (Eds.), *International responses to traumatic stress* (pp. 307–326). Amityville, NY: Baywood.

Sivard, R. L. (1996). *World military and social expenditures 1996.* Washington, DC: World Priorities.

Smith, D. (1997). *The state of war and peace atlas.* London: Penguin.

Straker, G. (1987). The continuous traumatic stress syndrome: The single therapeutic interview. *Psychology and Sociology, 8*(1), 48–79.

Straker, G., Mendelsohn, M., Moosa, F., & Tudin, P. (1996). Violent political contexts and the emotional concerns of township youth. *Child Development, 67*, 46–54.

Straker, G., Moosa, F., Becker, R., & Nkwale, M. (1992). *Faces in the revolution.* Cape Town, South Africa: David Philip.

Tempels, P. (1965). *La philosophie bantoue* [Bantu philosophy]. Paris: Presence Africaine.

UNICEF (1996). *The state of the world's children 1996.* Oxford, England: Oxford University Press.

Volkan, V. (1997). *Bloodlines.* New York: Farrar, Straus & Giroux.

Wessells, M. (1996). Assisting Angolan children impacted by war: Blending Western and traditional approaches to healing. *Coordinators' Notebook: An International Resource for Early Childhood Development, 19*, 33–37.

Wessells, M. (1997). Child soldiers. *Bulletin of the Atomic Scientists, 53*(6), 32–39.

Wessells, M. (2002). Recruitment of children as soldiers in sub-Saharan Africa: An ecological analysis. In L. Mjoset & S. Van Holde (Eds.), *The comparative study of conscription in the Armed Forces (Comparative Social Research, Vol. 20)* (pp. 237–254). Amsterdam: Elsevier.

Wessells, M., & Kostelny, K. (1996). *The Graça Machel/U.N. Study on the impact of armed conflict on children: Implications for early child development.* New York: UNICEF.

Wessells, M. G. (1998a). The changing nature of armed conflict and its implications for children: The Graça Machel/U.N. Study. *Peace & Conflict: Journal of Peace Psychology, 4*(4), 321–334.

Wessells, M. G. (1998b). Children, armed conflict, and peace. *Journal of Peace Research, 35*(5), 635–646.

Wessells, M. G. (1999). Culture, power, and community: Intercultural approaches to psychosocial assistance and healing. In K. Nader, N. Dubrow, & B. Stamm (Eds.), *Honoring differences: Cultural issues in the treatment of trauma and loss* (pp. 276–282). New York: Taylor & Francis.

Wessells, M. G., & Monteiro, C. (2000). Healing wounds of war in Angola: A community-based approach. In D. Donald, A. Dawes, & J. Louw (Eds.), *Addressing childhood adversity* (pp. 176–201). Cape Town, South Africa: David Philip.

Wessells, M. G., & Monteiro, C. (2001). Psychosocial intervention and post-conflict reconstruction in Angola: Interweaving Western and traditional approaches. In D. Christie, R. V. Wagner, & D. Winter (Eds.), *Peace, conflict, and violence: Peace psychology for the 21st century* (pp. 262–275). Upper Saddle River, NJ: Prentice-Hall.

Native Healing in Arab-Islamic Societies

Ihsan Al-Issa
The International Arab Psychological Association

Abdulla Al-Subaie
King Saud University
Riyadh, Saudi Arabia

Healing techniques have always reflected the human struggle for physical survival and psychological well-being in order to preserve a wholesome existence in the face of the mysteries of nature. Because illness is related to the interaction between the individual and both the physical and social environment, it is not surprising that there are commonalties across time and space regarding etiology and treatment. Possession by the spirits as an explanation of physical and mental illness has been with us throughout the history of human beings (Alexander & Selesnick, 1966). The evil eye as an etiological factor is found across cultures, including a number of European countries, India, and the Middle East (Dundes, 1981). Similarly, many universal factors are involved in the therapeutic process, such as the healer's shared worldview with his or her patients, labeling of the disease and the attribution of the cause, the expectations of the patient, and the importance of suggestion (Prince, 1980). Thus, the Arab-Islamic native healing systems share many characteristics with those of other cultures.

Nevertheless, these Arab-Islamic native systems also tend to have their own unique features. For orthodox Muslims, the Qur'an and the prophet-tradition (*hadith*) are the major sources of guidance in medical matters. They lay out the general outlines of lawful and unlawful healing practices: "We have revealed in the Qur'an that which is healing and mercy to the believers" (Qur'an 17:82). These two sources had become the basis of prophetic medicine after the death of the Prophet. However, when the Arabs later conquered many lands ranging from southern Spain to northern India, they were influenced by native supernatural beliefs, magical practices, and claims of miraculous healing which had nothing to do with orthodox Islam. The veneration of saints,[1] visits to shrines, the use of amulets and talismans, and many other magical practices and dealings with the *jinn* (spirits; jinni is singular) became popular in Islamic societies. Rejection of these practices by orthodox Muslims is based on the fundamental Islamic principle of *Tawheed*, "which means believing in His absolute knowledge and power of healing. Seeking help from diviners, magicians, astrologers or fortune-tellers is forbidden because it contradicts the principle of Tawheed" (Al-Subaie & Al-Hamad, 2000, pp. 214-215). Although the Qur'an itself is referred to as

---

[1] We use the word saint throughout the chapter to refer to various pious and venerated Muslims and holy men with no implication that they are comparable to Christian saints.

"healing and mercy to the believers" (17:82), it does not mention miraculous healing by the prophet Muhammad or other prophets except for Jesus who healed the blind and leprous and raised the dead (3:49; 5:113). Indeed, the Prophet himself did not claim miraculous powers and declared that he was only a mortal and a messenger of God (3:138; 17:95). Thus, most popular native healing in Arab-Muslim societies is regarded by orthodox Islam as a heretic innovation or *bid'a*.

The expansion of Islam also brought about an interchange of practices of religious healing between Muslims, Christians, and Jews, such as visitations to each other's healing shrines, veneration of each other's saints, and the wearing of each other's amulets and talismans. Early in this century, Lane (1954) stated that

> It is a very remarkable trait in the character of the people of Egypt and other countries of the East, that Muslims, Christians, and Jews adopt each other's superstitions, while they abhor the leading doctrines of each other's faiths. In sickness, the Muslim sometimes employs Christian and Jewish priests to pray for him: the Christians and Jews, in the same predicament, often call in the Muslim saints for the like purpose. Many Christians are in the frequent habit of visiting certain Muslim saints here; kissing their hands; begging their prayers, counsels, or prophecies; and giving them money and other presents. (Lane, 1908/1954, p. 241)

Although native healing is not accepted by Arab psychiatrists (El-Islam, 2000) who show little cooperation with native healers (Al-Subaie & Al-Hamad, 2000), it is sought by a large number of clients in Arab-Islamic countries. For example, in Egypt, 60 percent of patients at the University Clinic in Cairo, which serves persons from low socioeconomic backgrounds, had consulted traditional healers before coming to see a psychiatrist (Okasha, 1997). Algerian psychiatrists reported that native healing has been on the increase since independence in 1962 (Bensmail, Merdji, & Touari, 1984). It was suggested that acculturation and social change have made the new generation of educated young people so insecure that they reverted to traditional healing with which they have been familiar since childhood. In Lebanon, Jabir (1996) reported that the dramatic increase in the number of native healers and their clients is associated with trends toward development and modernity, to the extent that, in a survey, it was difficult to find a street in Beirut and its suburbs without a native practitioner! Ninety-five percent of clients of native healers were urban residents. In both Algeria and Lebanon, as well as in other Arab-Muslim countries, more recent increases in Islamic movements are expected to strengthen the belief in possession by the jinn and increase the practice of native healing. In Saudi Arabia, age, sex, social class, and education do not affect the choice between traditional healing and modern psychiatry (Al-Subaie & Al-Hamad, 2000). Saudi Arabia is the only Arab-Islamic country that recognizes two parallel medical systems, native healing and modern medicine (Al-Subaie & Al-Hamad, 2000). In two different outpatient psychiatric clinics, 49 to 53 percent of the patients had seen a native healer during the year before their visit (Al-Subaie, 1994; Hussein, 1991).

Although native healing is popular among the different strata of the Arab-Islamic communities, many magical beliefs and practices reported about these communities should not be generalized to all Arab-Muslim populations, and they should be considered within the context of a certain time and space. In this chapter, we first deal with the pluralistic medical system in the Arab-Islamic communities. Secondly, we describe the jinn (spirits) and sorcery as major perceived etiological factors in mental illness, the treatment of possession by the jinn, including exorcism, and the *Zar* and the *Hadra* carried out by the Zar cult and the Hamadsha brotherhood respectively. Third, the *dhikr*, or remembrance of God, as a method of meditation is also discussed. Fourth, in addition to the treatment of the effects of the evil eye, we shall present two methods of treatment: cautery (*al-kayy*) and visitations to the shrines (*al-ziyara*). Finally, some examples of the application of Islamic principles in psychotherapy are presented.

THE PLURALISTIC NATURE OF THE MEDICAL SYSTEM

In the Arab-Islamic countries, a pluralistic system reflects prophetic medicine developed after the death of the Prophet, Galenic[2] humoral medicine, pre-Islamic magico-religious traditions, and Western medicine. This pluralistic system also has a wide choice of healers. In all Muslim communities, people under distress turn to God to ask for His mercy and help. In almost all Arab-Muslim countries, the shrine of a *welly* (saint) or *sayid* (descendent of a prophet) is visited by patients to obtain *baraka* (blessings) and healing.

Table 19.1 lists native healers available in the Arab-Islamic countries. With the exception of the Zar treatment, which is a pagan African tradition, all other native healing methods are assumed to work through the baraka, "a mysterious wonder-working force" (Westermarck, 1926, p. 35) which is considered as a blessing from God channeled through the healer. The treatment may range from recitation of the Qur'an to carrying protective amulets or talismans, visiting a shrine, joining a cult, finding an exorcist, receiving prescriptions and medication from the *attar* (herbalist), and finally contacting a Western-trained medical practitioner.

Native etiological theories in this system do not differentiate between physical and mental illness. The emphasis tends to be on the social context. If the patient has enemies, he may have been bewitched by them. If the patient has more than one wife, he may have been poisoned by one of them; if he is better off than others in the community, he may have been influenced by the evil eye. All methods of treatment are used by patients and their families until the illness is cured; it is the success of treatment that eventually proves the etiology, as is demonstrated in the following Moroccan case of Fatima reported by Crapanzano (1973):

---

[2]The Galenic physiology of the four humors and the four qualities (blood is moist and hot, black bile is dry and cold, yellow bile is hot and dry, and phlegm is cold and moist) has been reduced to heat and cold in Arab-Islamic countries. An imbalance between hot food, such as aubergine, garlic, honey, and celery, and cold food, such as vinegar, citrus fruit, and turnips may result in different kinds of illnesses. However, both the etiology and treatment of illness are a mixture of Galenic medicine and religio-magical beliefs and practices. In Morocco, for example, the "bride" (*el-aroussa*) is a culture-specific illness that is explained both as cold or spirit illness (Greenwood, 1981). A patient inflicted by the bride first feels pain on one side of the head, face, body, or limb. This pain tends to subside after a few days, but the face or the limb remains paralyzed. The victim may also suddenly become dumb, deaf, or blind, or in some cases the pain may continue as a migraine or rheumatism without paralysis. The etiology and treatment of this illness could be both physical and spiritual. It is believed that the cause of the bride is a cold draft when going outside without sufficient clothing. The treatment involves letting out the cold through multiple cuts, applying heat with brands, and rubbing in garlic, which is considered a very hot substance. The same illness may be caused by a striking spirit and the sherif's baraka compels it to leave, but it may also be driven out through the cuts and its hate of heat and garlic.

TABLE 19.1
Native Healers in Arab-Islamic Societies

Algeria (Al-Issa, 1990)

Marabout literally means attached (to God). A marabout claims to be a descendent of some saintly ancestors and serves as an exorcist and healer. *Maraboutisme* in French refers to activities related to the worship of saints or cult of saints. During the patient's visit to a shrine of a *marabout*, his descendent may carry out a therapeutic session (Hadra) and exorcism.

A *taleb* functions as a religious teacher and a healer. His healing practice is more related to Muslim religion than that of the *marabout*. He recites verses from the Qur'an, gives amulets (*herz*) to carry around, or soaks a paper with religious writings in water for the patient to drink.

Egypt (Gawad, 1995)

A *sahir* or a witch puts a paper in water for a number of days. The patient uses the water for drinking and bathing. A sahir recommends a bird with special characteristics be killed; its blood should cover the head and body of patient.

A *kodia* (Sheika) is a Zar practitioner in Egypt who directs the ceremony, diagnoses the individual *Zar* (spirit) of patients, and finds out its demands.

Gulf and Saudi Arabia (Al-Subaie, 1989; Al-Subaie & Al-Hamad, 2000; El-Islam 1982)

A *mutawa'* reads Qur'anic verses over the patient, does *Maho*, which is writing verses from the Qur'an with saffron on a piece of paper to be soaked in water. The patient drinks the water or uses it to wash certain body parts. The *Mutawa'* tends to deal with behavioral and emotional rather than physical problems.

Iraq (Bazzoui & Al-Issa, 1966)

A *sayed* claims to be a descendant from the Prophet, recites a few verses from the Qur'an, and provides talismans or amulets to be worn by the patient.

Iraq, Lebanon (Bazzoui & Al-Issa, 1966; personal observation)

A *shawaf* (seer) or *kashaf al-fal* (fortune-teller) combines diagnosis and treatment. He or she may throw a pile of stone and inspect the pattern or look at the palm of the hand or the sediment of Turkish coffee poured in a plate to predict fortunes and misfortunes or explain current problems. Gypsies in Iraq combine it with cupping (*hejama*). This practitioner is found in almost all Arab-Islamic countries and serves mainly a diagnostic function.

Morocco (Crapanzano, 1973; Douki, Moussaoui, & Kacha, 1987; Greenwood, 1981)

A *sherif* claims to be a descendant from the Prophet and officiates at the shrine of his ancestral saint. He may be a member of a religious brotherhood and provide healing baraka (blessing) in the form of his saliva or shared food. He uses techniques of branding and bleeding.

A *faqih* is a Qur'anic or *hadith* expert who uses magic to influence spirits, prepares talismans (*hijab*) against misfortune, counteracts the evil eye and sorcery, and exorcises spirits.

A *muqaddam* is the caretaker of a saint's tomb and the leader of a Hamadasha lodge or team.

Palestine, Israel (Al-Krenawi, Graham, & Moaz, 1996; Canaan, 1927)

A *dervish* carries out exorcisms through individual and group therapy during *dhikr* sessions for the Negev Bedouins. He is initiated to provide healing through a dream and manifestations of abnormal behavior.

A *sheik* writes talismans, recites prayers, spits on the patient, and massages the body in order to force the jinn to leave. Found also in Egypt, Iraq, and Lebanon.

Yemen (Alzuhaidi & Ghanem, 1997)

A *walie* (or *welly*) combines religious rituals, hypnosis, suggestion, and native herbal medicine.

All Muslim communities

The *attar* (herbalist) sells traditional Arabic medicine produced locally or imported from India and the Far East. The *attar* may prescribe some of these mixtures of herbs, spices, and other plant products that have pharmacological effects.

An *imam* or *mullah* is a caretaker of a mosque who functions as a leader of group prayers or as a Qur'anic teacher. His treatment is similar to that of the *Mutawa'* (see Saudi Arabia and Gulf). In addition, he may serve as an exorcist in some Arab-Muslim countries.

One of my neighbors, a woman, had told me to go to that Faqih because he is especially good for children. I went to the house of the Faqih with the neighbor who recommended him. I said to him, "My daughter is sick. Can you write an amulet for her?" The Faqih looked at Fatima who was feverish, but he did not examine her. "It's all right. She will not die." Then he wrote a verse from the Koran. He told me to put the verse along with some herbs—rue (*fijil*), harmal (*hormal*), and a type of absinthe (*shiba*)—in a red cloth and hang it from Fatima's neck. He also gave me another verse from the Koran and told me to put it in a bowl with some water, olive oil, and garlic. I was to rub the mixture all over Fatima. All over her except the soles of her feet and the palms of her hands. I was to do this every morning and every night, twice a day, for three days. I was also to give Fatima a little of it to drink with every application. [Did the Faqih ask you anything?] The Faqih said absolutely nothing else. You go to him, really, only to know if the child will live or die. Three days later Fatima was still sick." (Crapanzo, p. 179)

After the Faqih's failure to cure Fatima's illness, the mother-in-law suggested that a mint should be pound into a powder, moistened with water, and put into a rag; then drops of it should be squeezed into the ears, mouth, and nostril of the child. But the mint treatment was not helpful. The mother remembered now that before Fatima was born, a neighbor had told her that she dreamt of her washing a sheepskin rug in the fountain. The hair of the sheepskin had been shaved and the skin was smooth. After the dream, the neighbor told Fatima's mother: "When you have your child, you must take it to Sidi 'Ali [a shrine] to have its head shaved by one of the children of the saint" (Crapanzano, 1973, p. 180). When Fatima was 40 days old, her mother took her to Sidi 'Ali where her head was shaved. She told the guardian of the shrine, "If all goes well with my child, I will return in a week's time with a chicken for you" (Crapanzano, 1973, p.180). Although the child was well, the mother did not go back to fulfill her vow. Now, everybody is telling the mother that "it is because of the chicken that Fatima is sick." After the visit to the saint's shrine, Fatima recovered from her illness.

Although herbal therapy usually starts in the home by an older female family member, the herbalist or attar (see Table 19.1) plays an important role in the diagnosis of illness and the prescription of treatment of minor complaints such as insomnia, headaches, and other physical pains. The attar may work closely with a native healer (e.g., a *Sheik*) and provide him or her with the required remedies. In many Arab-Islamic countries where the dispensing of medications is not regulated, the pharmacist may also provide patients with medication without prescription, saving patients the medical consultation fees.

A large number of patients combine native healing with psychiatric treatment or use the latter as a last resort. Native healers also tend to refer patients to psychiatrists when it is decided that certain causal factors such as the jinn are not involved (Baydoun, 1998; Crapanzano, 1973; Kennedy, 1978). They may integrate psychiatric treatment in their practice and try to provide a rational link with it. For example, a patient may be institutionalized in order to be secluded from the evil eye that caused the illness. On the other hand, when psychiatric treatment is ineffective and patients get worse, native healers believe that such treatment has caused the anger of the jinn.

MAJOR ETIOLOGICAL FACTORS OF MENTAL ILLNESS: THE JINN AND SORCERY

The jinn are supernatural creatures mentioned 22 times in the Qur'an (Yekun, 1994), which often differentiates them from human beings (*ūns*). God created them from smokeless fire, whereas human beings were created from clay. They live in communities, marry, and have children. Some are believers in Islam; others are infidels who are called *Shayateen* (Satans) and whose chief is Iblis. They are invisible even though they may appear in the form of cats, dogs, and other animals (Lane, 1908/1954). They could harm human beings and cause illness, including madness. *Al-junūn*, the word for madness in Arabic, literally means possessed by the jinn. The Prophet was accused by his enemies of being *majnūn* (mad), but God has defended him in the Qur'an: "Your companion is not *majnūn*" (81:22). As disease-spirits, Westermarck (1926) reported that the jinn are also called *riyah*, the plural of *rih*, or wind. This may explain the belief in some Arab countries that the wind, which may stand for a spirit, can be considered as a cause of mental illness (Bazzoui & Al-Issa, 1966).

One type of jinn, particularly popular in Egypt and North Africa, are the *afarit*, which are considered the aristocracy of the jinn because of their remarkable strength. The person becomes manic, strong, and brave when possessed by them (Blackman, 1927; Westermarck, 1926). The *Shaytan* (Satan), on the other hand, influences thinking and behavior and is responsible for distracting, obsessive thoughts or deviant behavior. His influence on sexual behavior is well expressed by the term *ja alayhi al-shaytan* (the Satan came upon him) for wet dreams.

However, the entrance of the jinn into the human body is doubted by some Muslim scholars. They go out in the streets at sunset when Muslims were instructed by the Prophet to keep children at home for protection. Satans are believed to share food with those who do not mention Allah before eating or who eat with their left hands.

It is believed that the jinn live under the earth and haunt springs, wells, and uninhabited areas (Blackman, 1927). They are so much feared by the general population that many precautions are taken to protect against their potential danger. In traditional Moroccan society in the nineteenth century, for example, nobody dared to live in a house alone or go out alone at night. Spirits tend to stay on the thresholds of doors and gates and nobody will then venture to remain at such spots. Sweeping the house at night is not permissible since the jinn might be struck and injured and so induced to revenge themselves. Similarly, cats are avoided as they may be disguised jinn (Klunzinger, 1878). In order to counteract their action, Moroccans burn candles in the dark, sprinkle salt in areas where the jinn gravitate, and utter atropaic phrases when crossing streams or thresholds, or entering caves, cars, and unfamiliar places. Salt is a very popular means of warding off or expelling the jinn (Crapanzano, 1973; Westermarck, 1926). Care should be taken not to injure them, particularly when they take the form of an animal such as a snake, a frog, or a cat.

In Saudi Arabia, jinn are believed to possess people for reasons of love or for reasons of hatred. Male jinn are believed to possess women, whereas female jinn possess men. When possession is for reasons of love, there is usually no harm to the possessed person, although he or she may not particularly enjoy the experience. When possession is for reasons of hatred, the person is usually believed to have harmed the jinni by dropping something or spilling something hot during sunset (Al Subaie & Al-Hamad, 2000).

The strong belief in the jinn in the Egyptian culture is well illustrated by the widely publicized court case in Cairo in 1980 of Abu Kaf as reported by Dols (1992). Abu Kaf was charged for practicing medicine without a license (the accusation was initiated by the Medical Association). Although a medical report stated that the man was suffering from various physical and mental disorders, he was acquitted not on the grounds of insanity but of deficiency of will (*ghayr kamil al-irada*) caused by spirit possession. The court decision was based on the case history of the accused. He was a soldier during the 1967 war and suffered from paralysis. He accepted a proposal from a *jinniya* (female of jinni) who had appeared to him and offered to cure him on the condition that he would obey her. Being cured from his paralysis, he was obliged to carry out her orders of curing the sick. The court recognized his healing abilities, but the doctors sought to overturn the court decision because it would legitimize unprofessional treatment. However, the medical association was unsuccessful in appealing the case.

Crapanzano (1973) observed that the jinn may be involved as etiological factors in the development of illness in two ways. One is called the explicative form of responsibility. The illness is not immediately attributed to the jinn; they only serve the function of stopping speculations about its etiology when it cannot be explained culturally or personally. In this case, the jinn are not involved in the treatment. Crapanzano gives the following discussion with one of his informants as an example of this form of involvement of the jinn:

> In discussing the reasons why a man goes crazy (*hamiq*), one of my informants told me that a man becomes crazy when he has lost all of his money or all of his children in some disaster. I then asked him about a particular man who was considered crazy. This man had neither lost all of his money nor all of his children, nor suffered any similar disastrous experience. "Ah," my informant said, "it is those people there" that chose to make the man crazy. It was written. Similarly, he had no idea of how the *jnun* [jinn] made the man crazy. There was nothing to be done, he said. The Hamadsha, the Gnawa, or even the Koranic teachers who specialize in exorcism could do nothing. True, the man's family could take him to a saint's tomb; there was always the chance that a saint could help him, but this was doubtful. The man was sure to end up in Berechid, the government's mental hospital. (Crapanzo, 1973, p. 151)

The other role of the jinn in illness is referred to as the "participational mode of responsibility" by Crapanzano (1973). In this case also, the illness cannot be explained culturally or personally, but no other explanations are offered at first and the jinn are not used as a last resort to stop speculation about the illness. The jinn not only cause the illness, but they must be appeased to bring about a cure. Unlike the explicative form of responsibility, the jinn are involved in the treatment of the patient. This second "participational mode of responsibility" is used by specific organized cults such as the Hamadsha cult in Morocco or the Zar cult in Egypt, which will be discussed later in this chapter.

Sorcery is mentioned 53 times in the Qur'an, but its practice is forbidden in Islam (Yekun, 1994). Magicians and sorcerers claim that they control the jinn by offerings and actions that violate Muslim law. For example, Westermarck (1926) reported that a Moroccan magician who wanted to summon a jinn did disgusting and forbidden things: He ate his own excrement, drank his urine and made his ablution with it, and prayed with his face not turned toward Mecca. Magicians may also write charms in which the name of the jinn is mentioned in order to harm people such as to cause illness or death, to make people crazy, and to make a husband hate or love his wife. Westermarck (1926) reported many magical methods of using charms to harm people in Morocco. For example, if one wants to have one's enemies quarrel among themselves, a black hen is killed, its head is shaved, and a charm containing the name of a jinn is written on the head of it with its own blood. Then the head is thrown into an enemy's house with the result that the jinn make the occupants quarrel and the house will be empty within three days. A case reported by Blackman (1927) is that of an illustration of madness caused by the use of magic in an Egyptian village in the early twentieth century.

In a small village in upper Egypt there lived a man and his wife, the latter being very good-looking. One day a certain *kadi* [judge] who was visiting the village in question saw her, and, falling in love with her on the spot, desired her as his wife. Knowing that she was already married, his only plan was to get rid of her husband, and so he determined to drive the unfortunate man mad. To accomplish this he induced a magician to write a charm on a piece of paper, which he tied to an inner branch high up on a palm-tree, where it could not easily be seen. The reason for his thus tying the charm to a palm-branch is the idea that, as the branches of the tree are blown this way and that in the wind in apparent confusion, so the brain of the man against whom the spell was concocted would be tortured and confused. Possibly the woman's husband got to know what had been done, but anyhow the poor man lost his reason. He tore off his clothes, tied a rope round his waist, and spoke at times in an unknown tongue. "You must say," so he told the village boys who congregated around him, "*kee ree bra ra kee ree bru.*"

He would also constantly mutter, "Kamaleh [his wife's name] went to the east, Kamaleh went to the east," repeating it over and over again. Finding that he got no better, his wife divorced him, whereupon the *kadi* asked for her in marriage, and was accepted. Meanwhile, the poor husband wandered aimlessly about, saying that he was king of his native village. He collected *bus*—dry *dura* (maize) stalks—each stalk of which he thought was a gun. With these he armed himself and the young lads of the village, and told them that he was their king, and that they must follow him to fight against the other villages. On the day of the weekly market he would repair to the market place, seize large pieces of meat hung up for sale, and eat them raw. He would also pounce upon the fish that the fishermen had caught in the pond adjoining the village. At last the "*omdeh*", or headman, of the village, finding that the poor fellow had become a disturbing element in the place, wrote to headquarters about him, and he was removed to an asylum. Here he died, but up to the last the one sensible word he was constantly uttering was his wife's name. (Blackman, 1927, pp. 191–192)

DEALING WITH POSSESSION BY THE JINN

In dealing with disorders caused by possession by the jinn, the treatment will aim at either exorcising the jinn or establishing symbiotic and working relationships with them (Crapanzano, 1973). Exorcism (*azima*, literally incantation) is usually employed when the attack is by an unnamed jinn, whereas forming a symbiotic relationship is the aim of treatment when one is attacked by a named jinn. Although exorcism is a procedure practiced in almost all Arab-Muslim countries, specific treatments that aim at forming symbiotic relationships with the jinn are popular mainly in Egypt and North Africa and are usually carried out by specific cults (Crapanzano, 1973; Westermarck, 1926). Exorcism also tends to be carried out in one session in contrast to the other treatments, which involve continuous sessions in which the patients become members of a cult and must go through the treatments periodically in order to placate the jinn, become their followers, and remain permanently dependent on them. In the following section, we first deal with exorcism, then with the Hadra, a Hamadsha brotherhood ceremony, and finally with the Zar. The last two illustrate how forming a symbiotic relationship with the jinn is an essential part of the treatment.

Exorcism

Although possession by the jinn is recognized in Islam, exorcism is not mentioned in the Qur'an. However, it seems to have been practiced in many Arab-Muslim communities. The exorcist (the *mu'azzim*) is not a specialist, but could be any of the healers reported in Table 19.1. The methods of exorcism also vary from one healer to another. In Palestine, Canaan (1927) reported that in carrying out exorcism the Sheik massages the body, moving his hands from the upper part of the body downwards so that the devil is to leave the important areas (heart and lungs) and is eventually thrown out of the body through the lower extremities (e.g., toes). The massage turns in most cases into violent beatings. Currently, the Dervish follows similar procedures among the Negev Bedouins of Israel (Al-Krenawi, Graham, & Moaz, 1996). Moreover, the Dervish employs music in exorcism in the belief that the jinn are attracted to it. Drums are used to convince the reluctant jinn to open a dialogue with the healer. The Dervish may also carry out exorcism during a dhikr ceremony, which will be discussed later. The belief in North Africa that the jinn detest salt has resulted in its use to expel them (Westermarck, 1926). However, forcing the possessed patient to drink large amounts of salty water may sometimes result in death.

Al-Subaie and Al-Hamad (2000) described a procedure of exorcism in Saudi Arabia as follows:

> One particularly unethical practice is beating the possessed patient so as to drive the jinni out of the body. When patients scream from pain, the healer believes that it is the voice of the jinni, since patients are believed not to feel physical pain when they are possessed. Some healers may go even further to strangle the patient with their hands until he/she loses consciousness which can be lethal. Under the pressure of beating and strangulation, patients may talk in a different voice indicating a jinni possession. Typically, the jinni is first asked by the healer about the reason and circumstances of possession and then he/she is asked about his/her religion and domicile. The typical answer of the jinni is that he/she is not a Muslim and lives far away. The jinni then says what he/she does to the patient and answers questions asked by the healer. Before the session ends the jinni is asked to convert to Islam (or else he/she will be beaten). This usually ends by acceptance of this proposal, in which case he/she will be educated about Islam and asked not to possess the patient again. If the jinni has any requests (usually things that the patient needs) he/she will make them before he/she agrees to leave. It seems that some patients go through a trance state facilitated by suggestion and perhaps brain hypoxia during strangulation leading to an abreaction. (pp. 212–213)

Many Christian shrines in Palestine and Lebanon were used for exorcism by both Christian and Muslim patients. Disturbed patients were brought to a Greek Orthodox Church of St. George in a village in Palestine. They were chained in front of the church, given a straw mattress, and bread and water with no hygienic provision or protection against the weather. This treatment was based on the belief that the jinn detest emaciated, ill-fed, and dirty persons. Patients were also beaten to drive out the devil (Canaan, 1927). Waldmeier (1897), as cited by Katchadourian (1980), described a cave dedicated to Saint Anthony of Padua in the Monastery of Kuzheya in Lebanon. The saint lived in the cave as a hermit and had bestowed special healing powers on the monastery monks. The person to be exorcised was led into the cave where water drippings formed stalactites, which were broken up and sold as amulets by the monks. The person sat on stone blocks and his neck was secured to the wall by a heavy collar and chain. The exorcism proceeded as follows:

> The initial treatment consisted of merely letting the afflicted person remain in the cave for three days. On the third night, the patron saint was expected to appear, cast out the demon, and restore him to reason. If the subject survived the wait but didn't recover, the monks then resorted to more forceful methods. He was made to face the priest who beat him on the head with a heavy boot while he read the text of exorcism: "Get thee away

from this person, accursed devil, and enter into the Red Sea and leave the temple of God. I force thee in the name of the Father, the Son, and the Holy Ghost to go to the everlasting fire . . . " In cases where the patient died while in the cave, the monks told his family that Saint Anthony had loosened his chains and had taken him straight to heaven which entitled the monastery to a donation. (Katchadourian, 1980, pp. 547–548)

The Hadra: A Ceremony of the Hamadsha Brotherhood in Morocco

The Hamadsha is a religious brotherhood in Morocco whose practices involve head shaving and various practices of self-mutilation. Their beliefs and practices reflect ancient Mediterranean religions and pagan influences from sub-Saharan Africa, even though they claim that their saints derive their baraka (blessing) from the Prophet and God. Crapanzano (1973) reported that the Hamadsha cult tends to deal with psychological disorders such as hysteria, depression, and schizophrenia rather than organic illnesses such as epilepsy. Their treatment results in dramatic cures for paralysis, muteness, sudden blindness, severe depression, palpitations, parasthesias, and possession. It is typically carried out during a ceremony called Hadra.

Before the start of the Hadra, an animal is sacrificed and the meat is used to make the *couscous* and the *tajin* (stew) that are usually served at the end of the ceremony. Then, the *sharif* or *muqaddam* (the caretaker of the saint's tomb) recites a *Fatha*, a term that usually refers to the opening *sura* of the Qur'an, but is used here for an invocation that may not contain Qur'anic verses. The muqaddam may massage or spit on the ailing part of the patient's body. A special prayer is usually said for the patient. The group then starts the praise of Allah (God) followed by a short break before the recitation of the dhikr begins: short phrases repeating the name of God, which are said more and more rapidly accompanied by hand-clapping and a gentle tapping of drums. The seated followers may start swaying back and forth more rapidly as they recite short dhikr phrases and also start to hyperventilate. Dancing and repeating the name of God will continue, which will induce in the performers and the patient altered states of consciousness or a trance. The ceremony culminates in two states called *hal* and *jidba*. The hal is an entranced state that the Sufis call *wajd* or ecstasy. It is a nonviolent trance similar to a somnambulistic state and is attributed to 'Aisha Qandisha[3] or another jinn rather than to a saint.

Just before the transition from the hal to jidba, a male participant described his state:

> My body tightens. It becomes more and more tight. Then I throw myself to the ground. I feel hot. I see only Aisha during the *Hadra*. She is in front of me. My head itches. My eyeballs do not move. I am not conscious of my body. I sweat a lot. I do not know where I am or what time it is. I remain this way for two minutes and then I begin *jidba*. (Crapanzano, 1973, pp. 199-200)

---

[3] 'Aisha Qandisha is a *jinniya* who is feared all over Morocco. She is especially named as causing harm and illness to those who seek help from the Hamadsha brotherhood. One popular story about Aisha is that she appears as a beautiful girl who seduces men when they are working alone in the fields. The men make love to her and may even marry her, but then she changes into an old ugly woman with long hair, a monkey's body, and the feet of a goat or a camel. "She becomes violent and demanding, and her victim may be struck with paralysis or deteriorate into a shambling, ragged, crazy outcast, wandering and helpless, the typical image of madness" (Greenwood, 1981, p. 230).

During the jidba, he may start dancing in a more frenetic fashion or fall to the ground in a cataleptic state, followed occasionally by convulsive movements and violent tremors of the limbs. In response to a particular tune, he will stand and charge wildly in the dance area screaming and frightening women and children in the audience. He may scratch his head and occasionally ask for a knife to slash his head until his face and shoulder are drenched in blood. This state during the jidba is an exaggeration of the hal condition. The participant hears nothing except the sound of the music and the blood throbbing in his head, which feels like exploding, and he is itching intensely "like a wasp under the skin." When his head itches, the dancer may "see" 'Aisha Qandisha before him, slashing at her head with a piece of iron and forcing the dancer to do the same. One dancer described his state as follows:

> I am hot and breathe heavily. I feel myself throbbing. There is much itching. I am not conscious of my body. I do not know what time it is; my body feels like boiling water. It is frightening. I see only 'Aisha. [How do you feel during the head hitting?] It is 'Aisha who makes me hit my head. I begin to hit my head also. I am not aware of the fact that I am hitting my head. There is itching and sweating, and my whole body is hot. When 'Aisha stops hitting her head, so do I. Then I continue to dance. My body and head continue to throb. I am not aware of my wounds. I am still hot. I am sweating a lot, and my breath is very fast. (Crapanzano, 1973, p. 201)

During the jidba, women also run around screaming and act as though they are seeing visions. They may fall to the ground in a convulsive state or suffer temporary paralysis of a limb or a contraction of the face. They may also scratch at their head or ask for a knife and slash at it. Their eyes will appear transfixed, their breath very rapid and rasping, their face flushed, and their movements are sudden and disorganized.

The flow of blood of participants seems to calm 'Aisha. If she is not "seen" by the dancer, it is believed that she has actually entered the body of the head slasher causing the itching. The dancers do not feel of the pain of their wounds during the jidba or after the dance; they only become aware of their wounds when they discover the blood stains on their cloths. The wounds tend to heal without treatment.

The patients who take part in the Hadra are encouraged to fall into jidba and show its "symptoms," except that they are not required to slash their head in order to be cured. Sometimes, the muqaddam or sharif walks on the patients' backs or just spits at them. This part of the Hadra ends suddenly and the muqaddam starts to recite a Fatha or invocation for anybody who wishes to obtain a blessing (baraka), including the patient. When the recitation is over, the second part of the Hadra begins. This part is designed for those who did not dance during the first part or those whose jinn have not been satisfied. It is quieter and patients dance until their jinn are placated when the appropriate tune is played. The ceremony usually ends with a meal.

The Zar

The Zar cult has been described in Egypt (Blackman, 1927; Fakhouri, 1968; Kennedy, 1978; Okasha, 1966), Iraq (Bazzoui & Al-Issa, 1966), Kuwait (Kline, 1963), Saudi Arabia (Prince, 1980), and Sudan (Baasher, 1967). The cult is well developed in Ethiopia but became popular in the Arab countries through the influence of African slaves in the nineteenth century. Although it has been suggested that the word Zar is derived from the word ziyara (a visit to a shrine) or from the town Zara in northern Iran, its origins are more likely to be in Ethiopia from where it was introduced to Arab countries through African slaves (Fakhouri, 1968). The Zar is not a culture-specific syndrome as described in the DSM IV (APA, 1994), but rather refers to a ceremony or to a class of possessing spirits. Patients who attend the Zar in Egypt tend to have a variety of disorders or social problems, such as hysteria, anxiety, depression, psychoses (including hallucinations), sterility, chronic headache, extreme apathy, convulsive seizures, and the inability to find a spouse (Fakhouri, 1968; Kennedy, 1978). Egyptian religious authorities and professionals have opposed the Zar because of its pagan origins and the animosity of Egyptian psychiatry toward native healing methods (El-Eleymi, 1993; Okasha, 1966). It was actually forbidden by the Egyptian government in the nineteenth century (Klunzinger, 1878).

The Zar practitioners, who are called *Kodiyas* or *Sheikas* (*Sheik* for the male), do not use sainthood as the basis of their practice, as in the case of the Hamadasha brotherhood, but instead claim professional competence through the transfer of power and knowledge from their relatives through the call of a spirit in a dream (Fakhouri, 1968). They are described as "masters of drama who understand how to surprise and thrill their audiences—how to entertain, as well as how to satisfy desires for security and self-expression. They must not only be good musicians, but must also have self-confidence and inspire expectations of hope in others" (Kennedy, 1978, p. 213).

The clients are mostly women from the lower classes. Similar to membership of the Hamadsha cult in Morocco, the Zar cult raises the status of its members and gives them the opportunity to express themselves through the spirit without responsibility for their behavior (Kennedy, 1978; Messing, 1959). When a Zar is requested, the Sheika first asks questions about the patients such as their appetite and sleep, whether or not the eating and sleeping of patients are disturbed, and she may in some cases decide that the Zar is not needed. In order to establish the diagnosis, the Sheika asks for the *athar* (belongings) of her patients, such as a piece of their clothing, which is brought wrapped around money—the diagnosis fee. The article is placed under the Sheika's pillow and if, during the night, she is disturbed by discomfort, she will know that the client is possessed by a spirit that responds to the Zar. A Sheika may throw seven dates into a plate of sugar and their pattern will determine whether the Zar or other treatments are recommended.

The ceremony room is filled with the fragrance of incense and perfume. The patient usually wears a white gown, a white veil, and jewelry. Her hands and body are dyed with henna and her eyelids are blackened with *kohl*, and heavily perfumed. Music and dancing are part of the Zar. The Sheika begins the ceremony with songs and drumming. When a spirit associated with some person in the audience is called, that person begins to shake in her seat, and then makes her way to the central dancing area, sometimes dancing and trembling until she falls exhausted on the floor. Before the spirit consents to leave, it usually demands special favors such as jewelry, new clothing, and expensive food. Relatives and friends gather around the woman to pacify the spirit. The patient may lie for some minutes on the floor motionless with her hand twitching, before a special song by the Sheika brings her back to consciousness (Kennedy, 1978).

The Zar also involves animal sacrifices. If the sponsoring family is poor, the sacrifice is a single cock or two pigeons. The Sheika determines at the initial diagnosis the color of the sacrificial animal. Typically, a white or black cock (according to the type of illness) is killed over the patient's head and the blood is smeared over her face, hands, and legs. In the evening or following day, it is cooked and shared by the Sheika and the patient. A lamb is also slaughtered and its hot blood is rubbed all over the body and face of the patient, and some of it is mixed in potion with cloves, henna, and water. After drinking the potion, the sick person ritually steps across the dead animal's body seven times. At this stage, the Zar is pacified, but the music and dancing continue while the lamb is cooking for the final feast (Kennedy, 1978).

The healer herself is possessed by a Zar, but it is already pacified. She first calls upon her own Zar to possess her and then tries to discover the identity of the unknown Zar of the patient. When the Zar is satisfied by meeting its demands, the patient will be a member of the Zar cult for the rest of her life. Regular donations and participation in the ceremonies will prevent the return of the illness. Rather than expelling the spirit and finding a complete cure during the Zar, the spirit has become friendly and protective of the patient (Fakhouri, 1968).

Many sociocultural factors may be involved in the therapeutic effects of the Zar and the Hadra[4] in Egypt and Morocco respectively (Crapanzano, 1973). The patients are given the social support of the whole group, including the family, friends, and neighbors, as well as members of the cult. The group offers sympathy, encouragement, and hope for a cure. The time and money involved in the ceremony are a demonstration of the group's care and concern, which put patients under pressure not to let the group down. Indeed, it was observed by Boddy (1989) that female patients improve immediately when the group recognizes the illness and starts preparing for the Zar. The group also provides an interpretation of the illness that reduces the anxiety of the patients. Supernatural explanations absolve the patients from responsibility and the feelings of guilt and shame; they are not punished for unacceptable behavior before or during the ceremony. These therapies activate the patients and make them feel that they participate in their own cure. After recovery, cult membership requires patients to perform in the Zar or Hadra in order to please their jinn and remain healthy. Cult membership provides a new social status and expands the patients' social network. They are now more respected by their community as they are in contact with the jinn.

THE DHIKR: A SUFIST MEDITATION

Sufism is a Muslim cult of mystics who follow the path (*tariqa*) of a spiritual leader or a *Sheik*. The dhikr, a meditative practice of the Sufis, literally means remembrance or recollection. The repetition of the name of God by the Sufis is used as part of meditation to reach a spiritual ecstasy (wajd), which is a state that enables the individual to abandon the self so that the soul can communicate directly with God and become united with Him (Nicholson, 1969). The concept of dhikr is originally based on the Muslim religion. The recollection of God and his unity (*la illaha illa allah*) is an important part of Muslim prayers and confession and based on Qur'anic suras such as "and recollect God often" (33:4) or "the recollection of God makes the heart calm" (13:28).

Although the dhikr ceremony has many variations, it usually starts with recitation of the Qur'an and the Fatha, the opening sura of the Qur'an, followed by the invocation of God. Then, the leader and the group start repeating "la illaha illa allah" (there is no God but God), swaying rhythmically from side to side. This is associated with the beating of drums and dancing by some participants. Beyond this basic meditative

---

[4]Similar to the Hamadsha clients referred to earlier (see Footnote 3), the Zar patients are also possessed by named *jinn* such as Muhammad Al-Makawi, Sheik Al-Araabi, Al-Sayida Zeinab, and Abdul-Salam Al-Asmar (Nemr, 1996).

procedure, some of these ceremonies may include extraordinary feats such as eating fire, glass, and serpents (Klunzinger, 1878; Lane, 1908/1954).

Apart from the evidence reported in the West that those who report mystical experience also tend to have better mental health (Prince, 1980), there is no research on the individual benefits of joining the Sufi cult. Sufi hagiographic works report various miracles of Sufi leaders, such as the ability to read the minds of disciples (tell their secrets and moods) or to become invisible and to "appear in spiritualized form, at a sick person's bed in order to cure him or at least relieve him temporarily from his pain" (Schimmel, 1975, p. 205). However, the Sufi ceremony was originally designed for meditation; it is only rarely used for treatment or exorcism as reported among the Negev Bedouin in Israel by Al-Krenawi and Graham (1996) and by Al-Krenawi, Graham, and Maoz (1996). Al-Krenawi et al. (1996) pointed out that the purpose of the dhikr is "to cure mental illness by making contact with the spirits which overwhelm the person and which cause the illness" (Al-Krenawi & Graham Maoz, 1996, p. 19). When the dhikr ceremony is carried out for exorcism, it is unlikely that it is part of a Sufi mystic cult. Traditionally, the ceremony is a meditative religious exercise with mystical purposes involving an altered state of consciousness or a trance rather than possession by the spirit as in the Zar in Egypt or the Hadra in North Africa. However, the dhikr or remembrance of God, when used in meditation, could result in relaxation and the relief of distress (Naranjo & Ornstein, 1971).

THE EFFECTS OF THE EVIL EYE AND THEIR TREATMENT

The belief in the evil eye as an explanation of illness and other misfortunes is widespread in the Arab-Islamic culture. As a causal factor, it is said to lead to serious personal problems involving health, family life, and social functioning. It may also influence other daily matters, for example, if an object that has not been put in a secure position falls down, the accident is caused by the eye of some person who covets it; or it can cause the dates to fall down from trees and animals to die.

Both physical and mental symptoms are attributed to the evil eye. In a study by Alsughayier (1996) in Saudi Arabia, interviewees reported that multiple aches, dermatological and menstrual disturbances, and symptoms of anxiety and depression were caused by the evil eye. Academic or career failure and marital discords were also cited by the respondents. The study shows that Western education (only 7.2 percent of his interviewees were illiterate) has not eliminated the belief in the evil eye.

In his classic book titled *At tib al-nabawi* [Prophetic Medicine], Ibn Qayyin al-Jawzia (1957) discussed many beliefs related to the origins of the evil eye. The person possessing the evil eye may emit poisonous power and injure the victims or transmit ethereal, dangerous substances into their bodies. The effects of the evil eye may also occur through the spirit of the envier. Thus, the transfer of the evil is not necessarily by contact and not even by sight, for the possessors of the evil eye may be blind yet still be able to emit their spirit. It may be noted that the evil eye is referred to in Arabic as *nafas* (breath), which indicates the association between air /wind and the spirits referred to earlier.

It is believed that the power of throwing an evil glance upon anything is by no means always voluntary, for even a father may cause the death of his own child by looking at her or him with admiration (Klunzinger, 1878). The look of a person is more dangerous if it is accompanied by words of praise. There may even be danger in being praised without being looked at as when somebody speaks of another person's children in their absence (Westermarck, 1926).

Envy is the major emotion involved in the evil eye, which in Arabic is called *Ayn al-hassud* (the eye of the envier). However, Westermarck (1926) pointed out that in addition to envy, the danger of the evil eye is comparable to the magical law of association by contrast, in that the praise or admiration of something good may readily recall its opposite. The phenomenon reflects the uncertainty of the future in these cultures, and that one's present fortunes cannot and should not be relied on (Westermarck, 1926).

The fear of the evil eye may serve as a social control mechanism and as a means of sanction against anybody who exceeds the limits established by the community. In a collectivist society where cohesiveness is emphasized in contrast to discord or conflict, the evil eye discourages greed, ostentation, pride, and other manifestations of inequality (extreme wealth, beauty, large number of children, and so on). Instead, it encourages modesty, humility, and equality among members of the group (Al-Issa, 1990).

Many methods are resorted to in order to escape or counteract the harmful influence of the evil eye. The best protection for Muslims is to turn to God: "Say I take refuge with the Lord of the Daybreak, from the evil of what He has created, from the evil of darkness when it gathers, from the evil of women who blow on knots, from the evil of the envier when he envies" (113:I-5). The recitation of Qur'anic verses such as the throne verses or the Fatha are also recommended. Amulets[5] as preventive and curative measures may be used both before and after the destructive influence of the eye (Klunzinger, 1878). Blue beads and necklaces are worn by children and women as protective charms against it (Blackman, 1927).

A popular method used by native healers in Lebanon and Syria to counteract the influence of the evil eye and to detect its perpetrator is lead pouring or *sab al rasas*.[6] The basic procedure consists of melting a small piece of lead, which is poured in a bowl of water held over the head of the sufferer. When the lead touches the surface of the water, it makes a cracking sound, solidifies, and becomes molded into the shape of the person who caused the illness (e.g., male or female, young or old). In Egypt, lead pouring is used to counteract the effects of sorcery by frightening the victim with the sudden cracking noise of the lead (Nemr, 1996). This method is also used in Turkey (Tuncer, 1995) and perhaps also in Spain because the procedure is demonstrated in the opera, *Carmen*.

When admiring a child or a neighbor's possessions, it is important to say *masha' Allah* (what God will) for protection against the evil eye so that there be no suspicions that you are casting the evil eye and causing injury (Blackman, 1927; Klunzinger,

---

[5]The composition of amulets is based on magic. They consist of "certain passages of the Qur'an, and names of God [the ninety-nine *asma'llah al-hosna* or excellent names of God], together with those of angels, genii, prophets, or eminent saints, intermixed with combinations of numerals, and with diagrams, all of which are supposed to have great secret virtues" (Lane, 1908/1954, p. 253). They protect against disease, enchantment, the evil eye, and other evils.

[6]The following is the only case we are familiar with in which a native healer was involved in the treatment of animals: Our informer reported that in Mount Lebanon Nasr has treated a wide variety of cases affected by the evil eye, representing both human and animal victims. Nasr was called to treat a village bull that was suffering from extreme fatigue and was no longer able to plough the farm. This was the only bull in the village and many people envied its owner. Therefore, the common belief was that the symptoms that the bull exhibited were the result of various "evil eyes." The owner thus sought assistance of Nasr who immediately realized the cause of the bull's symptoms and used *sab-al-rasas* as a method of treatment. Much to the surprise of everyone, the bull soon regained its strength and returned to plowing the farm.

1878). If a person, for example, exclaims "how pretty" or uses similar words, it is often desired to say, "*masha' Allah*" (Lane, 1908/1954). Other habits related to protection against the evil eye include throwing dust after the person who is suspected of having cast the evil eye as he or she goes by in the street or on the road, and throwing salt in the fire after the departure of a suspected visitor (Blackman, 1927).

The safest precaution against the evil eye is to avoid exposure to it altogether. Infants, especially boys and twins, are not allowed to be seen by persons whose glance may be dangerous to them. A person who is reported to have an evil eye is shunned and is not allowed to take part in special gatherings (Westermarck, 1926). Many customs were developed to avoid the danger of the evil eye: the dirty state in which children are kept to conceal their beauty, the practice of carefully concealing provisions as they are being carried home, and the readiness with which an object is handed to the person that admires it in order to avoid disastrous consequences (Blackman, 1927; Klunzinger, 1878).

OTHER METHODS OF TREATMENT

Al-ziyara

Al-ziyara is a visit to a saint's shrine and should not be confused with the *haj*, the pilgrimage to Mecca that is required of all Muslims and forms one of the pillars of Islam. With the exception of the holy mosques of Mecca, Medina (the city of the Prophet), and in Palestine all visits to shrines are forbidden in Islam. However it has been reported that in Egypt, Algeria, and Palestine there is hardly a village that does not have at least one saint or a tomb for a favorite patron saint (Al-Issa, 1990; Canaan, 1927; Lane, 1908/1954). Kennedy (1978) observed that in the district of Kennz in Egypt there were 150 shrines within a few miles. Saints may have many sanctuaries to commemorate the place of their birth, their tomb or the place where they have appeared after death. Therefore, a shrine for the same saint may be seen in more than one country. El-Dasuqi's tomb, for example, lies in Egypt, but he has a shrine in Palestine (Canaan, 1927). Table 19.2 presents some of the well-known shrines in Arab countries. The table shows that Imam Husayn is believed to be buried in Cairo by Egyptians and in Karbella in Iraq by Iraqis. Similarly, Egyptians believe that Siti Zeneb is buried in Cairo, whereas the Syrians believe that she is buried in Damascus. In general, after the burial of the saints, they appear in a dream to some wealthy persons and command them to build a tomb, usually with a dome. Some of the shrines are shared by Christians and Muslims such as Al-Khader (St. George) and Al-Izer (from Ezra or Lazarus) found in Palestine (Canaan, 1927) and Iraq. Blackman (1927) pointed out that when a saint is claimed by both Copts and Muslims in Egypt, their candles may be seen burning side by side.

The rituals carried out by the visitors may vary from one shrine to another. The visit to the shrine of Sidi Ahmed in Morocco is described by Crapanzano (1973) as follows:

> The pilgrim removes his shoes before entering the mausoleum. He kisses the doorjambs, first the right and then the left one, and he may drop a few coins into the alms box standing just inside the tomb room. Sometimes he waits to give alms until he is about to leave. Women turn to the left and walk clockwise around the tomb; men turn to the right and make a counterclockwise circumambulation. Both men and women kiss the four sides of the catafalque. Once the single circumambulation is completed, the pilgrim sits down—women to the left of the entrance, men to the right—and mumbles a *Fatha* or a few verses

TABLE 19.2
Some of the Well-known Shrines in the Arab Countries

Country	Shrine
Egypt (Lane, 1908/1954; Frishkoff, 2001)	Imam Husayn
	Ash-shafi'i
	Siti Zenab
	Sidi Ibrahim Al-Dasuqi
	Shaykh Mohammad Uthman Al-Burhani
Iraq (Al-Issa, unpublished data)	Abdul-Kadir Al-Gaylani
	Al-Khadim
	Imam Husayn
Lebanon (Al-Issa, unpublished data)	Abd al-Rahman al Oza'i
Morocco (Crapanzano, 1973)	Sidi Ali Ben Hamada
	Sidi Ahmed Dghughi
Syria (Al-Issa, unpublished data)	Siti Zenab
	Ruquayya

from the Koran that he happens to know. At this time the pilgrim is said to experience the fear of God (*Khūshū*). Occasionally he will experience a trance-like state which he calls the *hal*, a term which is also employed for one level of trance in the *Hadra*. (p. 174)

Patients' visits may involve temple sleep in which the patients may receive instructions about their illness in a dream. The visitors might offer a sacrifice (a chicken) or take part in an ecstatic dance (Hadra) or receive a blessing from the caretaker. Canaan (1927) reported that in Palestine rags are taken from the shrine by the sick because they possess baraka. Other objects such as water, oil, or stones are taken to be used as prophylaxis or cures. A talisman (*hijab*) is often made in these holy places. Another practice associated with shrines is the *nidhr* (vow), which is a conditional request to the saints, asking for a favor with the promise that if it is given, the Sheik or the saint will be rewarded (Canaan, 1927; Kennedy, 1978). The reward itself is also called nidhr. The saints are regarded as intercessors with God, and visitors make routine offerings to them. Patients make a nidhr (vow) that if they recover from a sickness, or obtain a son, or any other specific object or desire, then they will give to their saint a goat, a lamb, or a sheep. If they attain their objective, they sacrifice the animal that they have vowed at the tomb of the saint and may make a feast with the meat for any person who may choose to attend (Lane, 1908/1954). If the petitioner does not keep his promise, he will suffer some misfortune. If he asks for the birth of a son, the child will become ill or mad or die if the nidhr is not fulfilled after the birth of the child (Westermarck, 1926). In Morocco, according to Westermarck (1926), if a sick person promises to give to a saint some money in case he gets well, he puts it beneath his pillow until he recovers, but, if he dies, it is also given to the saints. Not keeping a vow to a saint may sometimes be used as a last resort to explain illness (as described elsewhere in this chapter). These practices are clearly against the Tawheed principle since they indicate how much people believe in the healing powers of others, although in reality Allah is the only one who can heal ailments.

Al-kayy [Cautery]

The use of heat in treatment by burning parts of the body, particularly the head, is a popular native treatment in traditional Arab-Islamic countries (Al-Subaie & Al

Hamad, 2000; Bazzoui & Al-Issa, 1966). In Saudi Arabia, for example, "a glowing red heated iron rod is applied to different parts of the head depending on diagnosis and inclinations of the healer. The size of the area treated may range from 4 to 20 cm" (Al-Subaie & Al-Hamad, 2000). Al-Subaie and Al-Hamad pointed out that cautery is the treatment of choice for *Wishrah*, a culture-specific syndrome with psychotic symptoms such as incoherence and irrelevant speech. The generally accepted etiology of Wishrah includes a mixture of phrenology, Galenic medicine, and the use of modern technology. Al-Subaie and Al-Hamad (2000) explained that "Wishrah means a malformation or an improper healing of the skull bones leaving an opening that is discovered by sliding hands slowly over the patient's shaved scalp. Healers look for elevations or depressions of the skull bones. Some call the elevations "male Wishrah" and the depressions "female Wishrah." Others describe old Wishrah as being cold compared to the rest of the head temperature, whereas the more recent Wishrah is believed to be hot. Patients are encouraged to touch the Wishrah in order to prove its diagnostic validity. Patients may also be sent to a hospital to obtain a skull X-ray to help locate the believed abnormality (Al-Subaie & Al-Hamad, p. 210). It remains, however, unclear whether cautery is used for both the cold and hot Wishrah, or only for the cold one.

Swagman (1989) reported the use of cautery in Yemen for a variety of disturbances such as feelings of general weakness, shortness of breath, dizziness, chest pain, backache, sexual dysfunction, painful intercourse, and intestinal parasites. All these disorders are subsumed under the label *fija'*, which in Arabic means a sudden catastrophe. Cautery is used in the belief that a sudden fright causes a general imbalance within the body and could be corrected by a counter shock to prevent an illness. Another belief is that fright causes the displacement of the soul (*nafs*), which should be shocked back into position so that illness is avoided. The following case shows how a fija' developed after a fright experience and how it was treated at home by cautery:

> In the southern highlands a 30-year-old woman witnessed her husband's Toyota Landcruiser begin to roll towards a steep drop with her son in the back seat. The vehicle stopped just before reaching the edge, but the woman was so frightened that she became weak and dizzy. She rested for a while and seemed to recover from the shock but later that evening she had very disturbed sleep. The next day she began to complain of dizziness and dropped plates and bowls while preparing the noon day meal. She began to complain that she was suffering from fija' and after some discussion among her family, it was decided that her fright had brought on her illness. Later that evening she was suddenly grabbed from behind by her husband, and while she was held down, her brother applied a glowing hot iron to the back of her neck. After she stopped sobbing and wailing and began to recover from the second, counter-balancing shock, she went to bed and rested. The next day she had to contend with a severe burn, but was no longer suffering from the symptoms of fija'. (Swagman, 1989, p. 384)

APPLICATIONS OF SOME ISLAMIC PRINCIPLES IN PSYCHOTHERAPY

Some Muslim psychologists and psychiatrists reject psychoanalysis not only because of its unscientific stance, but also because of its negative view of human nature, which is against Islam (Al-Abdul-Jabbar & Al-Issa, 2000; Azhar & Varma, 2000). Instead, they have attempted to develop a psychotherapy based on Islamic principles and practices. Azhar and Varma (2000), for example, used religious therapy based on a combination of prayer and change in the patients' values in accordance with Islamic moral principles. In treating anxiety they found that patients tended to be more relaxed at the end of the prayer (as rated by the patients themselves); the more they concentrated during the prayer, the more they became relaxed. The values of the patients were examined and modified by using the Qur'an and the Hadith (the prophet's tradition) as guidance.

Al-Abdul-Jabbar and Al-Issa (2000) suggested the application of strictly Islamic principles and practices in the treatment of psychological disorders. For instance, one syndrome of compulsive washing and cleanliness associated with ablution before prayer is called *waswās* in which some individuals repeat the ritual washing over and over again. Islam allows the replacement of this ritual by *tayamūm*, in which the person taps his or her hand on clean sand as an act of spiritual cleanliness and then touches different parts of the body with the same hand as if using water. Individuals suffering from waswās, are advised to replace the ordinary ritual of ablution with tayamūm. This will prevent the carrying out of the compulsion of washing without breaking Islamic rules. Another aspect of waswās is the repetition of individual prayer or parts of it over and over again. Consistent with the collectivistic point of view of Islam, it is always preferable to do one's prayer as part of a group. Individuals who compulsively repeat prayers were advised to confine their prayer to the mosque in a group led by an Imam, the Muslim "priest." Since the compulsive behavior involves doubts relating to errors of omission, such as the introductory invocation and raising one's arms, group prayer releases the worshiper from this responsibility. Group prayer is also suggested to patients with social phobias as a method of desensitization. Going to the mosque to attend group prayer is integrated with behavior therapy procedures as part of exposing the patient to social situations.

In carrying out group therapy with a variety of patients, admitted to Shahar Hospital in Saudi Arabia including drug addicts, Al-Radi and Al-Mahdy (1989) used psychotherapy based on Islamic principles. They held their group sessions in the local mosque after prayers. The treatment was based on some aspects of Islamic worship as well as on some principles of Western schools of group therapy, such as Frankl's (1986) idea of "the will to meaning" as a basic human characteristic. For example, in one group in which 47 percent of the patients were diagnosed with social phobia, the sessions started with washing one's face, head, and extremities (the Muslim ablution), which was followed by a prayer: "My God, I beg you for a peaceful mind, I believe in your presence, I am contented with my fate and satisfied by your giving" (Al-Radi & Al-Mahdy, 1989, p. 274). The solidarity and cohesion of the Muslim community were emphasized by reciting religious phrases such as "Hold fast together by the rope of Allah (God) and be not divisible among yourself," or "Believers are like a building, strengthening and supporting each other." It was reported that 30 percent of the clients experienced symptom remission and another 17.6 percent showed improvement. No controls were used by the therapists, nor was the diagnosis established for the patients who benefited from treatment. However, this study, as well as others, demonstrates that Islamic religious beliefs and practices may be fruitfully used for the development of psychotherapeutic techniques in psychiatry and clinical psychology in Arab-Islamic communities.

SUMMARY AND CONCLUSION

The invocation of God and the recitation of the Qur'an are available to all Muslims as the first resort in cases of illness and other misfortunes. This is perhaps the most frequently used method of healing because it provides direct contact between the faithful and God without any need for the mediation of a healer. Certain verses of the Qur'an such as the Fatha (the opening sura of the Qur'an) and the crown verses are frequently used. Writing out verses from the Qur'an, soaking them in water, and giving the water to the sick to drink or wash with is also practiced by healers in almost all Muslim countries. The Mosque is an integral part of the life of Muslim communities and its caretaker (the Imam or Mullah who teaches the Qur'an) is always available at moments of distress. Carrying amulets and talismans for protection and treatment is widely practiced in all Arab-Muslim countries, even though this practice is not acceptable according to orthodox Islamic doctrine. With the expansion of the Arab-Islamic culture to Egypt and North Africa, many practices were introduced that reflected the influences of pagan African and pre-Islamic beliefs. The Zar ceremonies and the Hadra are good examples of such non-Islamic influences. The dhikr, a meditative technique used by the Sufi cult has a therapeutic potential, but it has only rarely been used with patients.

A belief in the jinn (spirits) and magic is widespread in Arab-Islamic communities because their existence is acknowledged in the Qur'an. Recitation of the Qur'an and amulets or talismans are used for counteracting and protecting oneself and others against the jinn's harmful effects. Although some native healers specialize only in exorcism (such as a Sheik in Beirut witnessed by one of the authors), it may nevertheless be practiced by any healer. An interesting practice during the Zar ceremonies in Egypt or the Hadra in Morocco is not to exorcise the jinn, but to placate them so that patients can form a symbiotic relationship with them for the rest of their life. Another popular healing practice in Arab-Islamic societies is Al-ziyara, a visit to the shrines of saints for purposes of healing. It is customary in these shrines to make a vow (nidhr), a petition addressed to the saint in which a request (i.e., cure of one's illness) is coupled with a promise (sacrifice of a chicken) conditional on the fulfillment of such a request. Medieval Islamic medicine emphasizing the two qualities of heat and cold still dominates the belief systems of many Arab-Islamic communities. Imbalance between cold and hot food is believed to cause illness. In almost all Arab-Islamic countries a herbalist (attar) also prescribes and sells medications produced locally or imported from India and other Asian countries.

For traditional Arab-Muslim populations, native healing enjoys many advantages over Western psychiatric services. The native healer shares the worldview of the patient, provides explanations related to popular folklore prevalent in the culture, and uses family and community resources (Al-Subaie & Al-Hamad, 2000; Al-Krenawi & Graham, 1996). The cultural gap between psychiatrists and patients is especially wide in those Arab countries where the majority of psychiatrists are foreigners, as is the case in Algeria, Saudi Arabia, and the other gulf countries (Al-Issa, 1990; Al-Subaie & Al-Hamad, 2000). Furthermore, psychiatric service tends to be more expensive and less available for the majority of the population than native healing. Indeed, many native healers ask for no fees or ask for donations rather than fixed fees. Even sacrifices demanded by the jinn or the healer are tailored to the income of the client (e.g., a chicken versus a sheep). In general, native healing is more available for the general population. For example, statistics reported in the Egyptian National Program for Mental Health indicate that while there is one physician for each 40,000 citizens, the equivalent ratio for native healers is 1:500 (Nemr, 1996).

There is little research evaluating the effects of native healing relative to psychiatric treatment in Arab-Islamic communities. Kennedy (1978) reported the remission of a case of a single woman with "apparent schizophrenia." Initially her speech was meaningless and jumbled, and she ran around frantically. After a seven-day Zar ritual, she recovered from her illness, got married, and had two children. It's difficult to know whether this was a true case of schizophrenia or an acute psychosis from which the patient had recovered "spontaneously." The case of a 15-year-old Algerian girl named Zahra living in Belgium, as reported by Pierre (1993) and summarized by Al-Issa and Tousignant (1997), provides an illustration of the contrast between psychoanalytically oriented therapy and drug therapy on one hand, and native healing on the other. Zahra was treated first by an ethnopsychoanalyst and then by an Imam. The ethnopsychoanalyst used psychoanalytical symbolism to interpret the behavior and native customs of the patient combined with drugs to deal with her visual hallucinations. Although the ethnopsychoanalyst succeeded in suppressing the patient's visions temporarily, a few sessions with the Imam resulted in a complete recovery. We end the chapter with a brief description of this case, hoping that future research will assess the processes and outcomes of various native healing methods in Arab-Islamic societies and perhaps compare them with psychiatric treatment.

Zahra contacted the ethnopsychoanalyst with the complaint that she was seeing flashes depicting a camera with a man taking her picture as if she were a prostitute. She reported the delusion that the psychiatrist she had seen previously knew everything about her and even read her thoughts. She also reported a dream during one therapeutic session: While she was in a garden, she escaped from some unknown danger by hiding herself in a pumpkin. In the traditional North African rural society, a pumpkin is not only used for food, but also for churning: A small opening is made and the milk is poured through it and churned by a pestle (mothers also tend to rock their babies while churning the milk). The ethnopsychoanalyst interpreted the pumpkin in Zahra's dream as representing the mother's stomach ready to receive the male semen and to bear babies. Such interpretation ignores the family and the social conflicts that may be the source of the problems of this young Algerian girl.

One conflict Zahra had with her father was that she could not participate in sports in school. The ethnopsychoanalyst was aware of the belief that exercises and other physical activities are forbidden for North African girls because they may interfere with their virginity. In contrast, sports were conceived by the ethnopsychoanalyst as symbolic of masturbation. For Zahra's father, however, sports did not exist in the rural Algerian environment and therefore they may have represented to him strange and unfamiliar practices with no (or other) symbolic connotations.

No cooperation exists between therapists and native Arab-Islamic healers in Belgium. However, on the insistence of her parents, Zahra went to see an Imam who dealt directly with the contents of her vision: "If the man in your vision asks you to marry him, you should say no. Surely, he intended to ask you to marry him since he was tapping his feet on the ground as if he was taking a marriage photo. You are stronger than him since you can escape from him by lowering your head when he tries to take your photo." The Imam also told her that she became sick because she walked in dirty water. Because it is believed by Algerians that dirty water is a preferred location for the jinn, the implication is that the man of her vision is a jinn, and the Imam can deal with him. In contrast to ethnopsychoanalysis, only a few consultations with the Imam were needed for the disappearance of the patient's visions (Al-Issa & Tousignant, 1997, p. 144).

The case of Zahra as well as others may draw the attention of professionals to the benefits of alternative native healing methods and to the possibility that religious healers and "witch doctors succeed where doctors fail" (Jilek & Todd, 1974).

REFERENCES

Al-Abdul-Jabbar, J., & Al-Issa, I. (2000). Psychotherapy in Islamic society. In I. Al-Issa (Ed.), *Al-Junun: Mental illness in the Islamic World* (pp. 277–293). Madison, CT: International Universities Press.

Alexander, F., & Selesnick, S. T. (1966). *The history of psychiatry*. New York: Harper & Row.

Al-Issa, I. (1990). Culture and mental illness in Algeria. *The International Journal of Social Psychiatry, 36,* 230–240.

Al-Issa, I., & Tousignant, M. (1997). The mental health of North Africans in France. In I. Al-Issa & M. Tousignant (Eds.), *Ethnicity, immigration and psychopathology* (pp. 135–146). New York: Plenum Press.

Al-Krenawi, A., & Graham, J. R. (1996). Social work and traditional healing rituals among the Bedouin of the Negev, Israel. *International Social Work, 39,* 177–188.

Al-Krenawi, A., & Graham, J. R. (2000). Culturally sensitive social work practice with Arab clients in mental health settings. *Health and Social Work, 25,* 9–22.

Al-Krenawi, A., Graham, J. R., & Maoz, B. (1996). The healing significance of the Negev's Bedouin Dervish. *Social Science and Medicine, 43,* 13–21.

Al-Radi, O. M., & Al-Mahdy, M. A. (1989). Group therapy: An Islamic approach (abstracted by R. Prince). *Transcultural Psychiatric Research Review, 26,* 273–276.

Al-Subaie, A. (1989). Psychiatry in Saudi Arabia. *Transcultural Psychiatric Research Review, 26,* 245–262.

Al-Subaie, A. (1994). Traditional healing experiences in patients attending a university outpatient clinic. *The Arab Journal of Psychiatry, 5,* 83–91.

Al-Subaie, A., & Al-Hamad, A. (2000). Psychiatry in Saudi Arabia. In I. Al-Issa (Ed.), *Al-Junun: Mental illness in the Islamic world* (pp. 205–233). Madison, CT: International Universities Press.

Alsughayier, M. A. (1996). Public view of the "evil eye" and its role in psychiatry: A study in Saudi society. *The Arab Journal of Psychiatry, 7,* 152–160.

Alzubaidi, A. S., & Ghanem, A. (1997). Perspectives on psychology in Yemen. *International Journal of Psychology, 32,* 363–366.

American Psychiatric Association. (1994). *Diagnostic and statistical manual of mental disorders* (4th ed.). Washington, DC: American Psychiatric Association.

Azhar, M. Z., & Varma, S. L. (2000). Mental illness and its treatment in an Islamic society: Malaysia. In I. Al-Issa (Ed.), *Al-Junun: Mental illness in the Islamic World* (pp. 163–186). Madison, CT: International Universities Press.

Baasher, T. A. (1967). Traditional psychotherapeutic practices in the Sudan. *Transcultural Psychiatric Research Review, 4,* 158–160.

Baydoun, A. S. (1998). *The mental health of women between the scientists and the religious: A survey in Great Beirut.* Beirut, Lebanon: Dar-Al-Jadid (in Arabic).

Bazzoui, W., & Al-Issa, I. (1966). Psychiatry in Iraq. *British Journal of Psychiatry, 112,* 827–832.

Bensmail, B., Merdji, Y., & Touari, M. (1984). Pensée magique et therapie traditionelle [Magical thinking and traditional therapy]. *Psychiatrie Francophone, 3–4,* 28–33.

Blackman, W. S. (1927). *The Fellahin of Upper Egypt.* London: George G. Harrap.

Boddy, J. (1989). Spirits and selves in North Sudan. *American Ethnologist, 15,* 4–27.

Canaan, T. (1927). *Mohammadan saints and sanctuaries in Palestine.* London: Luzac.

Crapanzano, V. (1973). *The Hamadsha: A study in Moroccan ethnopsychiatry.* Berkeley, CA: University of California Press.

Dols, M. W. (1992). *Majnūn: The madman in medieval Islamic society.* New York: Oxford University Press.

Douki, S., Moussaoui, D., & Kacha, F. (1987). *Manuel de psychiatrie du practicien Maghrebin* [Manual of psychiatry for the Maghreb practitioner]. Paris: Masson.

Dundes, A. (1981). *The evil eye.* New York: Garland.

El-Eleymi, A. C. (1993). *Al-Zar.* Egypt: Al-Hey'a Al-Masria lil kitab (in Arabic).

El-Islam, M. F. (1982). Arab cultural psychiatry. *Transcultural Psychiatric Research Review, 19,* 15–24.

El-Islam, M. F. (2000). Mental illness in Kuwait and Qatar. In I. Al-Issa (Ed.), *Al-Junun: Mental illness in the Islamic world* (pp. 121–137). Madison, CT: International Universities Press.

Fakhouri, H. (1968). The Zar cult in an Egyptian Village. *Anthropological Quarterly, 41,* 49–56.

Frankl, V. E. (1986). *Man's search for meaning.* London: Holder and Straugton.

Frishkoff, M. (2001). Changing modalities in the globalization of Islamic saint veneration and mysticism: Sidi Ibrahim Al-Dasuqi, Shaykh Mohammad Uthman Al-Burhani, and their Sufi orders. *Religious Studies, 20,* 1–49.

Gawad, M. S. A. (1995). Transcultural psychiatry in Egypt. In I. Al-Issa (Ed.), *Culture and mental illness: An international perspective* (pp. 53–63). Madison, CT: International Universities Press.

Gran, P. (1979). Medical pluralism in Arab and Egyptian history: An overview of class structure and philosophies of the main phases. *Social Science & Medicine, 13B,* 339–348.

Greenwood, B. (1981). Cold or spirits? Choice and ambiguity in Morocco's pluralistic medical system. *Social Science and Medicine, 15B,* 219–235.

Holy Qur'an, The. (1971). Translated by Muhammad Zafrulla Khan. London: Curzon Press.

Hussein, F. (1991). A study of the role of unorthodox treatments of psychiatric illness in Riyadh. *The Arab Journal of Psychiatry, 2,* 170–184.

Ibn Qayyim, al-Jawzia (1957). *At-tib al-nabawi* [Prophetic medicine]. Beirut, Lebanon: Dar al-cutup al-Amah.

Jabir, T. (1996). Psychological or somatic medicine: Alienation from treatment and the trend toward modernity. *University Papers, 12–13,* 273–310 (in Arabic).

Jilek, W. G., & Todd, N. (1974). Witchdoctors succeed where doctors fail: Psychotherapy among Coast Salish Indians. *Canadian Psychiatric Association Journal, 19,* 351–356.

Katchadourian, H. (1980). Historical background of psychiatry in Lebanon. *Bulletin of the History of Medicine, 54,* 544–553.

Kennedy, I. G. (1978). *Nubian ceremonial life: Studies in Islamic syncretism and cultural change.* Berkeley, CA: University of California.

Kline, N. S. (1963). Psychiatry in Kuwait. *British Journal of Psychiatry, 109,* 766–774.

Klunzinger, C. B. (1878). *Upper Egypt: Its people and its products.* London: Blake.

Lane, E. W. (1908/1954). *Manners and customs of the modern Egyptians.* London: The Alpine Press.

Messing, S. D. (1959). Group therapy and social status in the Zar cult in Ethiopia. In M. K. Opler (Ed.), *Culture and mental health* (pp. 319–332). New York: Macmillan.

Naranjo, C., & Ornstein, R E. (1971). *On the psychology of meditation.* New York: Viking.

Nemr, H. H. (1996). *Folk beliefs and practices related to psychological disorder.* Unpublished master's thesis, Higher Institute of Folk Arts, Ain Sham University, Cairo, Egypt (in Arabic).

Nicholson, R. A. (1969). *The mystics of Islam.* London: Routledge & Kegan Paul.

Okasha, A. (1966). A cultural psychiatric study of El-Zar cult in U. A. R. *British Journal of Psychiatry, 112,* 1217–1221.

Okasha, A. (1997). *Psychiatry in Egypt* (unpublished manuscript). Ain Shams University, Cairo, Egypt.

Pearson, A. C. (1992). Vows (Greek and Roman). In J. Hastings (Ed.), *Encyclopedia of religion and ethics* (pp. 652–654). New York: Charles Scribner.

Pierre, D. (1993). Approche psychothérapeutique de patients migrants de première ou deuxième generation: Apports de l'ethnopsychoanalyse de Tobie Nathan [A psychotherapeutic approach to patients of first and second generation immigrants: Contributions to the ethno-analysis of Tobie Nathan]. *Acta Psychiatrica Belgica, 93,* 97–117.

Prince, R. H. (1980). Variations in psychotherapeutic procedures. In H. C. Triandis & J. G. Draguns (Eds.), *Handbook of cross-cultural psychology: Psychopathology* (Vol. 6, pp. 291–349). Boston, MA: Allyn & Bacon.

Schimmel, A. (1975). *Mystical dimensions of Islam.* Chapel Hill, NC: The University of North Carolina Press.

Swagman, C. F. (1989). Fija': Fright and illness in highland Yemen. *Social Science and Medicine, 28,* 381–388.

Tuncer, C. (1995). Mental illness in an Islamic-Mediterranean culture: Turkey. In I. Al-Issa (Ed.), *Culture and mental illness: An international perspective* (pp. 169–182). Madison, CT: International Universities Press.

Waldmeier, T. (1897). *Appeal for the first home for the insane on Mt. Lebanon.* London: Headley Brothers.

Westermarck, E. (1926). *Ritual and belief in Morocco.* London: Macmillan.

Yekun, F. (1994). *Islamic judgment of sorcery and its derivatives.* Beirut, Lebanon: The Risala Establishment (in Arabic).

V

Outlook

From Speculation Through Description Toward Investigation: A Prospective Glimpse at Cultural Research in Psychotherapy

Juris G. Draguns
The Pennsylvania State University

CULTURAL VARIATIONS IN PSYCHOTHERAPY: A RESEARCHABLE TOPIC?

The foregoing chapters present a panorama of psychological healing as it is practiced in a variety of homogeneous cultural contexts and multicultural milieus. Some readers may feel overwhelmed by the richness and complexity of this documentation. Others may pose questions as to the effectiveness, generalizability, and comparability of these interventions. Overriding these abstract concerns, there is the issue of relevance of these sometimes exotic and esoteric techniques within the multicultural microcosm of the contemporary United States society. On a higher plane of generality, one may explore the possibility of the existence and nature of universal, worldwide ingredients of psychotherapy that may be revealed through the conceptual analysis and empirical comparison of culturally specific modes of intervention. Potentially, these challenges fall within the province of cross-cultural psychotherapy research, an enterprise that, at the time of this writing, has barely been initiated. Even within the multicultural setting in the United States, as Hall (2001) has pointed out, a dysjunction exists between culturally sensitive (CST) and empirically supported (EST) therapies. Many CSTs, as yet, lack sound empirical support, and most ESTs have not been systematically or conclusively demonstrated to be effective in the various culturally distinctive components of the United States population. Even less information on these issues is available across national cultures. Rehm (2002) has acknowledged that demonstrations of the effect of ESTs rest on research that has for the most part been conducted in the United States and other English-speaking countries. American psychologists know little about how well these procedures work elsewhere in the world, and questions about any cultural variations in style, technique, and context of ESTs in other countries have rarely been addressed (Draguns, 2002). Psychodynamic, existential-humanistic, cognitive behavioral, interpersonal systems, and several other modes of psychotherapy are all practiced in widely different contexts around the world. However, empirically based knowledge is sparse on any cultural differences in therapist's interventions, client's responses to, and then impact of psychotherapies, whether the theoretical framework is varied or held constant.

This chapter attempts to make a start at filling this major gap in our knowledge. To this end, the origins of this topic of inquiry, in both conceptualization and research, are first briefly addressed. The chapter then introduces the experiences of some of the current innovative practitioners of psychotherapy who have responded to the challenge of modifying and tailoring their interventions to fit their culturally distinctive clientele. On the basis of their contributions and the findings and concepts of cross-cultural psychology, hypotheses are formulated for the systematic and worldwide investigation of psychotherapy. The ultimate challenge is to convert this scheme into reality through empirical research. With this objective in mind, several kinds of possible studies are prepared, from modest to grandiose.

KRAEPELIN: A FORGOTTEN FOREFATHER OF CULTURAL PSYCHOTHERAPY RESEARCH

Emil Kraepelin, a pioneering German psychiatrist, is generally recognized as the father of scientific psychiatry (Jilek, 1995). The current diagnostic system, as embodied in the Diagnostic and Statistical Manual of the American Psychiatric Association (DSM-IV) and the International Classification of Diseases (ICD-10), owes much to Kraepelin. The concepts of schizophrenia, bipolar mood disorder, and major depression were first identified and described by him, albeit under somewhat different names. It is often overlooked, however, that Kraepelin was intensely interested in the manifestations of mental illness at remote and culturally different sites. He conducted firsthand observations on the behavior of mental patients in Algeria and Indonesia. His report on non-Western symptoms of depression (Kraepelin, 1904) has not disappeared from the citation circuit, although it may be more often invoked than read. Sections of this classical article sound surprisingly perceptive and contemporary, even a century later. Witness the following paragraph:

> If the characteristics of a people are manifested in its religion and its customs, in its intellectual artistic achievements, in its political acts and its historical development, then they will also find expression in the frequency and clinical formation of its mental disorders, especially those that emerge from internal conditions. Just as the knowledge of morbid psychic phenomena has opened up for us deep insights into the working of our psychic life, so we may also hope that the psychiatric characteristics of a people can further our understanding of its entire psychic character. In this sense comparative psychiatry may be destined to one day become an important auxiliary science to comparative ethnopsychology ("Voelkerpsychologie"). (as cited by Jilek, 1995, p. 231)

The idea that the culturally dominant values, attitudes, and outlooks affect symptoms of mental disorder was novel in 1904. Even now, this notion is not universally accepted, although it animates an emerging research enterprise on the intertwining of culture and the experience and expression of psychopathology. As far as we know, Kraepelin did not practice psychotherapy nor did he explicitly write about it. His statement, however, can be easily extrapolated to it. If psychopathology is influenced by culture, the techniques to counteract or alleviate it are also likely to be culturally shaped. In the course of the twentieth century, this assertion acquired an increasing plausibility and gained a relatively wide, although by no means general, acceptance. However, the specific role of culture in psychotherapy has not yet been pinpointed. To this end, two tasks must be tackled: clarifying the concept of psychotherapy, especially in reference to its putative links to culture, and describing the contributions of a number of contemporary psychotherapists who have not shied away from adapting their services to their clients of very different cultural backgrounds.

WHERE IS CULTURE IN PSYCHOTHERAPY?

Several Definitions

For the sake of the argument, let us start with the null hypothesis and boldly assert that the conduct and the experience of psychotherapy are determined by the therapist's theoretical orientation, the repertoire of techniques and interventions in which he or she is trained, the client's needs and his or her distress, and the vicissitudes of the relationship between the therapist and the client, and that none of the above four factors are appreciably influenced by culture. By contrast, a culturally oriented definition of psychotherapy asserts the following:

> . . . psychotherapy can be conceived as a series of reinitiation techniques for reentry in fuller, more efficient participation in society. Psychotherapy then is always a procedure that is sociocultural in its ends and interpersonal in its means, it occurs between two or more individuals and is embedded in a broader, less visible, but no less real cultural context of shared social learning, store of meanings, symbols, and implicit assumptions concerning the nature of social living. (Draguns, 1975, p. 273)

Within this framework, culture is regarded as a third, invisible yet essential participant in every psychotherapy encounter (Draguns, 1975). This view is consonant with Pedersen's (1999) position that multiculturalism constitutes the fourth force in contemporary counseling and psychotherapy, parallel to the established psychodynamic, humanistic, and behavioral frameworks. Determining the client's relationship to the culture or cultures within which he or she functions and lives is an indispensable task that must be tackled in the course of the therapeutic process. Proceeding from somewhat different conceptual antecedents, Prince defined psychotherapy as follows:

> I suffer. Psychotherapy may be defined as any psychological procedure that is aimed at relieving an individual with such a complaint. Suffering and psychological methods for the relief of suffering are ubiquitous. But the way individuals experience suffering, the interpretations of the meaning or cause of the suffering, and above all the methods of relieving it vary enormously according to culture. (Prince, 1980, p. 291)

This definition posits the experience of suffering and of its alleviation as the universal or pancultural hallmarks of psychotherapy. At the same time, Prince's formulation allows culture considerable latitude in making sense of the client's experience of distress, and in techniques for relieving the client from it. The modes of presenting, expressing, and communicating suffering are also subject to cultural shaping. Thus, culture may play a major role in some situations, but its part in shaping therapeutic encounters may be trivial or negligible in other instances.

One may ask, for example, whether the same necessary and sufficient conditions for personality change through psychotherapy are identical across culture. Rogers (1957), it may be recalled, posited five such conditions: incongruence in the client, congruence by the therapist, the therapist's unconditional positive regard, the therapist's experience of empathy toward the client, and his or her sensitive and realistic communication of it to the client. Are these conditions recognizable, let alone indispensable, for workable intervention in other cultures, such as in the ceremonial spirit dances of the Salish Indians of British Columbia (Jilek, 1982, and Chapter 9)? Following these procedures, depressive manifestations were reduced, alienation gave way to ethnic pride, and drug and alcohol abuse declined as did violent outbursts and suicidal ideation. However, one is hard put to discern either unconditional acceptance or communication of empathy in these rituals. Instead, a symbolic enactment of death and rebirth occurs in an altered state of consciousness. Conversely, does each culture devise its distinctive therapeutic process whereby distress is relieved and behavior changed? The current state of experiential, clinical, and research evidence does not provide an unequivocal answer to these questions. One may further ask whether widely accepted basic practices and attitudes by modern Western therapists are crucial for beneficial effects of psychotherapy. Specifically, five questions may be posed: Can psychotherapy produce positive consequences without a benevolent and helpful intent on the part of the therapist? Is a relationship between the therapist and the client indispensable for therapy to work? Is psychotherapy possible in the absence of verbal communication between the client and the therapist? Must the therapist know and understand the client as a person, and is the gathering of biographical and experiential information indispensable for therapy to take place? Does intervention conducted entirely in the form of command, suggestion, or advice constitute psychotherapy? In light of Prince's (1980) worldwide survey of contemporary and traditional psychotherapy practices, exceptions to every one of the preceding five conditions have been observed at some time somewhere around the world. And yet the characteristics listed, especially those pertaining to helpfulness, relationship, and communication, are widespread and encountered in a wide variety of cultural settings. It would appear that healers of different traditions have independently evolved interventions that include the triad of benevolence, personal bond, and dialogue, supplemented in many cases by personal knowledge of the help seeker and culturally meaningful explanations for the distress encountered.

Perhaps the more cross-culturally robust features of effective therapy can be more readily discerned in the goals rather than in the rationales or practices of psychotherapy. Fish (1996 and Chapter 4) had the opportunity of developing and implementing therapy services in the interior of the state of Sao Paulo in Brazil. On the basis of this experience, he proposed to restructure the cross-culturally applicable features of therapy as follows: pinpointing the goals toward which the client is striving rather than the problems that he or she is experiencing; encouraging talk about solutions instead of dwelling on problems; helping the client see the problem in a new, and less hopeless and uncontrollable, light; finding exceptions to the problems and encouraging the search for additional instances of such exceptions; and promoting clients' anticipations of desirable and beneficial change.

It is readily apparent that the concept of psychotherapy has fuzzy boundaries. Its defining features are extremely difficult to pin down. Subject to these caveats, the following definition may provide a flexible guide for encompassing many, though not all, of the procedures described in the preceding chapters of this volume. It may also be useful in capturing the core characteristics of the gamut of interventions. Psychotherapy then encompasses the following:

> ... modes of intervention that (1) involve differential and asymmetrical roles of at least two individuals, one distressed and the other allegedly equipped with expertise to remove or alleviate such distress; (2) by means of techniques that are principally verbal, interpersonal, and psychological in nature; (3) with general objectives of bringing about relief, reorganization of adaptive resources, and personality change. (Draguns, 1975, p. 273)

With this description in mind, let us turn our attention to a number of contemporary psychotherapists who have extended its scope and modified its operations in different sociocultural milieus.

CONTEMPORARY INNOVATORS: THEIR EXPERIENCES AND CONCLUSIONS

Expectations of Therapists and Clients

Wolfgang Pfeiffer, a German psychiatrist with extensive international clinical and research experience (Pfeiffer, 1994), immersed himself in the effort of providing culturally fitting psychotherapeutic services to Turkish guest workers in Germany (Pfeiffer, 1996). On the basis of this experience, he identified five clashes of expectations that obstruct the initiation and implementation of psychotherapy in dyads of Turkish clients and German therapists. First, the client usually comes seeking advice and direction, while the therapist expects the client to search for and to find his or her own solution to problems and challenges of living. Second, on the basis of cultural experience, the client is predisposed to turn to and seek help and participation from the members of his or her family. The therapist's cultural outlook and professional training lead him or her to emphasize individuality and privacy in personal decision making. Third, the Turkish client is imbued with respect and deference to the elders within her or his family. It is from them that advice, suggestion, and solution are sought for pending personal problems. The therapist's cultural approach tends to be egalitarian and task-oriented. In the process, the traditional experience and wisdom of the elders is dismissed as irrelevant for resolving any current personal or practical problems. Fourth, the client often expresses his or her suffering in bodily terms, whereas the therapist's interest is focused on the client's subjective personal experience and his or her thoughts and feelings. Fifth, the client embarks upon therapy with the expectations of prompt or even instantaneous relief; the therapist knows that gradual and uneven improvement is the rule and that sudden cures tend to occur infrequently.

The cogency of these formulations is highlighted by Fisek and Kagitçibasi (1999) who, also working with Turkish help seekers who were being seen by German professionals, independently identified several of the same divergent expectations. Moreover, similar incompatibilities may be observed in other cross-cultural encounters between the therapist and the client. The therapist's implicit ethos may be extended across the culture gulf, and an alien and baffling framework may be imposed upon migrants, sojourners, or refugees. Differences in conceptions of what is helpful, necessary, and effective for relieving distress pose a challenge to researchers and practitioners alike. How to overcome or circumvent these obstacles remains an urgent task.

Taking Cultural Beliefs and Practices Seriously

Tobie Nathan (1994), a Parisian psychoanalyst, has been a pioneer in devising appropriate and effective therapeutic services for distressed and distraught migrants and sojourners, mostly from Northern and Western Africa. He has proceeded from the realization that imposed Western interventions have a high failure rate with clients of a pronouncedly different cultural outlook. Instead, Nathan has evolved a radically different approach. It emphasizes the discovery of the meaning of symptoms within the cultural framework of symbols and beliefs. In the process, verbal communication receives less emphasis than the presentation and manipulation of artifacts and objects. Metaphors, proverbs, and sayings are prominently incorporated into therapy interventions. Instead of isolating the client in the culturally alien office, clinic, or hospital setting, Nathan actively involves family members who participate with the client in the search for understanding and solution of his and her problems of living. Insight in the traditional Western sense is deemphasized and quick reduction or elimination of psychic distress is sought. On the basis of his unique experiences, Nathan has offered a set of recommendations that, in paraphrase, are worth sharing. Specifically, he admonishes prospective therapists to respect their clients' religious beliefs, even if they appear to be strange and bizarre; accept the traditional ways of doing things and the customary modes of decision making within their clients' cultures; respect the cultural artifacts and take seriously the powers attributed to them; honor the cultural rules of hospitality and act in accordance with them in the therapy setting; recognize the distress that their clients experience as a result of feeling uprooted from their homes and separated from their families and communities; and convey this recognition both empathetically and in a culturally meaningful manner. More generally, Nathan recognizes that therapeutic change is powerfully facilitated by social influence, provided that it is embedded in the person's sociocultural belief system. Of course, in most therapy encounters in the United States and Canada, the cultural gulf is not as wide as that which Nathan had to bridge. However, his recommendations may still be relevant so as to avoid cultural misunderstandings and enhance cultural sensitivity, especially in working with psychologically distressed newcomers of radically different cultural backgrounds, as exemplified by the traumatized survivors of the killing fields of Cambodia.

Discovering the Subjective World in Therapy

Bin Kimura (1995), a Japanese psychiatrist steeped in the German tradition of phenomenological analysis, has applied his lifelong knowledge of his culture, his theoretical outlook, and his technical therapeutic skills in highlighting the interpersonal nature of Japanese subjectivity. In Kimura's view, the decisive and formative experience of the Japanese self is centered on what happens between two interacting human beings. The self is not harbored within the individual. Rather, it is expressed in the course of the social give-and-take between persons. Thus, guilt may be keenly felt, but not as a result of violating abstract immutable principles. Instead, such feelings are painfully experienced because the person thinks that he or she has let down or alienated specific persons. Similarly, morbid shyness or avoidance of people is traced to social hypersensitivity and the fear of giving offense to another person. Kimura's observations and formulations illustrate the potential of looking at psychotherapy as a reflection of subjective culture while at the same time making psychotherapeutic operations more personally sensitive and culturally appropriate. Several authors (Draguns, 1981; Kakar, 1978; Roland, 1988; Vassiliou & Vassiliou, 1973; Wachtel, 1977) have proposed that therapy is a mirror through which subtle, implicit, and easily overlooked features of culture are reflected. Kimura, however, has gone further than anybody else in using phenomenological psychotherapy as the source for the identification and description of the unverbalized, yet fundamental, notions that guide social interaction and personal conduct at a specific point in space and time. Emblematic of this orientation is the Japanese word *ki*, which ties together affect, cognition, and volition and does so invariably in relation to another person. Experiencing *ki* in isolation, intrapsychically, is a semantic impossibility. Kimura's approach is worthy of emulation as an avenue of exploring culturally shaped experience through psychotherapy.

Developing and Applying Mental Health Services Across Cultures: Blending Approaches from Within and Outside of Culture

Karl Peltzer (1995), a German clinical psychologist, has described his unique experiences in inaugurating and developing mental health services in several African countries, from Ghana to Malawi. In all cases, he tried to respond to the preexisting and pressing mental health problems on the basis of an informal need assessment on site. As a result, he succeeded in blending standard Western intervention techniques, such as guided imagery, with culture-specific treatment methods, such as codified healing rituals. Dream interpretation was modified by blending Western principles and African symbols. In many cases, Western treatment approaches were changed and adapted in order to respond more effectively to a specific local problem, such as depressive reactions and posttraumatic stress disorders sustained in Malawi as a result of incarceration and torture by an oppressive (and eventually overthrown) regime (Peltzer, 1996). Specifically, he admonished therapists faced with similar tasks of instituting urgently needed intervention programs in radically different sociocultural settings as follows:

> Detect indigenous coping strategies and culturally mediated protective factors. This includes operational research on the cultural dimension of the psychosocial mechanisms that determine how people cope with trauma. The objective of this research is threefold: a) formulate guidelines for a community-based mental health care approach and for the counseling of victims which takes the context of the local culture in account, b) formulate guidelines for preventive actions both on community and individual level, and c) involve local healers in the programme and achieve that they work side by side with health workers. (Peltzer, 1996, p. 18)

Peltzer (1995) identified three distinctive components within the present day African population: (a) traditional persons who are functioning within the established framework of their respective cultures, little affected by the currents of social change; (b) transitional persons, shuttling between modern and traditional worlds; and (c) modern persons immersed in the contemporary, industrial or postindustrial, processes of modernization and globalization. Therapy needs and outlooks for these three categories tend to be different, and in designing and implementing services, where the person stands in this tripartite division must be taken into account. Peltzer (1995) has presented excerpts from clinical interactions between a traditional healer and a traditional patient, a European therapist with a transitional patient, and a European therapist with a European patient. He concluded that healer-patient interactions tend to be generally shorter and less continuous than Western therapist-patient interactions. Peltzer's therapeutic activities are characterized by flexibility, pragmatism, and willingness to combine and adapt techniques of local and imported derivation.

Modifying Psychotherapy to Fit Cultural Reality

Alba Nyda Rivera-Ramos (1984), a Puerto Rican clinical psychologist trained in the mainland United States, was impressed by the disparity between her training and the clinical and social realities in Puerto Rico. One of these discrepancies pertains to social and familistic emphasis prevalent in Puerto Rico. As Rivera-Ramos (1984, p. 6) put it: "In contrast to North Americans, Puerto Ricans place a special emphasis upon their families and their host of relatives."[1] The other divergence is especially keenly felt when psychotherapy is applied across class as well as cultural lines. Many Puerto Ricans of working class backgrounds, and especially those who are poor, perceive standard psychotherapy as not only irrelevant, but condescending. In Puerto Rico, greater weight in determining personal status is accorded to ascription than achievement. A person's respect rests more on his or her age and family reputation than on wealth or success. These considerations may be glossed over by the often youthful therapists trained on the U.S. mainland and eager to intervene in the most efficient and expeditious fashion. Their pragmatism and disregard of the nuances of cultural sensitivity may be perceived as offensive to the client's sense of dignity, a key value in Puerto Rican and other Latin American cultures. In response to this recognition, Rivera-Ramos has proposed a model of psychotherapy based on mutuality and cooperation between the therapist and client. In the process, she eschews paternalism and protectionism. Instead, both parties to the therapy transaction are united in their striving for the attainment of the mutually agreed therapy objectives. In fact, she objects to the designation of the help seeker as client and prefers to look upon her or him as a companion in a shared task or an "interacter" (interactuante). Rivera-Ramos fuses her collaborative orientation, problem-solving focus, and family and community emphasis in a conception of the human being as the following:

> . . . an integral, necessary, and indispensable component of society, that is, as a social being who cannot attain his or her goals. This position stands in diametric contrast to the traditional view of psychotherapy, in older as well as more recent models, which consider the individual as responsible for and capable of everything."[2] (Rivera-Ramos, 1984, p. 71)

In this respect, Rivera-Ramos' formulation converges with and anticipates an important trend in theory and research on culture and therapy.

Ethnographic Observations of Intercultural Therapy Dyads

Karen Seeley (2000), an American psychotherapist with training in anthropology, social work, and cultural psychology, brought the strands of her interdisciplinary background to bear upon the intensive qualitative study of clients in psychodynamic therapy. The six clients investigated in her study were of varied ethnic and cultural backgrounds, and in all cases their psychotherapists were of different ethnicity from their own. Culture then had to be encountered and crossed in therapy. Seeley was interested in exactly how culture impinges upon therapy and affects its experience within the client's framework and outlook. To this end, she explicitly adopted the ethnographer's modus operandi. Therapy clients became her informants who described what happened to them in therapy and the meaning that they attributed to these experiences in the same manner as an indigenous resource person elucidates the practices and rituals of his or her culture to a curious but naïve anthropologist. Indeed, the question of how psychotherapy is perceived and conceptualized across the culture gulf has rarely been asked, and the clients' reactions have rarely been given a voice, except in relation to the possible complication in the therapy process that they engendered. For this purpose, the roles of the therapist and the interviewer had to be

---

[1]Translated from Spanish.
[2]Translated from Spanish.

separated. Traditionally, the accounts of intercultural therapy are provided by the therapist and are incidental to the conduct of therapy. Seeley's research is unique in that she interviewed other therapists' patients and thereby provided another perspective to the experience of the therapy process.

Seeley's interviews explored the intertwining of therapy and culture. She concluded that all aspects of therapy experience are affected by the clients' cultural background, even in those cases where the person appears to be indistinguishable from his or her "mainstream" American counterparts in speech, dress, and demeanor. Specifically, clients' cultures affect the therapy relationship including self-disclosures, the construction of their selves, the expression of their emotions, the reconstruction of their developmental experience, and the idiom of distress (see Seeley, in preparation). Seeley cautioned practicing therapists against the widespread tendency of underestimating the distinctiveness of their foreign and ethnic clients' experience. Converging with findings from other sources, she emphasized the experience of selfhood of her ethnic and foreign interviewees. "The subjects described selves that were differently bounded and individuated than Western selves. Often their self-other boundaries were indistinct, so that self, family, and community representations, identifications, and interests were fused" (Seeley, 2000, p. 221). "Further, the subjects described selves which devalued the independent action, self-expression, and self-assertion that Western selves commonly prize" (p. 221). Thus, Seeley's unique data provide valuable glimpses into her interviewees' subjective culture. They also highlight the need for combining personal anamnesis with a cultural exploration in order to avoid distortions and misunderstandings by the therapist as well as constant cultural and personal sensitivity throughout the therapy process.

Culturally Sensitive Therapy: Its Common Features

On the basis of these six innovators' efforts, it is possible to provide a provisional composite sketch of culturally sensitive and flexible therapist's practices under the following seven headings:

1. Formulate mutually agreeable objectives and relate various therapy techniques to these agreed-upon goals.
2. Share information on the means for attaining these goals; demystify the therapy experience and reduce its ambiguity.
3. Identify the stereotypes of various groups that the therapist may harbor and work actively in order to transcend or eliminate them.
4. Experience and communicate empathy on the basis of shared experience and express and convey sympathy by extending human compassion beyond the range of the therapist's personal experiences (Stewart, 1981).
5. Cultivate culturally fitting modes of communication (e.g., by means of metaphors and analogies, fables, and storytelling or "Cuento" [Zuniga, 1991] therapy).
6. Exercise maximal flexibility consistent with the agreed-upon therapy goals.
7. Guard against construing cultural differences in terms of alleged deficits and/or disorders; any difference from or perceived violation of the prevailing in-group norms is never a sufficient indicator for the diagnosis or inference of a mental disorder.

Interim Conclusions

The six contemporary pioneers have provided rich "raw material" based on the conduct of psychotherapy across cultures. Such information is invaluable in the early, exploratory stages of investigating a phenomenon. Practitioners of naturalistic observation, which all six of these cultural innovators are, have to record realistically and truthfully their observations and to separate rigorously observations from inference. In their accounts of venturing across culture lines in therapy, these six explorers have successfully accomplished these objectives. Indispensable though recording and description are at the early stages of scientific inquiry, they must eventually be supplemented by more elaborate methods if the cause and effect nexus is to be disentangled and functional relationships between independent and dependent variables are to be established. Thus, the stage is set for more formal psychotherapy research across cultures.

TOWARD SYSTEMATIC INVESTIGATION OF PSYCHOTHERAPY WITHIN AND ACROSS CULTURES

Psychotherapy appears in a great many cultures in a dazzling variety of guises. What is essential and effective in psychotherapy and what is irrelevant? How can demonstrably effective features of psychotherapy vary with cultural characteristics? In this section, such relationships are proposed on the basics of linking the results of cross-cultural investigation on personality and social behavior with the research still to be conducted on cross-cultural variations in psychotherapy.

Hofstede's Cultural Dimensions

In one of the largest psychological studies ever undertaken, in terms of the number of both participants and countries represented, Hofstede (1980) in the Netherlands succeeded in identifying four factorially based dimensions by means of work-related attitudes. The sample on which this study was based was made up of the employees of IBM, a multinational corporation, which in the 1970s was represented in all regions of the world, except for the so-called Socialist countries led by the Soviet Union and the People's Republic of China. The number of participants in this research set world records; a total of 116,000 questionnaires was collected in 50 countries and 3 regions. By means of sophisticated multivariate statistical techniques, four factors were extracted from this array of data. They constitute the dimensions by means of which cultures around the world can be meaningfully compared. In the ensuing decades, these four factors have been extensively studied not only in industrial-organizational settings, but in family, community, and other interpersonal contexts.

Of the four constructs, individualism-collectivism has been most intensively investigated, not only by Hofstede (1980, 1991, 2001), but by Triandis (1995) and others. In brief, individualism refers to the extent that a person experiences himself or herself as a self-contained and autonomous human being. Collectivism is described as the experience of being integrated into a cohesive group, from birth to death. In Hofstede's worldwide study, the United States was found to exceed all other nations in individualism. This finding parallels the importance accorded to individualism by Katz (1985) in her analysis of the values, conceptions, and techniques of American counseling and, by extension, those of psychotherapy. From a hermeneutic point of view,

Christopher (2001) recently proposed to show "how we as therapists are shaped by culture and how much of psychological theory, research, and practice is influenced by our dominant outlook, individualism" (p. 116).

Power distance refers to the general acceptance within a culture of the unequal distribution of power. Uncertainty avoidance is indexed by the unease or discomfort in situations that are unclear, unstructured, or unpredictable. This discomfort is commonly reduced by rules and rituals. Masculinity-femininity is a bipolar construct. The masculine end of the continuum is exemplified by those cultures in which there is high differentiation of gender roles and little overlap between them. In such settings achievement and productivity are highly valued. Femininity prevails in those societies in which gender roles exhibit extensive overlap and in which such values as tenderness and care are prized.

On the basis of a very different methodology, a fifth dimension was added by Hofstede and Bond (1988) and by Chinese Culture Connection (1987). The items on the scale for the measurement of this construct were explicitly based on Confucian tenets. Subsequently, the instrument came to be used in a variety of countries in different geographic and cultural regions. Hofstede and Bond initially labeled this dimension "Confucian dynamism." Confucian values are focused on the promotion of individual striving at the service of the ingroup, such as family, clan, community, or nation. In his current formulation, Hofstede (2001) considers long-term versus short-term orientation to be the cardinal feature of this construct. In his words, "Long Term Orientation stands for the fostering of virtues oriented towards future rewards, in particular perseverance and thrift" (Hofstede, 2001, p. 359). Five East Asian countries historically imbued with Confucian values, China, Hong Kong, Taiwan, Japan, and South Korea, have been found to have the highest scores on a measure of long-term orientation.

A somewhat different version of Confucian dynamism as a cultural dimension was proposed by Cheng (1990, 1998). Cheng's concept stresses the values of filiality, propriety, and concordance; emphasizes social approval and acceptance; posits the objectives of self-subordination and social integration; and envisages harmony as a social ideal.

It should be emphasized that all five of Hofstede's constructs were explicitly designed to characterize cultures and not individuals. Hofstede (2001) endeavored to develop a broad theoretical framework relevant to the basic problems of human society. Such a conceptualization was envisaged as "an exploration into new territory; specifically, the territory that lies between the various rather neatly defined disciplines of the science of man: anthropology, sociology, psychology, economics, political science, law, and medicine" (Hofstede, 2001, p. 461). Ascertaining the impact of Hofstede's dimensions upon a specific domain of human interaction and experience, such as psychotherapy, involves a complex process. Hermeneutics (e.g., Christopher, 2001), psychoanalytic self-psychology (e.g., Roland, 1988), and social psychology (e.g., Triandis, 1995) converge in positing the self as the nodal concept tying culture and persons. To that end, cultural variations in self-experience must be introduced.

Cultural Dimensions Within the Self

Western psychologists construe the self as the core of personality. William James's (1891, 1952) classical definition describes the self as all that which the person "is tempted to call by the name of me" (James, 1952, p. 188). A century later, Landrine (1992, p. 402) referred to the "separated, encapsulated self of the Western culture . . .

that is presumed to be the originator, creator, and controller of behavior." At another point, she stated, "The self is presumed to be [the] cognitive and emotional universe, the center of awareness, emotion, judgement, and action" (Landrine, 1992, p. 402). A host of converging formulations (Chang, 1988; Kimura, 1995; Markus and Kitayama, 1991; Roland, 1988; Triandis, 1989) have joined Landrine in challenging the universality of this conception of the self. The alternative, sociocentric self is expressed through the person's characteristic interactions with other human beings, especially those with whom the person is involved in close and enduring personal relationships. Chang (1988) articulated the main distinction between the Western individualist self and the sociocentric self prevalent elsewhere. The sociocentric self is composed of bonds with other individuals; the individualistic self separates the person from other people by means of a firm, virtually impermeable boundary. Not surprisingly, Hofstede (1991), Triandis (1994), and others have posited a relationship between individualism-collectivism as a cultural trait and individualistic versus sociocentric self-experience. Draguns (1998) has hypothesized that socialization by means of a small number of intense relationships promotes the development of an autonomous, private, and differentiated self. This combination of experiences is likely to be found in individualistic cultures. In sociocentric cultures, the development of a more flexible self is promoted by a greater number of agents of socialization, with somewhat less intense, but more numerous, formative relationships.

Less thought has been given to the characteristics of the self associated with power distance, uncertainty avoidance, masculinity-femininity, and long-term or short-term orientation. On the basis of extrapolations from Hofstede's (1991) writings, tentative expectations (Draguns, 1998) have been formulated as follows:

1. High power distance would foster the development of an encapsulated self, prominently concerned with status and wealth; conversely, low power distance would be associated with a more permeable self, and a greater importance attached to personal relationships.

2. In settings of high uncertainty avoidance, emphasis would be placed on the consistency and explicitness of self-experience; with low uncertainty avoidance, more inconsistency within the self would be tolerated, and greater portions of self-experience would remain unverbalized.

3. Masculinity would favor the development of a task- and action-oriented, pragmatic, and practical self, whereas an altruistic, feeling-centered self would be associated with femininity.

4. Long-term orientation would emphasize self-restraint, modesty, and humility; short-term orientation would place a premium on self-assertion.

From Cultural Dimensions Through the Self to the Characteristic Modes of Therapy Intervention

The previous considerations suggest a number of links between the five cultural characteristics and therapeutic interventions. The entire set of predictions is contained in Table 20.1. The assumption on which these hypotheses are based is that socially characteristic modalities of behavior are reflected in the psychotherapy experience, through its goals, techniques, and patterns of interaction.

Given the large number of predictions advanced, there is a virtual certainty that not all of them will be confirmed. How many of these expectations are likely to receive

TABLE 20.1
Five Cultural Dimensions in Psychotherapy

INDIVIDUALISM:	COLLECTIVISM:
Insight, Self-understanding	Alleviation of Suffering
Guilt, Alienation, Loneliness	Relationship Problems, Shame
Therapist as Father Figure	Therapist as Nurturant Mother
Development of Individuality	Social Integration
Development of Responsibility	Acceptance of Controls
Conflict and Resolution	Harmonious Relationships
Feelings More Important than Relationships	Relationships More Important than Feelings
Individual Expression Through Behavior	Role Determines Behavior

HIGH POWER DISTANCE:	LOW POWER DISTANCE:
Directive Psychotherapy	Person-Centered Psychotherapy
Therapist as Expert	Therapist as Sensitive Person
Conformity and Social Effectiveness	Self-Discovery and Actualization
Differentiation of Therapist & Client Roles	Dedifferentiation of Therapist &
Emphasis Upon Professional Credentials	Client Roles
Expertise Through Interpretation and Direction	Promotion of Self-Improvement

HIGH UNCERTAINTY AVOIDANCE:	LOW UNCERTAINTY AVOIDANCE:
Biological Explanations	Psychological Explanations
Behavioral Techniques	Experiential Psychotherapy
Medical Orientation	Multiprofessional Orientation
Few Schools of Therapy	Many Schools of Therapy
Tightly Regulated Therapy Practice	Loosely Regulated Therapy Practice
Technique Adhered To	Spontaneity Promoted

MASCULINITY:	FEMININITY:
Society's Needs Paramount	Person's Goals Paramount
Responsibility, Conformity, Adjustment	Expressiveness, Creativity, Empathy
Guilt	Anxiety
Enabling	Caring
Competition	Cooperation

LONG-TERM ORIENTATION:	SHORT-TERM ORIENTATION:
Interpersonal Therapy	Intrapsychic or Behavioral Therapy
Somatic Interventions	Psychological Interventions
Self-Control	Self-Assertion
Self-Subordination	Self-Actualization
Limited and Slow Change Expected	Rapid and General Change Expected

support? That question does not admit even a speculative answer a priori. What can be said with reasonable certainty is that a program of investigations can put to the test the construct validity and the relevance of Hofstede's five dimensions for therapist/client interactions across cultures. The null hypothesis would assert that culture is not a significant determinant of therapist's intervention, client's self-presentation, or therapy's outcome. In the current discourse on psychotherapy and culture, virtually no one upholds this position. However, the issue is open as to whether Hofstede's five constructs, which originated in the industrial-organizational context, are applicable to psychotherapy. Specific predictions about these dimensions have been derived and tested in school milieus (Hofstede, 1986), intercultural encounters

(Hofstede, 1991, 2001; Triandis, Brislin, & Hui, 1988), intrafamily relationships (Hofstede, 1991), economic and political behavior (Hofstede, 1991, 2001), and human motivation (Hofstede, 1991, 2001). Of even greater relevance, Hofstede's constructs have been applied both to human distress (Draguns, 1990) and subjective well-being (Arrindell, Hatzichristou, Wensink, Van Trillert, Stedema, & Meijer, 1997). These developments spark the expectation that Hofstede's dimensions may be relevant to psychotherapy as well. If this expectation is supported, the specific points in Table 20.1 can be generalized as follows. Individualism fosters self-exploration and search for insight as the ultimate goal in psychotherapy, whereas collectivism primarily promotes a quest for harmony within and integration into the family and other primary groups. High power distance prizes expert intervention as a vehicle of therapeutic change, whereas low power distance capitalizes upon human sensitivity. High uncertainty avoidance promotes the reliance upon goal-oriented interventions of demonstrated scientific validity; low uncertainty avoidance is characterized by a greater readiness to try new avenues of therapy, even if they are as yet unproven. In masculine cultures, therapists are primarily regarded as the agents of society whose task is to enable their clients to restore their earning capacity and to enhance their social competence. Feminine cultures view psychotherapists as basically the client's helpers, and interventions are primarily animated by a caring attitude. Finally, long-term orientation is expected to capitalize on self-control and self-subordination, whereas short-term orientation is hypothesized to focus on self-assertion and self-actualization.

From Hypotheses to Results: A Promising Beginning

How can these predictions be tested? Ideally, one might envisage a Hofstede-type multinational investigation in which the rankings of the cultural dimensions, already ascertained, would serve as predictors of therapist's and client's behavior. For a host of practical reasons, this objective remains unrealized. However, a major step toward this goal has been taken by an international team of researchers who have embarked upon an international study of psychotherapists' development (Orlinsky et al., 1999). The Collaborative Research Network (CNR) of the Society for Psychotherapy Research has initiated the collection of self-descriptive data by means of standardized and equivalent scales across countries and languages. The object of this effort is to follow the changes in the experience of psychotherapists in the course of their careers. Orlinsky et al. report that 3,795 protocols have been collected on samples ranging from 100 to 1,059 participants, in Belgium, Denmark, France, Germany, Israel, Korea, Norway, Portugal, Russia, Sweden, Switzerland, and the United States. Smaller samples ranging from 32 to 67 persons have been gathered from among the psychotherapists in Argentina, India, Italy, Mexico, and the United Kingdom. The researchers are also international, encompassing, in addition to the 17 countries enumerated, Colombia, Finland, the Netherlands, Poland, and Taiwan. Beyond this information, CNR has the potential for elucidating relationships between a variety of cultural indicators and therapists' self-characterization. Once therapists' characteristics in various cultures are ascertained, they can be investigated in relation to cultural dimensions, e.g., individualism—collectivism or masculinity—femininity. That this expectation is not entirely unrealistic is attested by the CRN findings in Korea, as reported by Joo (1998). She found that "Korean therapists did differ from their Western counterparts in respects that appear to reflect traditional Korean values concerning interpersonal behavior" (p. 53). More dimly on the horizon, one may envisage the utilization of this unique data set for the exploration of ethnocultural nuances of therapy within countries. For example, are there detectable differences between French-speaking and German-speaking therapists in Switzerland and Flemish and Walloon therapists in Belgium?

The fundamental objective of the CNR investigators was to develop a comprehensive model of psychotherapists' development based on their unique store of international data. As reported by Orlinsky and Rønnestad (in press), three second-order factors pertaining to therapeutic work experience were extracted from self-descriptive data: healing involvement, stressful involvement, and controlling involvement. Future research may ascertain whether these three facets of therapists' interaction with their clients vary across social and situational parameters, including national cultures.

The general finding that has emerged from CNR indicates that, across the participating countries, therapists do not perceive themselves as mere technicians administering a series of impersonal interventions (Orlinsky, in press). Instead, they view themselves as participants in a meaningful and complex interpersonal encounter. Therapists' personalities then are bound to impinge upon the clients' experiences in therapy, and these personality characteristics are formed and expressed in a distinctive cultural context. Relevant in this respect is the report by Beutler, Mohr, Grawe, Engle, and McDonald (1991), who found that independently oriented clients consider nondirective therapy congenial, whereas less independent persons tend to be more acceptant of therapist's guidance and direction. Across cultures, these and other potentially relevant characteristics may vary in distribution and may serve as indicators of clients' preferences for and aversions against specific avenues and styles of therapeutic intervention.

In Australia, Snider (2003) explicitly tested the hypotheses advanced here about the association of individualism-collectivism and vertical collectivism, a concept that overlaps with power distance (Triandis, 1995), with expectations about counseling. Snider compared three samples of students: Chinese studying in Australia, and Australians and Americans in their respective home countries. Snider's findings indicated that individuals with collectivistic attitudes exhibited a pronounced preference for direct, expert-like, and practically oriented interventions. Snider also found that the individual's endorsement of collectivism or individualism was a stronger predictor of preference for counselor intervention, compared with his or her cultural background. On a higher plane of generality, Snider concluded that the dominant influence upon counseling preferences was verticalism or power distance among the Chinese, egalitarianism among the Australians, and individualism among Americans.

Other Research Possibilities Waiting to Be Explored

Beyond these innovative projects, a wide range of opportunities exists for studying psychotherapy within and across sociocultural contexts. Some of them have been only sparingly utilized, and others not at all. They involve a variety of research approaches, often to be applied piecemeal, gradually, and in several stages. In a few words, this section offers a sampling of such available yet rarely applied research strategies.

At the most modest and virtually universally realizable level, there is value and merit in providing accounts of culturally distinctive therapy in the multicultural settings in North America and elsewhere, and at various sites around the world. The more detailed and factual these case reports are, the greater their evidential value. Quantification is an additional feature that enhances the usefulness of such documentation.

As Kimura's (1995) and Seeley's (2000) research demonstrates, qualitative, case-based projects can also yield a rich store of novel and otherwise inaccessible information, especially about the subjective experience of therapy. To this end, the approaches practiced by anthropologists, ethnographers, and biographers deserve to be emulated and extended to the exploration of sociocultural contexts of therapy.

Brislin, Cushner, Cherrie, and Young (1986) have compiled distinctive critical incidents that illustrate the often hidden assumptions governing actions and choices in a specific culture. This approach can be extended to devising open-ended vignettes whose content is focused on client-therapist interactions in therapy sessions. Any cultural differences or contrasts could be construed as indirect expressions of expectations and preferences in therapy, such as for therapist's directive interventions (e.g., Folensbee, Draguns, & Danish, 1986) or his or her sensitivity to subtle nonverbal clues (e.g., Roland, 1988). Subsequently, these features could be further studied in relation to the culturally characteristic attitudes or features of self-experience.

More directly, studies may be conducted of both clients and therapists across cultures and ethnicities in order to establish the culture's impact upon their attitudes toward various aspects of therapy intervention. Along the same lines, inquiries could be focused on the experiences, events, and interventions considered by clients and/or therapists to be crucial for therapy to produce beneficial effects. These issues could be explored prospectively and retrospectively.

The National Institute of Health has inaugurated a policy that mandates the inclusion of ethnic minority members in federally supported research projects (cf. Hall, 2001). In the several comprehensive research projects on psychotherapy such as the Pennsylvania Practice Research Network (Borkovec, Echemendia, Ragusea, & Ruiz, 2001), that have recently been initiated, participants' ethnicity should be noted and incorporated as one of the potentially relevant indicators to therapy process and outcome.

In a more focused manner, investigators may set their sights on a remarkable research opportunity that has so far gone unutilized. At a number of points at the linguistic, cultural, and national borders, psychotherapists and clients meet on both sides of the divide. Are there any detectable differences in their operations and experiences? And, if so, do they match the expectations formulated in this chapter? In Canada, such a situation exists in the bicultural and bilingual city of Montreal, and between Mexico and the United States in the border cities on the two banks of the Rio Grande, such as El Paso; Ciudad Juarez; Nogales, Arizona; and Nogales, Sonora; and several others where Mexican and United States therapists and their respective clients could be compared. In Europe, Fribourg in Switzerland offers similar opportunities, with the French-German language boundary cutting right through the city. So far, no such studies appear to have been conducted anywhere. It is high time that they be initiated.

Archival sources have not yet been used in global explorations of therapeutic services. The Human Research Area Files (HRAF) (Barry, 1980) are a unique repository of coded ethnographic information about the cultures from all regions of the world. Although few ethnographies contain descriptions of psychotherapy in the narrow sense of the term, many of the accounts provide copious information about healing practices that could be related to data on socialization, emotional expression, social relationships, and other relevant characteristics. Perhaps a subsample within HRAF could even be coded for some or all of Hofstede's dimensions using an approach by which modern national cultures have so far been compared.

Finally, meta-analyses of psychotherapy in several countries, exemplified by Smith, Glass, and Miller (1980) for the United States and by Wittmann and Matt (1986) for Germany, may be scrutinized for any detectable national/cultural trends. In fact, a comparison of these two sets of results was undertaken by Matt (1993). It yielded significant differences however, that were realistically traced to artifactual sources. The results were further complicated by the fact that the languages in which the studies were published were being compared, rather than the populations of therapists and clients. In the Smith et al. (1980) meta-analysis in particular, investigations from outside the United States were included. Still, the complications so far encountered should not discourage the pursuit of meta-analyses of psychotherapy across cultures and nations. As the number of such studies increases and methodological challenges are faced and overcome, one may even envisage, in a grandiose and utopian manner, a global meta-analysis of meta-analyses. The implementation of such a project would enable the investigators to sift the array of data for the contributory influences of culture not only to the therapy outcome, but at other points of the therapeutic process.

CONCLUSION

The idea that psychotherapy encounters reflect the culture in which they occur can be traced to the beginnings of the twentieth century. Yet systematic descriptive information on what actually occurs in the course of psychotherapy in various cultures has been slow to accumulate. In the past two or three decades, there has been considerable acceleration in the growth of such documentation. This progression is reflected and exemplified in the chapters in this volume and in the contribution of pioneers and innovators introduced in this chapter. In the last few years, another trend has been gathering momentum, characterized by the advent and expansion of systematic research into the cultural and ethnic variations in therapy (e.g., Hall, 2001; Orlinsky et al., 1999). Advances in cross-cultural psychology (e.g., Hofstede, 2001) are moving toward coalescence with the fruits of progress in psychotherapy research. As yet, there is an incomplete mosaic composed of a host of clinical and a few research reports, suggesting that culture in psychotherapy matters. This recognition is intuitively shared by practicing psychotherapists who have ventured beyond their own cultural milieu and have looked across, or even scaled, cultural barriers. Many observers have concluded that culture permeates psychotherapy and that psychotherapy illuminates culture. However, there is little information on how culture influences psychotherapy, to what extent, and in what specific manner. The efforts of theoreticians, researchers, and clinicians should be directed at this ambitious issue, a both fascinating and urgently needed endeavor in the new millennium.

REFERENCES

Arrindell, W. A., Hatzichristou, C., Wensink, J., Rosenberg, E., van Twillert, B., Stedema, J., & Meijer, D. (1997). Dimensions of national culture as predictors of cross-national differences in subjective well-being. *Personality and Individual Differences, 23,* 37–53.

Barry, H. (1980). Description and uses of the Human Research Area Files. In H. C. Triandis & J. W. Berry (Eds.), *Handbook of cross-cultural psychology. Volume 2. Methodology.* (pp. 445–478). Boston: Allyn & Bacon.

Beutler, L. E., Mohr, D. C., Grawe, K., Engle, D., & MacDonald, R. (1991). Looking for differential treatment effects: Cross-cultural predictors of psychotherapy efficacy. *Journal of Psychotherapy Integration, 1,* 121–142.

Borkovec, T. D., Echemendia, R. J., Ragusea, S. S., & Ruiz, M. (2001). The Pennsylvania Practice Research Network and future possibilities for clinically meaningful and scientifically rigorous psychotherapy research. *Clinical Psychology: Science and Practice, 8*, 155–167.

Brislin, R. W., Cushner, K., Cherrie, S., & Yong, M. (1986). *Intercultural interactions: A practical guide.* Beverly Hills, CA: Sage.

Chang, S. C. (1988). The nature of self: A transcultural view. Part I: Theoretical aspects. *Transcultural Psychiatric Research Review, 25*(3), 169–204.

Cheng, S. K. (1990). Understanding the culture and behavior of East Asians: A Confucian perspective. *Australian and New Zealand Journal of Psychiatry, 24*, 510–515.

Cheng, S. K. (1998). *The need for approval: A psychological study of the influence of Confucian values on the social behaviour of East Asians.* Unpublished doctoral dissertation, Murdoch University, Perth, Western Australia.

Chinese Culture Connection (1987). Chinese values and the search for culture-free dimensions of culture. *Journal of Cross-Cultural Psychology, 18*, 143–164.

Christopher, J. W. (2001). Culture and psychotherapy: Toward a hermeneutic approach. *Psychotherapy, 38*(2), 115–128.

Draguns, J. G. (1975). Resocialization into culture: The complexities of taking a worldwide view of psychotherapy. In R. W. Brislin, S. Bochner, & W. J. Lonner (Eds.), *Cross-cultural perspectives on learning* (pp. 273–289). Beverly Hills, CA: Sage.

Draguns, J. G. (1981). Cross-cultural counseling and psychotherapy: History, issues, current status. In A. J. Marsella & P. B. Pedersen (Eds.), *Cross-cultural counseling and psychotherapy* (pp. 3–27). New York: Pergamon Press.

Draguns, J. G. (1990). Normal and abnormal behavior in cross-cultural perspective: Toward specifying the nature of their relationship. In J. J. Berman (Ed.), *Nebraska Symposium on Motivation 1989* (pp. 236–277). Lincoln, NB: University of Nebraska Press.

Draguns, J. G. (1998). Transcultural psychology and the delivery of clinical psychological services. In S. Cullari (Ed.), *Foundations of clinical psychology* (pp. 375–402). Boston: Allyn & Bacon.

Draguns, J. G. (2002). From empirically supported treatments around the world to psychotherapy as a mirror of culture: Tasks and challenges for international research on psychotherapy. *International Clinical Psychology, 4*(3), 7–9.

Fisek, G. O., & Kagitçibasi, Ç. (1999). Multiculturalism and psychotherapy: The Turkish case. In P. Pedersen (Ed.), *Multiculturalism as a fourth force* (pp. 77–92). Philadelphia: Brunner-Mazel.

Fish, J. (1996). *Culture and therapy: An integrative approach.* Northvale, NJ: Jason Aronson.

Folensbee, R. W., Jr., Draguns, J. G., & Danish, S. J. (1986). Impact of two types of counselor intervention on Black American, Puerto Rican, and Anglo-American analogue clients. *Journal of Counseling Psychology, 33*, 446–458.

Hall, G. C. N. (2001). Psychotherapy research with ethnic minorities: Empirical, ethical, and conceptual issues. *Journal of Consulting and Clinical Psychology, 69*, 502–510.

Hofstede, G. (1980). *Culture's consequences: International differences in work related values.* Beverly Hills, CA: Sage.

Hofstede, G. (1986). Cultural differences in teaching and learning. *International Journal of Intercultural Relations, 10*, 301–320.

Hofstede, G. (1991). *Cultures and organizations: Software of the mind.* London: McGraw-Hill.

Hofstede, G. (2001). *Culture's consequences: Comparing values, behaviors, institutions, and organizations across nations* (2nd ed.). Thousand Oaks, CA: Sage.

Hofstede, G., & Bond, M. H. (1988). The Confucius connection: From cultural roots to economic growth. *Organizational Dynamics, 16*(4), 4–21.

James, W. (1952/1891). *The principles of psychology.* Chicago: Encyclopedia Brittanica.

Jilek, W. G. (1982). *Indian healing: Shamanistic ceremonialism in the Pacific Northwest.* Vancouver, BC: Hancock House.

Jilek, W. G. (1995). Emil Kraepelin and comparative sociocultural psychiatry. *European Archives of Psychiatry and Clinical Neuroscience, 245*, 231–238.

Joo, E. (1998). The psychotherapeutic relationship in Korea compared to Western countries. *Korean Journal of Clinical Psychology, 17*, 39–56.

Kakar, S. (1978). *The inner world: A psychoanalytic study of childhood and society in India.* Delhi, India: Oxford University Press.

Katz, J. H. (1985). The sociopolitical nature of counseling. *The Counseling Psychologist, 13*(4), 615–624.

Kimura, B. (1995). *Zwischen Mensch und Mensch* [Between one human being and another]. (H. Weinhendl, Trans.) Darmstadt, Germany: Akademische Verlaganstalt.

Kraepelin, E. (1904). Vergleichende Psychiatrie [Comparative psychiatry]. *Zentralblatt für Nervenheilkunde und Psychiatrie, 27*, 433–437.

Landrine, H. (1992). Clinical implications of cultural differences: The referential versus the indexical self. *Clinical Psychology Review, 12*, 401–415.

Markus, H. R., & Kitayama, S. (1991). Culture and the self: Implications for cognition, emotion, and motivation. *Psychological Review, 98*(2), 224–253.

Matt, G. E. (1993). Comparing classes of psychotherapeutic interventions. A review and reanalysis of English- and German-language meta-analyses. *Journal of Cross-Cultural Psychology, 24*, 5–25.

Nathan, T. (1994). *L'influence qui guérit.* [The healing influence]. Paris: Odile Jacob.

Orlinsky, D. (2003). Disorder-specific, person-specific, and culture-specific psychotherapy: Evidence from psychotherapy and social science. *Psychotherapeut, 48*, 403–108.

Orlinsky, D., Armbühl, H., Rønnestad, M. H., Davis, J., Gerin, P., Davis, M., et al. (1999). Development of psychotherapists: Concepts, questions, and methods of a collaborative international study. *Psychotherapy Research, 9*(2), 127–153.

Orlinsky, D. E., and Rønnestad, M. H. (in press). *Therapeutic work and professional development. The psychotherapist's perspective.* Washington, DC: American Psychological Association.

Pedersen, P. (1999). Culture-centered interventions as a fourth dimension in psychology. In P. Pedersen (Ed.), *Multiculturalism as a fourth force* (pp. 3–18). Philadelphia: Brunner/Mazel.

Peltzer, K. (1995). *Psychology and health in African cultures: Examples of ethnopsychotherapeutic practice.* Frankfurt/Main, Germany: IKO-Verlag für Interkulturelle Kommunikation.

Peltzer, K. (1996). *Counseling and psychotherapy of victims of organized violence in sociocultural context.* Frankfurt/Main, Germany: IKO-Verlag für Interkulturelle Kommunikation.

Pfeiffer, W. M. (1994). *Transkulturelle Psychiatrie* [Transcultural psychiatry] (2nd ed.). Stuttgart, Germany: Thieme.

Pfeiffer, W. M. (1996). Kulturpsychiatrische Aspekte der Migration [Cultural psychiatric aspects of migration]. In E. Koch, M. Özek, & W. M. Pfeiffer (Eds.), *Psychologie und Pathologie der Migration* (pp. 17–30). Freiburg/Breisgau, Germany: Lambertus.

Prince, R. H. (1980). Variations in psychotherapeutic procedures. In H. C. Triandis & J. G. Draguns (Eds.), *Handbook of cross-cultural psychology. Volume 6. Psychopathology* (pp. 291–350). Boston: Allyn & Bacon.

Rehm, L. P. (2002). Empirically supported treatments: Are they supported elsewhere? *International Clinical Psychologist, 4*(2), 1.

Rivera-Ramos, A. N. (1984). *Hacia una psicoterapia para el puertorriqueño* [Toward psychotherapy for Puerto Ricans]. San Juan, Puerto Rico: Centro para el Estudio y Desarollo de la Personalidad Puertorriqueña.

Rogers, C. R. (1957). The necessary and sufficient conditions of therapeutic personality change. *Journal of Consulting Psychology, 21*, 95–103.

Roland, A. (1988). *In search of self in India and Japan.* Princeton, NJ: Princeton University Press.

Seeley, K. L. (2000). *Cultural psychotherapy. Working with culture in the clinical encounter.* Northvale, NJ: Jason Aronson.

Seeley, K. L. (in preparation). *The listening cure: Patients' talk, cultural intersubjectivity, and listening for culture in interpersonal treatments.* Unpublished paper.

Smith, M. L., Glass, G. V., & Miller, T. I. (1980). *The benefits of psychotherapy.* Baltimore: Johns Hopkins University Press.

Snider, P. D. (2003). *Exploring the relationship between individualism and collectivism and attitudes towards counseling among ethnic Chinese, Australian, and American university students.* Unpublished doctoral dissertation, Murdoch University, Perth, Australia.

Stewart, E. D. (1981). Cultural sensitivities in counseling. In P. B. Pedersen, J. G. Draguns, W. J. Lonner, and J. E. Trimble (Eds.). *Counseling across cultures* (2nd ed.) (p. 61–86). Honolulu: University Press of Hawaii.

Triandis, H. C. (1989). The self and social behavior in differing cultural contexts. *Psychological Review, 96*, 506–520.

Triandis, H. C. (1994). *Culture and social behavior.* New York: McGraw-Hill.

Triandis, H. C. (1995). *Individualism and collectivism.* Boulder, CO: Westview.

Triandis, H. C., Brislin, R. W., & Hui, C. H. (1988). Cross-cultural training across the individualism-collectivism divide. *International Journal of Intercultural Relations, 15*, 65–84.

Vassiliou, G., & Vassiliou, V. G. (1973). Subjective culture and psychotherapy. *American Journal of Psychotherapy, 27*, 42–51.

Wachtel, P. L. (1977). *Psychoanalysis and behavior therapy: Toward an integration.* New York: Basic Books.

Wittmann, W. W., & Matt, G. E. (1986). Meta-Analyse als Integration von Forschungsergebnissen am Beispiel deutschsprachiger Arbeiten zur Effektivität von Psychotherapie [Meta-analysis as integration of research findings as exemplified by German-language studies on the effectiveness of psychotherapy]. *Psychologische Rundschau, 37*, 20–40.

Zuniga, M. E. (1991). "Dichos" as metaphorical tools for resistant Latino clients. *Psychotherapy, 28*, 480–483.

Appendix

Culture, Therapy, and Healing: A Selective Bibliography

Uwe P. Gielen
St. Francis College

Juris G. Draguns
The Pennsylvania State University

Jefferson M. Fish
St. John's University

This selective bibliography includes volumes, a few chapters, and some journals dealing with psychological healing, indigenous forms of healing, multicultural and transcultural counseling and therapy, culturally sensitive psychiatric treatment, altered states of consciousness, and related works. A variety of disciplinary traditions and fields are represented, including medical anthropology, psychological and cultural anthropology, cross-cultural psychology, clinical psychology, counseling psychology, abnormal psychology, health psychology, family psychology, transcultural psychiatry, alternative medicine, the history of medicine, religious studies, and area studies. Books are listed in only one section even when their contents are relevant to two or more sections.

HANDBOOKS, SURVEYS, INTRODUCTIONS, RELATED WORKS

Abel, T., Metraux, R., & Roll, S. (1987). *Psychotherapy and culture* (rev. ed.). Albuquerque, NM: University of New Mexico Press.

Adler, L. L., & Mukherji, B. R. (Eds.). (1995). *Spirit versus scalpel: Traditional healing and modern psychotherapy.* Westport, CT: Bergin & Garvey.

Albrecht, G. L., Fitzpatrick, R., & Scrimshaw, S. C. (Eds.). (1999). *Handbook of social studies in health and medicine.* Thousand Oaks, CA: Sage.

Andrews, M. M., & Boyle, J. S. (2003). *Transcultural concepts in nursing care* (4th ed.). Philadelphia, PA: Lippincott, Williams & Wilkins.

Dasen, P. R., Berry, J. W., & Sartorius, N. (Eds.). (1988). *Health and cross-cultural psychology: Towards applications.* Newbury Park, CA: Sage.

Eisenberg, D. (Ed.). (2002). *Complementary and alternative medicine: State of the science and clinical applications.* Cambridge, MA: Harvard Medical School.

Fabrega, H., Jr. (1997). *Evolution of sickness and healing.* Berkeley, CA: University of California Press.

Fabrega, H., Jr. (2002). *Origins of psychopathology: The phylogenetic and cultural basis of mental illness.* New Brunswick, NJ: Rutgers University Press.

Fish, J. (1996). *Culture and therapy: An integrative approach.* Northvale, NJ: Jason Aronson.

Foster, G. M., & Anderson, B. G. (1978). *Medical anthropology.* New York: Wiley.

Frank, J. D., & Frank, J. B. (1991). *Persuasion and healing: A comparative study of psychotherapy* (3rd rev. ed.). Baltimore, MD: John Hopkins University Press.

Hahn, R. A. (1995). *Sickness and healing: An anthropological perspective.* New Haven, CT: Yale University Press.
Higginbotham, H. N. (1984). *Third World challenge to psychiatry: Culture accommodation and mental health care.* Honolulu, HI: University of Hawaii Press.
Higginbotham, H. N., West, S., & Forsyth, D. (1988). *Psychotherapy and behavior change: Social, cultural, and methodological perspectives.* New York: Pergamon.
Jonas, W. B., & Levin, J. S. (Eds.). (1999). *Essentials of complementary and alternative medicine.* Baltimore, MD: Lippincott, Williams & Wilkins.
Kazarian, S. S., & Evans, D. R. (1997). *Cultural clinical psychology: Theory, research, and practice.* New York: Oxford University Press.
Kazarian, S. S., & Evans, D. R. (2001). *Handbook of cultural health psychology.* New York: Academic Press.
Kiev, A. (Ed.). (1974). *Magic, faith, and healing: Studies in primitive psychology today.* New York: Free Press.
Kinsley, D. (1996). *Health, healing and religion: A cross-cultural perspective.* Upper Saddle River, NJ: Prentice-Hall.
Kirsch, I. (Ed.). (1999). *How expectancies shape experience.* Washington, DC: American Psychological Association.
Koenig, H. G. (Ed.). (1998). *Handbook of religion and mental health.* San Diego, CA: Academic Press.
Lee, J., & Sue, S. (2001). Clinical psychology and culture. In D. Matsumoto (Ed.), *The handbook of culture and psychology* (pp. 287–305). New York: Oxford University Press.
Lévy-Strauss, C. (1963). *Structural anthropology.* New York: Basic Books.
Middleton, J. (Ed.). (1967). *Magic, witchcraft and curing.* New York: Doubleday.
Moyers, B. (1993). *Healing and the mind.* New York: Doubleday.
Nichter, M. (1992). *Anthropological approaches to the study of ethnomedicine.* Yverdon, Switzerland: Gordon and Breach Science.
O'Connor, B. (1995). *Healing traditions: Alternative medicine and the health professions.* Philadelphia, PA: University of Pennsylvania Press.
Porter, R. (1998). *The greatest benefit to mankind: A medical history of humanity.* New York: W. W. Norton.
Prince, R. (1980). Variations in psychotherapeutic procedures. In H. C. Triandis & J. G. Draguns (Eds.), *Handbook of cross-cultural psychology, Vol. 6: Psychopathology* (pp. 291–309). Boston: Allyn & Bacon.
Rivera-Ramos, A. N. (1984). *Hacia una psicoterapia para el puertoriqueno* [Toward a psychotherapy for Puerto Ricans]. San Juan, PR: Centro para el Estudia de la Personalidad Puertoriquena.
Romanucci-Ross, L., Moerman, E. E., Moerman, D. R., & Tancredi, L. R. (Eds.). (1997). *The anthropology of medicine: From culture to method* (3rd ed.). Westport, CT: Greenwood.
Sargent, C. F., & Johnson, T. M. (Eds.). (1996). *Medical anthropology: Contemporary theory and method* (rev. ed.). Westport, CT: Praeger.
Scheff, T. (1979). *Catharsis in healing, ritual, and drama.* Berkeley, CA: University of California Press.
Schumaker, J. F., & Ward, T. (Eds.). (2001). *Cognition, culture, and psychopathology.* Westport, CT: Praeger.
Sheikh, A. A., & Sheikh, K. S. (1989). *Healing East & West. Ancient wisdom and modern psychology.* New York: Wiley.
Sullivan, L. E. (Ed.). (1989). *Healing and restoring: Health and medicine in the world's religious traditions.* New York: Macmillan.
Tanaka-Matsumi, J. (2001). Abnormal psychology and culture. In D. Matsumoto (Ed.), *The handbook of culture and psychology* (pp. 265–286). New York: Oxford University Press.
Torrey, E. F. (1986). *Witchdoctors and psychiatrists: The common roots of psychotherapy and its future.* New York: Harper & Row.
Tseng, W. S., & Streltzer, J. (Eds.). (2001). *Culture and psychotherapy: A guide to clinical practice.* Washington, DC: American Psychiatric Press.
Wampold, B. E. (2001). *The great psychotherapy debate: Models, methods, and findings.* Mahwah, NJ: Erlbaum.

THE HISTORY OF PSYCHOLOGICAL HEALING IN THE WEST

Burton, R. (1948). *The anatomy of melancholy.* New York: Tudor.
Caplan, E. (1998). *Mindgames: American culture and the birth of psychotherapy.* Berkeley, CA: University of California Press.
Clebsch, W. A., & Jackle, C. R. (1975). *Pastoral care in historical perspective.* New York: Jason Aronson.
Crabtree, A. (1993). *From Mesmer to Freud: Magnetic sleep and the roots of psychological healing.* New Haven, CT: Yale University Press.
Cutten, G. B. (1911). *Three thousand years of mental healing.* New York: Charles Scribner's Sons.

Ellenberger, H. F. (1970). *The discovery of the unconscious: The history and evolution of dynamic psychiatry*. New York: Basic Books.

Entralgo, P. L. (1970). *The therapy of the word in classical antiquity*. (L. J. Rather & J. H. Sharp, Trans.). New Haven, CT: Yale University Press.

Freedheim, D. K. (Ed.). (1992). *History of psychotherapy: A century of change*. Washington, DC: American Psychological Association.

Grossinger, R. (1980). *Planet medicine: From Stone Age shamanism to post-industrial healing*. Garden City, NY: Anchor Press.

Hamilton, M. (1906). *Incubation or the cure of disease in Pagan temples and Christian churches*. London: Simpkin, Marshall, Kent.

Jackson, S. W. (1999). *Care of the psyche: A history of psychological healing*. New Haven, CT: Yale University Press.

McNeill, J. T. (1965). *A history of the cure of souls*. New York: Harper Torchbooks.

Meier, C. A. (1967). *Ancient incubation and modern psychotherapy*. Evanston, IL: Evanston.

Numbers, R. L., & Amundsen, D. W. (Eds.). (1986). *Caring and curing: Health and medicine in the western religious traditions*. New York: Macmillan.

Oppenheim, J. (1991). *Shattered nerves*. New York: Oxford University Press.

Papadakis, T. (1975). *Epidauros: The sanctuary of Asclepios*. Zurich, Switzerland: Verlag Schnell & Stener.

Shapiro, A. K., & Shapiro, E. S. (1997). *The powerful placebo: From ancient priest to modern medicine*. Baltimore, MD: John Hopkins University Press.

Tick, E. (2001). *The practice of dream healing: Bringing ancient Greek mysteries into modern medicine*. Wheaton, IL: Quest Books.

Tuke, D. H. (Ed.). (1892). *Dictionary of psychological medicine* (Vols. 1-2). Philadelphia, PA: Blakiston, Son.

Zilboorg, G., & Henry, G. W. (1941). *A history of medical psychology*. New York: Norton.

PSYCHOPATHOLOGY AND MENTAL HEALTH ACROSS CULTURES

Al-Issa, I. (Ed.). (1995). *Handbook of culture and mental illness: An international perspective*. Madison, WI: International Universities Press.

Desjarlais, R., Eisenberg, L., Good, B., & Kleinman, A. (1995). *World mental health: Problems and priorities in low-income countries*. New York: Oxford University Press.

Helman, C. G. (2000). *Culture, health and illness: An introduction for health professionals* (4th ed.). Oxford, UK: Oxford University Press.

Kleinman, A. M., & Good, B. (Eds.). (1985). *Culture and depression: Studies in the anthropology and cross-cultural psychiatry of affect and disorder*. Berkeley, CA: University of California Press.

Marsella, A. J., Friedman, M. J., Gerrity, E. T., & Scurfield, R. M. (Eds.). (1996). *Ethnocultural aspects of post-traumatic stress disorder: Issues, research, and clinical applications*. Washington, DC: American Psychological Association.

Marsella, A. J., & White, G. M. (Eds.). (1984). *Cultural conceptions of mental health and therapy*. Boston: Reidel.

Mezzich, J. E., & Berganza, C. E. (Eds.). (1984). *Culture and psychopathology*. New York: Columbia University Press.

Simons, R. C., & Hughes, C. C. (1985). *The culture-bound syndrome: Folk illnesses of psychiatric and anthropological interest*. Dordrecht, The Netherlands: D. Reidel.

Tanaka-Matsumi, J., & Draguns, J. (1997). Culture and psychopathology. In J. W. Berry, M. H. Segall, & Ç. Kagitçibasi (Eds.), *Handbook of cross-cultural psychology. Vol. 3: Social behavior and applications* (pp. 449–491). Boston: Allyn & Bacon.

Triandis, H. C., & Draguns, J. G. (1980). *Handbook of cross-cultural psychology. Vol. 6: Psychopathology*. Boston: Allyn & Bacon.

Wilson, J., & Raphael, B. (Eds.). (1993). *International handbook of traumatic stress syndromes*. New York: Plenum.

CULTURE AND ASSESSMENT

Dana, R. H. (Ed.). (1998). *Handbook of cross-cultural and multicultural personality assessment*. Mahweh, NJ: Erlbaum.

Mezzich, J. E., Kleinman, A., Fabrega, H., Jr., & Parron, D. L. (Eds.). (1996). *Culture and psychiatric diagnosis: A DSM-IV perspective*. Washington, DC: American Psychiatric Press.

Sodowsky, G. R., & Impara, J. (Eds.). (1996). *Multicultural assessment in counseling and clinical psychology.* Lincoln, NB: Buros Institute of Mental Measurements.

Suzuki, L. A., Meller, P. J., & Ponterotto, J. G. (Eds.). (1996). *Handbook of multicultural assessment: Clinical, psychological, and educational applications.* San Francisco: Jossey-Bass.

Tseng, W. S., & Streltzer, J. (Eds.). (1997). *Culture and psychopathology: A guide to clinical assessment.* New York: Brunner/Mazel.

TRANSCULTURAL PSYCHIATRY

Gaines, A. (Ed.). (1992). *Ethnopsychiatry: The cultural construction of professional and folk psychiatries.* Albany, NY: State University of New York Press.

Kiev, A. (1972). *Transcultural psychiatry.* New York: Free Press.

Kleinman, A. (1988). *The illness narratives: Suffering, healing and the human condition.* New York: Free Press.

Kleinman, A. (1988). *Rethinking psychiatry: From cultural category to personal expereience.* New York: Free Press.

Leff, J. (1987). *Psychiatry around the globe: A transcultural view.* London: Gaskell.

Murphy, H. B. M. (1992). *Comparative psychiatry.* Berlin, Germany: Springer-Verlag.

Okpaku, S. (Ed.). (1997). *Clinical methods in transcultural psychiatry.* Washington, DC: American Psychiatric Press.

Pfeiffer, W. M. (1994). *Transkulturelle Psychiatrie: Ergebnisse und Probleme* [*Transcultural psychiatry: Results and problems*] (2nd ed.). Stuttgart, Germany: Thieme.

Price, R. K., Shea, B. M., & Mookherjee, H. N. (Eds.). (1995). *Social psychiatry across cultures: Studies from North America, Asia, Europe, and Africa.* New York: Plenum Press.

Tseng, W. S. (Ed.). (2001). *Handbook of cultural psychiatry.* San Diego, CA: Academic Press.

Tseng, W. S., & McDermott, J. F., Jr. (1981). *Culture, mind, and therapy: An introduction to cultural psychiatry.* New York: Brunner/Mazel.

HEALERS

Brody, H. (1992). *The healer's power.* New Haven, CT: Yale University Press.

Dobkin de Rios, M. (1992). *Amazon healer: The life and times of an urban shaman.* Bridgeport, England: Arism Press.

Edelstein, E., & Edelstein, L. (1945). *Asclepius* (Vols. 1–2). Baltimore, MD: John Hopkins University Press.

Jones, D. (1972). *Sanapia, Comanche medicine woman.* New York: Hold, Rinehart, and Winston.

Keeney, B. (Ed.). (2000). *Gary Holy Bull, Lakota Yuwipi man.* Stony Creek, CT: Leete's Island Books.

Keeney, B. (Ed.). (2001). *Walking Thunder: Diné medicine woman.* Stony Creek, CT: Leete's Island Books.

Kleinman, A. (1980). *Patients and healers in the context of culture: An exploration of the borderland between anthropology, medicine, and psychiatry.* Berkeley, CA: University of California Press.

McCalin, C. S. (Ed.). (1989). *Women as healers: Cross-cultural perspectives.* New Brunswick, NJ: Rutgers University Press.

Perrone, B., Stockel, H., & Krueger, V. (1989). *Medicine women, curanderas, and women doctors.* Norman: University of Oklahoma Press.

Pringle, R. (1998). *Sex and medicine: Gender, power and authority in the medical profession.* Cambridge, UK: Cambridge University Press.

SHAMANISM AND INDIGENOUS HEALING

Achterberg, J. (1985). *Imagery in healing: Shamanism and modern healing.* Boston: Shambhala.

Atkinson, J. M. (1992). Shamanisms today. *Annual Review of Anthropology, 21,* 307–330.

Clottes, J., & Lewis-Williams, D. (1998). *The shamans of prehistory. Trance and magic in painted caves.* New York: Harry Abrams. (Originally published in French in 1951.)

Eliade, M. (1964). *Shamanism: Archaic techniques of ecstasy.* New York: Pantheon.

Elkin, A. P. (1977). *Aboriginal men of high degree.* New York: St. Martin's Press.

Halifax, J. (1982). *Shaman: The wounded healer.* London: Thames and Hudson.

Harner, M. J. (Ed.). (1973). *Hallucinogens and shamanism.* New York: Oxford University Press.

Heinze, R. T. (1991). *Shamans of the twentieth century*. New York: Irvington.

Hultkrantz, A. (1992). *Shamanic healing and ritual drama*. New York: Crossroads.

Kalweit, H. (1984). *Dream time and inner space: The world of the shaman*. Boston: Shambhala.

Kalweit, H. (1992). *Shamans, healers, and medicine men* (Translated by M. Kohn). London: Shambhala.

Larsen, S. (1988). *The shaman's doorway* (2nd ed.). New York: Station Hill Press.

Lommel, A. (1966). *Shamanism: The beginning of art*. New York: McGraw Hill.

Pratt, V. (Ed.). (in press). *An encyclopedia of shamanism. A comprehensive guide to the field of shawanism* (vols. 1–2). New York: Rosen Publishing Group.

Siikala, A. L. (1978). *The rite technique of the Siberian shaman*. Helsinki, Finland: Academia Scientiarum Fennica.

Taussig, M. (1987). *Shamanism, colonialism and the wild man: A study in terror and healing*. Chicago: University of Chicago Press.

Vitebsky, P. (1995). *The shaman. Voyages of the soul, trance, ecstasy, and healing from Siberia to the Amazon*. Boston: Little, Brown.

Winkelman, M. (1992). Shamans, priests and witches: A cross-cultural study of magico-religious practitioners. Anthropological Research Papers #44. Tempe, AZ: Arizona State University.

Winkelman, M. (2000). *Shamanism: The neural ecology of consciousness and healing*. Westpoint, CT: Bergin and Garvey.

ALTERED STATES OF CONSCIOUSNESS

Anderson, E. (1996). *Peyote, the divine cactus* (2nd ed.). Tucson, AZ: University of Arizona Press.

Barber, T. X. (1970). *LSD, marijuana, yoga, and hypnosis*. Chicago, IL: Aldine.

Beattie, J., & Middleton, J. (Eds.). (1969). *Spirit mediumship and society in Africa*. London: Routledge & Kegan Paul.

Belo, J. (1960). *Trance in Bali*. New York: Columbia University Press.

Bourguignon, E. (1976). *Possession*. San Francisco: Chandler & Sharp.

Bourguignon, E. (1994). Trance and meditation. In P. K. Bock (Ed.), *Psychological anthropology* (pp. 297–313). Westport, CT: Praeger.

Crapanzano, V., & Garrison, V. (Eds.). (1977). *Case studies in spirit possession*. New York: Wiley.

Danforth, L. (1989). *Firewalking and religious healing*. Princeton, NJ: Princeton University Press.

Devereux, P. (1997). *The long trip: A prehistory of psychedelia*. New York: Penguin/Arkana.

Dobkin de Rios, M. (1984). *Hallucinogens: A cross-cultural perspective*. Albuquerque, NM: University of New Mexico Press.

Eliade, M. (1958). *Yoga: Immortality and freedom*. Princeton: Bollington Foundation.

Goldman, D. (1977). *The varieties of meditative experience*. New York: Irvington.

Goodman, F. D. (1990). *Where the spirits ride the wind: Trance journeys and other ecstatic experiences*. Bloomington, IN: Indiana University Press.

Goodman, F. D., Henney, J. H., & Pressel, E. (1974). *Trance, healing and hallucination*. New York: John Wiley.

Grof, S. (1980). *LSD psychotherapy*. Pomona, CA: Hunter House.

Johansson, R. E. A. (1970). *The psychology of nirvana*. Garden City, NY: Doubleday/Anchor.

Lewis, I. M. (1989). *Ecstatic religion: An anthropological study of spirit possession and shamanism* (2nd ed.). New York: Routledge.

Price-Williams, D., & Hughes, D. J. (1994). Shamanism and altered states of consciousness. *Anthropology of consciousness*, 5(2), 1–15.

Rasmussen, S. (1995). *Spirit possession and personhood among the Kel Ewey Tuareg*. Cambridge, UK: Cambridge University Press.

Schultes, R. E., Hoffman, A., & Ratsch, C. (2001). *Plants of the gods: Their sacred healing and hallucinogenic powers*. Rochester, VT: Healing Arts Press.

Shannon, B. (2002). *The antipodes of the mind: Charting the phenomenology of the ayahusca experience*. Oxford, UK: Oxford University Press.

Sharp, L. (1993). *The possessed and the dispossessed: Spirits, identity, and power in a Madagascar migrant town*. Berkeley, CA: University of California Press.

Siegel, R. K. (1989). *Intoxication: Life in pursuit or artificial paradise*. New York: E. P. Dutton.

Stoler Miller, B. (Transl.). (1998). *Yoga: Discipline of freedom: The Yoga Sutra attributed to Pantanjali*. New York: Bantam.

Suryani, L. K., & Jensen, G. D. (1993). *Trance and possession in Bali*. Kuala Lumpur, Malaysia: Oxford University Press.

Suzuki, S. (1970). *Zen mind, beginner's mind: Informal talks on Zen meditation and practice.* New York: Weatherhill.

Ward, C. A. (Ed.). (1989). *Altered states of consciousness: A cross-cultural perspective.* Newbury Park, CA: Sage.

Wasson, R. G. (1968). *Soma: Divine mushroom or immortality.* New York: Harcourt, Brace and World.

Wolman, B. B. (Ed.). (1977). *Handbook of parapsychology.* New York: Van Nostrand Reinhold.

Wolman, B. B., & Ullman, M. (1986). *Handbook of states of consciousness.* New York: Van Nostrand Reinhold.

NEO-SHAMANISM AND ITS CRITICS

Churchill, W. (1992). *Fantasies of the master race.* Monroe, ME: Common Courage Press.

Clifton, J. (Ed.). (1990). *The invented Indians.* Somerset, NJ: Transaction.

Doore, G. (Ed.). (1988). *Shaman's path.* Boston, MA: Shambhala.

Harner, M. (1984/1990). *The way of the shaman.* San Francisco: Harper.

Ingerman, S. (1991). *Soul retrieval. Mending the fragmented self.* San Francisco, CA: Harper SanFrancisco.

Noel, D. C. (1997). *The soul of shamanism: Western fantasies, imaginal realities.* New York: Continuum.

Pinkson, T. S. (1997). *The flowers of Wiricuta: A journey to shamanic power with the Huichol Indians of Mexico.* Rochester, VT: Inner Traditions.

The Shaman's Drum. (Popular journal emphasizing experimenal accounts of shamanistic healing; good book reviews.)

CHARISMATIC HEALING, ECSTATIC RELIGION, AND THE CHRISTIAN TRADITION

Blum, R., & Blum, E. (1965). *Health and healing in rural Greece.* Palo Alto, CA: Stanford University Press.

Cranston, R. (1955). *The miracle at Lourdes.* New York: McGraw-Hill.

Csordas, T. (1994). *The sacred self: A cultural phenomenology of charismatic healing.* Berkeley, CA: University of California Press.

Davies, S. (1995). *Jesus the healer: Possession, trance, and the origins of Christianity.* New York: Continuum International.

Harpur, T. (1994). *The uncommon touch: An investigation of spiritual healing.* Toronto, Canada: McClelland & Stewart.

Harrell, D. E., Jr. (1975). *All things are possible: The healing and charismatic revivals in modern America.* Bloomington, IN: Indiana University Press.

Harrell, D. E., Jr. (1985). *Oral Roberts: An American life.* Bloomington, IN: Indiana University Press.

Hastings, A. (1991). *With the tongues of men and angels: A study of channeling.* Orlando, FL: Holt, Rinehart and Winston.

Howard, J. K. (2001). *Disease and healing in the New Testament: An analysis and interpretation.* Lanham, MD: University Press of America.

Kelsey, M. T. (1973). *Healing and Christianity in ancient thought and modern times.* New York: Harper & Row.

McGuire, M. (1987). *Ritual healing in suburban America.* New Brunswick, NJ: Rutgers University Press.

Pilch, J. J. (2000). *Healing in the New Testament: Insights from medical and Mediterranean anthropology.* Minneapolis, MN: Fortress Press.

Randi, J. (1987). *The faith healers.* Buffalo, NY: Prometheus Books.

Spraggett, A. (1970). *Kathryn Kuhlman: The woman who believes in miracles.* New York: World.

MULTICULTURAL THERAPY AND COUNSELING

Aponte, J. R., & Wohl, J. (Eds.). (2000). *Psychological intervention and cultural diversity* (2nd ed.). Boston: Allyn & Bacon.

Atkinson, D. R., Morton, G., & Sue, D. W. (1998). *Counseling American minorities: A cross-cultural perspective* (5th ed.). Boston: McGraw-Hill.

Comas-Díaz, L., & Greene, B. (Eds.). (1994). *Women of color: Integrating ethnic and gender identities in psychotherapy.* New York: Guilford Press.

Comas-Díaz, L., & Griffith, E. E. H. (1988). *Clinical guidelines in cross-cultural mental health.* New York: Wiley.

Cuellar, I., & Paniagna, F. A. (Eds.). (1999). *Handbook of multicultural mental health: Assessment and treatment of diverse populations.* San Diego: Academic Press.

Dana, R. H. (2000). *Multicultural intervention perspectives for professional psychology.* Upper Saddle River, NJ: Prentice Hall.

De Rios, M. D. (2000). *Brief psychotherapy with the Latino immigrant client.* Binghamton, NY: The Hawarth Press.

Fukuyama, M. A., & Sevig, T. D. (1999). *Integrating spirituality into multicultural counseling.* Thousand Oaks, CA: Sage.

Garcia, J. C., & Zea, M. C. (Eds.). (1997). *Psychological interventions and research with Latino populations.* Needham Heights, MA: Allyn & Bacon.

Gaw, A. C. (Ed.). (1993). *Culture, ethnicity, and mental illness.* Washington, DC: American Psychiatry Press.

Gopaul-McNicol, S. A., & Brice-Baker, J. (1998). *Cross-cultural practice: Assessment, treatment, and training.* New York: Wiley.

Hays, P. A. (2001). *Addressing cultural complexities in practice: A framework for clinicians and counselors.* Washington, DC: American Psychological Association.

Kareem, J., & Littlewood, R. (1992). *Intercultural therapy: Themes, interpretations, and practice.* London: Blackwell Scientific.

Lee, C. C. (Ed.). (1997). *Multicultural issues in counseling* (2nd ed.). Alexandria, VA: American Counseling Association.

Lee, E. (Ed.). (1997). *Working with Asian Americans. A guideline for clinicians.* New York: Builford.

Marsella, A. J., Friedman, M. J., Gerrity, E. T., & Scurfield, R. M. (Eds.). (1996). *Ethnocultural aspects of post-traumatic stress disorder: Issues, research, and clinical applications.* Washington, DC: American Psychological Association.

Marsella, A. J., & Pedersen, P. B. (Eds.). (1981). *Cross-cultural counseling and psychotherapy.* New York: Pergamon.

Murphy-Shigematsu, S. (2003). *Multicultural encounters: Case narratives from a counseling practice.* New York: Teachers College Press.

Nader, K., Dubrow, N., & Stamm, B. (Eds.). (1999). *Honoring differences: Cultural issues in the treatment of trauma and loss.* Philadelphia: Taylor & Francis.

Nathan, T. (1994). *L'influence qui guérit* [*The healing influence*]. Paris: Odile Jacob.

Paniagua, F. (1994). *Assessing and treating culturally diverse clients: A practical guide.* Thousand Oaks, CA: Sage.

Pedersen, P. B. (Ed.). (1987). *Handbook of cross-cultural counseling and therapy.* Chicago, IL: Greenwood.

Pedersen, P. B. (Ed.). (1999). *Multiculturalism as a fourth force.* Philadelphia, PA: Brunner/Mazel.

Pedersen, P. B. (2000a). *Handbook for developing multicultural awareness* (3rd ed.). Alexandria, VA: American Counseling Association.

Pedersen, P. B. (2000b). *Hidden messages in culture-centered counseling: A triad training model.* Thousand Oaks, CA: Sage.

Pedersen, P. B., Draguns, J. G., Lonner, W. J., & Trimble, J. E. (Eds.). (2002). *Counseling across cultures* (5th ed.). Thousand Oaks, CA: Sage.

Ponterotto, J. G., Casas, J. M., Suzuki, L. A., & Alexander, C. M. (Eds.). (2001). *Handbook of multicultural counseling* (2nd ed.). Thousand Oaks, CA: Sage.

Seeley, K. M. (2000). *Cultural psychotherapy: Working with culture in the clinical encounter.* Northvale, NJ: Jason Aronson.

Straussner, S. L. A. (2001). *Ethnocultural factors in substance abuse treatment.* New York: Guilford.

Sue, D. W., Ivey, A. E., & Pedersen, P. B. (1996). *Multicultural counseling theory.* Belmont, CA: Brooks/Cole.

Sue, D. W., & Sue, D. (1999). *Counseling the culturally different. Theory and practice* (3rd ed.). New York: Wiley.

Sue, S., Zane, N., & Young, K. (1994). Research on psychotherapy with culturally diverse populations. In A. Bergin & S. Garfield (Eds.), *Handbook of psychotherapy and behavior change* (4th ed.) (pp. 783–817). New York: Wiley.

Vega, W. A., & Murphy, J. W. (1990). *Culture and the restructuring of community mental health.* New York: Greenwood.

MULTICULTURAL THERAPY WITH CHILDREN AND ADOLESCENTS

Botvin, G. J., Schinke, S., & Orlandi, M. A. (1995). *Drug abuse prevention with multiethnic youth.* Thousand Oaks, CA: Sage.

Canino, I. A., & Spurlock, J. (2000). *Culturally diverse children and adolescents: Assessment, diagnosis, and treatment.* New York: Guilford.

Cramer-Azima, F. J., & Grizenko, N. (Eds.). (2002). *Immigrant and refugee children and their families: Clinical, research, and training issues.* Madison, CT: International Universities Press.

Fadiman, A. (1998). *The spirit catches you and you fall down. A Hmong child, her American doctors and the collision of two cultures.* New York: Farrar, Straus & Giroux.

Gibbs, J. T., Huang, L. N., et al. (Eds.). (1989). *Children of color: Psychological intervention with minority youth.* San Francisco: Jossey-Bass.

Ho, M. K. (1992). *Minority children and adolescents in therapy.* Newbury Park, CA: Sage.

Johnson-Powell, G., Yamamoto, J., Wyatt, G. E., & Aroyo, W. (1997). *Transcultural child development: Psychological assessment and treatment.* New York: Wiley.

Stiffman, A. R., & Davis, E. (Eds.). (1990). *Ethnic issues in adolescent mental health.* Newbury Park, CA: Sage.

Vargas, L. A., & Koss-Chioino, J. D. (1992). *Working with culture: Psychotherapeutic interventions with ethnic minority children and adolescents.* San Francisco: Jossey-Bass.

MULTICULTURAL AND INTERNATIONAL FAMILY THERAPY

Boyd-Franklin, N. (2003). *Black families in therapy: Understanding the African American experience* (2nd ed.). New York: Guilford.

Falicov, C. J. (1998). *Hispanic families in therapy.* New York: Guilford.

Gielen, U. P., & Comunian, A. L. (Eds.). (1998). *The family and family therapy in international perspective.* Trieste, Italy: Lint.

Gielen, U. P., & Comunian, A. L. (Eds.). (1999). *International approaches to the family and family therapy.* Padua, Italy: UNIPRESS.

Gopaul-McNicol, S. A. (1994). *Working with West Indian families.* New York: Guilford.

Ho, M. K. (1987). *Family therapy with ethnic minorities.* Newbury Park, CA: Sage.

Lee, E. (1998). *American Asian families: A clinical guide to working with families.* New York: Guilford.

McGoldrick, M., Giordano, J., & Pearce, J. K (Eds.). (1996). *Ethnicity and family therapy* (2nd ed.). New York: Guilford.

McGoldrick, M., & Green, R. J. (Eds.). (1998). *Re-visioning family therapy from a multicultural perspective.* New York: Guilford.

Mindel, C. H., Habenstein, R. W., & Wright, R., Jr. (Eds.). (1998). *Ethnic families in America: Patterns and variations* (4th ed.). Upper Saddle River, NJ: Prentice Hall.

REFUGEES AND IMMIGRANTS

Al-Issa, I., & Tousignant, M. (Eds.). (1997). *Ethnicity, immigration, and psychopathology.* New York: Plenum Press.

Bemak, F., Chung, C. Y., & Pedersen, P. B. (2003). *Counseling refugees: A psychosocial approach to innovative multicultural counseling interventions.* Westport, CT: Greenwood Press.

Koch, E., Özek, M., & Pfeiffer, W. M. (Eds.). (1995). *Psychologie und Pathologie der Migration: Deutsch-Türkische Perspektiven* [*Psychology and pathology of migration: German-Turkish perspectives*]. Frankfurt/M., Germany: IKO-Verlag für Interkulturelle Kommunikation.

Marsella, A. J., Bornemann, T., Ekblad, S., & Orley, J. (Eds.). (1994). *Amidst peril and pain: The mental health and well-being of the world's refugees.* Washington, DC: American Psychological Association.

Peltzer, K., Aycha, A., & Bittenbinder, E. (Eds.). (1995). *Gewalt und Trauma. Psychopathologie und Behandlung im Kontext von Flüchtlingen und Opfern organisierter Gewalt* [*Violence and trauma: Psychopathology and treatment in the context of refugees and victims of organized violence*]. Frankfurt/M., Germany: IKO-Verlag für Interkulturelle Kommunikation.

Van der Veer, G. (1992). *Counseling and therapy with refugees: Psychological problems of victims of war, torture and repression.* Chichester, UK: Wiley.

Westermeyer, J. (1989). *Mental health for refugees and other immigrants: Social and preventive approaches.* Springfield, IL: Charles C. Thomas.

Westermeyer, J. (1989). *Psychiatric care of migrants: A clinical guide.* Washington, DC: American Psychiatric Press.

ASIAN AND OCEANIC HEALING TRADITIONS

Cohen, K. S. (1997). *The way of qigong: The art and science of Chinese energy healing.* New York: Ballantine.

Desai, P. N. (1989). *Health and medicine in the Hindu tradition.* New York: Crossroad.

Dioszégi, V., & Hoppál, M. (Eds.). (1978). *Shamanism in Siberia.* Budapest, Hungary: Akadémiai Kiadó.

Frankel, S., & Lewis, G. (Eds.). (1989). *A continuing trial of treatment: Medical pluralism in Papua New Guinea.* Dordrecht, The Netherlands: Kluwer.

Kakar, S. (1982). *Shamans, mystics, and doctors: A psychological inquiry into India and its healing traditions.* New York: Alfred A. Knopf.

Kapferer, B. A. (1983). *A celebration of demons: Exorcism and the aesthetics of healing in Sri Lanka.* Bloomington, IN: Indiana University Press.

Keeney, B. (Ed.). (2003). *Balians: Traditional healers of Bali.* Stony Creek, CT: Leete's Island Books.

Keeney, B., & Osumi, I. (Eds.). (2000). *Ikuko Osumi, Japanese master of Seiki Jutsu.* Stony Creek, CT: Leete's Island Books.

Kimura, B. (1995). *Zwischen Memsch und Mensch [Between one human being and another]* (H. Weinhendl, translator). Darmstadt, Germany: Akademische Verlaganstalt.

Laderman, C. (1991). *Taming the wind of desire: Psychology, medicine, and aesthetics in Malay shamanistic performance.* Berkeley, CA: University of California Press.

Laugani, P. (in press). *Asian perspectives in counselling and psychotherapy.* London, UK: Sage.

Leslie, C. (Ed.). (1976). *Asian medical systems: A comparative study.* Berkeley, CA: University of California Press.

Leslie, C., & Young, A. (Eds.). (1992). *Paths to Asian medical knowledge.* Berkeley, CA: University of California Press.

Lin, T. Y., Tseng, W. S., & Yeh, E. K. (Eds.). (1995). *Chinese societies and mental health.* Hong Kong: Oxford University Press.

Lock, M. (1980). *East Asian medicine in urban Japan: Varieties of medical experience.* Berkeley, CA: University of California Press.

Michael, H. N. (Ed.). (1963). *Studies in Siberian shamanism.* Toronto, Canada: University of Toronto Press.

Rahman, F. (1987). *Health and medicine in the Islamic tradition.* New York: Crossroad.

Reynolds, D. (1980). *The quiet therapies: Japanese pathways to personal growth.* Honolulu, HI: University of Hawai'i Press.

Reynolds, D. K. (1983). *Naikan psychotherapy: Meditation for self-development.* Chicago: University of Chicago Press.

Thacz, V., Zhambalov, S., & Phipps, W. (2002). *Shaman: Dedication ritual or a Buryat shaman in Siberia.* New York: Parabola Books.

Vitebsky, P. (1993). *Dialogues with the dead: The discussion of mortality among the Sora of Eastern India.* Cambridge, UK: Cambridge University Press.

Zysk, K. G. (1985). *Religious healing in the Veda.* Philadelphia, PA: American Philosophical Society.

TIBETAN BUDDHISM AND THE HIMALAYAN TRADITIONS

Birnbaum, R. (1989). *The Healing Buddha.* Boston: Shambhala.

Clifford, T. (1984). *Tibetan Buddhist medicine and psychiatry: The diamond healing.* York Beach, ME: Samuel Weiser.

David-Neel, A. (1932/1971). *Magic and mystery in Tibet.* New York: Dover.

Desjarlais, R. R. (1992). *Body and emotion. The aesthetics of illness and healing in the Nepal Himalayas.* Philadelphia, PA: University of Pennsylvania Press.

Kuhn, A. S. (1988). *Heiler and ihre Patienten auf dem Dach der Welt. Ladakh aus ethnomedizinischer Sicht [Healers and their patients on the roof of the world. Ladakh in ethnomedical perspective].* Frankfurt/M., Germany: Peter Lang.

Mumford, S. R. (1989). *Himalayan dialogues: Tibetan lamas and Gurung shamans in Nepal.* Madison, WI: University of Wisconsin Press.

Schenk, A. (1994). *Schamanen auf dem Dach der Welt [Shamans on the roof of the world].* Graz, Austria: Akademische Druck- und Verlagsanstalt.

Shrestha, R., & Baker, I. A. (1997). *The Tibetan art of healing.* San Francisco, CA: Chronical Books.

PSYCHOANALYSIS AND ASIAN TRADITIONS

Doi, T. (1981). *The anatomy of dependence*. Tokyo: Kodansha International.

Epstein, M. (1995). *Thoughts without a thinker. Psychotherapy from a Buddhist perspective*. New York: BasicBooks.

Fromm, E., Suzuki, D. T., & Martino, R. (Eds.). (1960). *Zen Buddhism and psychoanalysis*. New York: Harper and Row.

Magid, B. (2002). *Ordinary mind: Exploring the common ground of Zen and psychotherapy*. Boston, MA: Wisdom Publications.

Roland, A. (1988). *In search of self in India and Japan: Toward a cross-cultural psychology*. Princeton, NJ: Princeton University Press.

Roland, A. (1996). *Cultural pluralism and psychoanalysis: The Asian and North American experience*. New York: Routledge.

Rosenbaum, R. (1999). *Zen and the heart of psychotherapy*. Philadelphia, PA: Brunner/Mazel.

Rubin, J. B. (1996). *Psychotherapy and Buddhism: Toward an integration*. New York: Plenum.

Safran, J. (Ed.). (2003). *Psychoanalysis and Buddhism. An unfolding dialogue*. Boston: Wisdom Publications.

Segal, S. (Ed.). (2003). *Encountering Buddhism: Western psychology and Buddhist teachings*. Albany, NY: State University of New York.

INDIGENOUS HEALING TRADITIONS IN LATIN AMERICA AND THE CARIBBEAN

Brodwin, P. (1996). *Medicine and morality in Haiti: The contest for healing power*. New York: Cambridge University Press.

Brown, K. M. (1991). *Mama Lola: A Voodoo priestess in Brooklyn*. Berkeley, CA: University of California Press.

Crandon-Malamud, L. (1991). *From the fat of our souls: Social change, political process, and medical pluralism in Bolivia*. Berkeley, CA: University of California Press.

Deren, M. (1953/1970). *Divine horsemen: The living gods of Haiti*. New Paltz, NY: McPherson/Documentext.

Dobkin de Rios, M. (1972/1984). *Visionary vine: Hallucinogenic healing in the Peruvian Amazon*. Prospect Heights, IL: Waveland.

Fabrega, H., Jr., & Silver, D. B. (1973). *Illness and shamanistic curing in Zinacantan*. Stanford, CA: Stanford University Press.

Finkler, K. (1985). *Spiritualist healers in Mexico: Successes and failures in alternative therapeutics*. South Hadley, MA: Bergin & Garvey.

Harwood, A. (1977). *Rx: Spiritist as needed*. New York: Wiley.

Hurbon, L. (1995). *Voodoo: Search for the spirit*. New York: Harry N. Abrams.

Keeney, B. (Ed.). (2000). *Gurani shamans of the forest*. Stony Creek, CT: Leete's Island Books.

Keeney, B. (Ed.). (2002). *Shakers of St. Vincent*. Stony Creek, CT: Leete's Island Books.

Keeney, B. (Ed.). (2003). *Hands of faith: Healers of Brazil*. Stony Creek, CT: Leete's Island Books.

Kiev, A. (1968). *Curanderismo*. New York: Free Press.

Koss-Chioino, J. D. (1992). *Women as healers, women as patients: Mental health care and traditional healing in Puerto Rico*. Boulder, CO: Westview Press.

Langdon, J. M., & Baer, G. (1992). *Portals of power: Shamanism in South America*. Albuquerque, NM: University of New Mexico Press.

Langguth, A. J. (1975). *Macumba: White and black magic in Brazil*. New York: Harper & Row.

Luna, L. E. (1986). *Vegetalismo: Shamanism among the Mestizo population of the Peruvian Amazon*. Stockholm, Sweden: Almquist & Wiksell International.

Luna, L. E., & Amaringo, P. (1991). *Ayahuasca visions: The religious iconography of a Peruvian shaman*. Berkeley, CA: North Atlantic Books.

Métraux, A. (1959/1972). *Voodoo in Haiti*. New York: Schocken Books.

Pérez y Mena, A. I. (1991). *Speaking with the dead: Development of Afro-Latin religion among Puerto Ricans in the United States*. New York: AMS Press.

Reichel-Dolmatoff, G. (1975). *The shaman and the jaguar: A study of narcotic drugs among the Indians of Colombia*. Philadelphia, PA: Temple University Press.

Rubel, A. J., O'Neill, C. W., & Collado, A. R. (1984). *Susto: A folk illness*. Berkeley: University of California Press.

Voeks, R. A. (1997). *Sacred leaves of Candomblé*. Austin, TX: University of Texas Press.

INDIGENOUS NORTH AMERICAN HEALING TRADITIONS

Devereux, G. (1969). *Mohave ethnopsychiatry: The psychic disturbances of an Indian tribe.* Washington, DC: Smithsonian Institute Press. (Original work published 1961).

Farris, J. C. (1990). *The Nightway: A history and a history of documentation of a Navajo ceremonial.* Albuquerque, NM: University of New Mexico Press.

Grim, J. A. (1983). *The shaman: Patterns of Siberian and Ojibway healing.* Norman, OK: University of Oklahoma Press.

Hammerschlag, C. A. (1988). *The dancing healers: A doctor's journey of healing with Native Americans.* New York: Harper and Row.

Hultkranz, A. (1992). *Shamanic healing and ritual drama: Health and medicine in native North American religions.* New York: Crossroad.

Jilek, W. G. (1974). *Salish Indian mental health and culture change. Psychohygienic and therapeutic aspects of the guardian spirit ceremonial.* Toronto, Canada: Holt, Rinehart & Winston.

Jilek, W. G. (1982). *Indian healing: Shamanic ceremonialism in the Pacific Northwest today.* Blaine, WA: Hancock House.

Kunitz, S. J. (1983). *Disease, change, and the role of medicine: The Navajo experience.* Berkeley, CA: University of California Press.

Lame Deer, J., & Erdoes, R. (1972). *Lame Deer, seeker of visions.* New York: Simon and Schuster.

Lyon, W. S. (1996). *Encyclopedia of Native American healing.* Santa Barbara, CA: ABC-CLIO.

Neihardt, J. G. (1932/1973). *Black Elk speaks.* New York: Washington Square Press.

Rasmussen, K. (1952). *Intellectual culture of the Hudson Bay Eskimos. Report of the Fifth Thule Expedition, 1921–1924, Vol. 7* (Transl. by W. E. Calvent). Copenhagen, Denmark: Gyldenval.

Spicer, E. H. (Ed.). (1977). *Ethnic medicine in the Southwest.* Tucson, AZ: University of Arizona Press.

St. Pierre, M., & Soldier, T. L. (1995). *Walking in the sacred manner: Healers, dreamers, and pipe carriers—medicine women of the Plains Indians.* New York: Touchstone.

Trotter, R. T., & Chavira, J. A. (1981). *Curanderismo: Mexican American folk healing.* Athens, GA: University of Georgia Press.

Witherspoon, G. (1977). *Language and art in the Navajo universe.* Ann Arbor, MI: University of Michigan Press.

Wolfson, E. (1992). *From the earth to beyond the sky: Native American medicine.* Boston: Houghton Mifflin.

Vogel, V. J. (1973). *American Indian medicine.* New York: Ballantine.

HEALING TRADITIONS AND PSYCHOTHERAPY IN AFRICA AND THE ISLAMIC WORLD

Ahmed, R. A., & Gielen, U. P. (1998). *Psychology in the Arab countries.* Menoufia, Egypt: Menoufia University Press.

Al-Issa, I. (2000). (Ed.). *Al-Junun. Mental illness in the Islamic world.* Madison, CT: International Universities Press.

Boddy, J. (1989). *Wombs and alien spirits: Women, men, and the Zar Cult in Northern Sudan.* Madison, WI: University of Wisconsin Press.

Crapanzano, V. (1973). *The Hamadsha: A study in Moroccan ethnopsychiatry.* Berkeley, CA: University of California Press.

Field, M. J. (1962). *Search for security: An ethnopsychiatric study of rural Ghana.* Chicago: Northwestern University Press.

Fierman, S., & Jansen, J. M. (1992). *The social basis of health and healing in Africa.* Berkeley, CA: University of California Press.

Good, C. M. (1987). *Ethnomedical systems in Africa: Patterns of traditional medicine in urban and rural Kenya.* New York: Guilford.

Hammond-Tooke, D. (1989). *Rituals and medicine. Indigenous healing in South Africa.* Johannesburg, South Africa: Donker.

Isaacson, R. (2003). *The healing land: The Bushmen and the Kalahari desert.* New York: Grove Press.

Janzen, J. M. (1992). *Ngoma: Discourses of healing in central and southern Africa.* Berkeley, CA: University of California Press.

Katz, R. (1982). *Boiling energy: Community healing among the Kalahari !Kung.* Cambridge, MA: Harvard University Press.

Katz, R., Biesele, M., & St. Denis, V. (1997). *Healing makes our hearts happy.* Rochester, VT: Inner Traditions.

Keeney, B. (Ed.). (2000). *Kalahari bushmen healers.* Stony Creek, CT: Leete's Island Books.

Keeney, B. (Ed.). (2001). *Vusamazulu Credo Mutwa: Zulu high sanusi.* Stony Creek, CT: Leete's Island Books.

Keeney, B. (Ed.). (2003). *Ropes to God: Experiencing the Bushman spiritual universe.* Stony Creek, CT: Leete's Island Books.

Leighton, A. H., Lambo, C. G., Hughes, C. G., Murphy, J. M., & Macklin, D. B. (1963). *Psychiatric disorder among the Yoruba.* Ithaca, NY: Cornell University Press.

Lewis, I. M., Al-Safi, A., & Hurreiz, S. (Eds.). (1991). *Women's medicine. The Zari-Bori cult in Africa and beyond.* Edinburgh, Scotland: Edinburgh University Press for the International African Institute.

Mullings, L. (1984). *Therapy, ideology, and social change: Mental healing in urban Ghana.* Berkeley, CA: University of California Press.

Nathan, T., & Hounkpatin, L. (1996). *La guérison Yoruba* [Yoruba healing]. Paris: Odile Jacob.

Ngubane, H. (1977). *Body and mind in Zulu medicine. An ethnography of health and disease in Nyuswa-Zulu thought and practice.* London: Academic Press.

Peltzer, K. (1987). *Some contributions of traditional healing practices towards psychosocial health care in Malawi.* Eschborn bei Frankfurt am Main, Germany: Fachbuchhandlung für Psychologie Verlagsabteilung.

Peltzer, K. (1995). *Psychology and health in African cultures: Examples of ethnopsychotherapeutic practice.* Frankfurt/M., Germany: IKO-Verlag für Interkulturelle Kommunikation.

Peltzer, K., & Ebigbo, P. O. (1989). *Clinical psychology in Africa.* Enugu, Nigeria: Work Group for African Psychology.

Rasmussen, S. (2001). *Healing in community: Medicine, contested terrains, and cultural encounters among the Tuareg.* Westport, CT: Greenwood.

Simpson, G. E. (1980). *Yoruba religion and medicine in Ibadan.* Ibadan, Nigeria: Ibadan University Press.

Turner, E. (1992). *Experiencing ritual: A new interpretation of African healing.* Philadelphia: University of Pennsylvania Press.

Westermarck, E. (1926). *Ritual and belief in Morocco.* London: Macmillan.

JOURNALS CONTAINING ARTICLES ON TRANSCULTURAL HEALING, THERAPY, AND COUNSELING

American Journal of Community Psychology

Cultural Diversity and Ethnic Minority Psychiatry [Previously: *Cultural Diversity and Mental Health* (1995–1998)]

Culture, Medicine and Psychiatry

International Journal of Social Psychiatry

Journal for the Psychoanalysis of Culture and Society

Journal of Transcultural Nursing

Medical Anthropology

Medical Anthropology Quarterly

Social Psychiatry

Social Science and Medicine

Transcultural Psychiatry [Previously: *Transcultural Psychiatry Research Review* (1963-1999)]

Zeitschrift für Ethnomedizin und transkulturelle Psychiatrie [*Journal for Ethnomedicine and Transcultural Psychiatry*]

Author Index

A

Abe, T., 285, 286, 287
Aber, J.L., 328
Abrams, A.I., 216
Abuasisha, B.B., 226
Achterberg, J., 175
Adair, J.G., 295
Ader, R., 89, 90, 92, 94
Agari, I., 283
Agee, E., 39, 54
Agurs, T., 53
Akesson, J., 227
Al-Abdul Jabbar, J., 360, 361
Alexander, C.M., 114
Alexander, F., 256, 262, 343
Algotsson, L., 227
Al-Hamad, A., 343, 344, 346, 348, 351, 360, 362
Al-Issa, I., 363, 346, 348, 353, 357, 358, 360, 361, 362
Al-Krenawi, A., 346, 351, 356, 362
Allen, D.I., 182, 185
Allen, J.J.B., 226
Al-Mahdy, A., 361
Al-Radi, O.M., 361
Alstad, D., 265, 270
Alstein, M., 227
Al-Subaie, A., 343, 344, 346, 348, 351, 360, 362
Altuna, P.A., 325
Alzuhaidi, A.S., 346
Amelsvoort, A.V., 121
American Psychiatric Association, 104, 112, 354
Anderson, D., 89
Anderson, J.A., 95
Anderson, L.P., 109
Anderson, M.B., 327
Anderson, P.M., 97
Anderson, S.R., 214
Angel, R., 106
Aponte, C.E., 103
Aponte, J.F., 103, 104, 105, 107, 108, 109, 110, 111, 112, 113, 114, 115
Appadurai, A., 73
Arar, N.H., 61
Arnett, J.J., 72
Arrindell, W.A., 382
Arroyo, W., 328
Askeroth, C., 215
Astin, J.A., 214, 242
Atkinson, D.R., 108, 114, 115
Attkisson, C.C., 114
Atwood, G., 271
Ayllon, T., 74
Azhar, M.Z., 360
Azrin, N.H., 74
Azuma, H., 281

B

Baasher, T.A., 353
Bagheri, A., 125
Bailey, E., 39, 42, 52, 53
Bailey, K.G., 22
Baker, R., 121
Bakhtin, M., 253
Balant, L.P., 89
Balant-Gorgia, E.A., 89
Balian, K., 121
Balodhi, J.P., 297, 298
Bandura, A., 279
Baptiste, D.A., 123
Barg, J., 227
Barlow, D.H., 105, 288

401

Subject Index